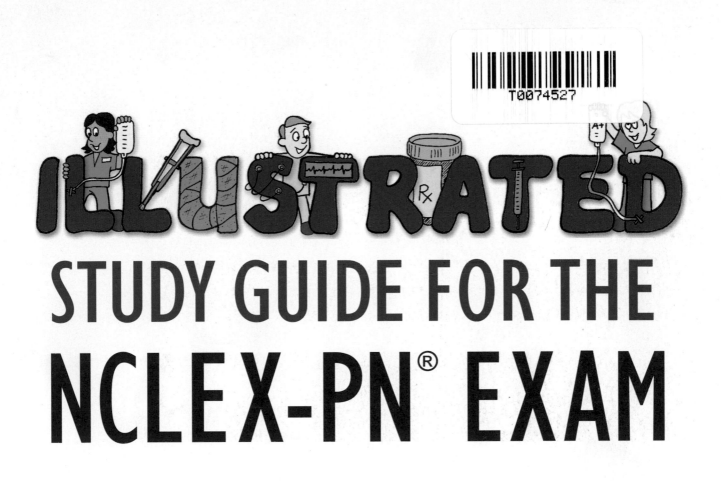

ILLUSTRATED
STUDY GUIDE FOR THE
NCLEX-PN® EXAM

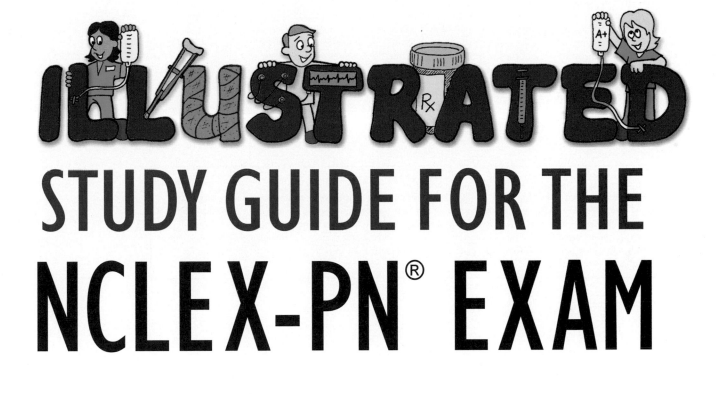

ILLUSTRATED
STUDY GUIDE FOR THE
NCLEX-PN® EXAM

10TH EDITION

JoAnn Zerwekh, EdD, MSN, RN

President/CEO
Nursing Education Consultants, Inc.
Chandler, Arizona

ELSEVIER

Elsevier
3251 Riverport Lane
St. Louis, Missouri 63043

ILLUSTRATED STUDY GUIDE FOR THE NCLEX-PN® EXAM, TENTH EDITION

Notice

ISBN: 978-0-443-11035-1

Content Strategist: Heather Bays-Petrovic
Senior Content Development Manager: Lisa P. Newton
Publishing Services Manager: Deepthi Unni
Senior Project Manager: Kamatchi Madhavan
Design Direction: Bridget Hoette

Printed in India

Last digit is the print number: 9 8 7 6 5 4 3 2 1

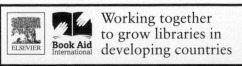

Contributors

Heather Ashby, MSN, RNC-OB, CNE
Assistant Clinical Professor
Nursing
Northern Arizona University
Flagstaff, Arizona

Chantelle Capeletti, MSN, RN, CPN
Assistant Academic Program Director
School of Nursing and Health Sciences
Capella University
Orlando, Florida

Ashley Garneau, PhD, RN
Nursing Faculty
Nursing
GateWay Community College
Phoenix, Arizona

Janis Longfield McMillan, PhD, MSN, RN, CNE
Clinical Professor
School of Nursing
Northern Arizona University
Flagstaff, Arizona

Reviewers

Heather Clark, DNP, RN
Penn State Practical Nursing Program
Director
Center Valley, Pennsylvania

Darla K. Shar, MSN, RN
Hannah E. Mullins School of Practical Nursing
Associate Director
Salem, Ohio

Linda Turchin, RN, MSN, CNE
Professor Emeritus of Nursing
Fairmont State University
Fairmont, West Virginia

Preface

The tenth edition of the *Illustrated Study Guide for the NCLEX-PN® Exam* continues to provide an up-to-date review, illustrated with graphics, pictures, and cartoon images to enhance your review and retention of critical nursing information. The book contains information specifically designed to assist you in preparing for the National Council Licensure Examination for Practical Nurses (NCLEX-PN®). This text emphasizes the integrated approach to nursing practice that the NCLEX-PN® is designed to test. The book's primary purpose is to assist you in thoroughly reviewing the facts, principles, and applications of the nursing process. It should alleviate many of the concerns you may have regarding what, how, and when to study.

I have spent a great deal of time studying the NCLEX-PN® test format and have incorporated that information into this book. Discussion and examples of alternate format questions and next-generation (NGN) test items are included. In my review courses, which I have taught across the country, I have identified specific student needs and correlated this information with the test plan to develop this study guide. Test questions are at the end of each chapter to help you check your level of comprehension. In addition, there is a companion Evolve website (http://evolve.elsevier.com/Zerwekh/illustratedstudyguidePN/) that provides questions for practicing your testing skills.

Graphics highlight important information make the book more visually appealing. They include:

ALERT This identifies important concepts that are reflected on the PN Practice Analysis from the National Council of State Boards of Nursing, Inc.

! This assists in distinguishing priorities of nursing care.

▯ Adult disease conditions are located by this design element.

♣ Pediatric disease conditions and implications are located by this design element.

🖎 Self-care and home care information can be found under the Nursing Interventions section.

Ⓡ Medication information is found in chapter appendixes.

▲ High-alert medications identified by The Joint Commission and the Institute for Safe Medication Practices are noted by this symbol.

The comments from review course participants and extensive content reviews have helped shape the development of this tenth edition. I hope this text will prove to be beneficial to nursing faculty, students, and graduate nurses. Thank you for allowing me to be part of your success in nursing.

Dr. JoAnn Zerwekh

ACKNOWLEDGMENTS

I truly appreciate the continuing support of my children – Tyler Zerwekh and Ashley Zerwekh Garneau – who have given me my wonderful grandchildren who brighten my day and make me smile – Maddie and Harper Zerwekh and Ben Garneau.

A special note of thanks to C.J. Miller, RN, BSN, and cartoonist, who has worked with me from the beginning of the *Memory Notebooks of Nursing*, through the many editions of *Nursing Today: Transition and Trends*, and more recently with the *Mosby's Memory NoteCard* series. She continues to bring her unique style to all of my books' recognizable images and cartoons.

This edition has offered me the opportunity to respond to nursing faculty and students who have utilized the book's previous editions. Their comments and suggestions for production of this 10th edition have been incorporated into the revision.

It is my pleasure to acknowledge the individuals who assisted me in the technical preparation and production of this edition. My sincere appreciation to the following:

Heather Bays-Petrovic, Content Strategist, with whom I have worked on many different projects, including the companion text to this book, the *Illustrated Study Guide for the NCLEX-RN® Exam* review book. You are the best!

Lisa Newton, Senior Content Development Manager, who provided assistance to me and the contributors from the beginning of the revision process throughout the entire production cycle of the book. It is always a pleasure to work with you.

Kamatchi Madhavan, Senior Project Manager, who monitored the production of this book and kept me on schedule. It is always a pleasure to work with you!

Thank you all!

Contents

CHAPTER ONE

Clinical Judgment and Testing Strategies for the NCLEX-PN® Examination

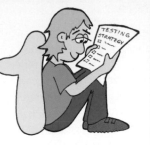

One of the first steps in being successful on the NCLEX-PN® (National Council Licensure Examination for Practical Nurses) is to understand how the test is developed. An important step in preparing for the examination is to find out as much as possible about the test. This will help reduce stress and anxiety. As you begin to prepare for the NCLEX-PN, it is important to consider who determines the content of the test plan and constructs the questions based on the test plan.

The National Council of State Boards of Nursing (NCSBN) is responsible for the development of the content and the construction of questions or items for the NCLEX-PN examination. A practice analysis is conducted by the NCSBN every 3 years to validate the test plan and to determine currency of nursing practice. Content experts are consulted to assist in the creation of the practice analysis. The practice of practical/vocational nursing requires application of knowledge, skills, abilities, and clinical judgment; therefore the majority of test items are written at the application or higher levels of cognitive ability. The percentage of test items on the test plan does not specifically address specialty areas. However, on review of the nursing activities, many of the test plan areas address specialty areas of nursing practice. This analysis provides the basis for development of the content to be included in the NCLEX-PN Test Plan.

The content experts are practicing nurses who work with or supervise new graduates in the practice setting. These content experts represent all geographic areas and are selected according to their area of practice; therefore all areas of nursing practice are addressed in the development of the test plan. Item writers are selected to create questions based on the content identified in the test plan. All new test items or questions are reviewed by item reviewers who are also nurses in current practice and who have been directly involved with supervision of new graduate nurses. Content experts and item reviewers not only create new items but are also involved in the continual review of items in the NCLEX test pool to ensure all items reflect current practice.

So, what does all this mean? It means that nurses in current practice and nursing faculty work together to identify the content and to develop questions for the NCLEX-PN. All geographic areas, as well as all areas of nursing practice, are included. The purpose of the examination is to assure the public that each candidate who passes the examination can practice safely and effectively as a newly licensed, entry-level practical nurse.

Every US state uses the NCLEX-PN to determine entry into nursing practice as a licensed practical/vocational nurse (LPN/LVN). Each state is responsible for the testing requirements, retesting procedures, and entry into practice within that state. Each state requires the same competency level or passing standard on the NCLEX. There is no variation in the passing standard from state to state.

CLINICAL JUDGMENT AND NCLEX-PN® EXAMINATION

Clinical Judgment and Next Generation NCLEX Items

The Next Generation NCLEX (NGN) exam began April, 2023. The NCSBN developed the NCSBN Clinical Judgment Measurement Model (NCJMM) to develop and measure clinical judgment with test items. A feature of the new NGN exam will be case studies commonly encountered in the real world that reflect the kinds of critical decisions nurses have to make in a variety of health care settings. They will start with a client scenario or case and will be either **stand-alone** (trend or bowtie) questions or be an **unfolding case study**, which involves six questions that correspond to the NCJMM. The case scenario will include part of a medical record or chart documentation (see Fig. 1.1). These are the steps and questions to consider, which are performed in a sequential manner, starting with number (1) recognize cues, (2) analyze cues, (3) prioritize hypotheses, (4) generate solutions, (5) take action, and (6) evaluate outcomes (Table 1.1). The new NGN exam is composed of current test item types (multiple-choice and alternate-item format) and 12 new NGN test item types (Table 1.2) along with the bowtie and trend item. The bowtie is a stand-alone item and addresses all six steps of the NCJMM in one test item. The trend item presents information over time in the medical record format or chart, and it can contain all new NGN item types except the bowtie. A more thorough discussion of all current and new NGN item types and examples can be found in the section "Types of Test Items."

Test Plan

The test plan is based on research (practice analysis study) conducted by the NCSBN every 3 years. The purpose of this research is to determine the importance, frequency, and clinical judgment relevancy of performing nursing care activities. The research indicates that the majority of newly licensed LPN/LVNs are caring most frequently for adult and older adult clients with stabilized chronic conditions, clients with behavioral/emotional conditions, and well clients. Each question reflects a level of the nursing process or an area of client needs, and each question is categorized according to a validated level of difficulty. The examination consists of questions that are designed to test the candidate's ability to use clinical judgment in applying the nursing process, prioritizing client care, and determining appropriate nursing responses and interventions to provide safe, effective nursing care at the entry level.

Integrated Processes

Integrated throughout the test plan are principles that are fundamental to the practice of nursing. There are six integrated processes in the NCLEX-PN exam: caring, clinical judgment, communication and documentation, culture and spirituality, and teaching and learning.

Caring

The interaction of the client and the nurse occurs in an atmosphere of mutual respect and trust. To achieve the desired outcome, the nurse provides hope, support, and compassion to the client.

> **TESTING TIP** *Always keep in mind that the NCLEX is about nursing care, so the concept of caring should be considered when selecting an option. Be sure to address and acknowledge the client's feelings and provide support.*

Clinical Judgment

The observed outcome of critical thinking and decision making is clinical judgment, which is a process involving multiple steps where nursing knowledge is used to observe and assess clinical situations, identify client care priorities, and generate the best possible evidence-based solutions to deliver safe, effective client care.

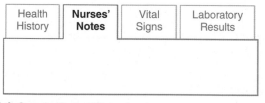

FIG. 1.1 Sample Medical Record.

Table 1.1 **SIX COGNITIVE SKILLS OR PROCESSES**	
NCSBN Clinical Judgment Cognitive Skills	**Description**

Recognize Cues	*What is important or matters the most?*
	• Cues are client findings or assessment data
	• Four major types of ***cues***
	   1. Environmental cues – presence of a family member; emergency department, clinic
	   2. Client observation cues – signs and symptoms
	   3. Medical record cues – flow sheets, vital signs, nurses' notes, laboratory results
	   4. Time pressure cues – onset and severity of symptoms
	• Need to identify important and relevant information from the four types of cues (assessment)

Analyze Cues	*What does the information mean and how do I interpret it?* • Organize and link the recognized cues to the client's condition or problem, which could be actual or potential (analysis) • Is the data expected or unexpected • Need to understand pathophysiology and signs and symptoms
Prioritize Hypotheses	*What is a priority and where do I start?* • Rank client conditions or problems according to immediacy, likelihood, risk, difficulty, and time constraints • Think about the *most likely* priority (analysis)
Generate Solutions	*What are possible options and what can I do?* • First identify expected or desired outcomes and interventions, which can include additional assessment data (planning)
Take Action	*What is the most appropriate action to take and what will I do?* • Implement the nursing interventions that address the client's priority conditions or problems (implementation)
Evaluate Outcomes	*Was the action effective and did it help?* • Compare observed outcomes against expected outcomes to determine effectiveness of care (evaluation)

From Dickison, P., Haerling, K. A., & Lasater, K. (2019). Integrating the National Council of State Boards of Nursing clinical judgment model into nursing educational frameworks. *Journal of Nursing Education, 58*(2), 72–78; National Council of State Boards of Nursing. (2020, Spring). The NGN case study. *Next Generation NCLEX NEWS*, pp. 2–6.

Table 1.2   A CLOSER LOOK AT NGN ITEM TYPES

Highlight	Drag and Drop	Drop Down	Matrix	Extended Multiple Response	Bowtie	Trend
Highlight						
• Highlight in Text	• Drag and Drop Cloze	• Drop Down Cloze	• Matrix Multiple Response	• Multiple Response Select All That Apply	• One Condition Most Likely Experiencing response in the middle	• Presents information over time in a medical record • Can use any NGN type, except bowtie
• Highlight in Table	• Drag and Drop Rationale	• Drop Down Rationale	• Matrix Multiple Choice	• Multiple Response Select N	• Two Actions to Take on the left	
		• Drop Down in Table		• Multiple Response Grouping	• Two Parameters to "Monitor" on the right	

From Betts, J., Muntean, W., Kim, D., & Kao, S. (2022, Winter). Next Generation NCLEX: Test design. *Next Generation NCLEX NEWS*, p. 3; National Council of State Boards of Nursing. (2021, Spring). Next Generation: Stand-alone items. *Next Generation NCLEX NEWS*, p. 2.

TESTING TIP *On the NCLEX clinical judgment will be tested by questions that involve critical thinking and decision making using the six cognitive skills or processes in the NCSBN's Clinical Judgment Measurement Model, which are (1) recognize cues, (2) analyze cues, (3) prioritize hypotheses, (4) generate solutions, (5) take action, and (6) evaluate outcomes.*

Communication and Documentation

Events and activities—both verbal and nonverbal—that involve the client, the client's significant others, and the health care team are documented in handwritten or electronic records. These records reflect quality and accountability in the provision of client care. Principles of documentation and provision of client confidentiality are important considerations in any area of nursing practice.

TESTING TIP *Communication-focused questions will be about effective or therapeutic communication techniques, which involve focusing on the client's feelings and concerns. Always acknowledge the client's feelings. When answering a question about documentation, remember the nurse's ethical and legal responsibilities and specific guidelines for the computerized documentation system.*

Culture and Spirituality

The interaction between the nurse and the client (individual, family, or group, including significant others and population), which recognizes and considers the client-reported, self-identified, unique, and individual preferences to client care, relates to the integrated processes of culture and spirituality.

TESTING TIP *Cultural awareness and sensitivity are a nursing responsibility. Be sure to ask the client about their cultural and spiritual beliefs and practices.*

Nursing Process

The nursing process is a scientific approach to problem solving; it has been a common thread in your nursing curriculum since the beginning of school. There is nothing new about the nursing process on the NCLEX. Assessment data are obtained, the data are analyzed, a plan is formulated, nursing actions are implemented, and the results of that intervention are evaluated. It is important to keep the steps of the nursing process in mind when you are critically evaluating an NCLEX question. See Box 1.1, Key Words for Identifying the Nursing Process.

TESTING TIP *When answering a test question, data collection or assessment is the first step of the nursing process. Keep in mind if the question involves an emergency situation, taking action may be the priority instead of assessment. Questions that are about planning will most often revolve around nursing care rather than medical treatment plans. Watch for questions about goal statements and questions that focus on actual problems rather than possible problems. Implementation is about nursing interventions or actions and monitoring the client's response to them. Evaluation questions may be written to address a client's response to treatment measures (e.g., medication response, oxygen therapy, hot/cold packs, etc.) or to determine a client's understanding of the prescribed treatment measures.*

Teaching and Learning

Nurses provide or facilitate knowledge, skills, and attitudes that promote a change in clients' behavior through teaching

The following words and phrases have the same meaning and are often interchangeable. The words are associated with activities in the practice analysis.

- **Data collection (assessment):** gather objective and subjective, determine, observe, identify findings, recognize changes, notice, detect, find data, verify data, gather information, describe status, assess client
- **Analysis:** interpret data, identify a nursing diagnosis, collect additional data, examine client data, consider nursing data, examine client data for priority
- **Planning:** establish goals, plan interventions, create plan, generate goals, prioritize outcomes of client care, arrange priorities and interventions, formulate short-term goal or long-term goals, prepare list of client outcomes, develop and modify nursing plan of care
- **Implementation:** implement nursing interventions, delegate nursing care, offer alternatives, teach, give, administer, chart, document, explain, inform, encourage, advise, provide, prepare, counsel, teach, perform or assist with client care and needs
- **Evaluation:** evaluate nursing care, question results, monitor findings, repeat assessment, compare outcomes with expected nursing care outcomes, reestablish, consider alternatives, determine changes and response, appraise findings, modify plan of care, evaluate plan of care based on client compliance

and learning. Nurses provide education to clients and to their significant others in a variety of settings. Identifying critical learning needs for clients and their significant others and providing information in a manner that promotes the health and safety of clients are important across all levels of nursing practice.

TESTING TIP   *The LPN/LVN reinforces the teaching initiated by the registered nurse (RN). A client's motivation and readiness to learn are priorities when it comes to client education.*

AREAS OF CLIENT NEEDS

The National Council Examination Committee has identified four primary areas of client needs, which provide a structure to define nursing actions and competencies across all practice settings and for all clients. These areas reflect an integrated approach to the testing content; no predetermined number of questions or percentage of questions pertain to any area of practice (e.g., medical-surgical, pediatric, obstetric, psychiatric).

Table 1.3 lists the areas of client needs, along with the subcategories and the specific percentages associated with each subcategory. The range of percentages for each category reflects how important that area is on the test plan. Coordinated care, safety and infection control, and pharmacologic therapies are the subcategories with the highest

emphasis on the test plan with psychosocial integrity and reduction of risk potential being the next highest.

Let's take a moment to see how a traditional multiple-choice test item might be written to address the eight categories of client needs across the life span in a variety of settings.

Safe and Effective Care Environment

This area consists of two subcategories, which are coordinated care and safety and infection control.

Coordinated Care

Example: A nurse is charting at the nurses' station. Which situation would be considered a priority and should be taken care of **first**?

1. A family member who is very angry regarding the quality of nursing care.
2. A health care provider on the phone with changes to a client's postoperative orders.
3. A request from a client for pain medication as soon as they can have it.
4. The postanesthesia recovery department calling to give a report on a client returning to the unit.

The correct answer is 1. Notice the words "priority" and "first," which asks the nurse to decide which situation should be addressed first. The family member would take priority over the other clients. The family member is angry and if they are put off, more than likely they will become angrier and more difficult to communicate with. There is no jeopardy placed on clients in the other options. The health care provider can either talk to another nurse, or you can politely tell them you have an urgent matter and you will call them back. Recovery can wait to give the report without jeopardizing the client's safety. The client complaining of pain is not an urgent situation because the client has asked for pain medication when it is available.

Safety and Infection Control

Example: The nurse is caring for a client diagnosed with a methicillin-resistant *Staphylococcus aureus* (MRSA) infection. What infection control procedure will the nurse implement when working with this client?

1. Remove any soiled linens from the room to prevent a reservoir for bacteria.
2. Cleanse the blood pressure cuff before removing it from the room.
3. Keep gloves on until out of the room and in an area in which they can be disposed.
4. Place specimens in a container that is clean and labeled on the outside for transport.

The answer is 4. All specimens, whether infectious or non-infectious, should be transported to the laboratory in a container that is clean on the outside of the container. The label should be on the outside of the bag or container. Linens should be placed in a bag and removed when necessary. When removed, linens should be placed in a waterproof linen bag and marked as contaminated. Blood pressure cuffs, stethoscopes, thermometers, dressing supplies, and irrigation fluids should remain in the client's room. Gloves should be removed before the nurse leaves the client's room.

Table 1.3   NCLEX-PN TEST PLAN—EFFECTIVE APRIL 2023 TO MARCH 2026ᵃ

Safe and Effective Care Environment

Coordinated care (18%–24%)	Concepts of coordinated nursing care—assignment, supervision, continuity of care, establishing priorities in client care; legal and ethical responsibilities; client rights; informed consent; confidentiality; information technology
Safety and infection control (10%–16%)	Prevention of errors and accidents, implementation of standard precautions, asepsis, use of least restrictive restraints and safety devices, safe use of equipment, ergonomic principles, emergency response plan, handling hazardous and infectious materials, security plan

Health Promotion and Maintenance

(6%–12%)	Aging process and developmental stages, lifestyle choices, high-risk behaviors; ante/intra/postpartum and newborn; health promotion and disease prevention, data collection techniques

Psychosocial Integrity

(9%–15%)	Mental health concepts and interventions; end-of-life care; grief and loss; sensory and perceptual alterations; cultural, religious, and spiritual influences; behavioral intervention/crisis intervention; chemical and substance use dependency; abuse and neglect; therapeutic communication and environment

Physiologic Integrity

Basic care and comfort (7%–13%)	Assistive devices, mobility/immobility, nutrition and oral hydration, personal hygiene, elimination, nonpharmacologic comfort measures, rest and sleep
Pharmacologic therapies (10%–16%)	Medication administration; expected medication actions, side effects/contraindication/outcomes; dosage calculation; pharmacologic pain management
Reduction of risk potential (9%–15%)	Nursing implications for and nursing care to minimize potential complications of diagnostic tests/procedures/surgery; potential for alterations in body systems (tubes, pacemakers, hyper/hypoglycemia, specimens, bleeding, wounds, positions); laboratory values; changes in and/or abnormal vital signs; therapeutic procedures
Physiologic adaptation (7%–13%)	Alterations in body systems: fluid and electrolyte imbalances, medical emergencies (CPR, airway, hemorrhage), unexpected response to therapies (seizures, changes in vital signs); basic pathophysiology

ᵃTest plan information is presented as examples only and is not intended to be a complete or thorough representation of information included in any specific category.

CPR, Cardiopulmonary resuscitation.

Adapted from the *2023 NCLEX-PN Test Plan for the National Council Licensure Examination for Registered Nurses*. (2023). Chicago: National Council of State Boards of Nursing.

Health Promotion and Maintenance

Example: In performing an assessment on a 4-month-old, what would the nurse expect the infant to be able to do?
1. Sit steadily without support.
2. Turn from back to abdomen.
3. Grasp for objects.
4. Hold head erect.

The correct answer is 4. When performing a wellness assessment on an infant, the nurse needs to understand growth and development milestones. Head in alignment with no support occurs around 4 to 5 months of age. At 8 months, infants should be able to sit steadily unsupported. Turning from back to abdomen occurs around 6 months of age, as does grasping for objects.

Psychosocial Integrity

Example: A client is crying and anxious and tells the nurse that their partner has recently asked for a divorce. Which is the **best** response for the nurse to make?

1. "Now, now, stop crying so that we can discuss your feelings about the divorce."
2. "How long were you and your partner together?"
3. "I can see how upset you are. Let's talk about what happened."
4. "Let's discuss how we can secure social services and a lawyer to help you look out for your interests."

The third comment is a therapeutic response, which is the "best" response. Acknowledging the client's feelings helps validate the personal distress and provides an opportunity for the client to talk about their feelings. The client is experiencing a crisis and needs to discuss their feelings. Discussing long-range plans, such as securing social services and a lawyer, is not an appropriate nursing intervention at this time. How long the relationship has existed is not relevant and telling the client to stop crying is a denial of their feelings.

Physiologic Integrity

This area has four subcategories, which are basic care and comfort, pharmacologic therapies, reduction of risk potential, and physiologic adaptation.

Basic Care and Comfort

Example: The nurse caring for a client diagnosed with Parkinson disease is now assisting with discharge planning. What would be a **priority** home care goal for this client?
1. Maintain proper positioning to prevent contractures.
2. Promote daily activity and independence.
3. Encourage use of laxatives to prevent constipation.
4. Decrease fluid intake to prevent aspiration.

Clients with chronic, neurogenerative diseases, such as Parkinson disease, need to maintain independence, which would be a priority home care goal for this client (option 2). It is important to plan for daily activity and to promote as much independence in activities of daily living (ADLs) and independent activities of daily living (IADLs) as much as possible. Positioning should not be an emphasis now, but active and passive range of motion should be. Fluid intake should be increased to maintain good hydration. Constipation can be prevented or alleviated with increased fluids and dietary fiber.

Pharmacologic Therapies

Example: What important point should the nurse remember when administering multiple medications via a feeding tube?
1. Administer each medication individually, followed by flushing the tube.
2. Maintain asepsis by using sterile gloves for the procedure.
3. Obtain vital signs before giving any medications via a tube.
4. Crush and mix all medications together to facilitate administration.

The correct answer is 1. Medications should be prepared separately followed by flushing the tube. This ensures that the medications do not mix with each other. Crushing and mixing medications together can cause interactions because the medications may be incompatible. Whether or not the vital signs are checked depends on the type of medication administered. This is a clean procedure, not a sterile procedure.

Reduction of Risk Potential

Example: An older adult client diagnosed with peripheral vascular disease (PVD) is being discharged. The nurse is assisting with the discharge instruction. Which of the client's risk factors would be **most important** to discuss regarding the client's medical history?
1. Orthostatic hypotension.
2. Age.
3. Smoking.
4. Hypoglycemia.

The correct answer is 3. Smoking causes vasoconstriction, which increases the complications brought about by PVD. This is a modifiable risk factor that will assist in increasing circulation. Age cannot be modified. Clients with diabetes are at increased risk for the development of PVD, but it is not due to hypoglycemia, instead hyperglycemia. These clients need to maintain good control of diabetes to avoid PVD as a complication of the disease process. Orthostatic hypotension is not a relevant condition unless the client is on antihypertensive medication or is dehydrated.

Physiologic Adaptation

Example: The nurse is caring for a client diagnosed with chronic kidney disease. What observations would indicate kidney failure is progressing?
1. Lethargy, hypertension, proteinuria.
2. Hypotension, tachycardia, increased irritability.
3. Increased urinary concentration, weight loss.
4. Diarrhea, hypovolemia.

Lethargy, hypertension, and proteinuria (option 1) are classic symptoms that may occur as kidney failure progresses. The urine has decreased concentration. There is increased weight gain and fluid overload. Other changes occur throughout the body, which may include confusion, bleeding, and an increase in serum potassium level, along with an increase in BUN and creatinine. Diarrhea and hypovolemia are not indicators of advancing kidney failure.

When you are studying for the NCLEX, these are concepts that should be identified across the scope of nursing practice. Table 1.3 has been adapted and summarized; it does not reflect the entire test plan content. The National Council's Detailed Test Plan for the NCLEX-PN may be obtained from the NCSBN (https://www.ncsbn.org). What was great new information in last month's nursing journals will not be immediately reflected on the NCLEX. New information or new practices must be established as a standard of practice across the nation before being included on the NCLEX.

ALERT boxes can be found throughout this book that call your attention to areas of the test plan. Pay attention to these boxes and think about how each concept or principle can apply to different types of clients.

> **TEST ALERT** The NCLEX-PN is a licensure test that requires use of the nursing process and application of nursing concepts and principles across the life span and to use clinical judgment in providing client care.

As client conditions or nursing principles are presented, the NURSING PRIORITY boxes call your attention to critical information regarding a client with a specific condition or situation being presented.

> **❗ NURSING PRIORITY** This is critical information to consider in providing safe nursing care for a client with a specific problem and assists you in making clinical judgments.

Classification of Questions

The majority of questions on the NCLEX are written at the level of *application* or a higher level of cognitive ability. This means a candidate must have the knowledge and understanding of concepts to be able to apply the nursing process to the client situation presented in the question. NCLEX questions are based on critical thinking concepts that demonstrate a candidate's ability to make decisions and solve problems. NCLEX questions are not fact, recall, or memory-level questions. The questions and answers have been thoroughly researched and validated. The standardization of information is important because the NCLEX is administered nationwide to determine entry level into nursing practice. This ensures that regional differences in nursing care will not be a factor in the examination.

All questions presented to a candidate taking the NCLEX have been developed according to the test plan and the integrated processes fundamental to nursing practice and have been categorized according to their level of difficulty. The questions have been researched and documented as pertaining to entry-level nursing behaviors.

COMPUTER ADAPTIVE TESTING

Computer adaptive testing (CAT) provides a method for generating an examination according to each candidate's ability. Each time a candidate answers a question, the computer then selects the next question based on the candidate's answer to the previous question. A candidate cannot skip questions or go back to previously answered questions. As the examination progresses, it is interactively assembled. The examination continues to present test items based on the test plan and identified level of difficulty to provide an opportunity for each candidate to demonstrate competency. The NCLEX-PN is graded in a manner different from the grading of conventional school examinations. A candidate's score is not based on the number of questions answered correctly but rather on the standard of competency as established by the NCSBN.

A test bank of questions is loaded into the candidate's computer at the beginning of the examination. With CAT, each candidate's test is unique. Different candidates receive different sets of questions, but all test banks contain questions that are developed according to the same test plan. For example, standard precautions are a critical element of the test plan. Many situations and clients can be presented to test this concept: One candidate may have a question based on standard precautions required for a client in labor; someone else may have a situation with implications for a client with a respiratory problem; and still, someone else may have a situation involving a newborn. All the questions are different, but they are all based on the test plan's critical element of standard precautions.

The questions to be presented to the candidate are determined by the candidate's response to previous questions. Every time the candidate answers an item, the computer reestimates the candidate's ability. With each additional answered item, the ability estimate becomes more precise. Items are selected that the candidate will find challenging. Based on the candidate's answers up to that point and the difficulty of those items, the computer estimates the candidate's ability. Next, an item is selected that the candidate should have a 50% chance of answering correctly. This way, the next item should not be too easy or too hard, and the examination can get maximum information about the candidate's ability from the item. The computer will continue to present questions that are based on the test plan and on the level of ability of the candidate until a level of competency has been established.

TAKING THE NCLEX-PN EXAMINATION
Application

An application must be submitted to the state board of nursing in the state in which the candidate wants to be licensed. The contact information for the state boards of nursing is available on the NCSBN website. After the candidate's application and registration fees have been received and approved by the state, the candidate will receive an authorization to test (ATT) from the NCSBN. After the examination fee has been paid, it will not be refunded, regardless of how the candidate registered. The candidate may register for the NCLEX at the NCLEX Candidate website (listed in the ATT) or by telephone (also listed in the ATT). The Candidate Bulletin (CB) is available on the NCSBN website; be sure to print this bulletin for future reference. The CB provides critical information, including addresses and phone numbers for registration and specific details regarding the registration process.

If you are an *internationally educated nurse*, it is most important for you to contact the board of nursing where you will be residing to obtain information about licensure. The state board of nursing will require you to provide specific documents as part of the application process to become eligible to take the NCLEX-PN exam.

Scheduling the Examination

After you have been declared eligible to take the NCLEX and have received an ATT via email, you may schedule an examination date. You *must have an ATT* before you can schedule your examination. The ATT email contains your authorization number, candidate identification number, and an expiration or validity date. Even though you will **not** need to bring a paper copy of the ATT for admittance to the NCLEX, take a few moments and print a copy of your ATT email, so it doesn't get lost in all your emails, because it contains important information. The CB lists the phone number to call to schedule the examination. Once the ATT has been emailed to the candidate, the state stipulates a period of time within which you must take the examination. This ranges with the average being 90 days; this period *cannot* be extended. You must test within the validity dates noted on your ATT. You are encouraged to schedule the appointment to take the examination as soon as possible after receiving the ATT, even if you do not plan to take the test immediately. This will increase the probability of getting the testing date you want.

Pearson Vue is the company that provides the testing facility and computers for the examination. An NGN tutorial is available at https://www.nclex.com/next-generation-nclex.htm. Go to the site and review the tutorial. It should be familiar to you when you see it on NCLEX. This same tutorial will be presented to you at the beginning of your examination.

Testing Accommodations

The candidate should contact their respective board of nursing to inquire and request testing accommodations **before** submitting the NCLEX registration to Pearson VUE or scheduling the testing appointment. The board of nursing will provide the candidate with the process for requesting accommodations. If the request is approved, the candidate will be notified and the procedure for registering for the NCLEX will be provided.

Changing Your Appointment

Life happens and you may need to change your scheduled appointment. Please review the CB for the process on how to change your appointment date, time, or location. If you fail to arrive for your examination appointment or fail to reschedule/unschedule without giving the appropriate notice, you will forfeit your examination fee (and scheduling fee, if applicable), and your ATT will be invalidated. You will be required to reregister and pay another examination fee.

Testing Center Identification

An acceptable form of identification is required at the testing site. If you arrive without your identification, you will be turned away and required to reregister and repay the examination fee. The first and last name printed on your identification must match exactly the first and last name provided when registering (name printed on the ATT email). If the name with which you have registered is different from the name on your identification, you must bring legal name change documentation with you to the test center on the day of your test. The only acceptable forms of legal documentation are a marriage license, divorce decree, and/or a court action legal name change document. Identification must be in English, cannot be expired, and must contain your signature. Acceptable forms of identification are a US driver's license, a passport book or passport card, a US state-issued identification, a permanent residence card, or a US military-issued identification. At the testing site before testing, each candidate is digitally fingerprinted, a photo is taken, and a signature and palm vein reader scan are required.

Day of the Examination

You should plan on arriving at the center approximately 30 minutes before the scheduled testing time. If you arrive more than 30 minutes late, the scheduled testing time will be cancelled, and you may have to reapply and repay the examination fee. An erasable note board will be available at your computer terminal. You are not allowed to take any books, personal belongings (watches, large jewelry), hats, coats, scarves, blank tablets, or scratch paper into the testing area. Cell/mobile/smartphones, pagers, or other electronic devices may not be accessed during the examination, including during breaks. Candidates will be provided a plastic bag to store their cell/mobile/smartphones and electronic devices, which will be collected by the testing center agent and sealed. Secure storage will be provided; however, candidates are not allowed to access any of the prohibited personal items at any time during the exam, including breaks. Storage space is small, so candidates should plan appropriately. Upon completion of the examination, the testing center agent will break the seal on the plastic bag and return the devices to the candidate.

Testing

There have been some modifications to the testing since the COVID-19 pandemic and now occurring since NGN launched in April 2023. Be sure to always check the CB for the most up-to-date information. You will have a maximum of 5 hours to complete the examination. After 2 hours of testing, you have a preprogrammed break; another optional break occurs after 3½ hours of testing. If you need a break before that time, raise your hand to notify one of the attendants at the testing center. The computer will automatically signal when a scheduled break begins. All of the break times and the tutorial are considered part of the total 5 hours of testing time. A palm vein scan will be taken when you leave the testing area and will be taken to reenter the testing area after each break.

The examination will stop when one of the following occurs:

1. Beginning in April 2023 on the NGN, 85 questions have been answered and a minimum level of competency has been established, or a lack of minimum competency has been established.
2. The candidate has answered the maximum number of 150 questions on the NGN.
3. The candidate has been testing for 5 hours, regardless of the number of questions answered.

Each candidate will receive between 85 and 150 questions. The number of questions on the NGN is not indicative of the level of competency. The majority of candidates who complete all 150 questions will have demonstrated a level of minimum competency and therefore pass the NGN. A mouse is used for selecting answers, so candidates should not worry about different computer keyboard function keys. An onscreen calculator is also available to use for math problems. If any problems occur with the environment or with the equipment, someone will be available to provide assistance.

On the minimum-length exam consisting of 85 items, 52 of the items will come from the eight content areas of client needs listed in Table 1.3 based on the percentages identified. Eighteen of the items will be three clinical judgment case studies (six items for each case study measuring the six clinical judgment skills). The remaining 15 items will be unscored, pretest items. The pretest items can be composed of clinical judgment case studies or standalone items. The total number of scored items on the new NGN will be 70 to 135.

The statistics on these items are evaluated to determine whether the item is a valid test item to be included in future NCLEX test banks. All of the items that are scored, or counted, on a candidate's examination have been pretested and validated. It is impossible to determine which questions or items are scored items and which are pretest items. While testing, it is important to treat each question as a scored item.

The Candidate Bulletin from the NCSBN is important; read the information carefully and keep it until the results from NCLEX have been received. The CB will provide dirrctions and will answer most of your questions regarding the NCLEX. The CB is available online (from the NCSBN at https://www.ncsbn.org or from Pearson Vue at https://www.pearsonvue.com/nclex).

Test Results

Each examination is scored twice, once at the testing center and again at the testing service. The test results are electronically transferred to the state boards of nursing. Test results are *not* available at the testing center, from Pearson Vue, or from the NCSBN. Check the information received from the appropriate state board of nursing to determine how and when your results will be available. Test results may be available online. In some states, results may be available within 2 to 3 days; in others, the results will be mailed, which will require a longer notification period. Do *not* call the Pearson Professional Center, NCLEX Candidate Services, the National Council, or the individual state board of nursing for test results. Follow the procedure found in the information from the state board of nursing where the license will be issued.

PARTIAL CREDIT SCORING

One of the significant changes in the NGN exam initiated in April 2023 is the introduction of **partial credit scoring**. This type of scoring will be used on the new, more complicated and involved NGN item types and include today's traditional alternate-item format of "select all that apply." Prior to the NGN exam, items were scored as either all correct or all incorrect, with no partial credit for partial understanding as noted by some correct responses. Partial credit scoring will not apply to single-option multiple-choice questions where one option is the correct answer. Instead, partial understanding will be evaluated by polytomous scoring models that allow a test item to be scored for individual credit. Although this type of scoring is a more complicated model, it provides better information about the candidate's ability.

Pass or Fail Decisions

The NCSBN has three scenarios that guide a decision on passing or failing the exam.

1. *95% confidence interval rule.* This is the most common for NGN candidates. The computer will stop administering items when it is 95% certain that the candidate's ability is either clearly above or clearly below the passing standard.
2. *Maximum-length exam.* The candidate's ability levels will be very close to the passing standard. The computer continues to administer questions until the maximum number of items is reached. When the final ability estimate is above the passing standard, the candidate passes and, likewise, when the final ability estimate is at or below the passing standard, the candidate fails.
3. *Run-out-of-time rule (ROOT).* The exam ends because the candidate runs out of time before reaching the maximum number of items; the computer does not have sufficient information to decide whether the candidate passed

or failed with 95% certainty. When the candidate has not answered the minimum number of items, the result will be a failing exam. When the candidate has answered the minimum number of items, then the exam is scored by using the final ability estimate, which if it is above the passing standard, the candidate passes.

Candidate Performance Report

When candidates fail, the state board of nursing will send a candidate performance report. This report provides the number of items administered to the candidate and a summary of the candidate's relative strengths and weaknesses based on the test plan. This information can be a helpful guide for studying as the candidate prepares to retake the exam. Each state has its own policy on the number of exam retakes; however, the NCSBN requires at least 45 days between each exam.

Nurse Licensure Compact

When you are making application to the state board of nursing for initial licensure, please check out whether your state is a member of the nurse licensure compact, which allows a nurse to have one multistate license with the ability to practice in their home state (legal residency state) and other compact states.

TYPES OF TEST ITEMS

According to the NCSBN (2022), the new NGN exam will have multiple-choice items, case studies, and items written in alternate formats. There may be multimedia such as charts, tables, and graphics in the different item formats. The new NGN item types are listed in Table 1.2.

This section provides an example of all of the previous test item formats. Let's start out with the multiple-choice item and its characteristics.

Multiple Choice

This is the type of test question that is the most familiar to you. It has three parts: the stem or situation, the question, and the options. The *stem or situation* of the question presents information or describes a client situation. Next, the *question* will ask you about the information that was presented. With this type of item there will be four *options* and one must be selected as the correct answer.

QUESTION 1.1 MULTIPLE CHOICE

A nurse is planning to irrigate a nasogastric tube prior to administering a tube feeding. What nursing measure is most reliable when confirming the placement of the nasogastric tube prior to the administration of a tube feeding?

- ○ Instill about 30 mL of air and listen for air over the gastric area.
- ○ Hold the end of the tube in a cup of water and observe for bubbles.
- ○ Ask the client if they are having any difficulty breathing.
- ● Aspirate fluid into the syringe and determine the pH.

Test-Taking Strategy: The correct answer is 4. The question is asking what the **most reliable method** is to confirm placement, which is to aspirate contents and determine the pH of the aspirated fluid using blue litmus paper. If the aspirated fluid is acidic (stomach contents), the litmus paper will turn blue. It is not recommended to insert air and listen for the air movement into the stomach because it is unreliable, as are the second and third options.

Alternate Item Format

The following are types of alternate format questions and include multiple response, fill in the blank, hot spot, ordered response (drag-and-drop), chart or exhibit, graphic options, and audio.

Examples of each type of question will be presented and additional questions can be found on the companion Evolve site. *All item types may include multimedia such as charts, tables, and graphics.*

Multiple Response: Select All That Apply (SATA)

Multiple-response items require you to select all of the options that apply to the question. Essentially, they are formatted like a multiple-choice item; however, there will be more than four options from which to select answers and the question will clearly state, "**Select all that apply.**" Using the mouse, you will select each item to be included in the answer. Consider each item and make a decision whether it is to be included in the correct answer. The options are preceded by square boxes, and you can check more than one box; however, there can be just one correct answer.

QUESTION 1.2 MULTIPLE RESPONSE: SELECT ALL THAT APPLY (SATA)

The nurse is caring for an 85-year-old client who has a diagnosis of vancomycin resistant enterococci (VRE) pneumonia. What precautions will the nurse implement in assisting the client with morning care? **Select all that apply.**

- ■ Wear clean gloves.
- □ Remove all extra suctioning supplies from the room.
- □ Dispose of the gown and mask in the container outside client's door.
- ■ Wear face mask when working within 3 feet of the client.
- ■ Put on a gown prior to entering the room.
- □ Remove the stethoscope from the room if it did not come in contact with the client.

Test-Taking Strategy: Think about the client's condition. Standard plus droplet precautions will be used for this client. What is added to standard precautions when droplet precautions are included? Go through all of the options and decide which options are true and are something the nurse should do; then select all of the true options that apply to this client. Options 1, 4, and 5 are correct. In option 1, yes (true), the nurse is going to provide morning care and have direct contact with the client; therefore gloves should be worn. Option 2, no (false), the suctioning supplies should be left in the room. Option 3, no (false), the gown and mask

are disposed of in the client's room. Option 4, yes (true), a mask is necessary if the nurse is to come within 3 feet of the client, which the nurse can expect to do when providing or assisting with morning care. Option 5, yes (true), a gown should be worn because the nurse is going to be close to and have direct contact with the client. Option 6, no (false), the stethoscope should not be taken into the client's room; if it is taken into the room, it should be left in the room.

Fill-in-the-Blank

Fill-in-the-blank questions are frequently presented for medication dosage calculations, IV drip calculations, or intake and output calculations, just to name a few. A drop-down calculator is provided on the computer screen. With calculation questions, the final unit of measurement is always provided. *Only the number is placed in the answer box.* Check the items necessary to make this calculation. For example, is it necessary to make conversions from grams to milligrams or from liters to milliliters? Make sure all of the units of measurement needed in the final answer are in the same system of measurement.

Memorize the formulas necessary to calculate the drug dosages and conversions. The number of decimal places to be included in the answer is indicated in the question. *Do not round any numbers until you have the final answer.* You should not enter any other characters except those necessary to form a number.

QUESTION 1.3 FILL-IN-THE-BLANK

The health care provider calls the unit and leaves an order for cefaclor 0.1 gm PO, every 6 hours. The dose available on the unit is 125 mg/5 mL. How many milliliters will the nurse give?

Answer: [4] mL

Test-Taking Strategy: The correct answer is 4 mL. Use your calculator and consider what formula you will use for the dosage calculation.

First convert gm to mg.

1 gm = 1000 mg, therefore 0.1 gm = 100 mg

$$\text{Formula: } \frac{\text{Desired dose}}{\text{Available dose}} \times \text{Volume} = \text{mL}$$

$$\frac{100 \text{ mg}}{125 \text{ mg}} \times 5 \text{ mL} = 5 \times 100 = 500 \text{ X} = 500/125 = 4 \text{ mL}$$

Hot Spot

In a hot-spot question, you will be presented with a graphic or picture and asked to identify a specific item, area, or location on the graphic or picture by clicking on it with the mouse.

QUESTION 1.4 HOT SPOT

The nurse is caring for a client who is receiving 0.25 mg digoxin each morning. On the picture, identify the correct location where the nurse should place the stethoscope to determine the client's apical pulse.

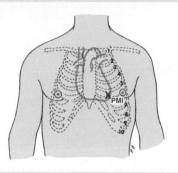

Test-Taking Strategy: The "hot spot" (in this case, the correct area to assess the apical heart rate) is at the PMI, or point of maximum impulse, which is located at the fifth intercostal space, just to the left of the sternal border. To answer this question, you would simply click the area on the graphic. The correct location is noted in the figure with a red X.

Ordered Response (drag-and-drop)

In an ordered response or drag-and-drop question, several steps or actions are listed, and your job is to place them in a correct sequence. All of the options will be used, but you must place them in the correct order. The first thing to do is to decide in what order you want to place the options or rank the actions. After you have determined your answer, click on the option you want to place first, "drag" that option over, and place it in the first box. Then select the option you want to place second, drag that option over, and place it in the next box. Continue this process until you have used all of the options present.

QUESTION 1.5 ORDERED RESPONSE (DRAG-AND-DROP)

The nurse is caring for a client diagnosed with pneumonia. The client is dyspneic and has a temperature of 102 °F (38.9°C) orally. The client is reporting chest pain. In what order would the nurse provide care for this client?

Place all of the nursing actions below in the order of priority for nursing care. Use all the options.

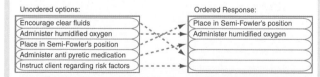

Unordered options:	Ordered Response:
Encourage clear fluids	Place in Semi-Fowler's position
Administer humidified oxygen	Administer humidified oxygen
Place in Semi-Fowler's position	
Administer anti pyretic medication	
Instruct client regarding risk factors	

Test-Taking Strategy: Think about what your first action would be. Remember independent actions should be done first. The client should be placed in a semi-Fowler position before oxygen administration is started; an antipyretic medication could be given next. This action addresses current needs. Next, encourage intake of clear liquids to decrease viscosity of secretions. Finally, provide instruction regarding risk factors (psychosocial need).

Chart/Exhibit

In this type of question, a client situation or problem and client information are provided in a chart or an exhibit, which is part of a medical record. To begin, click on the tab on the bottom of the screen to see the exhibit; then click on the tabs within the exhibit to find the information needed to answer the question. There may be several tabs to click on; check the information included within each tab and determine whether it is pertinent to the situation.

QUESTION 1.6 CHART/EXHIBIT

After a postoperative client reports pain, the nurse assesses the client and determines the pain is in the abdomen around the area of the incision; pain level is 7 on a scale of 10. The time is 2000 and the nurse is determining what can be done regarding the client's pain. **Select the best answer based on the information in the chart.**

1. Give morphine sulfate 15 mg IM now.
2. Medication cannot be administered.
3. Give morphine sulfate 10 mg IM now.
4. Give hydrocodone 10 mg PO.

Chart:

NURSES' NOTES	MEDICATION RECORD	ORDERS
0800: Reporting abdominal pain around area of incision. Reports pain level of 7 on a scale of 10. Pain medication administered. **1100:** Sleeping, easily aroused. **1600:** Reporting pain level 5 on scale of 10. Pain medication administered. **1800:** Client remains comfortable. **2000:** Beginning to report return of abdominal incision pain.	**0800:** Morphine sulfate 10 mg IM administered. **1600:** Hydrocodone 10 mg PO administered.	**0700:** Morphine sulfate 10–15 mg q 3–4h PRN severe pain. Hydrocodone 10 mg PO, every 3–4 hours moderate pain.

Interpretation of chart information: Client received morphine 10 mg IM at 0800 for severe pain, became lethargic, and slept for the next 5 hours. The client received hydrocodone PO at 1600 and was comfortable for the next 4 hours. The health care provider's orders are current for both the IM and the PO medication for pain.

Test-Taking Strategy: The correct answer is 4. Give the hydrocodone, PO, for the moderate pain being reported at this time. It is preferable to give a client a PO pain medication than a parenteral pain medication. The hydrocodone provided effective pain relief for 4 hours when it was administered the last time, and the health care provider's order is current.

Graphic Options

In this type of question, pictures or graphics instead of text are used for the options. You will need to select the appropriate picture or graphic. This is like a multiple-choice question; the only difference is viewing pictures or graphics as the answer options.

QUESTION 1.7 GRAPHIC OPTIONS

Which ECG rhythm strip would require immediate nursing intervention?

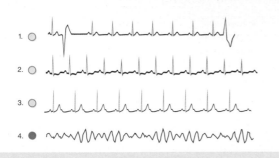

Test-Taking Strategy: The question is asking you to select the option with the ECG strip that represents your answer choice. The correct answer is 4. The nurse will need to intervene immediately if a client demonstrates ventricular fibrillation, which is indicative of a life-threatening dysrhythmia. The priority for this client will be defibrillation and cardiopulmonary resuscitation (CPR). Option 1 is normal sinus rhythm with multifocal premature ventricular contractions (PVCs). Option 2 is sinus tachycardia. Option 3 is sinus bradycardia.

Audio

Audio questions will tell you to put on the headphones to listen to the audio clip of information. You will need to click on the "play" button to hear the information. The information may be replayed, if necessary. After listening to the information, you will select an answer from the options presented.

QUESTION 1.8 AUDIO

A client is postoperative after an abdominal exploratory laparoscopy procedure. The nurse auscultates the abdomen and hears the following:

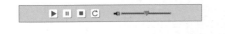

Listen to the audio clip. What would be an appropriate nursing intervention?
- Begin clear liquids, as ordered.
- ○ Notify the surgeon.
- ○ Reinsert nasogastric tube.
- ○ Keep client NPO.

Test-Taking Strategy: First, listen to the audio clip and consider should this postoperative client have bowel sounds. The correct answer is 1. Bowel sounds are noted on the audio clip, which means that peristalsis has returned to the gastrointestinal tract

and the client can begin a clear liquid diet. If bowel sounds are present, there is no need to notify the surgeon. If bowel sounds are *not* present, keep the client NPO or reinsert the nasogastric tube. Laparoscopic procedures are associated with lower rates of postoperative complications, earlier diet progression, and shorter hospital stays.

NGN Item Types

Let's look at the new NGN item types.

Extended Multiple Response: Select All That Apply

In the **select all that apply** question type, there are one or more correct options and information is presented with a chart. There will be a minimum of five options and a maximum of 10 options.

Question 1.8 shows an example of this type of item to measure the clinical judgment skill of *Take Action* about reinforcing teaching with a client about their medications.

QUESTION 1.9 EXTENDED MULTIPLE RESPONSE: SELECT ALL THAT APPLY

A 56-year-old client with history of obesity has been diagnosed with hypertension and prescribed hydrochlorothiazide (HCTZ) 12.5 mg, PO, daily and lisinopril 10 mg, PO, daily. The client is returning to the clinic for follow-up.

Health History	Nurses' Notes	Health Care Provider Orders	Laboratory Results

1030: Client reports taking his medication most of the time and dislikes that he urinates a lot after taking the medication and stopped taking the lisinopril because it caused a nagging cough. States he has been following a low-calorie, low-fat diet and has lost only 2 lb (1 kg) in the past month. Reports it is difficult to stay on the diet with the traveling that he must do as part of his job.

- Temperature: 98°F (37°C)
- BP: 188/100 mm Hg
- Heart rate: 76 beats/min and regular
- Respirations: 20 breaths/min
- SpO2: 98% on room air

Health Care Orders	Nurses' Notes	Vital Signs	Laboratory Results

- Discontinue the lisinopril.
- Continue HCTZ, 12.5 mg, PO daily.
- Start losartan, 25 mg, PO daily.
- At home BP monitoring.
- Return to clinic in 1 month.

Which of the following information provided in previous teaching about the client's medication does the nurse reinforce? **Select all that apply.**
1. "Staying on your medications is very important; you may be on these medications for your lifetime."
2. "Maintain your BP log so we can track how well your BP medications are working."

3. "Put the losartan under the tongue and leave until fully dissolved."
4. "Make sure to maintain a low-cholesterol diet and use sea salt instead of table salt."
5. "Don't stop your losartan suddenly, it can cause rebound hypertension."
6. "Even though you are not a diabetic, you'll need to monitor your blood glucose levels daily."
7. "Make sure you get up slowly to avoid your blood pressure dropping suddenly when you stand up."
8. "Flushing is a common side effect, so take your medication with breakfast."
9. "Keep appointments with your health care provider to monitor your blood pressure."

Note: The correct answers are in *red color*.

Test-Taking Strategy: Read each statement and determine whether it is accurate information that the nurse would reinforce with the client. Long-term compliance is important to prevent complications of hypertension. It is helpful for health care personnel if the client monitors and records home blood pressure and brings the log to health care provider visits. Rebound hypertension can occur if the client stops taking an antihypertensive medication suddenly. Orthostatic hypotension, a drop in blood pressure with a change in position, can occur with clients taking antihypertensives so the client should get up or change positions slowly. Appointments should be kept with the health care provider to monitor the client's progress and adjust the treatment as needed. Nitrates are placed under the tongue, but not losartan, which is taken orally. Sea salt has the same sodium levels as table salt and counts the same as sodium consumption. Clients should be instructed on a low-sodium, low-calorie, and low-fat diet to reduce weight. It is not necessary for this nondiabetic client to check blood glucose levels daily. Flushing is a common side effect of nicotinic acid, not HCTZ or losartan, and taking it with meals does not affect flushing.

Extended Multiple Response: Select N

This item type is similar to select all that apply; however, you are told the number of options to select. Again, there will be a minimum of 5 options and a maximum of 10 options to *select a given N* (number). Question 1.10 shows an example of this type of item to measure the clinical judgment skill of *Take Action* about preventing pressure injury and reducing pressure points in an older adult client. The question asks the nurse to select four nursing interventions.

⚡ QUESTION 1.10 EXTENDED MULTIPLE RESPONSE: SELECT N

The nurse is caring for an 85-year-old client who is transferred from a nursing home to the medical-surgical unit. The client has a history of chronic obstructive pulmonary disease and bilateral hip replacement. The nurse reviews the client's admission assessment.

| Health History | Nurses' Notes | Vital Signs | Laboratory Results |

0800: Client is alert, oriented, and cooperative. Client used a walker to ambulate until recently. After several episodes of dizziness, the client has been reluctant to get out of bed for fear of falling and injuring her hips. Client reports staying in bed for the past week and has episodes of incontinence daily due to inability to get from the bed to the bathroom. Client prefers to lay on the back. Skin in the coccyx area is a deep reddish-pink that does not blanche with fingertip pressure. Skin is warm and tender to touch. Braden Scale score is 16.

Which nursing interventions will assist in reducing pressure points and prevent further pressure injury? **Select four nursing interventions.**
1. Position the client directly on the trochanter when side-lying.
2. Turn every 2 hours.
3. Massage bony prominences.
4. Elevate the head of the bed no more than 30 degrees when possible.
5. When the client is side-lying, use the 30-degree lateral inclined position.
6. Use a pressure-reducing mattress.
7. Use the Braden Scale risk assessment weekly.
8. Restrict fluids to eliminate incontinence.
9. Use a donut-shaped cushion in the coccyx area.

Note: The correct answers are in *red color*.

Test-Taking Strategy: This question is asking for a specific number of correct options. The client is at risk (Braden Scale of 16) and preventative nursing interventions are important. A standard of nursing care to prevent pressure injury is to turn the client every 2 hours when in bed using a written schedule; however, some clients may require more frequent repositioning. Elevating the head of the bed to 30 degrees or less will decrease the chance of pressure injury from shearing forces. When placing the client in a side-lying position, use the 30 degrees lateral inclined position. Do not place the client directly on the trochanter, which can create pressure over the bony prominence. Avoid the use of donut-shaped cushions because they reduce blood supply to the area. Bony prominences should not be massaged because this increases the risk for capillary breakage and injury to underlying tissue. The Braden Scale risk assessment tool should be administered immediately upon admission and while in the hospital every 8 hours. The client should have adequate fluids and nutrition to promote healing and prevent further pressure injury.

Extended Multiple Response: Multiple-Response Grouping

In the *multiple-response grouping*, the options are located in a table. There will be a maximum of four options in each grouping. You will need to select at least one option from each grouping, although more than one option may be correct in each grouping. Question 1.11 shows an example of this type of item to measure the clinical judgment skill of *Recognize Cues* in a child who has fallen with injuries.

⚡ QUESTION 1.11 EXTENDED MULTIPLE RESPONSE: MULTIPLE-RESPONSE GROUPING

A school-age child is at recess and swinging on the playground. The child falls off the swing and is taken immediately to the emergency department.

| Health History | Nurses' Notes | Vital Signs | Laboratory Results |

1330: A 9-year-old child fell while swinging at the school playground and is accompanied to the emergency department by a teacher who relates that the child lost consciousness momentarily after the fall. The child's parents are notified and in transit to the emergency department. Child alert and oriented × 3 with PEERLA. Child is crying and states pain in the left arm and left leg to be 8 on a scale of 10. Severe tissue damage noted on left wrist with bone protrusion. Extensive bruising noted on the left lower leg. Left side of face has a 3 × 1 inch abrasion. Able to move right arm and leg; bruising noted on right lower leg.

For each body system/function below, select the current assessment finding that needs *immediate* follow-up. More than one client finding may be selected for each body system/function.

BODY SYSTEM/ FUNCTION	CURRENT ASSESSMENT FINDING
Neurologic	• PERRLA • Pain 8 on a scale of 10 • Alert and oriented
Musculoskeletal	• Bone protruding from wrist • Moving right arm and leg • Difficulty moving left leg

Note: The correct answers are in *red color*.

Test-Taking Strategy: The immediate assessment findings for the child is pain, protruding bone from the wrist, difficulty in moving the left leg, abrasions on the face, and the concern for a potential head injury due to the momentary loss of consciousness after the fall. With difficulty in moving the left leg, there could be a fracture as noted by the bruising in the lower leg area. It will be important nursing management to monitor for any neurologic changes and prevent infection in the left wrist area until the child is taken to surgery to treat the compound fracture.

Matrix Multiple Choice

With the *matrix multiple choice* item type, the test item is structured in a matrix or table type format with at least four rows and two columns. You can only select one option in each row as the correct answer. Question 1.12 shows an example of this type of item to measure the clinical judgment skill of *Take Action* about discharge instructions for the postpartum client.

⚡ QUESTION 1.12 MATRIX MULTIPLE CHOICE

A nurse is reviewing the postpartum chart of a client who had a term vaginal delivery of a viable female infant 22 hours ago. The nurse is coordinating care with the RN and is preparing to assist with discharging this client and newborn to home. The nurse is reviewing the client's chart.

| Health History | Nurses' Notes | Provider Orders | Laboratory Results |

0800: Client is finishing breakfast. Reports having intermittent sleep through the night while caring for newborn. Client denies perineal discomfort at this time, states she has had some mild uterine cramping with breastfeeding. Examination of the perineum shows mild edema. Uterine placement is one finger breadth below the umbilicus and at midline. Client states lochia discharge remains small but increases when getting up from the bed to walk in the room. Client reports voiding frequently but has not had a bowel movement yet. Client appears loving and attentive toward newborn and verbalizes excitement for discharge home later this morning. Supportive partner is at the bedside. Verbally reports intermittent cramping pain with breastfeeding as 2 out of scale of 10.

- Temperature: 98.6°F (37°C)
- BP: 124/68 mm Hg
- Heart rate: 74 beats/min
- Respirations: 20 breaths/min
- SpO2: 99% on room air

Use an X to indicate which teaching is indicated or contraindicated for the postpartum client being discharged. Each row must have only one response option selected.

CLIENT DISCHARGE TEACHING	INDICATED FOR DISCHARGE TEACHING	CONTRAINDICATED FOR DISCHARGE TEACHING
Coitus should be avoided until 2 weeks postpartum		X
A fever higher than 100.4°F (38°C) should be reported to your provider	X	
Bright red vaginal bleeding is normal in the second week postpartum		X
Any localized breast tenderness or redness should be reported to your provider	X	
Feeling emotional in the first weeks after delivery is common, if it persists or worsens, notify your provider	X	
Afterpains or backaches are common for several weeks after delivery		X

Test-Taking Strategy: Teaching that is indicated includes having the mother report a fever of 100.4 °F (38°C) to the health care provider along with any localized breast tenderness or redness as this can indicate infection. The regulation of hormones after delivery can cause a new mother to feel intense emotions, which is common. If the client has feelings that are persistent and pervasive, the health care provider should be notified. It is contraindicated to have coitus prior to the cessation of lochia discharge, healing of the episiotomy, and clearance from the health care provider; this clearance usually occurs at the first postpartum visit, which can be between 2 and 6 weeks. A return to bright red vaginal bleeding in the postpartum period once lochia flow has become serosa or alba is not common and needs to be further assessed by the health care provider. If afterpains or backaches persist into the weeks postpartum, this could be indicative of an infection.

Test-Taking Strategy: Think about what you know of the signs and symptoms of the three conditions. The client most likely has a form of leukemia because bleeding episodes do not occur with anemia. Hemophilia would have been diagnosed early in the client's life, as it is a hereditary sex-linked disorder. Chronic lymphocytic leukemia (CLL) represents the most common form of leukemia in adults (>55 years old) and is characterized by fever, bleeding tendencies, weight loss, frequent infections, swollen lymph nodes, hepatomegaly, and splenomegaly. Signs and symptoms of hemophilia include persistent or prolonged bleeding, bleeding into the joint cavities (hemarthrosis), spontaneous hematuria, and hematomas. Petechiae are uncommon because the platelet count is normal. Clients with anemia have pale skin (pallor), shortness of breath, dyspnea on exertion, tachycardia, fatigue, weight loss, headache, sore tongue (glossitis), and dizziness.

Matrix Multiple Response

The *matrix multiple-response* item type is structured like the matrix/grid multiple-choice item; however, there can be more than one option correct in each row but at least one option must be selected. Question 1.13 shows an example of this type of item to measure the clinical judgment skill of *Analyze Cues* for an adult client with bleeding problems and fatigue.

⚡ QUESTION 1.13 MATRIX MULTIPLE RESPONSE

A client is seen in the clinic for bleeding problems and fatigue. The client has been seen twice in the last month for an upper respiratory infection and has been prescribed antibiotics.

| Health History | Nurses' Notes | Provider Orders | Laboratory Results |

1230: A 69-year-old client reports having frequent nosebleeds over the past couple weeks, along with bruising on the arms. Client reports fatigue, night sweats, and a weight loss of 3 lb (1.4 kg) since the last clinic visit. On assessment, there is bleeding around the gums and multiple bruising and petechiae on the upper extremities. Pallor noted.

- Temperature: 100.6°F (38.1°C)
- BP: 128/78 mm Hg
- Heart rate: 80 beats/min
- Respirations: 22 breaths/min
- SpO2: 97% on room air

For each client finding, use an X to specify whether the finding is consistent with the disease process of hemophilia, chronic lymphocytic leukemia (CLL), and anemia. Each finding may support more than one disease process.

CLIENT FINDING	HEMOPHILIA	CLL	ANEMIA
Bleeding	X	X	
Dyspnea on exertion			X
Fatigue		X	X
Hemarthrosis	X		
Pallor		X	X
Persistent infections		X	
Sore tongue (glossitis)			X

Drop-Down Cloze

The *drop-down cloze* and the drop-down rationale formats are similar. There will be blanks in a sentence for which you will select options provided in the drop-down menu in the blank area. You will have a minimum of one sentence or a maximum of five sentences with this item type. Each sentence will have a minimum of one drop-down menu in the blank area. Question 1.14 shows an example of this type of item to measure the clinical judgment skill of *Prioritize Hypotheses* in a postoperative client following a laparoscopic cholecystectomy.

⚡ QUESTION 1.14 DROP-DOWN CLOZE

The client is a 46-year-old with no known history and no known allergies who presented to the emergency department with reports of increasing upper right quadrant pain. A nurse is working on a medical-surgical unit and receives the client from the recovery room.

| Health History | Nurses' Notes | Provider Orders | Laboratory Results |

1100: Received client from recovery room to unit via bed following an open cholecystectomy. Jackson-Pratt drain in place with 10 mL of serosanguineous drainage. Abdominal dressing in place with scant amount of serosanguineous drainage. IV in left forearm running ½ NS at 100 mL/hr without difficulty. Client opens eyes, holds hands over abdomen, and grimaces.

Choose the *most likely* options for the information missing from the statement below by selecting from the drop-down list of options provided.

The nurse will use a _____1_____ to assess the client's pain level. The nurse will plan to use _____2_____ and/or _____2_____ based on the pain level and client's preferences.

OPTIONS FOR 1	OPTIONS FOR 2
Wong-Baker FACES pain rating scale	Palliative pain relief
Recent BP and pulse reading	Nonpharmacologic methods
Standardized 0–10 pain rating scale	Analgesic medications

Drag-and-Drop Rationale

Similar to the drop-down rationale, the *drag-and-drop rationale* item uses a cloze format in a cause-and-effect sentence. Instead of clicking on the blank for the selection of options, you will need to drag or click on the options and move them to complete the blanks in the sentence. The sentence may have one cause and one effect or one cause and two effects. Question 1.18 shows an example of this type of item to measure the clinical judgment skill of *Prioritize Hypotheses* for a client who is postoperative.

⚡ QUESTION 1.18 DRAG-AND-DROP RATIONALE

A 62-year-old client is admitted for severe lower abdominal pain, history of diverticulitis, and surgery for a colectomy. Due to peritonitis on 3rd postop day, subsequent surgery with temporary loop ileostomy placed, unable to close abdomen, midline abdominal wound vac in place. Transferred to medical-surgical unit day 10 postop; plan for transfer to rehab hospital for reconditioning when stable.

Health History	Nurses' Notes	Provider Orders	Laboratory Results

0830: Orders received to get client out of bed to chair twice daily for minimum of 30 minutes. Chart blood pressure lying down and standing before getting client to chair. Client states feels very weak after so long in bed and days in the ICU. States hardly able to hold arms over head to comb hair after UAP washed hair. Client alert and oriented × 4, heart regular rate and rhythm, lungs clear to auscultation, abdomen distended, wound vac in place, pedal and radial pulses 2+ bilaterally, grips 5/5 bilaterally, feet push/pulls 4/5 bilaterally. Client states pain level 3 on a scale of 10.

- Temperature: 98.0°F (36.6°C)
- Heart rate: 78 beats/min
- Respirations: 18 breaths/min
- BP: 130/78 mm Hg (lying down); 112/60 mm Hg (standing)
- SpO2: 97% on room air

Drag one condition and one client assessment finding to fill in each blank in the following sentence.

The client *most likely* has _____ based on the client findings of _____.

CONDITION	ASSESSMENT FINDINGS
Pneumonia	Muscle weakness in arms and legs
Orthostatic hypotension	Blood pressure 130/78 (lying down); 112/60 (standing)
Urinary tract infection	Lungs clear to auscultation

Note: The correct answers are in *red color* and would be dragged to the blanks in the sentence.

Test-Taking Strategy: Review the assessment data first. The nurse should immediately be concerned with the change in blood pressure as the decrease indicates orthostatic hypotension, a drop of 20 mm Hg in systolic BP or a 10 mm Hg drop in the diastolic BP, along with an increase in the client's pulse when the client stands. Additionally, this client also reports dizziness, which is a common subjective symptom of hypotension. The client does not have pneumonia because the lungs are clear to auscultation and respiratory rate and SpO2 are within normal limits. Urinary tract infection can be a complication of immobility; however, the client is not showing common symptoms of frequency, urgency, or dysuria. Muscle weakness may be associated with immobility.

Highlight in Text

A case scenario is presented most often in the medical record format where client assessment data, health history, vital signs, etc., is provided. You will use the mouse and *highlight in the text* the information based on what the question is asking. Question 1.19 shows an example of this type of item to measure the clinical judgment skill of *Recognize Cues* for a client with a foot infection.

⚡ QUESTION 1.19 HIGHLIGHT IN TEXT

A young adult client presents to urgent care with a suspected foot infection. **Highlight in the assessment findings in the nurse's notes that require follow-up by the nurse.**

Health History	Nurses' Notes	Provider Orders	Laboratory Results

2000: The client states that he cut his foot while swimming a couple days ago. The cut went unnoticed until yesterday when the client's foot became too painful to walk and began oozing thick, yellowish discharge. Client is responsive to questions but is lethargic and complains of nausea. The client's foot is edematous, very warm to touch, and has red streaks spreading out from the wound. Pain noted as 8 out of 10 on a scale.

- Temperature: 100°F (37.8°C)
- BP: 98/68 mm Hg
- Heart rate: 94 beats/min and regular
- Respirations: 24 breaths/min
- SpO2: 99% room air

Test-Taking Strategy: Are the client findings normal or abnormal? The client has a localized infection due to an infectious organism. Assessment findings for the foot infection include a change in skin color (redness), increase in skin temperature, swelling and pain, drainage (pus, odorous), restricted movement, and fever.

Highlight in Table

Using the same process as highlight in text, *highlight in table* will have a table of information with two columns and up to five rows. Question 1.20 shows an example of this type of item to measure the clinical judgment skill of *Recognize Cues* for a client who is having a laboratory test prior to starting a new medication.

⚡ QUESTION 1.20 HIGHLIGHT IN TABLE

The nurse is reviewing the client's laboratory results for a client who is going to begin to take lovastatin. The client has a history of coronary artery disease and has several alcoholic beverages each day. Baseline liver function studies are drawn. **Highlight the findings in the laboratory results that the nurse would need to notify the health care provider.**

LABORATORY TEST	RESULT	REFERENCE RANGE
Lactate dehydrogenase (LDH)	1.1 mg/dL	0.6–1.2 mg/dL (53–106 μmol/L)
Albumin (Alb)	4.5 g/dL	3.5–5.0 g/dL (35–50 mg/L)
Total Protein (TP)	5.3 g/dL	6.4–8.3 g/dL (64–83 mg/L)
Alanine Transaminase (ALT)	40 U/L	4–36 U/L (4–36 U/L)
Aspartate Transaminase (AST)	33 U/L	0–35 U/L (0–35 U/L)
Total Bilirubin	0.9/dL	0.3–1.0 mg/dL (5.1–17.1 μmol/L)
Gamma-Glutamyl-transferase (GGT)	55 U/L	5–40 U/L
Prothrombin time (PT) INR	12 sec; 97% INR 0.9	11–12.5 sec; 85–100% 0.8–1.1

Test-Taking Strategy: First determine which laboratory results are normal or abnormal. Clients who are taking lovastatin, which is a statin for hyperlipidemia, need to have their liver enzymes checked before starting on the medication. The statin medications may cause liver enzymes to rise. Statins rarely cause liver damage, and health care providers no longer routinely check liver enzymes for people on statins; however, a baseline of liver function is usually drawn. The client's low protein could indicate dehydration, malnourishment, or chronic liver disease. The GGT test is used to detect liver cell dysfunction and can accurately indicate even the slightest degree of cholestasis including detecting biliary obstruction, cholangitis, or cholecystitis, along with chronic alcohol ingestion. Prothrombin time measures the clotting mechanism and can monitor hepatocellular disease and obstructive biliary disease.

Bowtie

The *bowtie* item is called this because the test item looks like a bowtie and can address all six steps of the NCJMM. A case scenario is presented. Correct answers are inserted using drag-and-drop technology to select two actions to take (on the left), two parameters to monitor (on the right), and a single most likely condition the client is experiencing in the middle. You will need to identify from the case scenario what condition the client is most likely experiencing first, then select the two actions to take and the two parameters to monitor. Question 1.21 shows an example of this type of test item, which measures all six clinical judgment skills for a postoperative client.

QUESTION 1.21 BOWTIE

The following is the postoperative nurses' notes for a 63-year-old client who had an exploratory laparotomy. Client has a history of type 2 diabetes and is morbidly obese.

Health History	Nurses' Notes	Provider Orders	Laboratory Results

1130: Client reports discomfort in abdominal incision area and continuing nausea with two episodes of vomiting. For the past 2 hours, the client has been unable to urinate. Incision area reddened and lower edge slightly separated with a large amount of serosanguinous drainage noted. Fine crackles noted in lower lobes.

- Temperature: 100.8°F (38.2°C)
- BP: 162/88 mm Hg
- Heart rate: 108 beats/min and regular
- Respirations: 26 breaths/min
- SpO2: 97% on room air

Complete the diagram by dragging from the choices below to specify what condition the client is most likely experiencing, two actions the nurse should take to address that condition, and two parameters the nurse should monitor to assess the client's progress.

ACTION TO TAKE		PARAMETER TO MONITOR
Position the client supine with knees flexed.		Incision site

ACTION TO TAKE	CONDITION MOST LIKELY EXPERIENCING	PARAMETER TO MONITOR
Cover wound with sterile dressing moistened with sterile normal saline.	Wound dehiscence	Position

ACTIONS TO TAKE	POTENTIAL CONDITIONS	PARAMETERS TO MONITOR
Administer pain medication.	Wound evisceration	Vital signs
Position the client supine with knees flexed.	Wound infection	Fluid volume status
Assess for abdominal distention.	Urinary retention	Incision site
Cover wound with sterile dressing moistened with sterile normal saline.	Wound dehiscence	Pain level
Obtain an order for a straight catheterization for urinalysis.		Position

Test-Taking Strategy: The nurse needs to monitor the postoperative client for complications following surgery. This client is most at risk for dehiscence (separation or disruption of the incision site) and evisceration (complete wound separation with viscera protruding through the incision) because the client is a type 2 diabetic and is obese, which contribute to poor healing. Wound healing tends to be delayed in clients with diabetes and the incidence of infection in surgical wounds is also higher. Wound dehiscence and evisceration create an emergency, which requires immediate surgery to prevent serious complications. After dehiscence and evisceration occur and before reparative surgery, the client should lie supine with the knees flexed. The nurse should cover the wound with a sterile towel or sterile dressings moistened with sterile normal saline. The rationale for positioning the client with the knees flexed prevents further abdominal muscle strain. Urinary retention is a common problem following surgery but is not the priority in this instance. Although the client has an elevated temperature, which is indicative of postoperative infection, it is not the priority at this time.

Trend

The *trend* item is a standalone item that presents *data gathered over a period of time* rather than at one point in time in the case scenario and can measure more than one cognitive skill in the item. You will examine trends in data over time to determine changes in the client's condition. The information is presented in the format of a medical record and can include any of the following medical record tabs: nurses' notes, history and physical, laboratory results, flow sheet, intake and output, progress notes, medications, vital signs, etc. Keep in mind that a trend item can use any of the previous formats discussed, except the bowtie. Question 1.22 shows an example of this type of test item, which measures *Evaluate Outcomes* for a client with heart failure. This is a matrix multiple-choice item style.

⚡ QUESTION 1.22 TREND

A 66-year-old client with history of hypertension and heart failure is discharged from hospital to home with home health visits scheduled. Discharge medications include bumetanide 1 mg PO daily, enalapril 5 mg PO daily, metoprolol XL 25 mg PO daily, and ASA 81 mg PO daily. The nurse reviews the home care chart and documents the findings.

| Health History | Nurses' Notes | Provider Orders | Laboratory Results |

Visit 1 Home health (1 day after discharge from hospital): Client states is good to be home. Has walked around the house but not ventured outside, still fatigued. Client teaching regarding medications reinforced.

Visit 2 Home health (visit 1 week later): Client states has more energy and has walked to the mailbox daily without shortness of breath. Client reports weight is up 1 pound since yesterday. Client verbalizes understanding the need to take medications per schedule and states is happy to know medications will cure the heart failure. Regular heart rate and rhythm, lungs clear to auscultation, abdomen soft and nontender, no peripheral edema noted.

Vital Signs	Visit 1 1100	Visit 2 0900
• Temperature	98.4°F (36.8°C)	98°F (36.6°C)
• Heart rate (beats/min)	82	86
• Respirations (breaths/min)	16	18
• BP (mm Hg)	132/76	154/90

For each assessment finding listed below, use an X to specify whether the finding indicates whether the interventions were Effective (helped to meet expected outcomes), Ineffective (did not help meet expected outcomes), or Unrelated (not related to the expected outcome).

ASSESSMENT FINDING	EFFECTIVE	INEFFECTIVE	UNRELATED
Temperature: 98.0°F (36.6°C)			X
Client verbalizes understanding the need to take medications per schedule	X		
Lungs clear to auscultation	X		
Client reports weight is up 1 pound since yesterday		X	
No peripheral edema present	X		
Client states is happy to know medications will help the heart failure		X	
BP: 154/90 mm Hg		X	
Client states has more energy	X		
Client states has walked to the mailbox daily without shortness of breath	X		

Test-Taking Strategy: This test item is evaluating outcomes between the first and second home care visit. On the second visit, the client's assessment findings of lungs clear to auscultation and negative edema are evidence of the effectiveness of treatment. Improvement in the client's condition is shown with increased energy and the ability to ambulate short distances without shortness of breath, dizziness, or tachycardia. Additionally, the client demonstrated understanding of the importance of taking medications as prescribed. Medications and other treatments can reduce or eliminate symptoms but do not provide a cure for heart failure, which is an ineffective outcome of the discharge teaching. Other ineffective outcomes include an increase in weight of 1 to 2 lb overnight or 3 to 5 lb over a week and increased blood pressure. This information will need to be reported to the health care provider. The client's temperature remains within normal limits and is unrelated to the client's treatment for heart failure.

Unfolding Case Study

The *unfolding case study* is a group of six test items each addressing the six areas of clinical judgment. As the case study changes, or "unfolds," NGN test items require you to make multiple clinical decisions. You will use all of the information, including the information in the current phase of the client's care, to answer each test item. The case study will be available to you as you move through the six test items. Questions 1.22-1 through 1.22-6 show examples of the unfolding case study test item.

TEST ALERT Remember that 18 of the items on NCLEX will be three clinical judgment case studies (six items for each case study measuring the six clinical judgment skills).

⚡ QUESTION 1.23 UNFOLDING CASE STUDY

Note: This case study applies to the following six questions.

Question 1.23-1 Recognize Cues: Item type – Drag-and-Drop Cloze

The following is the nurses' notes for a newly admitted client experiencing dyspnea. The client has a history of arteriosclerotic heart disease and hypertension.

Health History	Nurses' Notes	Provider Orders	Laboratory Results

Day 1, 0900: A client is admitted to the emergency department with severe dyspnea and anxiety and reports experiencing a weight gain of 4 pounds over the last 2 days. The client also noted that the swelling in the lower legs present for the past 2 years has worsened over the past month, making it difficult to wear shoes comfortably. In the past week, the client reports having a decreased appetite, some nausea and vomiting, and tenderness in the right upper quadrant of the abdomen. The client says to the nurse, "You've got to help me. I cannot get enough air." On physical examination, slight jugular neck vein distention noted, 3 + pitting edema in both lower legs, lungs clear to auscultation.

- Temperature: 97.8°F (36.6°C)
- BP: 160/98 mm Hg
- Heart rate: 100 bpm and regular
- Respirations: 26 breaths/min
- SpO2: 95% on room air

Drag the assessment findings from the choices below to fill in the blanks in the following sentence.

The assessment findings that require *immediate* follow up include _____, _____, and _____.

ASSESSMENT FINDINGS

SpO2: 95% on room air
Nausea and vomiting
3 + pitting edema of lower extremities
BP 160/98; pulse 100; respirations 26
Anorexia
Weight gain of 4 lb

Test-Taking Strategy: The nurse needs to *Recognize Cues* in the client's assessment findings. The client is experiencing symptoms of chronic heart failure, which most often is the result of coronary artery disease and long-standing hypertension. The nurse needs to immediately report to the health care provider the 3 + pitting edema of the lower extremities, elevated BP, pulse, respirations, and recent weight gain. These symptoms of right-sided chronic heart failure include dyspnea, murmurs, jugular venous distention, edema (e.g., pedal, scrotum, sacrum), weight gain, tachycardia, ascites, anasarca (massive, generalized body edema), hepatomegaly (liver enlargement), fatigue, anxiety, depression, dependent bilateral edema, right upper quadrant pain, anorexia, nausea, and GI bloating.

Question 1.23-2 Analyze Cues: Item type – Extended Multiple Response: Select N

What other assessment findings would the nurse expect to identify to support this client's probable diagnosis? **Select three assessment findings.**

1. Heart murmur
2. Ascites
3. Flushed skin
4. Fatigue
5. Urinary retention
6. Constipation
7. Dry, hacking cough
8. Frothy, pink-tinged sputum

Test-Taking Strategy: To *Analyze Cues,* look at the bigger picture of the overall client's condition. The nurse would expect additional symptoms as the client's heart failure progresses to include heart murmur, ascites, and fatigue, along with the other symptoms previously mentioned for right-sided heart failure. Dry, hacking cough, nocturia, orthopnea, and frothy, pink-tinged sputum are signs of left-sided chronic heart failure.

Question 1.23-3 Prioritize Hypotheses: Item type – Drop-Down Rationale

The following is an updated nurses' note.

Health History	Nurses' Notes	Vital Signs	Laboratory Results

Day 1, 1030: Furosemide 40mg, PO STAT dose ordered and administered. Client reports feeling tired and having no energy.
Day 1, 1200: 850mL urine output following furosemide. Breathing easier and dozing on and off since admission.

Choose the most likely options for the information missing from the statements below by selecting from the drop-down list of options provided.

Fatigue is a/an _____1_____ symptom of chronic heart failure. Clients may experience _____2_____, which is associated with poor kidney perfusion and function. The development of _____3_____ or a sudden weight _____4_____ of more than 3 lb (1.4 kg) in 2 days is often a sign of decompensating heart failure.

OPTIONS FOR 1	OPTIONS FOR 2	OPTIONS FOR 3	OPTIONS FOR 4
early	nocturia	dyspnea	gain
late	polyuria	dependent edema	loss
intermediate	anuria		
	pyuria	nausea	
		polyuria	

Test-Taking Strategy: When the nurse *prioritizes hypotheses,* you are considering what client problems require immediate attention and what *most likely* is occurring. Clients who have chronic heart failure often have poor renal perfusion and function and develop increased peripheral and systemic edema. At night when lying flat, extravascular fluid is reabsorbed from the interstitial spaces back into the circulatory system. This results in increased perfusion to the kidneys. The increased renal blood flow results in diuresis. The client often reports of having to urinate frequently throughout the night (nocturia). Fatigue is caused by decreased cardiac output, impaired perfusion to vital organs, decreased oxygenation of the tissues, and anemia. Edema is a common sign of right-sided heart failure and characterized by weight gain due to retention of fluid. It may occur in dependent body areas (peripheral edema), liver (hepatomegaly), and abdominal cavity (ascites) and with left-sided failure in the lungs (pulmonary edema and pleural effusion).

Question 1.23-4 Generate Solutions: Item type – Matrix Multiple Choice

The health care provider has written a series of orders for the client described in the scenario.

For each prescriber order listed, use an **X** to specify whether the order would be Indicated (appropriate or necessary), Non-Essential (makes no difference or not necessary), or Contraindicated (could be harmful) for *planning* the client's care at this time. Select only one response for each prescribed order.

PRESCRIBER ORDER	ANTICIPATED	NON-ESSENTIAL	CON-TRAINDI-CATED
Furosemide	X		
Unrestricted sodium diet			X
Oral fluid restriction (1000 mL/day)	X		
Passive range of motion twice daily		X	
Captopril 25 mg, PO, 3 times/day	X		
Metoprolol extended release, 25 mg, PO, daily	X		
Supplemental oxygen via nasal cannula, 3–4 L/min as needed	X		

Test-Taking Strategy: Think about what a safe plan of care would be for this client. When the nurse *generates solutions,* you

need to look at what would be appropriate and inappropriate interventions and identify expected outcomes in *planning* the client's care. For routine therapy, heart failure (HF) is treated with three types of drugs: (1) diuretics (furosemide, HCTZ), (2) angiotensin-converting enzyme inhibitors (captopril), and (3) beta blockers (metoprolol). Medications are started at small doses. Previously, HF was considered an absolute contraindication to administering a beta blocker. Other agents (e.g., digoxin, dopamine, hydralazine) may be used as well. Digoxin, which had been used widely in the past, may be added as indicated. A commonly ordered diet for a client with HF is a 2-gm low-sodium diet. A structured exercise program, such as cardiac rehabilitation, should be considered for all clients with chronic HF. In moderate to severe HF and renal insufficiency, fluids are limited to less than 2 L/day.

Question 1.23-5 Take Action: Item type – Drop-Down Table

The nurse is planning nursing interventions for the client described in the scenario.

For each body system listed below, drop down to select the potential nursing intervention that would be appropriate for the client at this time. Each body system may support more than one potential nursing intervention, but a least one option in each category needs to be selected.

BODY SYSTEM	POTENTIAL NURSING INTERVENTIONS
Respiratory	
Cardiovascular	

RESPIRATORY POTENTIAL NURSING INTERVENTIONS	CARDIOVASCULAR POTENTIAL NURSING INTERVENTIONS
Weekly pulmonary function studies. Assess lung sounds. Position in low Fowler. Administer supplemental oxygen PRN.	Check daily weight. Limit exercise activities. Monitor electrolytes. Check for pedal edema daily.

Test-Taking Strategy: When the nurse *Takes Action,* nursing interventions are performed. Symptom management in heart failure is controlled by the client with self-management tools (e.g., daily weights, drug regimens, diet, and exercise plans); salt and, at times, water must be restricted; and energy must be conserved. The client is on furosemide, which causes hypokalemia and the need to monitor electrolytes. Supplemental oxygen will assist clients who have dyspnea, along with high Fowler position in bed to improve ventilation. Assessing lung sounds can monitor for possible progression to left-sided heart failure, which requires early recognition of symptoms (i.e., pulmonary edema). Clients need to report immediately any of the following signs of worsening heart failure to the primary health care provider, which include weight gain of 3 lb (1.4 kg) in 2 days or 3 to 5 lb (2.3 kg) in a week; difficulty breathing, especially with activity or when lying flat; waking up breathless at night; and frequent dry, hacking cough, especially when lying down.

Question 1.23-6 Evaluate Outcomes: Item type – Highlight in Text

The following is an updated nurses' note occurring on day 2 following the client's admission. The client's medications include the following: metoprolol, furosemide, and captopril.

Highlight the findings in the Nurses' Notes that would indicate that the client is improving.

| Health History | Nurses' Notes | Provider Orders | Laboratory Results |

Day 2, 1500: Client reports feeling tired all day, uninterested in eating, and has refused to meet with the cardiac rehabilitation specialist this afternoon. Tolerates semi-Fowler position with limited activity. On physical examination, slight jugular neck vein distention noted, 2 + pitting edema in both lower legs, lungs clear to auscultation.

- Temperature: 97.8°F (36.6°C)
- BP: 140/78 mm Hg
- Pulse: 80 beats/min
- Respirations: 20 breaths/min
- SpO2: 96% on room air
- Urine output 600mL in past 8 hr

Test-Taking Strategy: When the nurse *Evaluates Outcomes*, you need to see if the interventions were effective based on an updated status of the client. By day 2 the client's medications have begun to alleviate the dyspnea (respirations decreased from 26 to 20 breaths/min), SpO2 increased from 95% to 96%, elevated blood pressure and pulse decreased through diuresis (urine output 600 mL in past 8 hr). The client's edema is resolving as evidenced by a change in pitting of edema from 3 + to 2 + over the past 2 days. The rest of the assessment findings remain unchanged.

TESTING STRATEGIES

TEST ALERT Practicing test-taking strategies is critical if you are going to be able to use them effectively on the NCLEX. Practice test taking should be a component of your NCLEX preparation.

Test-taking strategies are beneficial during nursing school and on the NCLEX. Start using them on current examinations. Implementing testing strategies now will help increase test scores in school, in addition to being one more step toward success on the NCLEX (Box 1.2).

Being able to apply test-taking strategies effectively on an examination is almost as important as having the basic knowledge required to answer the questions correctly. Everyone has taken an examination only to find, on review of the examination, that questions were missed because of poor test-taking skills. Nursing education provides the graduate with a comprehensive base of knowledge; how effectively the graduate can *demonstrate* the use of this knowledge and make clinical judgments is a major factor in the successful completion of the examination.

The NCLEX-PN is designed to evaluate minimum levels of competency. The purpose of the examination is to determine whether a candidate has the knowledge, skills,

Box 1.2 APPLYING TESTING STRATEGIES

Check out the question!

- Read the question from beginning to end. Read all choices or options before answering the question.
- Check for **key** words that establish the question as asking for a priority: *first action, priority nursing action, most important, next, immediate, essential, primary,* or *best.*
- Is the answer going to be a correct, true, or positive statement? Or is the question asking for an answer that is incorrect or a negative or false statement? A positive question would be "What statement would be an effective communication response?" A negative question would be "Which statement indicates the client needs further teaching?"
- Rephrase the question in your own words. Do you understand what the question is asking?

Now go for the options

- Look at option 1: Is the statement true or false? Does it answer what the question is asking?
- Go through every option: Eliminate it if it is not a correct answer; keep it around if it is a possible right answer.
- When you have decided what option or options are correct, go back and reread the question and review the case scenario and/or client's chart. Make your selection(s) and move on.

abilities, and clinical judgment required for safe and effective entry-level nursing practice. Throughout the examination, questions are described as being based on clinical situations common in nursing; uncommon situations are not emphasized. NCLEX questions are not fact, recall, or memory-level questions; they are questions that require critical thinking, decision making, and clinical judgment to determine the correct answer. Clinical judgment requires an analysis of client data, an understanding of the client's condition or disease, and the ability to determine the best action that will most effectively meet the client's needs.

The following strategies are critical in evaluating and successfully answering NCLEX questions.

- **The NCLEX Hospital.** What a great place to work! Remember, on the NCLEX, all clients are being cared for in an ideal environment—the NCLEX Hospital. Questions ask for nursing care and decisions based on situations in which everything is available for client care. Nursing care provided on the examination is performed in the NCLEX Hospital, where the nurse always has adequate staff, supplies, and anything else required to provide the safest care for the client. This approach is necessary because this is a nationally standardized examination.
- **Calling the doctor (or anyone else).** Be cautious about passing the responsibility for care of the client to someone else. This is an examination on nursing care; evaluate the question carefully and see what nursing action should be taken before consulting or calling someone else. This includes the social worker, respiratory therapist, and hospital chaplain, as well as the health care provider. After you have carefully evaluated the question, if the client's

condition is such that the nurse cannot do anything to resolve the problem, then calling for assistance may be the best answer. Frequently, there is a nursing action to be taken before contacting someone for assistance. A specific item on the test plan states that the nurse will identify client data that must be reported immediately.

- **Health care provider's orders.** It should be assumed that a health care provider's order is available to provide the nursing care in the options presented in the question. If the question asks for administration of a specific medication for the client's problem, then assume that there is an order for it. If the focus of a question is to determine whether a nursing action is a dependent or an independent nursing action, then it will be stated in the stem of the question. For example, the question may ask what an independent nursing action would be to provide pain relief for a specific client.

- **Focus on the client.** Look for answers that focus on the client. Identify the significant or central person in the question. Most often, this is going to be the client. Wrong choices would be those that focus on maintaining hospital rules and policies, dealing with equipment, or solving the nurse's problems. Evaluate the status of the client first and then deal with the equipment problems or concerns. Other questions may ask the nurse to respond to a client's family or significant others. Determine the person to whom the question is directed.

- **Client's age.** Consider a client to be an adult unless otherwise stated. If the age of a client is important to the question, it will be stated in years or in months. Descriptions such as "elderly adult" and "geriatric client" are not commonly used. These terms have been established as negative descriptors of older clients. The description of such a client may be "older adult," or a specific age may be given.

- **Laboratory values.** It is important to understand normal values for common laboratory tests. Be able to identify laboratory values and/or diagnostic procedures that indicate a client's progress or lack of progress or indicate whether a client's status is getting better or worse. A normal range for laboratory values will be provided.

- **Positions.** Positioning a client may be an option to consider in the implementation of care. If a specific position for the client appears in the stem or scenario of the question, then consider whether the position is for comfort, for treatment, or to prevent a complication. Evaluate the question: What is to be accomplished by placing the client in the position, and why is the position important for this client? Consider whether positioning is important to the care of the client presented. See Appendix 3.1 for a further description of positions.

- **Mathematic computations.** Mathematic computations may include calculations of intravenous rate and drip factors, calculations of medication dosages, conversion of units of measurement, and calculation of intake and output. You should be able to apply the appropriate formula to the situation. Some of the questions may call for two computations, as in a question in which all items must be converted to one unit of measurement before a dosage is calculated. There will be an onscreen calculator; find the "calculator" button when you do the NCLEX Tutorial. The mathematic calculations may be presented in a multiple-choice format or in an alternate format question in which you are asked to fill in the blank. For fill-in-the-blank questions, calculate your answer and then type the answer or number into the box provided. The unit of measurement will be provided in the box.

STRATEGIES AND EXAMPLES

Read the question carefully, without reading into it

- *Read the question carefully before ever looking at or considering the options.* If you glance through the options before understanding the question, you may pick up distracting words that will affect the way you perceive the question.

 It is important to understand the question and not formulate an opinion about the answer before you understand the question.

- *Do not read extra meaning into the question.* The question is asking for specific information; if it appears to be simple "common sense," then assume it is simple. Do not look for a hidden meaning in a question. Avoid asking yourself, "what if ...?" or speculating about the future ("maybe the client will ..."). Do not make the client any sicker than the client already is!

Example (Take Action): A bronchoscopy was performed on a client at 0700. The client returns to their room, and the nurse plans to assist them with morning care. The client refuses the morning care. What is the **best** nursing action regarding the morning care for this client?

1. Perform all the morning care to prevent the client from becoming short of breath.
2. Avoid morning care and continue to monitor vital signs and assess swallowing reflexes.
3. Postpone the morning care until the client is more comfortable and can participate.
4. Cancel all the morning care because it is not necessary to perform it after a bronchoscopy.

Test-Taking Strategy: The correct answer is 3. The question is asking for a nursing judgment regarding morning care. Do not read into the question and make it more difficult by trying to put in information relating to respiratory care, such as checking for gag and swallowing reflexes.

Make sure you know what the question is asking

- *Make sure you understand exactly what information the question is asking.* Determine whether the question is stated in a positive (true) or negative (false) format.
- *Watch for words that provide direction to the question.* A positive or true stem may include the following: "indicates the client understands," "the best nursing action is," "the preoperative teaching would include," or "the best nursing assignment is." Also watch for words in the

stem that have a negative meaning so that the question is asking for a response that is *not* accurate or expected. Phrases such as "what indicates the client *does not understand*," "which order *would you question*," and "what indicates (medication, equipment, nursing action) is *not working*" are negative indicators. It may help rephrase the question in your own words to better understand what information is being requested.

Example (Evaluate Outcomes): The nurse is reinforcing teaching about body mechanics with a client who has had back surgery. What comment would indicate the client *did not understand* the principles discussed?

1. "I will bend at the knees to pick up an object from the floor."
2. "I will carry objects close to the body."
3. "I will place my feet apart when bending to pick up an object."
4. "I will bend from the waist to pick up an object on the floor."

Test-Taking Strategy: *The correct answer is 4. Rephrase the question: I need to identify what comment is incorrect regarding body mechanics. Bending from the waist does not represent good body mechanics; the client should bend with the knees (squatting), not from the waist. All other options represent good body mechanics.*

Consider information about timing

- *Watch where the client is in the disease process or condition the client is experiencing.* Examples of this are phrases such as "immediately postoperatively," "the first postoperative day," and "experienced a myocardial infarction this morning."

Example (Take Action): A client had a cardiac catheterization through the left femoral artery. During the first few hours after the cardiac catheterization procedure, which nursing action would be **most important**?

1. Check the temperature every 2 hours and monitor catheter insertion site for inflammation.
2. Elevate the head of the bed 90 degrees and keep affected extremity straight.
3. Evaluate blood pressure and respiratory status every 15 minutes for 4 to 6 hours.
4. Check pedal and femoral pulses every 15 minutes for first hour and then every 30 minutes.

Test-Taking Strategy: *The correct answer is 4. The phrase "during the first few hours after the procedure" is important in answering this question correctly. The danger of hemorrhage and hematoma at the puncture site is greatest during this time. The question also asks for the most important nursing care. In option 3, it is important to evaluate vital signs, but it is not required that they be evaluated every 15 minutes for 4 to 6 hours if the client is stable. Option 4 is critical in the first few hours after a cardiac catheterization. Positioning is important but is not the priority to monitor for potential complications.*

Consider characteristics of the condition

- *Before considering the options, think about the characteristics of the condition and critical nursing concepts.* What are the nursing priorities in caring for a client with this condition/procedure/medication/problem?

Example (Take Action): A woman who gave birth 3 days ago returns to the clinic reporting soreness and fullness in her breasts and states that she wants to stop breastfeeding her infant until her breasts feel better. What is the **best** nursing response?

1. Show the client how to apply a breast binder to decrease the discomfort and the production of milk.
2. Share with the client that breast fullness may be a sign of infection and she will not be able to continue breastfeeding.
3. Suggest to the client that she decrease her fluid intake for the next 24 hours to temporarily suppress lactation.
4. Explain to the client that the breast discomfort is normal, and that the infant's sucking will promote the flow of milk.

Test-Taking Strategy: *This is a positive question. The answer will be a true statement. Think about breastfeeding and the common discomforts and problems the client encounters. Do not look at the options yet. Think, "Is it normal to have fullness and soreness in the breasts during the first 3 days of lactation, and what happens if she stops breastfeeding the infant?" Option 4 is correct. Initially, breast soreness may occur for approximately 2 to 3 minutes at the beginning of each feeding until the let-down reflex is established. Options 1, 2, and 3 would decrease her milk production; the question did not state that she wanted to quit breastfeeding permanently.*

Identify the step in the nursing process

- *Identify the step in the nursing process being tested.* Remember, you must have adequate *assessment* data before you move through the steps of the nursing process. Is there adequate information presented in the stem of the question to determine appropriate planning or intervention? Is the correct nursing action to obtain further assessment data? Look for **key words** that can assist you in determining what type of information is being requested (Box 1.1).

Example (Prioritize Hypotheses): An 85-year-old client from a residential care facility is brought into the emergency department. Numerous bruises and abrasions in various stages of healing are present on the client's face and arms. The attendant from the residential facility explains that the client fell. What **priority** nursing action would the nurse take in planning this client's care?

1. Call the residential facility and ask for an incident report.
2. Put ice on the bruises and cover the abrasions with protective gauze.
3. Notify the supervisor regarding the possibility of an abusive situation.
4. Perform a head-to-toe assessment and determine the extent of the injuries.

their condition. Before the nurse provides instruction, what is **most important** to determine?

1. Required dietary modifications.
2. Understanding of carbohydrate counting.
3. Ability to administer insulin.
4. Present understanding of diabetes.

Test-Taking Strategy: Options 1, 2, and 3 are certainly important considerations in diabetic education. However, they cannot be initiated until the nurse evaluates the client's knowledge of their disease state, which is the reason that option 4 is the correct answer. When two options appear to say the same thing, only in different words, then look for another answer; that is, eliminate the options that you know are incorrect. Options 1 and 2 both refer to the client's understanding of nutrition.

Consider all information in the options

* *Some questions may have options that contain several items to consider.* After you are sure you understand what information the question is requesting, evaluate each part of the option. Is the option appropriate to what the question is asking? If an option contains one incorrect item, the entire option is incorrect. All the items listed in the option must be correct if that option is to be the correct answer to the question.
  Example (Take Action): The nurse is preparing a client's 0800 medications. The client has the following medications ordered: digoxin 0.125 mg, PO; furosemide 20 mg, PO; and captopril 25 mg, PO. The client's current vital signs are blood pressure 110/86 mm Hg, pulse 78 beats/min, respirations 18 breaths/min, and temperature 99°F (37.2°C) orally. What would be the **best** nursing action?

1. Administer all the medications, chart them as given, and document the client's apical heart rate.
2. Hold the digoxin and the captopril; recheck the heart rate and blood pressure in 30 minutes.
3. Hold the captopril, administer the other medications, and notify the nursing supervisor.
4. Hold the furosemide until the intake and output can be evaluated; administer all other medications.

Test-Taking Strategy: In the methodical evaluation of the items in the options, you can eliminate items. Review the client's vital signs. They are within normal limits, except for a slight temperature elevation. Option 2, there is no reason to hold the digoxin or the captopril. Option 3, there is no reason to hold the captopril or to notify the nursing supervisor. Option 4, there is no reason to hold the furosemide. Therefore option 1 is correct. Also note, the three incorrect options are to "hold" the medications while the correct answer is to "administer." Remember the strategy, three are similar and the different one may be the correct answer, which it is in this question!

Reread the question

* *After you have selected an answer, reread the question.* Does the answer you chose give the information the question

is asking for? Sometimes the options are correct but do not answer the question.
  Example (Prioritize Hypotheses): A client is 88 years of age and has previously been alert, oriented, and active. The nursing assistant reports that on awakening this morning, the client was disoriented and confused. What action would the nurse take to determine what is **most likely** the cause of this change in the client's behavior?

1. Review the history for any previous episodes of this type of behavior.
2. Call the health care provider and discuss the changes in the client's behavior.
3. Perform a thorough neurologic evaluation to evaluate the specific changes in behavior.
4. Assess for the presence of a urinary tract infection and for adequate hydration.

Test-Taking Strategy: Option 4 is the only answer that supplies what the question asked for ("determine the most likely cause of this change"). The most likely cause of a sudden change in the behavior of an older adult client is a significant physiologic change, often an infection (commonly in the urinary tract) or dehydration. Options 1 and 3 relate more to the gradual behavior changes seen in the progression of dementia and do nothing "to determine the most likely cause." Option 2 also does not provide any assistance in determining the most likely cause of the behavior change; further nursing assessment needs to be conducted before calling for assistance.

Management of client care

As the role of the PN has expanded, management of client care has become increasingly important. A large percentage of graduates surveyed on the last job analysis reported they had "charge nurse" responsibilities. The majority of the management responsibilities were in the long-term care facilities. LPNs may direct the care of the nursing assistants as well as other LPNs. However, LPNs are under the supervision of a registered nurse. There is a director of nurses or an administrator that is an RN that is ultimately responsible for nursing care delivered in that facility. Do not panic: pay close attention to what nursing action the question is focusing on and to whom the nurse is assigning the care or nursing activity—is it to another LPN, or is it to a less-qualified person? Let's review some specific management test-taking strategies.

* **Identify the most stable client.** The most stable client is the one who has the *most predictable outcome* and is *least likely* to have abrupt changes in condition that would require critical nursing judgments. When determining the stability of clients, Maslow's hierarchy of needs should be considered (see Chapter 3, Fig. 3.1). The most stable client is often the one for which some nursing activities can be delegated to a nursing assistant.
* **Assign tasks that have specific guidelines.** Those tasks that have specific guidelines that are unchanging and are used in the care of a stable client can often be assigned to the nursing assistant. Bathing, collecting urine samples, feeding, providing personal hygiene, and assisting with ambulation are just a few examples of these activities.

- **Identify your priority client.** The priority client is the one who is most likely to experience problems or ill effects if not taken care of first. Priority clients include those with respiratory compromise, those whose conditions are unstable and changing, and those who are at high risk for developing complications. NCLEX questions may present a typical nursing care assignment and ask which client the nurse would care for first, or a situation with a client may be presented and you will be asked to select the first nursing action. Review the testing strategies regarding priority questions. It is important to identify the most unstable client, to see that client first, and to determine what is necessary to do first for this client.

- **Carefully read the question** and determine which clients are in a *changing unstable situation*; these are clients that may require *contacting the RN or the health care provider.* This clinical judgment could be tested in a question where the LPN cannot meet the client needs and would need to obtain further assistance and/or direction.

- **Client care assignments.** Nursing care assignments should take into consideration the caregiver who is educationally prepared, experienced, and most capable of caring for the client. Unlicensed assistive personnel (UAP), patient care attendants (PCAs), and/or certified nursing assistants (CNAs) must be directly supervised in the provision of safe nursing care. Pay close attention to the person to whom the nurse is assigning the care or nursing activity: Is it to another LPN, or is a specific activity (bathing, ambulating, etc.) being delegated to a UAP?

Establishing nursing priorities

Almost all nurses will agree that the NCLEX is full of priority questions. These questions may be worded in a variety of ways and will have **key** words:

"What is the **priority** nursing action?"

"What should the nurse do **first**?"

"What is the **best** nursing action?"

In other words, the NCLEX wants to know whether the nurse can identify the most important nursing action to be taken to provide safe care for the client in the situation presented. This is where clinical judgment is necessary— *think like a nurse!* There are three areas to consider when determining priority nursing actions: Maslow's hierarchy of needs, the nursing process, and client safety.

- **Maslow's hierarchy of needs.** And you thought this was just for fundamentals! *Always consider Maslow's hierarchy of needs and remember that physiologic needs must come first.* When evaluating options, identify client needs that are physiologic and those that are psychosocial. Physiologic needs are a higher priority than psychosocial or teaching needs. A client's physical needs must be met before psychosocial or teaching needs are considered. Also remember that the ABCs (airway, breathing, and circulation) are the critical physiologic needs because these are at the base of Maslow's pyramid. However, be cautious; do not always select "airway" as the best answer. Sometimes the client does not have

an airway problem, so do not read into the question and give the client an airway problem! Remember, if performing CPR, then you need to follow the CAB (circulation, airway, breathing) process. Maslow's hierarchy of needs also applies to psychosocial questions (see the section in this chapter regarding answering psychosocial questions).

- **Nursing process.** The first step in the nursing process for the practical nurse is *data collection or assessment (Recognize Cues).* When evaluating a question, it is important to determine whether the question provides adequate data for the nurse to make a decision regarding nursing interventions. Obtaining more information (data collection) may be the first nursing action. However, do not automatically select an option that involves data collection. If client data are provided in the stem of the question, then it will be important to consider Maslow's hierarchy of needs when planning or selecting the best nursing action or implementation. If a nursing action has been implemented, then the question may focus on evaluating the effectiveness of the nursing action. Read the question carefully and determine what is being asked (see Box 1.1).

- **Safety issues.** These issues may include situations in the hospital or in the client's home environment. The first issue to consider is meeting basic needs of survival: oxygen, hydration, nutrition, elimination (in that order of priority!). Reduction of environmental hazards is also a concern and may include prevention of falls, accidents, and medication errors. Environmental safety also includes the prevention and spread of disease. This may include how to avoid contagious diseases or even activities such as handwashing. When you are critically evaluating questions that involve a client's safety and multiple options appear to be correct, determine which activity will be of most benefit to the client.

Example (Generate Solutions): The LPN is making assignments on a nursing care unit. What task could the LPN assign to the experienced certified nursing assistant?

1. Evaluate the skin in the sacral area for a client on bed rest.
2. Report on the quantity and characteristics of a client's urine output.
3. Assist a client to obtain a clean-catch urine specimen.
4. Evaluate the tolerance of client on tube feedings.

Test-Taking Strategy: *The correct answer is option 3. The CNA can be assigned activities that involve standard, unchanging procedures such as helping to obtain a clean-catch urine specimen from a client. The LPN should evaluate the skin on the sacral area for any evidence of a break in skin integrity. The characteristics of the urine should be evaluated by the LPN; however, the CNA can empty and measure the amount of urinary output. Dietary intake for clients who do not have a problem with nutrition can be reported by the CNA; however, the LPN needs to determine the tolerance of the tube feedings.*

Example (Prioritize Hypotheses): The LPN is working on a step-down nursing telemetry unit. A client tells the nurse they are beginning to have midsternum chest pain. What is the **first** nursing action?

1. Begin oxygen at 4 L/min per nasal cannula.
2. Request the charge nurse evaluate the cardiac rhythm.
3. Auscultate breath sounds and maintain airway.
4. Determine client activities prior to onset of chest pain.

Test-Taking Strategy: The correct answer is option 1. When a client complains of chest pain, oxygen should be started immediately, followed by determining the status of the vital signs. The client is on a telemetry unit and is experiencing chest pain—this is enough information for a nursing action. Data collection will determine the status of the vital signs and further action can be evaluated. If the vital signs are unstable or if the client is experiencing a dysrhythmia, then oxygen administration would still be the most important initial nursing action. Activity prior to the chest pain can be evaluated after the current physical status is determined. Option 3 assumes the client has airway problems, and there is no indication in the question stem that airway is a problem.

Example (Prioritize Hypotheses): The LPN received a shift handoff report for a group of assigned clients. When planning morning care, which client should the LPN see **first**?

1. A client who underwent a thoracotomy 3 days ago; vital signs are stable; and reports chest pain when coughing.
2. An 85-year-old client who has a fractured hip; in Buck traction and reporting of pain; scheduled for surgery in 4 hours.
3. An adult client admitted 3 hours ago for dehydration; vital signs are temperature 99°F (37.2°C), pulse 100 beats/min and irregular, and BP 118/80 mm Hg.
4. A client with a history of atherosclerosis and hypertension who was admitted 24 hours ago and is beginning to report increased chest pain.

Test-Taking Strategy: The correct answer is option 4. The client with atherosclerosis and hypertension is the most unstable and is beginning to exhibit symptoms that could be warning signs of cardiac ischemia. This client needs to be assessed immediately, and the nurse should anticipate administration of sublingual nitroglycerin. After assessment of vital signs, this client's change in condition may need to be reported to the charge nurse and/or to the health care provider. The client with a thoracotomy may be developing pneumonia secondary to surgery and immobility, but the situation does not require immediate attention. The client with a fractured hip is also not in an unstable situation, even though the client reports being uncomfortable. The client with dehydration is exhibiting symptoms related to dehydration but is not unstable at this time.

Therapeutic nursing process: Principles of communication

Throughout the examination, there will be questions requiring use of the principles of therapeutic communication. In therapeutic communication questions, do not assume the client is being manipulative or is in control of how they feel. Psychosocial problems or mental health problems are most often not under the conscious control of the client.

> **TEST ALERT** Use therapeutic communication techniques to provide support to the client and the family; establish a trusting nurse-client relationship; assess psychosocial, spiritual, cultural, and occupational factors affecting care; allow time to communicate with client/family and significant others; and provide a therapeutic environment.

- **Situations requiring use of therapeutic communication are not always centered on a psychiatric client.** Frequently, these questions are centered on the client experiencing stress and anxiety. There may be questions relating to therapeutic communication in the care of clients experiencing stress, anxiety related to a specific client situation, or a change in body image as a result of physiologic problems.
- **Look for responses that focus on the concerns of the client.** Do not focus on the concerns of the nurse, hospital, or health care provider. Determine whether the client is the central focus of the question or whether the question pertains to a spouse or significant other.
- **Watch for responses that are open-ended and encourage the client to express how they feel.** Clients frequently experience difficulty in expressing their feelings. Focus on responses that encourage a client to describe how they feel. These are frequently open-ended statements made by the nurse.
- **Eliminate responses that are not honest and direct.** To build trust and promote a positive relationship, it is important to be honest with the client. Options that include telling the client "don't worry" or "everything is going to be all right" or "your doctor knows best" are wrong answers.
- **Look for responses that indicate acceptance of the client.** Regardless of whether the client's views or moral values are in agreement with yours, it is important to respect their views and beliefs. Responses that involve telling clients what they *should* or *should not* be doing are often wrong answers (e.g., telling an alcoholic to quit drinking or telling a depressed client to not feel that way).
- **Be careful about responses that give opinions or advice on the client's situation.** Do not assume an authoritarian position. You should not insist that the client follow your advice (e.g., quit drinking, exercise more, quit smoking).
- **Do not select options or responses that block further interaction.** These options are frequently presented as closed statements or questions that encourage a yes-or-no answer from the client. Better responses are those that indicate an expectation of a more revealing verbal response from the client. For example, "Are you feeling better today?" The client can just answer no to this question. It is better to ask, "How are you feeling today compared with yesterday?" Likewise, it is better to ask, "How did you feel when your family visited today?" rather than "Did your family visit today?"

- **Look for responses that reflect, restate, or paraphrase feelings the client expressed.** Look for responses that encourage the client to describe how they feel—responses that reflect, restate, or paraphrase feelings the client expresses. An option such as "You should not feel that way" is bound to be a wrong answer. It is better to ask, "How did that make you feel?"
- **Do not ask "why" a client feels the way they do.** Most of the time, if a client understood why they felt a certain way, the client would be able to do something about it. The most common answer when a nurse asks a client why they feel a certain way is "I don't know," which does not help anyone.
- **Do not use coercion to achieve a desired response.** Do not tell clients that they cannot have their lunch until they get out of bed or bribe children to take their medicine with a promise of candy.

Example (Take Action): A client in a mental health facility has suddenly developed an intense fear of heights. During a group therapy session, the client makes the following statements: "I know my feeling of being terrified of heights is dumb. It doesn't make any sense. I just can't seem to do anything about it." Which response would be **most** appropriate for the nurse to make?

1. "Having a nurse accompany you while you climb a couple flights of stairs could help you overcome your fear."
2. "Knowing that your fears don't make any sense doesn't seem to help you feel better."
3. "Participating in several of our ward activities may help you feel better."
4. "Being frightened as a child by some particular event or incident probably caused these fears."

Test-Taking Strategy: The correct answer is option 2. This question uses the therapeutic communication technique of restating. Acknowledging the client's fear by restating what was said is a form of therapeutic communication. Progressive desensitization is a type of therapy that could be used for the client, but it is not appropriate to suggest treatment to the client at this time. Participating in activities does not allow the client to voice discomfort and fears, and a history of being frightened is not necessarily correct information.

- **See examples of therapeutic and nontherapeutic communication in Chapter 7 (Tables 7.1 and 7.2).**

TIPS FOR TEST-TAKING SUCCESS

- **Do not indiscriminately change answers.** On a paper-and-pencil test, if you go back and change an answer, you should have a specific reason for doing so. Sometimes you do remember information and realize you answered the question incorrectly. However, students often "talk themselves out" of the correct answer and change it to the incorrect one. The good news is that you cannot go back to previously answered questions on the NCLEX. At the point at which the examination asks you to confirm your answer, review the strategies used to answer the question, confirm your answer, and move on to the next question.
- **Watch your timing. Do not spend too much time on one question.** It is important to track your timing on practice examinations. This will help you to be more comfortable with timing on computer testing. The NCLEX will allow you a total of 5 hours to complete the examination. Some questions you will answer quickly; others may take some time. Do not spend more than 2 minutes deliberating the answer to a question. If you do not have a good direction for the right answer in 2 minutes, then you probably do not know the answer. Eliminate all of the options you can, pick the best one, and move on. (Remember, you are not supposed to know *all* of the right answers.) Plan for 2 to 3 hours of practice testing and answer the questions using testing strategies. After answering the questions, review the correct answers and focus on what and why you missed questions. Practice your timing and application of test strategies so you will be comfortable with timing and the progression of questions on the NCLEX.
- **The NCLEX is a nursing competency examination, and the correct answer will focus on nursing knowledge, safety, and clinical judgment in the provision of nursing care.** The examination does not focus on medical management or making a medical diagnosis.
- **Eliminate distracters that include the assumption that the client would not understand or would be ignorant of the situation and those distracters that protect clients from worry.** For example, "The client should not be told they have cancer because it would upset them too much" would almost certainly be an incorrect answer.
- **There is no pattern of correct answers.** The examination is compiled by a computer, and the position of the correct answers is selected at random.

STUDY HABITS

Study Effectively

1. **Use memory aids, mind mapping, and mnemonics.** Memory aids and mind mapping are tools that assist you in drawing associations from other ideas with the use of visual images (Fig. 1.2). Mnemonics are words, phrases, or other techniques that help you to remember information. Images, pictures, and mnemonics may stay with you longer than written text information.
2. **Develop 3 × 5 cards with critical information.** Do not overload the card; put a statement or question on one side and answers or follow-up information on the other side. For example, on one side you might write "low potassium" and, on the other side, you would list the relevant values. Another card might say "nursing care for hypokalemia" on the front and, on the back, you could list the nursing care. These cards are much easier for you to carry than a load of books or class notes. When you have developed and studied your set of cards with priority information,

REFERENCES

National Council of State Boards of Nursing. (2019, Fall). Approved NGN item types. *Next Generation NCLEX News*. https://www.ncsbn.org/NGN_Fall19_ENG_final.pdf

National Council of State Boards of Nursing. (2019, Winter). Clinical judgment measurement model. *Next Generation NCLEX News*. https://www.ncsbn.org/NGN_Winter19.pdf

National Council of State Boards of Nursing. (2019, Spring). The clinical judgment model and task model. *Next Generation NCLEX News*. https://www.ncsbn.org/NGN_Spring19_Eng_04_Final.pdf

National Council of State Boards of Nursing. (2020, Spring). The NGN case study. *Next Generation NCLEX News*. https://www.ncsbn.org/NGN_Spring20_Eng_02.pdf

National Council of State Boards of Nursing. (2021, Spring). Next Generation NCLEX: Stand-alone items. *Next Generation NCLEX News*. https://www.ncsbn.org/NGN_Spring21_Eng.pdf

National Council of State Boards of Nursing. (2022). *2022 NCSBN Annual Meeting: Business Book*. Author.

National Council of State Boards of Nursing. (2023). *NCLEX Examination Candidate Bulletin. Note: this publication changes yearly; navigate to* https://www.ncsbn.org/candidatebulletin.htm *for current bulletin.*

Nielsen, A. Gonzalez, L. Jessee, M. Monagle, J. Dickison, P. & Lasater, K. Current practices for teaching clinical judgment. *Nurse Educator*. 2023;48(1):7–12.

CHAPTER TWO

Health Implications Across the Life Span

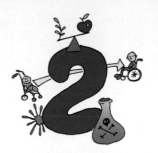

LONG-TERM CARE

Long-term care includes those services provided in institutional settings, such as a nursing home, rehabilitation center, or adult daycare program, after the acute phase of an illness has passed. This often involves restorative care for clients with chronic health care problems.

A. Types of long-term care or extended care facilities.
1. Nursing home or nursing center: provides 24-hour services ranging from maintenance to restorative care with skilled nursing, use of certified nursing assistants, licensed practical nurses, and registered nurses.
2. Adult daycare center: the client lives at home during the evening and night and spends the day in a facility that provides a range of care from skilled nursing to restorative care.
3. Palliative and hospice care: end-of-life care provided in the home and/or client care settings. (See Chapter 3, End-of-Life Care).
4. Respite care: a type of short-term care provided to give the primary caregiver (often a family member) a rest from the daily responsibilities of taking care of the client. This care may be provided in the client's home or in a facility.
5. Rehabilitation center: an inpatient rehabilitation facility (IRF) that provides multiple services for the client and family to adjust to daily living. It assists the client in achieving as much independence as possible in activities of daily living (ADLs).
6. Home care: nursing care provided in the home to clients who do not need hospitalization but do need additional assistance with medical problems.
7. Adult housing or assisted living centers: facilities for clients to live as independently as possible but still receive supervision, meals, housekeeping, 24-hour oversight, and other services.
8. Intermediate care or skilled nursing facility (SNF): offers skilled care from a licensed nursing staff, which often includes administration of intravenous (IV) fluids, wound care, long-term ventilator management, and physical rehabilitation.

B. For older adults in the United States, rehabilitation services for the first 100 days of inpatient care are paid by Medicare A.

REHABILITATION

Rehabilitation means the restoration of an individual to his or her optimal level of functioning. This includes physical, mental, social, vocational, and economic parameters.

A. Rehabilitation: term used when an individual has lost functional ability as a result of illness or injury and is working to get back or improve skills and functioning.
B. Habilitation: term used to refer to congenital problems or deficiencies where the person has not yet acquired or established skills.

Goals of Rehabilitation

For the client undergoing rehabilitation to achieve the highest level of productivity, the rehabilitation process must begin when the condition becomes evident or when the disease is diagnosed.

A. Prevention of deformities and complications.
1. Maintain function and prevent deterioration of unaffected organs or areas.
2. Prevent further injury to affected area or organ.
3. Prevent or reduce complications of immobility.
B. Encourage client to perform ADLs with minimum or no assistance, depending on his or her level of disability. *Examples of ADLs: eating, dressing, bathing*
C. Encourage client to perform independent activities of daily living (IADLs) with minimum or no assistance, depending on ability. *Examples of IADLs: shopping for groceries, paying bills, lawn care*
D. Promote continuity of care when the client is discharged or transferred.

Psychological Responses to Disability

Not every client will progress through all stages of grief in an orderly fashion. Clients will fluctuate between emotional crises.

A. Initial responses of *confusion, disorganization, shock, and denial* represent a state of internal conflict and emotional numbness that can last for a few hours or several days.
B. A period of depression may occur as the client mourns for the loss of or change in body function.
C. An anger stage may occur as the client projects blame and hostility on family and health care providers.

D. *Adaptation, adjustment,* and *acceptance* will come as the client begins to redirect his or her energy toward coping with the disability.

E. New situations (going home, new job, etc.) may precipitate emotional outbursts and trauma.

F. Some clients will refuse to accept their disability and will not put forth any effort to adapt to everyday living.

HOME HEALTH CARE

Home health care is the provision of health care to clients in the home environment.

A. Guidelines for home health care personnel.
   1. Respect client's religious, cultural, and ethnic background.
   2. As a caregiver/guest in the client's home, your behavior should reflect sensitivity to the client and family; a pleasant attitude and sense of humor are helpful.
   3. Gain family members and significant others as your advocates.
   4. Communication with other health care team members is vital to the maintenance of the client's well-being.
   5. Working with more autonomy without immediate hospital support is challenging and requires an increased level of nursing competence for decision making.
   6. A Patient's Bill of Rights is applicable in the home health care setting (i.e., client has the right to disclosure of information concerning his or her condition and care and the right to refuse or stop treatment, etc.).

CHRONIC ILLNESS

A chronic illness may be defined as an illness or condition that is present for more than 3 months in a year and interferes with daily function and lifestyle.

TEST ALERT   Help the client cope with life transitions.

Nursing Considerations

A. The majority of clients with extended health care needs have at least two chronic health conditions. These conditions may or may not be interrelated.

B. The focus of care for chronically ill clients is on assisting them to control their health problems and disease symptoms and manage their lifestyle.
   1. Prevention and management of medical crises.
   2. The control of disease symptoms, which may focus on pain control and comfort measures.
   3. Implementation of the prescribed therapeutic regimens.
   4. Psychosocial implications and adjustments to lifestyle; frequently, client must deal with social isolation.
   5. Adjustments to lifestyle as disease or condition changes.

6. Financial strain caused by paying for medical care and supplies.
   7. Coping with strain on marriage and family structure.

C. The majority of clients with chronic health care needs are older than 65 years of age. The developmental level of these individuals, according to Erikson, is ego integrity versus despair. The feeling of powerlessness is a common problem in the older adult.

D. The nursing process is directed toward identification of nursing actions to assist the older adult in maintaining independence and being as functional as possible.

Chronically Ill Pediatric Client

The diagnosis of a child's chronic illness is a major situational crisis in the family. Available support systems, perception of the problem, and coping mechanisms will ultimately determine the resolution of the crisis.

A. Focus care on the child's developmental age rather than chronologic age. Emphasis should be placed on the child's strengths rather than disabilities.

B. Assist the child and the family in returning to or establishing a normal pattern of living.

C. Promote the child's maximum level of growth and development. The current trend is to promote education within the child's peer group.

D. Assess the family's response to the child's illness and evaluate for parental overprotection. Overprotection by the parents prevents the child from developing self-esteem, independence, and self-control over the disease and ADLs. Look for the following parental characteristics that will impede development:
   1. Shows inconsistency in discipline; disciplinary measures often differ from those used with other children in the family.
   2. Attempts to protect the child from every discomfort, both physical and psychosocial. Frequently restricts play with peers based on fear of injury and/or rejection by peers.
   3. Makes decisions for the child without involving the child.
   4. Does not allow the child the opportunity to learn self-care; frequently, afraid the child cannot handle the requirements for self-care (e.g., a child with diabetes becoming responsible for administration of his or her own insulin).
   5. Continues to do things for the child, even when child is capable of doing them on his or her own.
   6. Shows self-sacrifice and isolation of family from social interactions.

GROWTH AND DEVELOPMENT

A. Normal growth and development progresses in a steady, predictable pattern across the life span.
   1. Development progresses in a cephalocaudal (head to toe) manner.
   2. Development progresses from proximal to distal, with a progression from gross to fine motor skills.

B. The developmental age of a client is critical to the planning of care in the hospital.
   1. Nurses need to be aware of the major developmental milestones.
   2. Nursing care is planned around the child's developmental level, not his or her chronologic age.
   3. Physical development is described in Table 2.1.

4. Developmental tasks and health promotion and maintenance needs are described in Table 2.2.

> **⚠ TEST ALERT** Provide care appropriate to developmental level (e.g., newborn, child, older adult), especially for the adult and older adult.

Table 2.1 GROWTH AND DEVELOPMENT

Birth–4 months	Consistently gains weight (5-7 oz; 142-198 g/week) Posterior fontanel closes Responds to sounds and begins vocalizing Gains head control → lifts chest → rolls over one way Smiles responsively → smiles when spoken to Teething may begin Coordination progresses from jerky movement to grasping objects Provide toys that increase hand-eye coordination
4–9 months	Doubles birth weight (gains 3-5 oz; 85-142 g/week) Teething begins with lower incisors Sits with support; begins crawling Turns over in both directions Laughs aloud Reaches for objects and grasps them Begins "stranger anxiety" Begins vocalizing with single consonants Provide brightly colored toys that are easy to grasp Enjoys noisemakers and mirrors; plays pat-a-cake
9–12 months	Birth weight triples Head and chest circumferences are equal Anterior fontanel begins to close Teething: has 6-8 teeth Sits alone → moves from prone to sitting position Crawls → pulls up → walks holding on to furniture May stand alone Has developed crude to fine pincer grasp Transfers objects from one hand to another Recognizes own name Enjoys playing alone (solitary) Explores objects by putting them in mouth
Toddler (12–24 months)	50% of height at 2 years Exaggerated lumbar curve Mobile: walks, runs, jumps Walks up and down stairs, one foot at a time Begins using eating utensils Obeys simple commands Begins to develop vocabulary Speech becomes understandable Thumb sucking may be at peak Solitary play at 12 months; parallel play at 18 months Beginning to develop bladder and bowel control Attention-seeking behavior: temper tantrums Enjoys activities that provide mobility: riding vehicles, wagons, pull toys
Preschool (3–5 years)	Birth length doubles at 4 years Coordination continues to improve Rides tricycle, throws a ball Walks up and down stairs with alternating feet Begins to demonstrate self-care abilities Knows own name Good verbalization: talks about activities Plays "dress up"; plays with cars, dolls, grooming aids

Continued

Box 2.1   OLDER ADULT CARE FOCUS

Age-related factors influencing older adult care

- Frequent absence of social and financial support
  Examples: Disease and/or loss of spouse, inadequate income from pension
- Presence of significant concurrent illness
  Examples: Dementia, chronic obstructive pulmonary disease, congestive heart failure, depression, diabetes, hypertension
- Altered pain perception
  Example: Increased incidence of referred pain
- Impaired homeostatic mechanisms
  Examples: Increased problems with dehydration, incontinence, decreased lymphocyte production, altered immune status
- Impaired mobility
  Examples: Dependence on assistive devices (e.g., walkers and canes), need for assistance with bed transferring, change in use of transportation, presence of parkinsonism or degenerative joint disease
- Increased frequency of adverse reactions to drugs
- Impaired equilibrium, resulting in falls

stairs, shoes in poor repair, and household items that are tripping hazards like rugs and extension cords).
E. Response to hospitalization will reflect moral and cultural values.
F. Hospitalization causes increased stress because of family and job responsibilities, in addition to being a threat to the client's well-being.
G. Direct nursing interventions to stabilize chronic conditions, promote health, and promote independence in basic and instrumental ADLs.
H. Concepts of death follow common sequence.
  1. Shock, anger, denial, disbelief.
  2. Development of an awareness, bargaining; may experience depression.
  3. Acceptance, reorganization, restitution.
I. Adults 18 to 65 years of age tend to have an abstract and realistic concept of death.
J. Older adult clients (aged 65 and older) have frequently lost a spouse, a child, or close friends. Attitudes toward death are realistic, but older adults tend to have a more philosophic concept of death.

NUTRITION

❗ TEST ALERT Monitor the client's nutritional and hydration status.

Nutritional Assessment: Recognize Cues

A. Assess nutritional and hydration needs.
B. Create client profile: age, sex, height, weight, socioeconomic status, and culture.

C. Determine nutritional status: note food habits; look for physical signs indicative of nutritional and hydration status.
D. Determine disease or pathophysiologic process.
E. Be alert to high-risk clients: those who are overweight or underweight; those with congenital anomalies of the gastrointestinal (GI) tract; those who have had surgery of the GI tract; those who have problems with ingestion, digestion, and/or absorption; and those receiving IV therapy for 10 days or more.

❗ TEST ALERT Intervene with the client who has an alteration in nutritional intake (adjust diet, change delivery to include method, time, and food preferences).

Dietary Considerations Throughout the Life Span
Infant

❗ NURSING PRIORITY A newborn will lose weight for the first few days but should not lose more than 10% of his or her birth weight or take longer than 10 to 14 days to regain it.

A. Growth.
  1. Birth weight doubles by 6 months and triples by 1 year.
  2. Infant gains only another 4 (1.81 kg) to 6 lb (2.72 kg) until 2 years of age.
  Birth weight 7 lb (3.17 kg); at 6 months, should be 14 lb (6.36 kg); at 1 year, should be 21 lb (9.54 kg) (birth weight tripled).
B. Diet.
  1. Ideal food is breast milk because it is nutritionally superior to alternatives, is easier to digest, and contains maternal antibodies. Breastfeeding exclusively until 6 months of age is recommended.
  2. Bottle-fed infants need to be on a formula that is iron fortified.
  3. Breastfed infants do not need additional water.

❗ NURSING PRIORITY A newborn has a higher fluid requirement in relation to body size than an adult.

  4. Breastfed infants should receive 400 international units (IU) of vitamin D as a daily supplement.
  5. Bottle-fed infants should receive 400 IU of vitamin D until the infant is consuming greater than 1 L/day (or 1 quart) of vitamin D-fortified formula.
  6. Whole cow's milk, low-fat cow's milk, skim milk, and imitation milks are not recommended for infants younger than 12 months of age.
  7. Iron-fortified cereal is often the first solid food introduced and is recommended around age 6 months.
  8. Strained meats, vegetables, and fruits are introduced one at a time to determine infant's tolerance of each food.
  9. Chopped foods are introduced at 6 to 9 months.

10. Before adding another food item, wait 3 to 5 days to ensure no allergic or adverse reaction has occurred from a previously added food item.

> ❗ **NURSING PRIORITY** Breastfed infants may gain weight at a slower rate than formula-fed infants. Breastfed infants are leaner and often have less body fat than formula-fed infants.

C. Nursing implications.

> ❗ **TEST ALERT** Monitor and provide for nutritional needs of client at all ages.

1. Newborns cannot swallow voluntarily until 10 to 12 weeks of age.
2. Extrusion reflex (pushing food out of mouth with tongue) lasts until 4 to 6 months; therefore solids are not introduced until around 6 months.
3. When solids are being introduced, offer only one new food per week; avoid multigrain cereals until tolerance is established.
4. Usual progression of food textures is strained to mashed to minced to chopped to cut-up table foods.
5. Increase the use of small-sized finger foods as pincer grasp develops (9 months). Be alert for choking hazards.
6. Texture of food becomes increasingly important from 6 months to 1 year, but the food must be easily dissolved (e.g., crackers or zwiebacks).
7. Teach parents *not* to warm frozen breast milk in the microwave; this may change the composition of the milk and cause oral burns.

> ❗ **NURSING PRIORITY** Infants should not be given honey until after their first birthday. Raw carrots, celery, popcorn, nuts, and hard foods should not be given until the toddler stage because of problem with choking.

Toddler

A. Growth.
   1. Steady increases in growth.
   2. Legs grow more rapidly than the trunk.
B. Diet.
   1. Needs 16 oz of milk daily; more than 24 oz can lead to refusal of other foods and development of a milk anemia (peak incidence at 18 months).
   2. Whole milk is recommended between 1 and 2 years of age; switch to 2% milk after age 2.
   3. Prefers finger foods (e.g., vegetables he or she can pick up, crackers, macaroni).
   4. Tends to refuse casseroles, salads, and mixed dishes.
   5. Use of 100% fruit juice in limited quantities; offer fruit snack, not juices.
C. Nursing implications.
   1. Struggle for autonomy may be manifested by refusal of food, mealtime negativism, and ritualism.

2. Bribery and rewards for eating should be avoided.
3. Around 18 months of age, a decreased appetite is normal; toddler may become a picky eater.
4. Do not mix foods on plate or overfill the plate.

Preschooler

A. Growth.
   1. Growth rate slows and appetite decreases.
   2. Activity level and nutrient requirements remain high.
B. Diet.
   1. *Food jags* are common; the child may refuse to eat anything except one food at each meal.
   2. Three meals and two snacks/day; begin to encourage five servings of fruits and vegetables.
   3. Finger foods remain popular.
C. Nursing implications.
   1. Do not bribe the child to eat or tell him or her to "clean your plate."
   2. Serve smaller portions; if sufficient amounts are not eaten during mealtimes, eliminate snacks.
   3. Recognize that refusing to eat is a way to attract attention.

School-Age Child

A. Growth.
   1. Growth is slow and steady.
   2. Food intake gradually increases while energy needs per unit of body weight decline.
   3. There is a yearly gain of 1.36 to 2.26 lbs (3-5 kg) in weight and 2.36 inch (6 cm) in height, ending with a growth spurt in puberty.
B. Diet.
   1. Food intake is more varied.
   2. Child enjoys most foods, with vegetables being the least favorite.
C. Nursing implications.
   1. After-school snack: encourage healthy choices such as fruits, raw vegetable sticks, and peanut butter sandwiches.
   2. Child learns good table manners from imitating parents.
   3. Appetite is usually good, but a child often does not want to take the time to eat. Sometimes it is helpful to spend a specific amount of time at the table (15-20 min) to prevent the child from forming the habit of gulping food down.
   4. Avoid using food as a reward for behavior.
   5. Begin teaching child to recognize high-fat foods.

Adolescent

A. Growth.
   1. Rapid growth rate and maturation changes make the adolescent vulnerable to nutritional deficiencies.
   2. Girls' peak growth occurs between 10 and 14 years of age.
   3. Boys' peak growth occurs between 12 and 15 years of age.

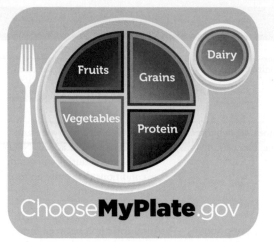

FIG. 2.1 MyPlate Food Guide. (From the U.S. Department of Agriculture. [Based on the *Dietary Guidelines for Americans*, 2020-2025]. https://www.ChooseMyPlate.gov.)

b. Milk: includes milk, soymilk, yogurt, and cheese (select no-fat or low-fat).
c. Oils: use selected fish, nut, and vegetable oils; limit butter, margarine, shortening, and lard (select oils with no *trans* fats).
d. Fruits and vegetables: eat a variety; 100% fruit juice is acceptable; eat more dark green and orange vegetables. (Fruits and vegetables should make up half the plate.)
e. Grains, breads, and cereals: whole-grain products should make up half the daily grain.
4. Drink water and unsweetened beverages instead of sugary drinks (energy drinks, sport drinks).
5. Balance calories: find out how many calories are needed to manage weight; stay physically active.
6. Enjoy food but eat less and avoid oversized portions.
a. Eating too fast may lead to eating too many calories.
b. Pay attention to hunger and fullness cues before, during, and after meals.
c. Use a smaller plate, bowl, and glass.
d. When eating out, choose a smaller size portion, share a dish, or take-home part of the meal.

Therapeutic Meal Plans

A therapeutic meal plan or prescription diet is a modification of an individual's normal nutritional requirements based on the changes in his or her physiologic needs as a result of an illness or disease state (Table 2.4).

> ❗ **TEST ALERT** Collect data on the client's nutrition or hydration status; identify client's ability to eat (chew, swallow); provide for nutritional needs by encouraging the client to eat, feeding the client, or assisting with menu.

CHILDHOOD DISEASES

> ❗ **TEST ALERT** Understand communicable diseases and modes of organism transmission (airborne, droplet, contact). Apply principles of infection control.

A. Incubation period: time from exposure to the pathogen until clinical symptoms occur.
B. Communicability: period of time in which an infected person is most likely to pass the pathogens to another person.
C. Prodromal period: begins with early manifestations of the disease or infection and continues until there are overt clinical symptoms characteristic of the disease.
D. Immunizations (Boxes 2-2, 2-3, and 2-4).
1. *Immunization* is the process whereby a person is made immune or resistant to an infectious disease, typically by the administration of a vaccine.
2. *Vaccination* is when a vaccine is administered. A *vaccine* is a product that stimulates a person's immune system to produce immunity to a specific disease, protecting the person from that disease (i.e., it is what initiates the immunization process).
3. The CDC updates the recommended immunization schedule yearly. The schedule needs to be read along with the explanatory notes. A copy of both child and adult schedules can be downloaded at: https://www.cdc.gov/vaccines/schedules/index.html.

> ❗ **NURSING PRIORITY** General contraindications to receiving an immunization include a severe febrile and/or an anaphylactic reaction to a previously administered immunization or to a substance in the immunization.

Varicella (Chicken Pox)

Characteristics

A. Herpes virus: varicella zoster; highly contagious, usually occurs in children younger than 15 years of age.
B. Maculopapular rash with vesicular scabs in multiple stages of healing.
C. Incubation period: 14 to 16 days.
D. Transmission: contact, airborne.
E. Communicability: 1 day before lesions appear to time when all lesions have formed crusts.

Assessment: Recognize Cues

A. Prodromal: low-grade fever, malaise, anorexia.
B. Acute phase: red maculopapular rash, which turns almost immediately to vesicles, each with an erythematous base; vesicles ooze and crust.
C. New crops of vesicles continue to form for 3 to 5 days, spreading from trunk to extremities.
D. All three stages are usually present in varying degrees at one time; pruritus.

Table 2.4   THERAPEUTIC MEAL PLANS

Diet	Purpose/Use	Foods Allowed	Foods Restricted
Clear liquid	To begin introduction of food after removal of NG tube, after GI surgery, and/or before GI diagnostics	Liquids that are clear, such as tea and coffee without cream, apple juice, ice pops, broth, clear sodas	Milk products, juice with pulp, any solid food; anything that is not liquid at room temperature
Full liquid	To begin introduction of food; used after removal of NG tube or after GI surgery	Any food that is liquid at room temperature	Any solid food
Soft diet	To progress diet as tolerated; food should be easy to chew and swallow	Soft, tender foods easy to swallow and digest; eggs	Highly seasoned foods, whole grains, fruits, vegetables, nuts, fried foods
Mechanical soft diet	To assist clients who cannot chew effectively	Soft foods that are easy to chew and swallow	Tough foods that are difficult to digest and swallow; steak
Bland diet	To eliminate foods irritating to the digestive system; used in clients after GI surgery and those with peptic ulcer disease and GI inflammatory problems	Milk, custards, refined cereals, creamed soups, potatoes (baked or broiled); all foods are white; no bright-colored food	Highly seasoned or strong-flavored foods; tea, colas, coffee, fruits, whole grains, raw fruit
Low-residue diet	To decrease fiber or stool in GI tract; acute episodes of enteritis, diarrhea; before and/or after GI surgery	Clear liquids, meats, fats, eggs, refined cereals, white bread, peeled white potatoes, small amount of milk	Cheeses; whole grains; raw fruits and vegetables; high-carbohydrate foods, which are usually high in residue and fiber
High-residue diet (also known as high-fiber)	To prevent constipation and acute diverticulitis; recommended for clients with irritable bowel syndrome (IBS)	Raw fruits and vegetables; whole grains; high-carbohydrate foods, which are high in residue and fiber	Indigestible fibers: celery, whole corn; seeds such as sesame and poppy; foods with small seeds
Lactose-free diet	To prevent GI effects of lactose intolerance	Nonmilk products, yogurt	Milk and milk products, processed foods that may have dried milk as filler
PKU diet	To control intake of phenylalanine, an essential acid; affected children cannot metabolize it	Specially prepared infant formula if infant is not breastfed, vegetables, fruits, juices, some cereals, and breads; may allow 20–30 mg of phenylalanine per kilogram of body weight to fulfill normal growth needs	Most high-protein foods, including meat and dairy products, are significantly reduced
Low-fat/low-cholesterol diet	To prevent gall bladder spasms, clients with increased cholesterol levels, or problems with malabsorption of fat (cystic fibrosis)	Low-fat or fat-free milk, fruits, vegetables, breads, cereals, reduced amounts of red meat	Egg yolks, whole milk, fried foods, processed cheese, shrimp, avocados, pastries, butter
Low-sodium diet	To reduce sodium intake to decrease retention of fluids, especially in clients with cardiac disease or hypertension	Salt-free preparations, fresh fruits, vegetables with no added salt	Processed foods, smoked or salted meats, prepared foods, frozen and canned vegetables, breads and pastries
High-potassium diet	To replace lost potassium in clients taking diuretics and/or digitalis	Dried fruits, fruit juices, fresh fruits (e.g., bananas, apricots, grapefruit, oranges, and tomatoes); sweet potatoes, legumes	No specific restrictions
Renal diet	Control potassium, sodium, and protein levels in clients with renal problems	High biologic protein (limited intake): eggs, milk, meat; decreased sodium products and decreased potassium (cabbage, peas, cucumbers are low in potassium)	High-potassium foods (dried fruits), high-sodium foods (processed foods), salt substitutes with high-potassium content
Low-purine diet	To decrease serum levels of uric acid; prescribed for clients with gout and high levels of uric acid	Vegetables, fruits, cereals, eggs, fat-free milk, cottage cheese	Glandular meats, fish, poultry, nuts, beans, oatmeal, whole wheat, cauliflower

GI, gastrointestinal; NG, nasogastric; PKU, phenylketonuria.

D. Dim lights to decrease photophobia.

E. Tepid baths and lotion to relieve itching.

F. Encourage intake of fluids to maintain hydration; temperature may spike 2 to 3 days after rash appears.

Rubella (German Measles)

Characteristics

A. An acute, mild systemic viral disease that produces a distinctive 3-day rash and lymphadenopathy.

B. Incubation: 14 to 21 days.

C. Transmission: nasopharyngeal secretions, direct contact.

D. Communicability: from up to 7 days before rash until 5 days after rash.

Assessment: Recognize Cues

A. Prodromal: low-grade fever, headache, malaise, symptoms of a cold, mild conjunctivitis.

B. Rash first appears on face and spreads down to neck, arms, trunk, and then legs; lasts an average of 3 days.

C. Diagnostics: persistent rubella antibody titer of 1:10 to 1:20 usually indicates immunity.

D. Complications: can have teratogenic effects on a fetus.

Nursing Interventions: Take Action

A. Primarily symptomatic; bed rest until fever subsides; droplet precautions.

B. Preventive: MMR immunization; *MMR should not be given to severely immunosuppressed clients.*

C. Pregnant women should avoid contact with children who have rubella. If not immunized before pregnancy, vaccination should not be given until completion of pregnancy.

Roseola Infantum (Exanthema Subitum)

Characteristics

A. A common, acute benign viral infection, usually occurring in infants and young children (ages 6 months to 3 years), characterized by sudden onset of a high temperature, followed by a rash.

B. Incubation period: usually 5 to 15 days.

C. Transmission: unknown, generally limited to children age <3 years but peak age is 6 to 15 months.

D. Communicability: unknown.

Assessment: Recognize Cues

A. Sudden onset of high fever: 103°F (39.5°C).

B. As fever drops, a maculopapular, nonpruritic rash appears abruptly; rash blanches or fades under pressure and disappears in 1 to 2 days.

C. Complications: febrile seizures.

Nursing Interventions: Take Action

A. Symptomatic: provide tepid baths, offer fluids frequently, dress child in cool clothing.

B. Acetaminophen and/or ibuprofen for fever control.

Erythema Infectiosum (Fifth Disease)

Characteristics

A. A common, acute benign viral infection, usually occurring in school-age children.

B. Incubation period: usually 4 to 14 days; may be as long as 21 days.

C. Transmission: respiratory secretions, blood, blood products.

D. Communicability: uncertain.

Assessment: Recognize Cues

A. Rash appears in 3 stages.

1. Erythema on face ("slapped cheek or face" appearance); disappears in 1 to 4 days.

2. About 1 day after rash appears on face, maculopapular red spots appear, symmetrically distributed on upper and lower extremities; rash progresses from proximal to distal surfaces and may last ≥1 week.

3. Rash subsides but reappears if skin is irritated or traumatized (sun, heat, cold, friction).

B. Complications: arthritis, arthralgia, anemia.

Nursing Interventions: Take Action

A. Isolation is not necessary.

B. There is no specific antiviral therapy.

C. Pregnant health care workers should avoid contact with children who have Fifth disease, as this may place the fetus at risk.

Diphtheria

Characteristics

A. An infection caused by *Corynebacterium diphtheriae*.

B. Incubation period: 2 to 5 days.

C. Transmission: direct contact, contaminated articles (fomites).

D. Communicability: variable, usually 2 weeks, or after 4 days of antibiotics; three negative cultures required.

Assessment: Recognize Cues

A. Nasal discharge, anorexia, sore throat, low-grade fever.

B. Smooth, white or gray membrane over tonsillar region; hoarseness and potential airway obstruction.

C. Frequently, tachypnea, dyspnea, stridor, or airway obstruction may occur if condition goes untreated.

D. Complications: cardiomyopathy, neuropathy.

Nursing Interventions: Take Action

A. Maintain isolation from other children.

B. Antibiotic and IV diphtheria antitoxin are common medications.

C. Humidified oxygen with respiratory problems; have tracheostomy set available.

D. Provide adequate humidification to allow for liquefaction of secretions.

E. Preventive: DTaP immunization.

Pertussis (Whooping Cough)

Characteristics

A. An acute inflammation of the respiratory tract caused by *Bordetella pertussis*, most severe in children younger than 2 years of age.
B. Incubation period: 6 to 20 days; average, 7 days.
C. Transmission: droplet and direct contact.
D. Communicability: highly contagious.

Assessment: Recognize Cues

A. Begins with symptoms of an upper respiratory tract infection, fever.
B. Cough occurs primarily at night; it consists of a series of short rapid coughs, followed by a sudden inspiration that is a high-pitched, crowing sound or a "whoop." Coughing may continue until a thick mucus plug is expelled.
C. Complications: pneumonia, atelectasis, seizures, myocarditis.
D. Preventive: DTaP immunization; adults (19-64 years of age) should receive one dose Tdap booster to reduce transmission of pertussis to infants.

Nursing Interventions: Take Action

A. Droplet precautions are recommended; continue bed rest as long as fever is present.
B. Antibiotic therapy started to limit spread of infection.
C. Provide oxygen and humidification and look for signs of increasing respiratory distress.
D. Maintain nutrition with small frequent feedings.
E. Avoid use of cough suppressants and sedatives.
F. Report cases to local public health department.

Tetanus (Lockjaw)

Characteristics

A. An acute, serious, potentially fatal disease characterized by painful muscle spasms and convulsions caused by the anaerobic gram-positive bacillus *Clostridium tetani*.
B. Incubation period: generally, from 3 days to 3 months; average, 8 days.
C. Transmission: through a puncture wound that is contaminated by soil, dust, or excreta that contain *C. tetani* or by way of burns and minor wounds (e.g., infection of the umbilicus of a newborn).

Assessment: Recognize Cues

A. Progressive stiffness and tenderness in the muscles of the neck and jaw (lockjaw).
B. Spasm of facial muscles produces the so-called sardonic smile.
C. Progressive involvement of trunk muscles causes opisthotonos positioning.
D. Paroxysmal muscular contractions occur in response to stimuli (noise, touch, light).

E. Client remains alert; mental status is not affected.
F. Complications: laryngospasm and tetany of the respiratory muscles cause contractions that may precipitate atelectasis and pneumonia.

Nursing interventions: Take Action

A. Preventive.
  1. Careful cleansing and debridement of wounds.
  2. Immunization: DTaP for child; adult tetanus toxoid (Td) every 10 years.
B. Maintain seizure precautions: quiet, nonstimulating environment; monitor vital signs, muscle tone, etc.

Poliomyelitis

Characteristics

A. An acute, contagious viral disease affecting the central nervous system.
B. Incubation period: 5 to 35 days; average, 7 to 14 days.
C. Transmission: fecal-oral or pharyngeal-oropharyngeal contact.
D. Communicability: virus in throat for 1 week after onset; in feces, present for 4 to 6 weeks.

Assessment: Recognize Cues

A. Nonparalytic type: pain and stiffness in the neck, back, and legs.
B. Paralytic type: initial symptoms are similar to those of nonparalytic poliomyelitis, followed by recovery, then signs of central nervous system paralysis.

Nursing Interventions: Take Action

A. Preventive: inactivated polio virus vaccine (IPV).
B. Bed rest during acute phase; standard and droplet precautions.
C. Physical therapy with warm moist packs and range of motion.
D. Position to maintain body alignment.
E. Complications: teach family and client early symptoms of respiratory distress.

Scarlet Fever

Characteristics

A. Group A beta-hemolytic streptococcal infection that often follows acute *streptococcal* pharyngitis.
B. Incubation period: 1 to 7 days; average, 3 days.
C. Transmission: direct contact or droplet of nasopharyngeal secretions; indirect contact with contaminated objects or ingestion of contaminated food.
D. Communicability: variable, approximately 10 days.

Assessment: Recognize Cues

A. Sudden onset of high fever and tachycardia.
B. Enlarged edematous tonsils covered with exudate; nausea, vomiting; "strawberry" tongue.

Goal: To reduce circulating volume and cardiac workload

A. Carefully monitor all IV fluids and evaluate tolerance of hydration status.

B. Maintain client in semi-to-high Fowler's position but allow legs to remain dependent.

Goal: To provide psychological support and decrease anxiety

A. Approach client in a calm manner.

B. Explain procedures.

C. Remain with client in acute respiratory distress.

Goal: To prevent recurrence of problems and preventive measures

A. COVID-19 vaccination and booster.

B. Recognize early stages and obtain medical treatment.

C. Maintain client in semi-Fowler's position.

D. Decrease levels of activity.

E. Wear a face mask; cough in the elbow area of arm; hands away from eyes, nose, and mouth.

F. Avoid close contact with others by keeping a distance of at least 6 feet.

G. Clean and disinfect frequently touched surfaces daily; wash hands frequently.

POISONING

General Principles (Remember SIRES)

A. *S*tabilize the client's condition.

B. *I*dentify the toxic substance.

C. *R*emove the substance to decrease absorption.

D. *E*liminate the substance from the client's body.

E. *S*upport the client both physically and psychologically.

Salicylate Poisoning

A. Toxic dose levels: 300 to 500 mg/kg (1086-2172 μmol/L) of body weight. For a 30 lb (13.6 kg) child, 12 adult-strength aspirin or 48 baby aspirin would be toxic.

B. In severe toxic overdose, metabolic acidosis eventually occurs because of the change in body processes.

C. Chronic use causes a deficiency in platelets, leading to bleeding tendencies.

Assessment: Recognize Cues

A. Acute *early* symptoms: hyperventilation, nausea, vomiting, tinnitus.

B. Acute *later* symptoms: hyperactivity, fever, confusion, seizures (metabolic acidosis), renal failure, respiratory failure.

C. Chronic poisoning: same as above but subtle onset and nonspecific, often mistaken for a viral illness, bleeding tendencies.

Nursing Interventions: Take Action

A. Administer activated charcoal.

B. Administer vitamin K to decrease bleeding tendencies.

C. Provide oxygen and ventilatory support for respiratory depression; provide IV fluids and sodium bicarbonate to treat acidosis.

D. Administer cooling activities and treatments for hyperthermia.

E. In severe cases, hemodialysis may be performed.

Acetaminophen Poisoning

A. Definition of toxicity in children is 150 mg/kg or greater.

B. Primary toxic effects are on the liver.

C. Antidote: N-acetylcysteine.

D. Most common poisoning in children.

Assessment: Recognize Cues

A. Clinical manifestations: four stages.
   1. Stage 1 (0-24 hours).
      a. Nausea and vomiting.
      b. Sweating and pallor.
   2. Stage 2 (24-72 hours); child improves.
   3. Stage 3 (72-96 hours; hepatic involvement).
      a. Right upper-quadrant pain.
      b. Coagulation abnormalities, confusion.
      c. Jaundice, vomiting.
   4. Stage 4 (more than 5 days; recovery if hepatic damage is not severe).

Nursing Interventions: Take Action

A. Early administration of activated charcoal – preferably within 30 minutes to 1 hour after ingestion.

B. Antidote is N-acetylcysteine: one loading dose and multiple maintenance doses.

Lead Poisoning

A. Ingestion of lead from hand to mouth and exposure to lead-contaminated dust, eating from improperly glazed glassware (leaded glass) or lead-based pottery or chewing on furniture with lead-based paint.

B. Increased risk in children younger than 6 years of age because they absorb 40% to 50% of lead, whereas adults absorb only 5% to 10%.

Assessment: Recognize Cues

A. Renal: problem in adults with occupational exposure; renal impairment will delay excretion of the lead from the body.

B. Hematologic: anemia, blue lead line on gums and "lead lines" on x-rays of the long bones noted in chronic conditions.

C. Neurologic: hyperactivity, increased distractibility, seizures.

Nursing Interventions: Take Action

A. Chelation therapy process for removing lead from the circulating blood; aids in secretion by the kidneys.

B. Encourage high fluid intake.

C. Seizure precautions.

CHARACTERISTICS OF CANCER

Cancer must be regarded as a group of disease entities with different causes, manifestations, treatments, and prognoses.

The basic disease process begins when normal cells undergo change and begin to proliferate in an abnormal manner.

Major Dysfunction in the Cell

A. Cellular proliferation: cancer cells divide in an indiscriminate, unregulated manner and exhibit significant variations in structure and size.

B. Loss of contact inhibition: cancer cells have no regard for cellular boundaries; normal cells respect boundaries and do not invade adjacent areas or organs.

C. Cancer can arise from any cell in the body that can evade the normal regulatory controls of proliferation or growth and cellular differentiation.

D. Tumors (neoplasms).
   1. Benign: encapsulated neoplasm that remains localized in the tissue of origin and is typically not harmful.
      a. Exerts pressure on surrounding organs.
      b. Will decrease blood supply to the normal tissue.
   2. Malignant: nonencapsulated neoplasm that invades surrounding tissue. Depends on the stage of the neoplasm as to whether metastasis (spreading to distant body parts) occurs. The neoplasm spreads by means of four primary mechanisms:
      a. Vascular system: cancer cells penetrate vessels and circulate until trapped. The cancer cells may penetrate the vessel wall and invade adjacent organs and tissues.
      b. Lymphatic system: cancer cells penetrate the lymphatic system and are distributed along lymphatic channels.
      c. Implantation: cancer cells implant into a body organ. Certain cells have an affinity for particular organs and body areas.
      d. Seeding: a primary tumor sloughs off tumor cells into a body cavity, such as the peritoneal cavity.
   3. Common sites for metastasis: brain, liver, lungs, adrenals, spinal cord, and bone.

Etiology

A. Viruses: incorporate into the genetic structure of the cell, causing mutations.

B. Radiation: exposure to sunlight and radiation (e.g., bone cancer in radiologists, ultraviolet [UV] radiation, and melanoma).

C. Chemical agents: produce toxic effects by altering.

D. Genetic and familial factors.

E. Hormonal agents: tumor growth is promoted by disturbances in hormonal balance of the body's own (endogenous) hormones or administration of exogenous hormones (e.g., prolonged estrogen replacement, oral contraceptives).

F. Idiopathic: many cancers – breast, colon, rectal, lymphatic, bone marrow, and pancreatic cancers – arise spontaneously from unknown causes.

Prevention

A. Cancer prevention.
   1. Eat a balanced diet that includes fresh fruits and vegetables, adequate amounts of fiber and whole grains,

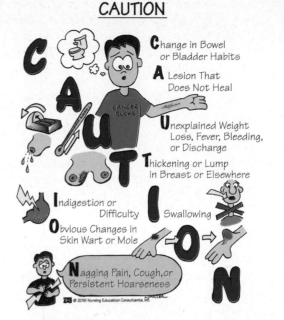

FIG. 2.3 Cancer Early Warning Signs. (From Zerwekh J, Garneau A, Miller CJ. [2017]. *Digital collection of the memory notebooks of nursing* [4th ed.]. Chandler, AZ: Nursing Education Consultants, Inc.)

and decreased fats and preservatives; avoid smoked and salt-cured foods containing increased nitrates.
   2. Avoid exposure to known carcinogens (e.g., cigarette smoke, tanning beds, and sun exposure).
   3. Keep weight in normal range; obesity is associated with cancer of uterus, gallbladder, breast, and colon.
   4. Get enough rest and sleep – at least 6 to 8 hours per night.
   5. Decrease stress, or perception of stress, and improve ability to effectively manage stress.
   6. Engage in at least 30 minutes of moderate to vigorous exercise 5 days a week.
   7. Limit alcohol use.

B. Screening guidelines – early detection is important. Know the seven warning signs of cancer and encourage early reporting of any change in an individual's normal body function (Figure 2.3).
   1. Cervical: screening should begin at age 21; between ages 21 and 29 should have a Pap test every 3 years; between ages 30 and 65 should have a Pap test plus a human papillomavirus (HPV) test every 5 years; if vaccinated against HPV, should still follow the screening recommendations.
   2. Prostate: The pros and cons of prostate cancer screening should be discussed with men beginning at age 50. Testing could include a digital rectal examination (DRE) or prostate-specific antigen blood test. African American men and those men with strong family history should have this talk beginning at age 45.
   3. Colorectal: For ages 50 to 75, all clients should have one of the following: a flexible sigmoidoscopy every 5 years, a colonoscopy every 10 years, a double-contrast barium enema every 5 years, computed tomography (CT) colonography (virtual colonoscopy) every 5

years, a yearly highly sensitive fecal occult blood test (FOBT), or a yearly fecal immunochemical test (FIT). Screening selection will be determined based on the client's history and the schedule that works best for the client.

4. Breast: Women should undergo annual screening mammography from ages 45 to 54. At 55 years, women may transition to biennial screening. Screening mammography should continue as long as life expectancy is 10 years or longer.

5. Testicular self-examination: monthly from ages 20 to 40.

Treatment of Cancer

A. Common cancer diagnostic studies.
1. X-ray.
2. Tissue biopsy.
3. Radiographic studies: mammography, ultrasonography, CT scans, or magnetic resonance imaging (MRI).
4. Radioisotopic scans: bone, liver, lung, brain.
5. Cytology studies (bone marrow aspiration, urine and cerebrospinal fluid analysis, cell washings, Pap smears, and bronchial washings).
6. Positron emission tomography (PET) scan.
7. Tumor markers; genetic markers.
8. Endoscopic examinations: upper GI, sigmoidoscopy, or colonoscopy examinations – including stool for occult blood.
9. Complete blood count (CBC), chemistry profile, liver function tests.
10. Bone marrow examination (if hematolymphoid malignancy is suspected).
11. Molecular receptor status (estrogen and progesterone receptors).

B. Biopsy.
1. Used for definitive diagnosis.
2. Needle: tissue samples are obtained by a small-gauge aspiration needle (fine-needle aspiration) or with a large-bore needle (large-core biopsy).
3. Incisional: scalpel or dermal punch is used to obtain a tissue sample.
4. Excisional: involves removal of the entire tumor.
5. Endoscopic biopsy: direct biopsy through an endoscopy of the area (GI, respiratory, genitourinary tracts).

Goals of Cancer Therapy

A. Prophylaxis: to provide treatment when no tumor is detectable but when client is known to be at risk for tumor development, spread, or recurrence.
B. Cure: client will be disease-free and live to normal life expectancy.
C. Control: client's cancer is not cured but controlled by therapy over long periods.
D. Palliation: to maintain as high a quality of life for the client as possible when cure and control are not possible (Figure 2.4).

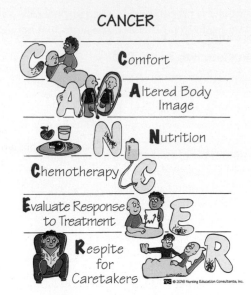

FIG. 2.4 Care of Cancer Patient. (From Zerwekh J, Garneau A, Miller, CJ. [2017]. *Digital collection of the memory notebooks of nursing* [4th ed.]. Chandler, AZ: Nursing Education Consultants, Inc.)

Modalities of Cancer Treatment

> **NURSING PRIORITY** Therapy generally involves using two or more modalities of treatment.

A. Surgery.
1. Evaluate any adverse effects of previous treatment and their implications for proposed surgery (e.g., poor nutritional status or fibrosis from effects of radiation therapy that may lead to poor wound healing, leukopenia from chemotherapeutic agents).
2. Evaluate extent of disfigurement or debilitation caused by surgery and consider its effect on client (e.g., ostomy formation, amputation).
3. Promote healthful self-image and return to normal lifestyle by recommending cancer support groups and other rehabilitation resources.

B. Chemotherapy: overall goal of chemotherapy is to destroy the cancer cells without excessive damage to normal cells.
1. Medications are highly toxic and destroy healthy cells in addition to cancer cells.
2. Combination chemotherapy is more effective than single-dose therapy.

> **TEST ALERT** Follow procedures for handling biohazardous materials (e.g., chemotherapeutic agents, radiation sources).

3. Nursing interventions in chemotherapy (Table 2.5).
a. Assess client for symptoms of bone marrow suppression (increased bruising and bleeding, sore throat, fever, increased fatigue).
b. Prevent exposure of client to people with communicable diseases or infections.

Table 2.5 NURSING IMPLICATIONS AND CHEMOTHERAPY

Problem	Nursing Implications
Bone Marrow Suppression • Thrombocytopenia (decreased platelets)	1. Initiate bleeding precautions (e.g., decrease invasive procedures; minimize injections). 2. Observe for bleeding tendency (bruising, hematuria, bleeding gums, etc.). 3. Monitor platelet counts.
• Anemia (decreased hemoglobin)	1. Fatigue is normal with chemotherapy; client should report any significant increase in fatigue. 2. Encourage diet high in protein, calories, and iron; administer iron supplements and erythropoietin. 3. Monitor hemoglobin level.
• Leukopenia (decreased white cells)	1. Advise health care provider regarding any unexplained temperature elevation greater than 100°F (37.7°C) or other signs of infection. 2. Protect client from exposure to infections (e.g., frequent hand hygiene, location of room, screen visitors, etc.). 3. Monitor WBC count, especially neutrophil levels. 4. Administer WBC growth factors.
Pneumonitis (pulmonary toxicity)	1. Monitor for persistent nonproductive cough, fever, exertional dyspnea, and tachypnea. 2. Most cases are cumulative-dose related and can be fatal.
Hyperuricemia (increased serum levels of uric acid)	1. Encourage fluid intake up to 3000 mL daily, if allowed. 2. Assess for involvement of the kidneys, ureters, and bladder. 3. Allopurinol may be used as prevention or as treatment.
Alopecia	1. Encourage client to wear something to cover the scalp (e.g., wig, scarf, turban, hat). 2. Avoid exposure of scalp to sunlight. 3. Do not rub scalp; do not use hair rollers, hair dryers, curlers, or curling irons. 4. Avoid excessive shampooing, brushing, or combing of hair. 5. Hair usually grows back in 3-4 weeks after chemotherapy; it is usually a different texture and color.

Stomatitis (mucositis)	1. Encourage good oral hygiene and frequent oral checks.
	  a. Encourage frequent mouth rinses of saline or salt and soda solution to keep mucous membranes moist.
	  b. Brush teeth with a small, soft toothbrush after every meal and at bedtime.
	  c. Remove dentures to prevent further irritation.
	2. Avoid alcohol and spicy or hot foods; a mechanical soft, bland diet may be ordered.
	3. Rinse mouth with topical anesthetics, such as viscous lidocaine, for pain control.

GI: anorexia, nausea and vomiting, diarrhea, and constipation	1. Assist client to maintain good nutrition.
	  a. Discuss food preferences with client and dietitian; encourage small, frequent meals.
	  b. Correlate meals with antiemetic medications.
	  c. Encourage family to provide client with favorite foods.
	  d. Increase calories, protein, and iron; encourage supplemental vitamins. Nutritional supplements may be indicated.
	2. Monitor weight, hydration status, and electrolyte imbalances.
	3. Evaluate skin around anal area in the client with diarrhea; prevent excoriation.
	4. If prone to constipation, maintain high-fluid and high-fiber intake; use stool softeners as needed.
	5. If experiencing diarrhea, encourage fluids, low-fiber, low-residue diet.

Tissue irritation, necrosis, ulceration from infusion therapy	1. Vesicant medications should be administered via a central line to promote dilution of medication. Monitor site for infection. 2. If multiple drugs are administered, flush between each administration.

> **🔋 NURSING PRIORITY** Observe client for side effects of a chemotherapeutic agent. If extravasation occurs with a vesicant medication in a peripheral site:
> 1. Stop the infusion: remove any remaining drug in the tubing or needle.
> 2. Contact physician and consult hospital policy and precautions for specific medication.
> 3. Antidote medication may be instilled directly into the infiltrated area.
> 4. Ice or heat may be applied to site, depending on the medication; the extremity may be elevated for the first 24-48 hrs after extravasation.

GI, gastrointestinal; IV, intravenous; WBC, white blood cell.

1. Maintain adequate fluid intake (at least 3000 mL/day).
2. Frequently assess for symptoms of cystitis.
3. Avoid bladder catheterization if possible.
4. Check urine for presence of hematuria.
5. Encourage frequent voiding.

Goal: To prevent and/or decrease infectious process (see Table 2.5)

A. Monitor temperature routinely.
B. Meticulous personal hygiene, including frequent handwashing.
C. Child should be isolated from others with communicable diseases.
D. Frequently assess for potential infectious processes.
E. Fresh fruits and vegetables should be eaten only after they have been cooked, peeled, or washed thoroughly.

Goal: To decrease hematologic complications

A. Evaluate for decreasing platelet levels and thrombocytopenia.

> **! NURSING PRIORITY** Institute bleeding precautions if platelet count is less than 50,000/mm3.

B. Administer platelets as indicated.
C. Evaluate areas of potential bleeding.
1. Mucous membranes, nosebleed (epistaxis).
2. Urinary tract (hematuria).
3. GI bleeding (hematemesis), stool (melena).
4. Implement bleeding precautions.

> **! NURSING PRIORITY** Advise client to use electric razor and a soft-bristle toothbrush.

D. Anemia.
1. Maintain adequate rest; encourage client to pace activities to avoid fatigue.
2. *Assess respiratory and cardiac systems and report changes to RN.*

Goal: To relieve pain (see Chapter 3)

A. Evaluate client and family responses to pain.
B. Evaluate characteristics of pain: determine whether pain control is to be palliative.
C. Administer medications for pain relief.
D. Use nonpharmacologic approaches to pain relief (positioning, imagery, hypnosis, etc.).

Goal: To recognize complications specific to radiation and chemotherapy

A. Alopecia.
B. Hemorrhagic problems.

C. GI distress (anorexia, ulcerations, nausea, vomiting).
D. Bone marrow depression (myelosuppression) – thrombocytopenia, anemia, neutropenia.
E. Skin reactions.
F. Decreased immune response.

Home care

Goal: To effectively manage pain to provide client optimal rest and pain relief

A. Assist client to identify provoking and alleviating factors and adjust environment accordingly.
B. Assess other psychological factors affecting pain tolerance (fear, anxiety, agitation, and past experiences with pain).
C. Assist client with nonpharmacologic pain therapies.
D. Layer pain management strategies as needed; medicate with opioids, nonsteroidal antiinflammatories, and adjuvant pain medications as necessary.
E. Assess effectiveness of therapies and medications and modify as necessary.
F. Provide a calm, healthy environment with appropriate lighting and personal belongings as warranted by disease progression.

Goal: To decrease or limit exposure to infection

A. Limit number of people having direct contact with the client.
B. Good oral hygiene: regular flossing if there is no bleeding problem and no tissue irritation; soft toothbrush; avoid irritating foods.
C. Client should avoid coming in direct contact with animal excreta (cat litter boxes, bird cages, etc.).
D. Teach client to take his or her temperature daily and report temperature over 100.4°F (38°C).
E. Use antipyretics cautiously, as they tend to mask infection.
F. Teach client that the highest risk for infection occurs within 7 to 10 days after the administration of chemotherapy.
G. Teach client importance of frequent handwashing.

Goal: To maintain optimum psychosocial function

A. Assess coping mechanisms.
B. Assess family/significant other resources.
C. Provide opportunities for client to express feelings, concerns, and fears.
D. Encourage activity; one of the best activities is walking for about 30 minutes at a rate that is comfortable.

Appendix 2-1 CANCER CHEMOTHERAPY

General *Nursing Implications*
- Observe for adverse effects (see Table 2.5).
- Monitor client and laboratory values for evidence of bone marrow suppression: infection from loss of neutrophils, bleeding from loss of thrombocytes, and anemia from loss of erythrocytes.
- **Chemotherapy is only administered by the RN. The LPN/LVN does not administer chemotherapy. The LPN/LVN should assist with monitoring the client during administration.**
- General side effects of antineoplastic agents are nausea, vomiting, diarrhea, anorexia, alopecia, hyperuricemia, nephrotoxicity, and bone marrow suppression.
- Monitor renal and hepatic function to evaluate ability of client to break down and excrete chemotherapeutic agents.

MEDICATION	SIDE EFFECTS	NURSING IMPLICATIONS
Alkylating Agents **Kill cells by alkylation of the DNA; all are dose limiting by bone marrow suppression.**		
Cyclophosphamide	Renal, hepatotoxic	1. Monitor for hemorrhagic cystitis; encourage high fluid intake.
Mechlorethamine (nitrogen mustard)	Blood dyscrasias	1. Strong vesicant; prevent extravasation and direct contact with the skin.
Chlorambucil	Pulmonary infiltrates and pulmonary fibrosis, hepatotoxic	1. Monitor respiratory status and maintain good respiratory hygiene.
Busulfan	Pulmonary infiltrates and pulmonary fibrosis, sterility	1. Monitor respiratory status and maintain good respiratory hygiene.
Ifosfamide	Hemorrhagic cystitis	1. High risk for cystitis; urinalysis done before each dose.
Platinum Compounds **Have a similar action as the alkylating agents and are cell-cycle nonspecific.**		
Cisplatin Carboplatin	Neurotoxicity, ototoxicity	1. Produces nausea and vomiting within an hour of administration. 2. Assess for tinnitus and hearing loss. 3. Encourage high fluid intake.
Antimetabolites **Disrupt critical cellular metabolism; cell-cycle specific; dose limited by bone marrow suppression.**		
Methotrexate sodium	Pulmonary infiltrates and fibrosis; oral and GI ulceration High doses can damage kidneys Teratogenic	1. Leucovorin may be administered to increase uptake; it can be potentially dangerous, especially if the right dose is not administered at the right time, in which case it could be fatal. 2. Monitor GI status; potential of intestinal perforation; nausea and vomiting occur early. 3. Encourage high fluid intake to promote drug excretion. 4. Avoid pregnancy for at least 6 months. 5. Do not take folic acid.
Pemetrexed	Teratogenic GI toxicity – stomatitis and diarrhea may be dose limiting	1. Vitamin B12 and folic acid to decrease bone marrow and GI toxicity. 2. Avoid in pregnancy.
Cytarabine	High doses may cause pulmonary edema and cerebellar toxicity	1. Nausea and vomiting after bolus administration. 2. Monitor pulmonary status and fluid balance.
5-Fluorouracil	Stomatitis, GI ulceration	1. Monitor and report early GI symptoms; may be discontinued.
Mercaptopurine	Hepatotoxicity common, GI ulceration Mutagenic – avoid in pregnancy	1. Monitor for jaundice. 2. Allopurinol increases risk for toxicity.
Thioguanine	Hepatic dysfunction; GI ulceration	1. Monitor for jaundice.

Continued

Practice & Next Generation NCLEX (NGN) Questions

1. The nurse finds the client's radiation implant in the bed. What is the **priority** nursing action?
   1. Using tongs, replace the implant in the lead container in the room.
   2. Immediately evacuate the client and all others from the room.
   3. Wearing gloves, replace the implant into the body cavity.
   4. Call radiation control to pick up the implant.

2. The mother of a newborn asks when the infant can be given solid food. What is an appropriate response?
   1. Begin fortified cereals at 3 months; then begin fruits at 6 months.
   2. Start fruits as the first solids at 6 months, then vegetables at 8 months.
   3. Start fruits at 3 months, followed by fortified rice cereal.
   4. Begin fortified cereals at 6 months, followed by fruits.

3. In reviewing the client's plan of care, what is important to reinforce when teaching a client about self-care during radiation therapy?
   1. Remove skin dye markings between treatments.
   2. Avoid exposure to the sun and do not remove dye markers.
   3. Reduce carbohydrate and protein intake during treatments.
   4. Decrease fluid intake and increase carbohydrate intake after treatment.

4. A client undergoing chemotherapy is experiencing nausea and vomiting. What is the **best** nursing action?
   1. Give antiemetics and monitor hydration.
   2. Administer oral care and assess for mouth lesions.
   3. Decrease fluid intake and monitor renal function.
   4. Record daily weight and encourage small meals.

5. A client is on furosemide for his heart condition. What foods would the nurse encourage the client to eat?
   1. Breads and fortified cereals.
   2. Fresh fruits and vegetables.
   3. Leafy green vegetables.
   4. Lean red meat and whole grains.

6. A client arrives in the emergency department with a penetrating wound he received while chopping trees. What is a **priority** nursing action?
   1. Cleanse the wound with antibacterial solution.
   2. Administer gamma globulin intramuscularly.
   3. Anticipate notifying poison control for plant toxicology.
   4. Determine when client received last tetanus injection.

7. The nurse is discussing nutrition with a woman who is 50 years of age, perimenopausal, and has a history of hypertension. What food choices would be **best** to help meet the dietary needs of this woman?
   1. Cheese and macaroni, fresh fruit, and milkshake.
   2. Cottage cheese, glass of skim milk, and fresh spinach salad.
   3. Roast beef with whole wheat bread, potato, and lettuce salad.
   4. Cheeseburger, French fries, and milkshake.

8. The mother of a 3-month-old infant is concerned because the baby seems to sleep most of the time. The nurse's response is based on the knowledge that a 3-month-old infant usually spends:
   1. 10 hours sleeping in a 24-hour period.
   2. 15 to 16 hours sleeping in a 24-hour period.
   3. 18 to 19 hours sleeping in a 24-hour period.
   4. Most of the 24 hours sleeping, waking only to eat.

9. What is the **most** serious effect of long-term exposure to lead in children?
   1. Anemia.
   2. Glycosuria.
   3. Impairment of the central nervous system.
   4. Constipation.

10. A 5-year-old child is diagnosed with chickenpox. The mother is concerned about how long the child will be contagious. On what principle will the nursing response be based?
    1. The child will be contagious until the fever has subsided, and all lesions are healed.
    2. The contagious period will extend to approximately 1 week after the lesions have healed.
    3. One day before appearance of the lesions until all lesions have crusted is considered the most contagious period.
    4. The most contagious period is approximately 7 to 10 days after onset or until the lesions are dried.

11. The clinic nurse is reviewing the immunization record of a 1-year-old who is in for a well-baby exam. The nurse notes the child's immunization record (shaded gray boxes on electronic MAR). **Highlight the immunization(s) that would be administered at this visit.**

MAR										
IMMUNIZATION	BIRTH	1MO	2MOS	4MOS	6MOS	12-15MOS	15-18MOS	4-6YRS	11-12YRS
Hep B	░	░	░						
IPV			░	░	░				
DTaP			░	░	░				
Hib			░	░	░				
PCV13			░	░	░				
RV			░	░	░				
MMR									
VAR									
Hep A									
HPV									

Hepatitis B vaccine (HepB); Inactivated poliovirus vaccine (IPV); diphtheria, tetanus, acellular pertussis vaccine (DTaP); *Haemophilus influenzae* type b conjugate vaccine (Hib); pneumococcal conjugate vaccine (PCV13), rotavirus vaccine (RV); measles, mumps, rubella vaccine (MMR); hepatitis A vaccine (Hep A); varicella vaccine (VAR); human papillomavirus vaccine (HPV).

12. The long-term care nurse is reviewing the health history of an 85-year-old woman who was newly admitted to the unit. **Highlight the statements or clinical findings that require follow-up.**

| Health History | Nurses' Notes | Provider Orders | Laboratory Results |

1300: Client is alert and oriented x3. Weight 98 lbs (44.5 kg); Height 5ft 6in. Reports having all three COVID-19 vaccinations and a yearly flu vaccination. Does not remember whether she had a pneumonia vaccination or when she had the last tetanus booster. States that she has not had a shingles vaccination because she had a case of shingles when her husband died about 15 years ago. Takes only one prescribed medication for hypertension, which is HCTZ, 12.5 mg, PO, daily.

- Temperature: 98°F (37.7°C)
- BP: 138/88 mm Hg
- Heart rate: 78 bpm and regular
- Respirations: 20 breaths/min
- SpO2: 97% on room air

Answers to Practice & Next Generation NCLEX (NGN) Questions

1. **1**
Client Needs: Safe and Effective Care Environment/ Safety and Infection Control
Clinical Judgment/Cognitive Skill: Prioritize Hypotheses
Item Type: Multiple Choice
Rationale & Test-Taking Strategy: Note the **key** word, "priority." This test item focuses on the priority nursing intervention for a client with a radiation implant. Safety is always a priority with clients who have a radiation implant. If there is dislodgement of a radiation implant, there should always be tongs and a lead container in the room to place the radiation source. Getting the client away from the radiation source is most important to prevent skin irradiation. The room does not need to be evacuated. If gloves are ever used, they must be lead-lined. After the radiation implant is secured in the lead container, notify radiation control.

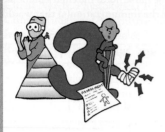

CHAPTER THREE

Nursing Care Concepts

BASIC HUMAN NEEDS

A. Maslow's hierarchy of basic human needs.
   1. Human behavior is motivated by a system of needs.
   2. Clients will focus on or attempt to satisfy needs at the base of the pyramid before focusing on those higher up in the pyramid (Fig. 3.1).
   3. Human needs are *universal;* however, some may be modified by cultural influence.
   4. The nursing process is always concerned with physiologic needs first; it then progresses to safety, teaching, decreasing anxiety, etc. This is also true for the client with psychosocial needs; the client's physiologic and safety needs must be met before they can progress to the next level.

> **NURSING PRIORITY** Maslow's hierarchy of needs is useful in answering test questions related to setting priorities. Always remember that the physiologic needs at the base of the pyramid must be satisfied first, before turning to focus on other needs – and remember that oxygenation (think ABC's – airway, breathing, circulation) is always the first physiologic need or priority.

MASLOW'S HIERARCHY OF BASIC HUMAN NEEDS

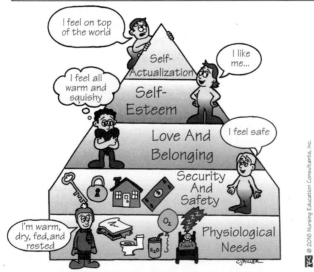

FIG. 3.1 Maslow's Hierarchy of Needs. (From Zerwekh J, Garneau A, Miller CJ. [2017]. *Digital collection of the memory notebooks of nursing* [4th ed.]. Chandler, AZ: Nursing Education Consultants, Inc.)

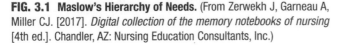

STEPS OF THE NURSING PROCESS

The categories of the nursing process and the activities in each category vary somewhat according to nursing authors. The nursing process as presented here correlates with the categories of the NCLEX-PN®.

Data Collection (Assessment)

1. Collecting data.
   Objective data (signs) are nursing observations.
   Example: Client weighs 125 lb; 50 mL of green drainage via the nasogastric tube.
2. Subjective data (symptoms) are information provided by the client.
   Example: "My stomach hurts; I am scared about my upcoming surgery."
3. Client data is collected using physical examination techniques.
   a. Inspection: what can be seen.
      Example: Is the client awake or asleep; is the client obese or underweight; is the client smiling or frowning?
   b. Auscultation: what can be heard.
      Example: Is the client coughing; are lung sounds clear; do you hear hyperactive bowel sounds?
   c. Palpation: what can be felt.
      Example: Is the client's skin warm and dry; can you feel the client's pedal pulses; is the client's abdomen soft?
   d. Percussion: tapping body surfaces to produce sound; it is also used to identify organ borders.
      Example: Is the client's abdomen hyperresonant; does the client have an enlarged liver?

Planning

A. Assign priority to the nursing care activities.
B. Specify goals reflecting desired outcome of nursing care.
   1. Develop short-term and long-term goals.
   2. Identify nursing interventions for goal attainment.
   3. Establish outcome criteria.
C. Contribute to developing and/or updating the client's plan of care.
   1. Involve client and family in all aspects of planning.
   2. Keep client's plan of care current and flexible.

Implementing

A. Initiate and carry out planned nursing activities.

B. Coordinate activities of client and family members along with health team members.

C. Document client's responses to nursing actions.

Evaluating

A. Collect objective and subjective data and determine whether goals were achieved.

B. Identify and revise the nursing care plan.

HEALTH ASSESSMENT

TEST ALERT Collect baseline physical examination data on admission.

Health History

The health history is a primary source of client information. The source of the information can be the client, relatives, friends, medical records, or any combination of these. A predetermined format should be used as a guide for the interview.

A. Demographic data.
1. Name, address, phone, age, sex, marital status.
2. Race, religion, usual source of medical care.

B. Chief complaint/reason for visit.
1. Chief complaint (CC): main reason client sought health care.
2. CC is recorded in client's own words.
Example: "I have been vomiting blood since this morning."

C. History of the present illness.
1. Descriptive narrative of client's reason for seeking care.
Remember **PQRST** for obtaining data on the client's present pain or (problem) illness.
P – What is the current problem? What provokes or palliates the problem?
Q – Describe the quality of the problem or pain.
R – What region of the body is involved?
S – If experiencing pain, how would you rate your pain on a scale of 0 to 10?
T – When did the problem or pain start?

D. Past health history.
1. Childhood diseases, immunizations.
2. Allergies.
3. Relevant family history (heart disease, diabetes, cancer).
4. Hospitalizations and serious illnesses.
5. Accidents and injuries.
6. Prescribed medications and over the counter (OTC) supplements or medications.
7. Activities of daily living (ADLs).
8. Psychosocial history.
9. Prenatal, labor and delivery, or neonatal history (recorded for all children younger than age 5 and older children with a congenital anomaly or developmental delay).

E. Review of systems.
1. Brief account from the client regarding any recent signs or symptoms associated with each body system.
2. Contains subjective data given by the client; *does not* contain objective data from the physical examination.
3. Review of system progresses from head to toe. The pertinent information to include is located in the assessment section at the beginning of each system.

Nursing Assessment

A. *Comprehensive health assessment* completed by registered nurse.

B. *Focused assessment* is limited to the current need, health care problem, or health risk the client is experiencing.

TEST ALERT Collect data as part of a focused assessment (neurologic checks, neurovascular checks, bowel sounds, etc.). Gather data on client health history and risk factors for disease (e.g., lifestyle, family, and genetic history).

1. Frequently used for bedside assessments.
2. Data collection on specific characteristics of the problem.
3. Determine what type of nursing intervention is necessary.
4. Determine when the intervention should be implemented: immediately, later in shift, before client's discharge, etc.

C. *Follow-up assessments are performed throughout the shift, as warranted by any change in the client's status.*

HEALTH PROMOTION

Levels of Prevention

Preventive health care is more dynamic than health maintenance; it focuses on health enhancement and health promotion, whereas health maintenance is concerned with maintaining the client's current health status.

A. Primary: prevention of disease.
1. The goal is to achieve maximum functioning in each health potential area.
Examples: Smoking cessation, practice safe sex, maintain body weight, limit alcohol intake, follow a regular exercise program and a healthy diet. Immunizations (e.g., influenza, pneumococcal, COVID-19, and shingles vaccine) and occupational/environmental safety (e.g., wearing protective goggles or earplugs) are included in primary prevention.

B. Secondary: early screening, diagnosis, and treatment.
1. Emphasis is on determining intervention priorities.
Examples: Screening for tuberculosis, glaucoma test, Pap smear, mammography, colorectal cancer screening, and breast and testicular self-examination.

C. Tertiary: prevention of complications and maximize functional capabilities.

Box 3.3 CULTURAL SENSITIVITY WITH SEXUAL ORIENTATION AND GENDER IDENTITY

Provision of Care, Treatment, and Services Checklist

- Create a welcoming environment that is inclusive of LGBT patients.
  - Prominently post the hospital's nondiscrimination policy or patient bill of rights.
  - Waiting rooms and other common areas should reflect and be inclusive of LGBT patients and families.
  - Create or designate unisex or single-stall restrooms.
  - Ensure that visitation policies are implemented in a fair and nondiscriminatory manner.
  - Foster an environment that supports and nurtures all patients and families.
- Avoid assumptions about sexual orientation and gender identity.
  - Refrain from making assumptions about a person's sexual orientation or gender identity based on appearance.
  - Be aware of misconceptions, bias, stereotypes, and other communication barriers.
  - Recognize that self-identification and behaviors do not always align.
- Facilitate disclosure of sexual orientation and gender identity but be aware that disclosure or "coming out" is an individual process.
  - Honor and respect the individual's decision and pacing in providing information.
  - All forms should contain inclusive, gender-neutral language that allows for self-identification.
  - Use neutral and inclusive language in interviews and when talking with patients.
  - Listen to and reflect patients' choice of language when they describe their own sexual orientation and how they refer to their relationship or partner.
- Provide information and guidance for the specific health concerns facing lesbian and bisexual women, gay and bisexual men, and transgender people.
  - Become familiar with online and local resources available for LGBT people.
  - Seek information and stay up to date on LGBT health topics. Be prepared with appropriate information and referrals.

From The Joint Commission. (2011). *Advancing effective communication, cultural competence, and patient- and family-centered care for the lesbian, gay, bisexual, and transgender (LGBT) community: a field guide.* The Joint Commission.

Assessment of Cultural Aspects

> ❗ **NURSING PRIORITY** Avoid stereotyping and generalizing. Clients are individuals who are unique, with beliefs, values, and traditions that deserve a personalized nursing assessment.

A. Communication styles.
  1. Does the client speak English fluently? If not, what language is preferred?
  2. What are considered signs of respect or disrespect? Attentiveness or inattentiveness?

Box 3.4 GUIDELINES FOR WORKING WITH INTERPRETERS

A. For those with limited English proficiency, a professional medical interpreter is needed whenever serious decisions are needed (e.g., end-of-life care, informed consent, treatment changes, discharge planning).
B. It is not recommended to use family, children, or support staff as interpreters.
C. Guidelines for working with interpreters:
  1. Before an interview, instruct interpreter to use client's own words; avoid paraphrasing and inserting their ideas or omitting any information.
  2. During interview, look and speak with client, not interpreter or client's family if present.
  3. Use brief, concise sentences, and simple language—avoid technical terms and slang language.
  4. If you feel an interpretation is not correct, stop and address the situation directly with the interpreter.
  5. Watch and listen to the client's nonverbal communication when client is talking.

3. Is touch part of the communication process?
4. What practices are considered appropriate greetings or farewells?
5. How is silence used in communication?
6. What is the use of nonverbal communication?
7. Is language assistance (e.g., written translation services or medical interpreter) needed? (Box 3.4)

> ❗ **NURSING PRIORITY** Use a medical interpreter from the health care facility and avoid using family members for clients with limited English proficiency (LEP).

B. Ethnic or religious group.
  1. With what particular group does the client identify?
  2. What cultural practices are important?
C. Nutrition.
  1. What does the client and their family like to eat?
  2. Are there certain ethnic or religious preferences about the selection or preparation of foods?
  3. Who prepares meals in the client's home?
D. Family relationships.
  1. Is the family matriarchal or patriarchal?
  2. What role in the family does the client hold?
  3. What is the role and attitude toward children and older family members (extended family)?
E. Health beliefs about health and illness.
  1. What does the client most fear about the illness?
  2. What are the problems the illness has caused the client to experience?
  3. Does the client rely on folk medicine practices or complementary and alternative therapies (e.g., acupuncture, healing touch, Ayurveda, etc.)?
  4. Has the client been recently treated by any traditional healers?
  5. Does the client take any herbal supplements or over the counter (OTC) medications?

F. Health practices.
   1. What are the strategies used to maintain health (e.g., hygiene, self-care)?
   2. Who does the client contact when ill?
   3. Does the client prefer to have a health professional of the same gender, age, ethnic, and/or racial background?
G. Time orientation.
   1. What is the client's orientation to time? Are they future oriented, present oriented, or past oriented?
   2. What are the client's views on being punctual and wasting time?
H. Personal space preferences.
   1. What is the personal space preference?
   2. Territoriality or personal space is the distance that a client prefers to maintain from another.
   3. Large personal space is usually more than 18 inches.
I. End-of-life care.
   1. What are the spiritual and religious practices that ease the client during end-of-life care?
   2. Are there any garments, religious items, or rituals that are important during end-of-life care?
   3. What are the practices about care of the body after death? How should the body be treated?
   4. Does the client prefer a visit from a religious leader or clergy member?
   NOTE: The Joint Commission has a publication divided into two sections: cultures and religions, which is detailed and provides a handy resource for health care providers. (Galanti GA. [2018]. *Cultural and religious sensitivity: A pocket guide for health care professionals* (3rd ed.). Oakbrook, IL: The Joint Commission.)

BASIC NURSING SKILLS
Comfort Measures and Hygiene

TEST ALERT Assist with ADLs.

A. Beds and comfort measures.
   1. Avoid shaking linens.
   2. Hold all soiled linens away from your uniform.
   3. Specialty beds.
      a. Air-fluidized bed.
         (1) Provides a continuous shift of pressure by alternating inflation and deflation of air every 2 to 5 minutes.
         (2) Used to prevent development of or to treat pressure injuries.
      b. Pressure-relieving mattress.
         (1) Foam, air, gel, or water mattress that is built-in to the bed unit.
         (2) Used to prevent pressure areas from developing in a bedridden client.
B. Bathing.
   1. Types of baths.
      a. Bed bath.
      b. Partial bath.
      c. Shower.
      d. Therapeutic bath: sitz bath or medicated bath.
   2. Nursing implications: Take action.
      a. Room should be kept warm, bath should begin with clean areas and progress to dirty areas.
      b. To prevent dry skin, irritation, and infection, carefully rinse all surface areas and dry them.
      c. Keep client warm by using a bath blanket and controlling room temperature.
      d. Ensure privacy and only expose the area of the body that is being cleaned.
      e. Moisturize skin with lotion.

! NURSING PRIORITY Clients who are receiving external radiation therapy should not be bathed with soap over the area of the radiation, which will be marked. Lotions, oils, and powders should not be used on the area.

   3. Levels of personal care.
      a. Complete care: Client requires total assistance from nurse because client is able to do little or nothing without assistance.
      b. Partial care: Client performs as much of their own care as possible; nurse usually completes remaining care.
      c. Nighttime care (bedtime or hour of sleep): Is provided to prepare client for a relaxing, uninterrupted period of sleep; includes oral care, possible partial bathing, skin care, soothing back massage, straightening or changing the bed linen, and offering the bedpan or urinal.
C. Oral hygiene.
   1. Includes care of the client's teeth or dentures, gums, tongue, and lips.
   2. When providing oral care to unconscious client, turn the client's head to the side and facing downward to prevent aspiration.
D. Hair care.
   1. Newborn infants need scalp scrubbed daily to prevent cradle cap.
   2. Adolescents usually require more frequent shampooing because of increased oil production.
   3. Older adult clients will need to shampoo less often.

Vital Signs

TEST ALERT Take client's vital signs. Compare changes in vital signs to client's baseline. Notify supervisor or health care provider about a change in client's status.

A. Normal values (Table 3.1).
B. Assessment: Recognize cues.
   1. Respirations.
      a. Evaluate an infant's respiratory pattern before stimulating them.
      b. Check thoracic cavity for symmetric thoracic excursion.

4. To reduce effects of gravity on the vascular bed and reduce edema formation.

Adverse Physical Effects of Immobility

Goal: To prevent complications

A. Cardiovascular system.
   1. Assessment of physical effects: Recognize cues.
      a. Orthostatic hypotension.
      b. Decrease in cardiac reserve.
      c. Venous stasis.
      d. Formation of thrombi.
      e. Increase in cardiac workload.
   2. Nursing implications: Take action.
      a. Position body to decrease venous stasis.
      b. Change position frequently.
      c. Passive and active range of motion (ROM).
      d. Begin activity gradually; allow client to sit before standing and to rise slowly to standing position.
      e. Have client use bedside commode when possible to decrease effects of Valsalva maneuver.
B. Respiratory system.
   1. Assessment of physical effects: Recognize cues.
      a. Decrease in thoracic excursion.
      b. Decrease in ability to mobilize secretions.
      c. Decrease in oxygen/carbon dioxide exchange.
      d. Increase in pulmonary infections.
   2. Nursing implications: Take action.
      a. Elevate head of bed.
      b. Maintain adequate hydration: 2400 to 3000 mL/day if tolerated.
      c. Have client turn, cough, and breathe deeply at regular intervals (every 2 hours while awake); use incentive spirometry 10 times/hour while awake.
      d. Promote increase in activity as soon as possible: have client sit up in chair at bedside.
      e. Evaluate pulmonary secretions for infection.
C. Urinary system.
   1. Assessment of physical effects: Recognize cues.
      a. Urinary stasis.
      b. Increased calcium level, stasis, and infection precipitate stone formation.
      c. Urinary tract infections.
   2. Nursing implications: Take action.
      a. Have client sit or stand to void if possible.
      b. Establish and maintain a voiding schedule.
D. Musculoskeletal system.
   1. Assessment of physical effects: Recognize cues.
      a. Demineralization of bones: decrease in bone strength.
      b. Muscle weakness and atrophy.
      c. Loss of motion in joints leads to fibrosis and contractures.
      d. Loss of height secondary to vertebral fractures associated with osteoporosis.

   2. Nursing implications: Take action.
      a. Perform ROM exercises.
      b. Active contraction and relaxation of large muscles.
      c. Position body to maintain proper alignment.
      d. Encourage daily weight-bearing exercise when possible.
E. GI system.
   1. Assessment of physical effects: Recognize cues.

      a. Anorexia.
      b. Ineffective movement of feces through colon: constipation and fecal impaction.
      c. Fecal incontinence caused by impaction.
   2. Nursing implications: Take action.
      a. Establish bowel program: every other day or three times a week.
      b. Encourage diet with adequate protein, fiber, and fluids.
      c. Check for fecal impaction.
F. Integumentary system.
   1. Assessment of physical effects: Recognize cues.

      a. Decrease in tissue perfusion leading to pressure injury development.
      b. Decreased sensation in area of increased pressure.
   2. Nursing implications: Take action.
      a. Maintain cleanliness.
      b. Promote circulation through frequent repositioning.
      c. Protect bony prominences when turning.
      d. Prevent creation of pressure areas by tight clothing, cast, or braces.
      e. Perform frequent visual inspection of pressure prone areas.

Body Alignment and Range of Motion

A. Characteristics of correct body alignment in bed.
   1. Head up with eyes looking straight forward.
   2. Neck and back straight.
   3. Arms relaxed and supported at sides.
   4. Legs parallel to hips with knees slightly flexed.
   5. Feet separated and parallel to the legs with the toes pointed upward and slightly outward.
B. ROM. (Fig. 3.2)
   1. Active ROM.
      a. Client performs exercise without assistance.
      b. Used for client who independently performs ADLs but for some reason is immobilized or limited in terms of activity.
      c. Purpose is to maintain muscle tone, decrease venous stasis, prevent muscle atrophy, and prevent contracture.
   2. Passive ROM.
      a. Client cannot actively move and requires assistance.

RANGE OF MOTION

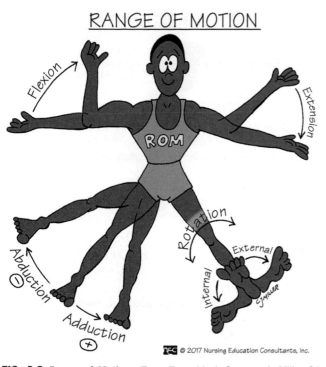

FIG. 3.2 Range of Motion. (From Zerwekh J, Garneau A, Miller CJ. [2017]. *Digital collection of the memory notebooks of nursing* [4th ed.]. Chandler, AZ: Nursing Education Consultants, Inc.)

b. Client cannot contract muscles; therefore muscle strengthening *cannot* be accomplished.

c. Purpose is to maintain joint flexibility, prevent contractures, and promote venous return.

C. Principles of ROM exercises.
1. Stretch muscles by moving the body part; avoid movement to the point of discomfort.
2. Perform ROM at least twice daily for immobile clients, with a minimum of four to five repetitions of each exercise.
3. Always support extremity above and below the joint when performing passive ROM on extremities.
4. Involve the client in planning the exercise program.

D. Client positions (see Appendix 3.1).

> **TEST ALERT** Monitor and provide for mobility needs – mobility aids, ambulation, ROM, transfers, positioning, and use of assistive and adaptive devices.

SAFETY AND INFECTION CONTROL

Asepsis

> **TEST ALERT** Always apply principles of infection control (handwashing/hand hygiene, room assignment, isolation, aseptic/sterile technique, and standard precautions).

A. Medical asepsis.
1. Designed to reduce the number of pathogens in an area and decrease the likelihood of their transfer (e.g., by handwashing/hand hygiene).

Box 3.7   STERILE TECHNIQUE: PROCEDURES AND GUIDELINES

Procedures Requiring Sterile Technique
- Surgical procedures in the operating room (e.g., transurethral prostatectomy [TURP], appendectomy)
- Biopsies in the operating room, treatment room, or client's room
- Catheterizations of the heart, bladder, or other body cavities
- Injections: intramuscular (IM), subcutaneous (subQ), intradermal
- Infusions: intravenous (IV), instillations, or infusions of medication or radioactive isotopes into body cavities
- Dressing changes:
- Usually, first postoperative dressing change done by using sterile technique
- Dressings over catheters inserted into body cavities (e.g., Hickman catheter, subclavian lines, dialysis access sites, peripherally inserted central venous catheter [PICC])
- Dressings of clients with burns, immunologic disorders, skin grafts, and dressings involving the abdomen or cranium.

Guidelines for Sterile Field
- Never turn your back on a sterile field. The front of the sterile gown is considered sterile.
- Do not reach across a sterile field.
- Avoid talking.
- Keep all sterile objects within view (e.g., below waist and above shoulders are not within sterile field; the outer 1-inch perimeter is not considered sterile, avoid placing objects in this area).
- Moisture will carry bacteria across/through a cloth or paper barrier.
- Transfer of objects from sterile to contaminated (not sterile) = contaminated.

2. Often referred to as *clean technique;* wash hands between visits with individual clients.
3. Included in this category are daily hygiene practices and administration of oral medications, enemas, and tube feedings.

B. Surgical asepsis.
1. Designed not simply to *reduce* the number of pathogens but to make the object *free* of all microorganisms.
2. Also known as *sterile technique.*
3. Surgical asepsis is reserved primarily for sterile dressing changes, sterile catheterizations, and surgical procedures in the operating room (Box 3.7).

> **TEST ALERT** Set up a sterile field. Use appropriate supplies to maintain asepsis (gloves, mask, sterile supplies); evaluate whether aseptic techniques are performed correctly.

📋 Wound Care

A wound is a disruption in normal tissue caused by traumatic injury or created surgically.

PAIN

- Clients have the right to appropriate assessment and pain management.
- Physiologic and behavioral signs of pain should not replace the client's ability to report the pain unless client is unable to communicate verbally.
- Pain can exist even when there is no identifiable cause; pain is always a subjective personal experience.
- Different clients experience different pain levels, even in response to the same type of pain stimulus.
- Pain is an early warning system; its presence triggers awareness that something is wrong in the body.
- Unrelieved pain causes adverse physical and psychological responses.

TEST ALERT Plan measures to care for clients with anticipated or actual alterations in comfort.

Classification of Pain

- *Acute pain:* has an identifiable cause; is protective; short, predictable duration (lasting less than 3 months); immediate onset; reversible or controllable with treatment. It most often has an identifiable source such as postoperative pain that disappears as the surgical site heals.
- *Chronic pain:* lasts more than 6 months; continual or persistent and recurrent. Pain may not go away; periods of decreased and increased pain. Origin of pain may not be known.
- *Cancer pain:* pain arising from cancer (tumor compressing on nerve(s) or organ involvement) and treatments (chemotherapy, surgery, radiation) associated with treating cancer.
- *Breakthrough pain:* pain experienced in individuals with cancer and chronic pain. Pain medication that normally controls the cancer or chronic pain does not relieve breakthrough pain. Therefore the client may experience intense pain that requires additional pain-relief measures.
- *Nociceptive pain: somatic* pain that affects skeletal muscles, joints, and ligaments; generally diffuse and less localized; *visceral* pain arises from internal organs and may be caused by a tumor or obstruction.
- *Neuropathic pain:* caused by damage to peripheral nerves or to the central nervous system; can result from trauma, metabolic disease, or neurologic disease.
- *Referred pain:* pain that does not occur at the site of injury. For example, pain related to myocardial ischemia may be felt in the left arm or shoulder only; cholecystitis may be felt as shoulder pain.
- *Phantom pain:* pain that follows the amputation of a body part; it may be described as throbbing, cramping, or burning in the body part amputated.

Pain Characteristics

TEST ALERT Monitor and document client's discomfort and pain levels. Evaluate pain using standardized rating scales.

Box 3.8	MNEMONIC TO EVALUATE PAIN
O:	Onset
P:	Provoking or palliative factors
Q:	Quality
R:	Region or radiation; relieving factors
S:	Severity
T:	Timing

A. Pattern of pain (Box 3.8).
   1. Pain onset and duration: when it started, precipitating causes, and how long it lasts.
   2. Pain pattern: continuous, intermittent, and timing of when pain occurs (morning, evening, after activity).
B. Area of pain.
   1. Ask the client to identify the pain site.
   2. Pain may be referred from the precipitating site to another location—shoulder pain with cholecystitis, left arm pain with myocardial infarction (MI).
   3. Radiating pain involves pain traveling along a nerve pathway from the pain origination site to another region of the body. Sciatica pain follows a nerve pathway of the sciatic nerve, generally down the back of the thigh and inside the leg.
C. Intensity of pain: use a pain scale to help the client communicate the pain intensity.
D. Pain quality/type.
   1. Neuropathic pain may be burning, numbing, electric/shock-like, shooting.
   2. Somatic pain may be superficial, sharp, throbbing, cramping.
   3. Visceral pain may be sharp, dull, deep, aching.
E. Determine any activities and situations that increase the level of the pain—movement, ambulation, coughing.
F. Client responses to pain (Box 3.9).
   1. Increased blood pressure, pulse, and respiration, diaphoresis, increased muscle tension, nausea, and vomiting (acute pain).
   2. Withdrawn, insomnia, decreased activity, hypersomnia, anxiety (chronic pain).
   3. Client's interpretation and meaning of the pain experience.

⊞ NURSING PRIORITY In addition to the pain and discomfort associated with a surgical procedure, it is important to assess other possible sources of discomfort, such as a full bladder, occluded catheter or tube, gas accumulation, intravenous (IV) infiltration, or compromised circulation caused by position or prolonged pressure over a bony prominence.

Cultural Implications of Pain

A. Cultural beliefs and values affect how a client responds to pain.

B. Assess attitudes and beliefs that may affect effective treatment of the pain. Some clients may believe that taking pain medications will cause "addiction"; other clients may believe that complaining of pain is a sign of weakness.

C. Avoid stereotyping clients by assuming that members of a specific cultural group will or will not exhibit more or less pain.

D. Nursing considerations of pain control associated with a client's culture.

1. Identify what the pain means to the client; for example, a woman in labor may perceive the pain differently from a client who experiences pain as an indication of advanced disease.

2. Identify cultural implications regarding how a client responds to or expresses pain; some clients moan and cry; others may be quiet and stoic.

3. Individualize pain control based on client's response to pain.

4. Establish a communication method for the client to express the level of pain and effectiveness of pain control (e.g., pain rating scale, FACES scale, pictures, images) (Fig. 3.6).

5. Expression of pain is subjective; accept the client's perception of pain and expression of pain and facilitate nursing care to meet the client's cultural needs when providing pain control.

TEST ALERT Assess importance of client culture/ethnicity when planning, providing, and evaluating care.

Nonpharmacologic Pain Relief Measures

A. Relaxation techniques.

❗ NURSING PRIORITY Low levels of anxiety or pain are easier to reduce or control than higher levels. Consequently, pain relief measures should be used *before* pain becomes severe.

1. Relaxed muscles result in a decreased pain level.

2. Relaxation response requires quiet environment, comfortable position, and a focus of concentration.

3. Identify the relaxation method that is most effective for the client—music, guided imagery, therapeutic massage, and meditation for progressive muscle relaxation.

4. Rhythmic breathing: method of relaxation and distraction focusing on the breath.

TEST ALERT Monitor the need for pain management and intervene using nonpharmacologic comfort measures. Recognize differences in client perception and response to pain. Evaluate client response to nonpharmacologic comfort measures.

B. Hypnosis produces a state of altered consciousness characterized by extreme responsiveness to suggestion.

C. Biofeedback provides client with information about changes in bodily functions of which they are usually unaware (e.g., blood pressure, pulse rate).

D. Cutaneous stimulation alleviates pain through stimulation of skin.

1. Use of pressure, massage, bathing, and heat or cold therapy to promote relaxation.

2. Therapeutic touch: holistic approach in which touch is used to realign energy fields (laying on of hands).

Box 3.9	ASSESSING THE HARMFUL EFFECTS OF PAIN

Acute Pain	*Chronic Pain*
Disturbs sleep	Fatigue
Appetite decreases	Weight gain
Fluid intake decreases	Poor concentration
Decreased diaphragmatic movement, decreased alveolar expansion, and avoidance of coughing	Decreased use of thoracic muscles, decreased chest expansion, and avoidance of coughing
Increased pulse rate, increased systolic blood pressure, facial grimacing	Job loss Divorce Depression
Nausea and vomiting	

❗ NURSING PRIORITY The nurse should administer pain medication to clients experiencing acute pain without fear of the client becoming addicted to the medication..

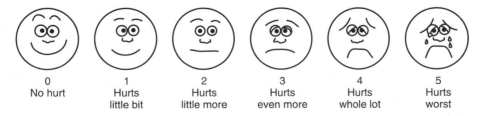

0	1	2	3	4	5
No hurt	Hurts little bit	Hurts little more	Hurts even more	Hurts whole lot	Hurts worst

FIG. 3.6 Wong-Baker FACES Pain Rating Scale. FACES Pain Rating Scale consists of six cartoon faces ranging from a smiling face for "no pain" to a tearful face for "worst pain." The FACES scale provides three scales in one: facial expressions, numbers, and words. The numbering system can be based on a 0-to-5 or a 0-to-10 pain scale. The nurse points to each face using the words to describe the pain intensity and then asks the child to choose the face that best describes their own pain and documents the appropriate number. (From Hockenberry MJ, Wilson D. [2015]. *Wong's nursing care of infants and children* [10th ed.]. Mosby.)

Box 3.10   OLDER ADULT CARE FOCUS

Preoperative and postoperative considerations

Older clients are at increased risk for developing postoperative complications because of the decreased response of the immune system (which delays healing) and the increased incidence of chronic disease.

- *Cardiovascular*: decreased cardiac output and peripheral circulation, along with arrhythmias and increased incidence of arteriosclerosis and atherosclerosis, can lead to hypotension or hypertension, hypothermia, and cardiac problems.
- *Respiratory*: decreased vital capacity, reduced oxygenation, and decreased cough reflex can lead to an increased risk for atelectasis, pneumonia, and aspiration.
- *Kidney*: decreased kidney excretion of wastes and renal blood flow, along with increased incidence of nocturia can lead to fluid overload, dehydration, electrolyte imbalance, and drug toxicity.
- *Musculoskeletal*: increased incidence of arthritis and osteoporosis can lead to bone and joint trauma with positioning in the operating room if pressure points and limbs are not padded.
- *Sensory*: decreased visual acuity and reaction time can lead to safety problems associated with falls and injuries. Decreased sense of touch, pain, temperature, and smell can also pose safety concerns.
- *Integumentary*: Decreased subcutaneous tissue and increased capillary permeability can contribute to the development of pressure-related injuries, skin tears, and bruising.
- The older client may require repeated explanation, clarification, and additional time when providing teaching. Older clients often have a reduced thirst mechanism and decreased protein intake, which can delay wound healing and postoperative recovery.

TEST ALERT Provide care that meets the needs of the older adult client..

  5. Medications may predispose client to operative complications.
  6. Check results of routine diagnostic laboratory studies.
     a. Blood studies: complete blood count, serum electrolytes, coagulation studies, serum creatinine, blood urea nitrogen, lipid panel, and fasting glucose.
     b. Urinalysis.
     c. Chest x-ray.
     d. Electrocardiogram for clients over 40 years of age.
     e. Coagulation studies for clients with known problems or to establish a baseline.
B. Preoperative teaching: the goal is to decrease the client's anxiety and prevent postoperative complications.

TEST ALERT Anticipate questions regarding basic pre- and postoperative nursing care in addition to questions that apply to a specific surgical condition or procedure. Nursing implications for specific surgical procedures may be found under the major systems in the care of the medical-surgical client.

  1. Evaluate the client's current understanding of his/her illness and of the anticipated surgical intervention.

  2. Use terminology the client will understand.
  3. Do not overwhelm the client with too much information at one time; allow adequate time for client to ask questions.
  4. Involve the client's significant others in the preoperative teaching.
  5. Reinforcement of preoperative teaching content.
     a. Deep breathing and coughing exercises.
     b. Turning and extremity exercises.
     c. Pain medication administration policy.
     d. Adjunct equipment used for breathing: nebulizer, oxygen mask, spirometer.
     e. Explanation of (nothing by mouth) NPO policy.
     f. Antiembolism stockings and/or pneumatic compression device to decrease venous stasis and reduce risk of developing deep vein thrombosis (DVT).
  6. Pediatric implications in preoperative teaching.
     a. Plan the reinforcement of teaching content around the child's developmental level and previous experiences.
     b. Use correct terms for body parts and clarify terms with which the child is unfamiliar.
     c. Fear of anesthesia is common in children.
C. Physical preparation of client.
  1. Skin preparation: the purpose is to reduce bacteria on the skin (may be done in surgical suite or in the preoperative holding area).
     a. Area of preparation is always longer and wider than area of incision.
     b. Antiseptic soap/agent (2% chlorhexidine gluconate) is used to cleanse area.
     c. Assess for allergies before using, especially tape allergies.
  2. GI preparation.
     a. Food and fluid restriction: NPO orders may be individualized for each client. Client may be NPO for 6 to 8 hours before surgery or NPO from midnight on the night before surgery.
     b. Enemas or cathartics may be administered the evening before surgery to prevent fecal contamination in the peritoneal cavity for GI surgeries.
  3. Promote sleep and rest: sleep-aid medication and anti-anxiety medication may be given to promote rest and reduce anxiety (e.g., benzodiazepine, alprazolam).
  4. In older adults, evaluate status of teeth, presence of bridges and dentures; in children, evaluate for presence of loose teeth.
D. Informed consent.
  1. Each surgical procedure must have the voluntary, informed, and written consent of the client or the person legally responsible for the client.

TEST ALERT Identify appropriate person to provide informed consent for client (e.g., client, parent, legal guardian). Provide written materials in client's spoken language. Describe components of informed consent (purpose of procedure, risks of procedure). Participate in obtaining informed consent as a witness. Ensure that the client has given informed consent for treatment.

2. Health care provider: gives the client a full explanation of the procedure, including complications, risks, and alternatives.

3. Client's informed consent record (permit) must be signed by the client or legal guardian. A witness signs to validate this is the client's signature, that the client has voluntarily given consent, and that the client is competent to give consent. The witness is frequently a staff nurse. Depending on facility policy, the surgeon also may be required to sign the consent form.

> **❗ NURSING PRIORITY** Determine that the client understands relevant information before procedure/surgery; do not witness the client's signature on an informed consent form until you verify that the client has received the relevant information and document findings. The informed consent record (permit) must be signed before the client receives the preoperative medication.

4. The signed consent record (permit) is part of the permanent chart record and must accompany the client to the operating room.

Day of Surgery

> **TEST ALERT** Monitor a client before, during, and after a procedure or surgery.

A. Nursing responsibilities (Fig. 3.7).
  1. Vital signs within 1 hour before "on call" to surgery, or per agency policy.

2. Remove jewelry, including piercing jewelry; wedding bands may be taped on finger.

3. Remove contact lenses, fingernail polish, depending on agency policy.

4. Dress client in surgical gown.

5. Determine whether dentures and removable bridgework need to be removed before surgery.

6. Instruct client and document disposition of glasses, dentures, bridgework, jewelry, and valuables before the administration of preoperative anesthetic.

7. Continue NPO status.

8. Check client's identification for two identifiers.
  a. The first identifier should reliably identify the client for whom service or treatment is intended, for example, the client's first and last name.
  b. The second identifier is used to match the service or treatment to that individual, for example, the date of birth and/or client's medical record number.

9. Identify family and significant others who will be waiting for information regarding client's progress.

10. Instruct client about what to expect in operating room, for example, skin preparation, cold room, availability of warm blankets, bright lights, time-out procedure, to decrease patient anxiety.

11. Check the chart+ for completeness regarding drug allergies, laboratory reports, consent form, significant client observations, history, and physical examination records (Fig. 3.8).

12. Allow parent to accompany the child as far as possible.

B. Preoperative medications (see Appendix 3.2).

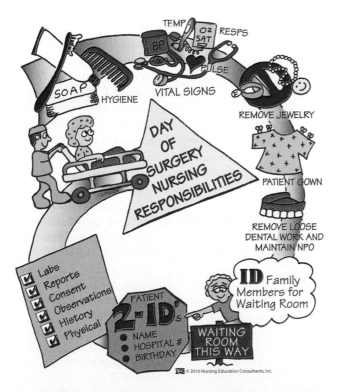

FIG. 3.7 Day of Surgery Nursing Responsibilities. (From Zerwekh J, Garneau A, Miller CJ. [2017]. *Digital collection of the memory notebooks of nursing* [4th ed.]. Chandler, AZ: Nursing Education Consultants, Inc.)

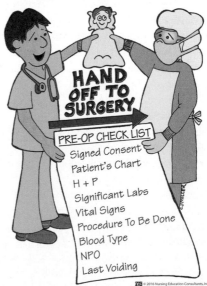

FIG. 3.8 Handoff to Surgery. (From Zerwekh J, Garneau A, Miller CJ. [2017]. *Digital collection of the memory notebooks of nursing* [4th ed.]. Chandler, AZ: Nursing Education Consultants, Inc.)

! **NURSING PRIORITY** Explain to client the purpose of preoperative medications and advise client not to get out of bed. Side rails should be up and the call light within reach.

1. Purpose.
   a. Induce anesthesia rapidly.
   b. Reduce anxiety.
2. Nursing responsibilities.
   a. Confirm that all consent forms are signed, and that the client understands the procedure.
   b. Ask client to void before administration of medication.
   c. Obtain baseline vital signs.
   d. Administer medication 45 minutes to 1 hour before surgery or as ordered. *Many institutions are administering the medication in the operative suite so the client can participate in the "time-out" process for identification of operative site.*
   e. Raise the side rails and instruct the client not to get out of bed.
   f. Observe for side effects of medication.
C. The Joint Commission established Universal Protocol guidelines for preventing wrong site, wrong procedure or surgery, wrong person must occur prior to the procedure or surgery.
   1. The Universal Protocol includes the following three criteria:
      a. Preoperative verification of required documents (e.g., lab results, client chart, signed consent form).
      b. Marking the operative site with indelible ink.
      c. A "time-out" just before the procedure.
   2. The surgical team is involved in conducting a "time-out" just before beginning the procedure. The "time-out" involves positive identification of the client, the intended procedure, and the site of the procedure is marked with indelible marker by the surgeon before entering the surgical suite.
   3. The operative site marking and "time-out" occur in the location where the procedure or surgery will take place.

Anesthesia

A. General anesthesia: used as an IV induction agent before the inhalation agent is administered.
B. Regional anesthesia: used to anesthetize one region of the body; client remains awake and alert throughout the procedure.
   1. Spinal or epidural blocks are typically used for high-risk clients undergoing pelvic or lower extremity surgery.
   2. Epidural blocks are widely used in obstetric procedures.
   3. Nerve block used for foot surgery and some orthopedic procedures.
   4. Local anesthesia is used for minor surgical procedures, e.g., suturing a laceration.
C. Nursing considerations for regional anesthesia (spinal/epidural) (Fig. 3.9).

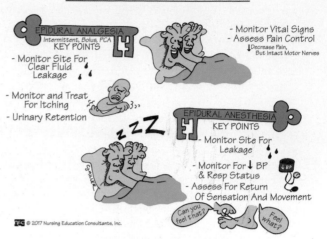

FIG. 3.9 Analgesia versus Anesthesia. (From Zerwekh J, Garneau A, Miller CJ. [2017]. *Digital collection of the memory notebooks of nursing* [4th ed.]. Chandler, AZ: Nursing Education Consultants, Inc.)

D. Conscious sedation or monitored anesthesia care: the administration of an IV medication to produce sedation, analgesia, and amnesia.
   1. Characteristics.
      a. Client can respond to commands, maintains protective reflexes, and does not need assistance in maintaining an airway.
      b. Amnesia most often occurs after the procedure.
      c. Slurred speech and nystagmus indicate the end of conscious sedation.
   2. Nursing implications: Take action.
      a. Client is assessed continuously; vital signs are recorded every 5 to 15 minutes.
      b. Monitor level of consciousness; client should not be unconscious, but relaxed and comfortable.
      c. Client should respond to physical and verbal stimuli; protective airway reflexes should remain intact.
      d. Potential complications include loss of gag reflex, aspiration, hypoxia, hypercapnia, and cardiopulmonary depression.
      e. Does not require extensive postoperative recovery time.

Immediate Postoperative Recovery

TEST ALERT Provide postoperative care (Fig. 3.10).

A. Admission of client to recovery area.
   1. Position client to promote patent airway and prevent aspiration.
   2. Perform baseline assessment.
      a. Vital signs, quality of respirations, pulse oximetry, pulse rate and rhythm, general skin color.
      b. Type and amount of fluid infusing.
      c. Special equipment; status of dressings.
   3. Determine specifics regarding the operation from the operating room nurse.

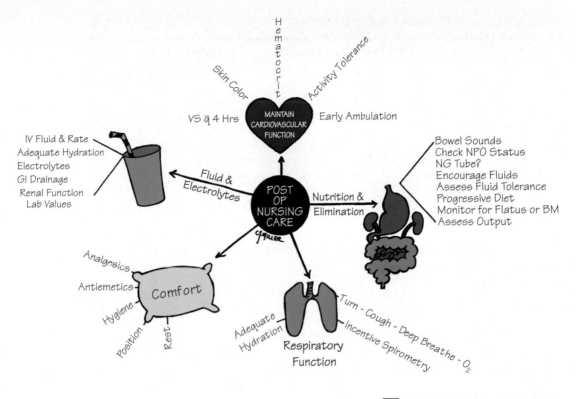

FIG. 3.10 Postop Nursing Care. (From Zerwekh J, Garneau A, Miller CJ. [2017]. *Digital collection of the memory notebooks of nursing* [4th ed.]. Chandler, AZ: Nursing Education Consultants, Inc.)

  a. Client's overall tolerance of surgery.
  b. Type of surgery performed and type of anesthetic agents used.
  c. Results of procedure: Was the condition corrected?
  d. Any specific complications to watch for.
  e. Status of fluid intake and urinary output.
  f. Common postoperative complications (Table 3.2).
B. Nursing management during recovery: Take action.

Goal: To maintain respiratory function

> ❗ **NURSING PRIORITY** The client's respiratory status is a priority concern on admission to the postoperative recovery area and throughout the postoperative recovery period.

1. Leave airway in place until pharyngeal reflex (gag reflex) has returned.
2. Position client on side (modified left lateral recumbent position) or on the back with the head turned to the side to prevent aspiration.
3. Suction excess secretions and prevent aspiration.
4. Encourage coughing and deep breathing.
5. Administer humidified oxygen.
6. Auscultate breath sounds.

Goal: To maintain cardiovascular stability
1. Check vital signs every 15 minutes until condition is stable.
2. Report blood pressure that is continually dropping 5 to 10 mm Hg with each reading.

3. Report increasing or persistent bradycardia or tachycardia.
4. Evaluate quality of pulse and presence of dysrhythmia.
5. Evaluate adequacy of cardiac output and tissue perfusion.

Goal: To maintain adequate fluid status
1. Evaluate blood loss in surgery and response to fluid replacement.
2. Maintain rate of IV infusion; maintain intake and output (I&O) record.
3. Monitor urine output and possible bladder distention.
4. Evaluate hydration and electrolyte status.
5. Observe amount and character of drainage on dressings or drainage in collecting containers.
6. Assess amount and character of gastric drainage if nasogastric tube is in place.
7. Evaluate amount and characteristics of any emesis.

> ❗ **NURSING PRIORITY** When a client is vomiting, prevent aspiration by positioning the client on the left side with head turned and facing downward; suction, if not contraindicated.

Goal: To maintain incisional areas
1. Evaluate amount and character of drainage from incision and drains.
2. Check and record status of Hemovac, Jackson-Pratt, Penrose, or any other wound drains.

Table 3.2 COMMON POSTOPERATIVE COMPLICATIONS

Complication	Signs and Symptoms	Nursing Intervention
Atelectasis – a collapse of a portion of the lung, producing an airless state in the alveoli	Dyspnea, decreased or absent breath sounds over affected area, asymmetric chest expansion, hypoxia	*Prevention:* have client turn, cough, and breathe deeply; provide adequate hydration; encourage early ambulation and incentive spirometer use. Position client on unaffected side. Maintain humidification with oxygen therapy.
Shock – a decrease in cardiac output resulting from a loss of circulating blood volume	Decreasing blood pressure, weak pulse, restless, confusion, oliguria	Initiate IV access, keep NPO, maintain bed rest. Position supine with legs elevated and knees straight. Monitor ventilation and vital signs frequently.
Wound infection – an infection of the surgical incision area	Delayed wound healing, redness, tenderness, fever, tachycardia, leukocytosis, purulent drainage	*Prevention:* identify high-risk clients; maintain sterile technique with dressing changes. Obtain wound culture to determine organism. Evaluate progress and prevent spread of infection.

TEST ALERT Monitor wounds for signs and symptoms of infection.

Complication	Signs and Symptoms	Nursing Intervention
Wound dehiscence –unintentional opening of the surgical incision	Unintentional opening of the surgical incision	Evaluate for hemorrhage; use measures to prevent further pressure at incision site.
Wound evisceration –protrusion of a loop of bowel through the surgical wound	Protrusion of a loop bowel through the surgical wound	Cover bowel with sterile saline solution–soaked dressing. Position client with knees flexed as this reduces pressure on incision site. Do not attempt to replace loop of bowel. Notify health care provider; client will most likely return to surgery for further exploration.
Urinary retention – inability to empty urinary bladder	Inability to void after surgery; bladder may be palpable; voiding small amounts, dribbling	Determine preoperative risks: medications, length of surgery, history of prostate problems. Determine amount of fluid intake and when to anticipate client to void – generally within 8 hr. Perform bladder ultrasound to evaluate residual urine volume. Palpate suprapubic area, perform bladder scan, run tap water, provide privacy. Catheterize if necessary.
Gastric dilation, postoperative nausea and vomiting (PONV), postoperative ileus (POI)	Nausea, vomiting, abdominal distention, decreased bowel sounds	*Prevention:* Older adult clients are at increased risk; encourage activity as soon as possible. Position client in semi-Fowlers to decrease risk of aspiration. Maintain client NPO status and NG tube suction if NG tube is in place.
Paralytic ileus – lack of intestinal peristalsis and bowel sounds	Decreased or absent peristalsis 24-36 hr after surgery with fewer than 5 sounds/min, gastric distention, intestinal obstruction, pain	*Prevention:* Maintaining NPO status until bowel sounds return. When permitted by the surgeon, chewing sugarless gum can speed bowel recovery after abdominal surgery. Gum chewing has also been shown to be effective for recovery from paralytic ileus. Monitor bowel sounds; encourage early ambulation; nothing by mouth as ordered.

IV, intravenous; *NPO*, nothing by mouth; *NG*, nasogastric.

Goal: To maintain psychological equilibrium
1. Speak to client frequently in calm, unhurried manner.
2. Continually orient client; it is important to tell client that surgery is over and where they are.
3. Maintain quiet, restful atmosphere.
4. Promote comfort by maintaining proper body alignment.
5. Explain all procedures, even if client is not fully awake.
6. In the anesthetized client, sense of hearing is the last to be lost and the first to return.

Goal: Client meets criteria to return to room
1. Vital signs are stable and within normal limits.

2. Client is awake; reflexes have returned.
3. Dressings are intact with no evidence of excessive bleeding or drainage.
4. Client can maintain a patent airway without assistance.

General Postoperative Care

Goal: To maintain cardiovascular function and tissue perfusion
1. Monitor vital signs every 4 hours or per agency guidelines.
2. Evaluate skin color and nail beds for pallor and cyanosis.
3. Assess client's tolerance to increasing activity.
4. Encourage early activity and ambulation.

Goal: To maintain respiratory function
1. Have client turn, cough, and breathe deeply every 2 hours.
2. Use incentive spirometry to promote deep breathing and prevent atelectasis.
3. Administer small-volume nebulizer (SVN) treatment and bronchodilator as needed.
4. Maintain adequate hydration to keep mucus secretions thin and easily mobilized.
5. Encourage deep breathing with ambulation.

Goal: To maintain adequate nutrition and elimination
1. Assess for return of bowel sounds, normal peristalsis, and passage of flatus.
2. Assess client with a nasogastric (NG) tube for return of peristalsis.
3. Assess client's tolerance of oral fluids; usually begin with clear liquids and advance as tolerated by client.
4. Encourage intake of fluids, unless contraindicated.
5. Progress diet as client's condition and appetite indicate or as ordered.
6. Record bowel movements; normal bowel function should return on the second or third postoperative day (provided that the client is eating).

7. Assess urinary output.
   a. Client should void within 8 to 10 hours after surgery.
   b. Assess urine output; should be at least 30 mL/h.
   c. Promote voiding by allowing client to stand or use bedside commode.
   d. Avoid intermittent or indwelling catheterization if possible.

Goal: To maintain fluid and electrolyte balance
1. Monitor IV infusions for correct fluid and rate of infusion.
2. Assess for adequate hydration.
   a. Moist mucous membranes.
   b. Adequate urine output with normal urine specific gravity.
   c. Good skin turgor – no evidence of skin tenting.
3. Assess character and amount of gastric drainage through the nasogastric tube.

Goal: To promote comfort
1. Determine nonpharmacologic pain relief measures.
2. Administer analgesics and/or monitor PCA.

> **⊞ NURSING PRIORITY** In addition to the pain and discomfort associated with a surgical procedure, it is important to assess other possible sources of discomfort, such as full bladder, occluded catheter or tube, gas accumulation, IV infiltration, or compromised circulation resulting from position/pressure.

📋 Postoperative Complications

Table 3.2 summarizes the major postoperative complications and the nursing interventions to prevent them. Some complications are immediately life-threatening.

Appendix 3.1 POSITIONING AND BODY MECHANICS

POSITION	PLACEMENT	USE
Fowler 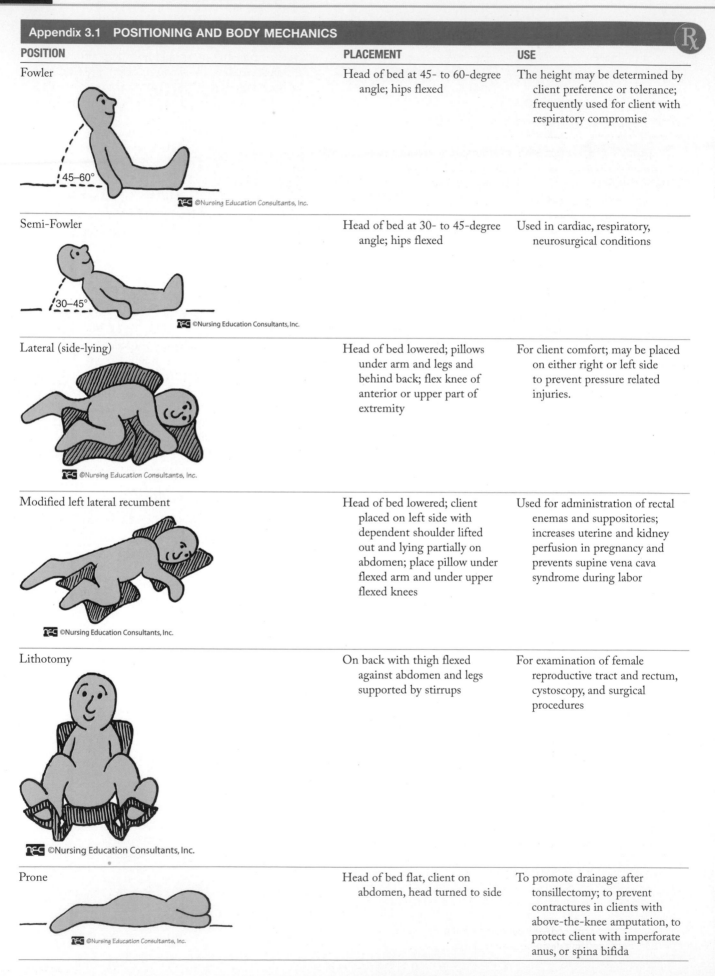	Head of bed at 45- to 60-degree angle; hips flexed	The height may be determined by client preference or tolerance; frequently used for client with respiratory compromise
Semi-Fowler	Head of bed at 30- to 45-degree angle; hips flexed	Used in cardiac, respiratory, neurosurgical conditions
Lateral (side-lying)	Head of bed lowered; pillows under arm and legs and behind back; flex knee of anterior or upper part of extremity	For client comfort; may be placed on either right or left side to prevent pressure related injuries.
Modified left lateral recumbent	Head of bed lowered; client placed on left side with dependent shoulder lifted out and lying partially on abdomen; place pillow under flexed arm and under upper flexed knees	Used for administration of rectal enemas and suppositories; increases uterine and kidney perfusion in pregnancy and prevents supine vena cava syndrome during labor
Lithotomy	On back with thigh flexed against abdomen and legs supported by stirrups	For examination of female reproductive tract and rectum, cystoscopy, and surgical procedures
Prone	Head of bed flat, client on abdomen, head turned to side	To promote drainage after tonsillectomy; to prevent contractures in clients with above-the-knee amputation, to protect client with imperforate anus, or spina bifida

45–60°

©Nursing Education Consultants, Inc.

30–45°

©Nursing Education Consultants, Inc.

©Nursing Education Consultants, Inc.

©Nursing Education Consultants, Inc.

©Nursing Education Consultants, Inc.

©Nursing Education Consultants, Inc.

Appendix 3.1 POSITIONING AND BODY MECHANICS—cont'd

POSITION	PLACEMENT	USE
Supine ©Nursing Education Consultants, Inc.	Bed in flat position, small pillow under head	For client comfort
Dorsal recumbent ©Nursing Education Consultants, Inc.	Bed flat, small pillow under head, patient's knees flexed and soles of feet flat on bed	Used for a variety of procedures and examinations (Foley catheter insertion, perineal care, abdominal assessment)
Knee-chest ©Nursing Education Consultants, Inc.	Variation of prone position; patient face down with head turned to side; chest elbows and knees rest on bed; thighs perpendicular to bed	Used for prolapsed cord during labor to prevent compression of the umbilical cord

TEST ALERT Position client to prevent complications after tests, treatments, or procedures.

Appendix 3.2 SAFE CLIENT HANDLING – PREVENTION OF INJURY

- Use lift equipment and ask for adequate assistance.
- Manual lifting of a client should be avoided. If it is necessary to manually lift most or all of the client's weight, obtain adequate assistance or use safe client handling equipment.
- Principles (ergonomics) and body mechanics of lifting:
  1. Avoid twisting; keep your head and neck aligned with your spine.
  2. Place feet wide apart for good base of support; knees should be flexed.
  3. Position yourself close to the bed or close to the client.
  4. Use arms and legs to assist in lifting client, not your back.
- Use friction-reducing device to move client to side of bed and/or to move up in bed.

TEST ALERT Use safe client handling techniques (e.g., body mechanics). Maintain correct body alignment.

✔ KEY POINTS: Assisting the Client to Move up in Bed

- Lower the head of the bed so that it is flat or as low as the client can tolerate; raise the bed frame to a position that does not require leaning.
- If more than one person is needed for assistance, obtain a lifting device.
- Determine the client's strong side and have them assist with the move.
- Instruct the client to bend legs, put feet flat on bed, and push.
- Use a friction-reducing device and draw sheet.

- Never pull a client up in bed by his arms or by putting pressure under his arms.

✔ KEY POINTS: Logrolling the Client

- Spinal immobilization – use a team approach (three nurses).
- Maintain proper alignment on head and back areas while turning.
- Before moving client, place a pillow or hip abduction pillow between client's legs and instruct client to cross arms over chest.
- Move client in one coordinated movement, using a turn/lift sheet.

✔ KEY POINTS: Moving from Bed to Chair

- Move client to the side of the bed (bed wheels locked) closest to the edge where the client will be getting up.
- Assist client out of bed on strongest side.
- Raise head of bed to assist client in pivoting to the side of the bed.
- Move client to edge of bed and place hands under legs and shift his weight forward; pivot the client's body so client is in sitting position and feet are flat on the floor.
- Have client reach across chair and grasp arm.
- Stabilize client by positioning your foot at the outside edge of client's foot.
- Pivot client into chair using your leg muscles instead of your back muscles.
- Assist client to move back and up in the chair for better position.

Continued

Appendix 3.2   SAFE CLIENT HANDLING – PREVENTION OF INJURY—cont'd   ℞

Tips for moving and positioning clients

- Use a transfer belt (gait belt) to support client with repositioning or ambulation.
- Encourage client to assist in move by using the side rails and strong side of their body.
- No-lift policy: use of equipment and assistance whenever a client requires most of his weight to be supported or lifted by someone.
- Obtain additional assistance and/or use lift equipment to help in moving the client.
- Use hip abduction pillow or trochanter roll made from bath blankets to align the client's hips to prevent external rotation.
- Use foam bolsters to maintain side-lying positions.
- Use folded towels, blankets, or small pillows to position client's hands and arms to prevent dependent edema.

Appendix 3.3   MEDICATIONS: ANALGESICS, NSAIDs, AND PREOPERATIVE   ℞

Analgesics

General Nursing Implications

- Assess pain parameters, blood pressure, pulse, oxygen saturation, and respiratory status before and periodically after administration.
- Use a pain rating scale to determine level of pain.
- Administer before pain is severe for better analgesic effect.
- Older or debilitated clients may require decreased dosage.

MEDICATIONS	SIDE EFFECTS	NURSING IMPLICATIONS
Opioid Analgesics:		
Bind to opiate receptors in the central nervous system (CNS), altering the perception of and emotional response to pain; controlled substances (Schedule II).		
Strong Opioid Analgesics		
▲ Morphine sulfate: PO, subQ, IM, IV, epidural, intrathecal, sublingual analgesia Meperidine: PO, subQ, IM, IV Fentanyl: IM, IV, transdermal, transmucosal, nasal spray	Respiratory depression Orthostatic hypotension Sedation, dizziness, lightheadedness, dysphoria Constipation Tolerance, physical and psychological dependence May decrease awareness of bladder stimuli Seizure with Demerol	1. Morphine is most commonly administered drug for PCA. 2. Meperidine: The American Pain Society does not recommend use as an analgesic; use with caution in children and older adult clients because of increased risk for toxicity and seizures. 3. Morphine is not commonly used after biliary tract surgery. 4. All opioids: Use with caution in clients who have respiratory compromise or are taking other CNS depressants. 5. Pediatric implications: Medication dosage is calculated according to body surface area and weight. 6. Assess bowel and urinary characteristics and encourage client to void every 4 hours. 7. Requires documentation as indicated by Controlled Substance Act. 8. Instruct client to change position slowly to minimize orthostatic hypotension.

> **！ NURSING PRIORITY** Advise clients using fentanyl patches not to expose patch to heat (hot tub, heating pad) because this will accelerate the release of the fentanyl.

> **！ OLDER ADULT PRIORITY** Prevent problems with constipation.

| Appendix 3.3 | SAFE CLIENT HANDLING – PREVENTION OF INJURY—cont'd | ℞ |

MEDICATIONS	SIDE EFFECTS	NURSING IMPLICATIONS
Moderate to Strong Opioid Analgesics		
Codeine: PO, subQ, IM Hydromorphone: PO, subQ, IM, IV Oxycodone: PO (combination with ibuprofen; combinations with acetaminophen) Hydrocodone: PO (combinations with acetaminophen; combination with ibuprofen)	Sedation, euphoria, respiratory depression, constipation, urinary retention, cough suppression	1. Usually administered by mouth. 2. Codeine is an extremely effective cough suppressant. 3. Do not confuse hydromorphone with morphine. 4. Warn client to avoid activities requiring alertness (operating machinery, driving, etc.) until effects of drug are known. 5. Medications are often in various strength combinations with acetaminophen and/or ibuprofen. Advise client not to take additional medication containing acetaminophen or ibuprofen.

> **⚠ NURSING PRIORITY** Concurrent administration with nonnarcotic analgesics may enhance pain relief because they act at different sites.

Moderate Opioids		
Butorphanol: IM, IV, nasal spray Nalbuphine: subQ, IV, IM	Dizziness, drowsiness	1. Monitor client for effective pain control. 2. Abrupt withdrawal after prolonged use may produce symptoms of withdrawal.

Opioid Antagonist
Antagonist that competitively blocks the effect of opioids, without producing analgesic effects.

Naloxone: IV, IM, subQ (most common routes in a hospital setting); auto-injector and nasal spray formulations are available for caregivers to administer to clients outside of the hospital setting	Hypotension, hypertension, dysrhythmias	1. Assess respiratory status, blood pressure, pulse, and level of consciousness until opioid effects wear off. Repeat doses may be necessary if effect of opioid outlasts the effect of the opioid antagonist. 2. Remember that opioid antagonists reverse analgesia along with respiratory depression. Titrate dose accordingly and assess pain level to prevent abrupt withdrawal reaction. 3. *Uses:* Used to reverse CNS effects (sedation, comma) and respiratory depression in opioid overdose. 4. *Contraindications and precautions:* Use with caution in opioid-dependent clients; may cause severe withdrawal symptoms.

Intravenous Anesthetic Agents: Used alone or in combination with an inhalation anesthetic, which permits a lower dose of inhalation agent or produces effects that cannot be achieved by inhalation agents.

| ▲ Propofol: IV | Unconsciousness develops within 60 secs and lasts for 3-5 min
Cardiovascular and respiratory depression
Bacterial infections | 1. Monitor for adverse effects of profound respiratory depression (including apnea) and hypotension.
2. Medication is administered only in settings where there is appropriate monitoring and resuscitation equipment available. |

> **⚠ NURSING PRIORITY** Rapid onset and short duration of action can lead to respiratory depression, so respiratory support should be immediately available.

Continued

R̲x̲

MEDICATIONS	SIDE EFFECTS	NURSING IMPLICATIONS

Nonsteroidal Anti-inflammatory Drugs (NSAIDs) and Acetaminophen

General Nursing Implications

- Give with a full glass of water, either with food or just after eating.
- Store in childproof containers and out of reach of small children.
- Do not exceed recommended doses.
- Discontinue 1-2 weeks before elective surgery.
- NSAIDs prolong bleeding time by decreasing platelet aggregation; may increase anticoagulant activity of warfarin products.
- Avoid in clients with history of peptic ulcer disease (PUD) or bleeding problems.
- Monitor for GI bleeding – black, tarry stools,
- May compromise renal blood flow and precipitate kidney impairment.
- Do not crush enteric-coated tablets; if available, administer as enteric or buffered tablets.

Uses: **Fever:** acetaminophen, aspirin, ibuprofen; **Inflammation:** aspirin, naproxen, ketorolac; **Arthritis:** aspirin, ibuprofen, naproxen, piroxicam, sulindac; **Dysmenorrhea:** ibuprofen, naproxen

MEDICATIONS	SIDE EFFECTS	NURSING IMPLICATIONS

Nonsteroidal Anti-inflammatory Drugs (NSAIDs) and Acetaminophen

Inhibit the enzyme cyclooxygenase (both COX-1 and COX-2), which is responsible for the synthesis of prostaglandins; suppress inflammation, relieve pain, and reduce fever.

Acetylsalicylic acid: PO	Salicylism: skin reactions, redness, rashes, ringing in the ears, GI upset, hyperventilation, sweating, and thirst Long-term use: erosive gastritis with bleeding; increases anticoagulant properties of warfarin	1. Most common agent responsible for accidental poisoning in small children. 2. Associated with Reye syndrome in children. 3. Assess for bleeding tendencies. 4. Prophylactic use for colon cancer. 5. Prophylactic use for cardiovascular problems due to the antiplatelet aggregation properties.

❗ NURSING PRIORITY Advise client that the Centers for Disease Control and Prevention warns against giving aspirin to children or adolescents with a viral infection or influenza.

❗ NURSING PRIORITY Aspirin is the only NSAID used to protect against MI and stroke.

Ibuprofen: PO, IV	Gastric ulceration, dyspepsia (heartburn, nausea, epigastric distress), bleeding, hypertension, dizziness, rash, dermatitis, kidney impairment	1. Do not exceed 3200 mg/day in adults and older adult clients. 2. Avoid taking with aspirin. 3. Increased risk of myocardial infarction and stroke.
Naproxen: PO	Headache, tinnitus, hearing loss, dyspepsia, dizziness, drowsiness	1. Avoid tasks requiring alertness until response is established. 2. Take with food to decrease GI irritation. 3. Primarily used for pain control.
Acetaminophen: PO, rectal, IV	Anorexia, nausea, diaphoresis Toxicity: vomiting, right upper quadrant tenderness, elevated liver function tests Antidote: N-acetylcysteine (Mucomyst, Acetadote)	1. Maximum dose of acetaminophen, 4000 mg/day. 2. Does not have antiinflammatory properties. 3. Overdose can cause severe liver injury; client should consult health care provider if they drink more than three alcoholic beverages daily. 4. Has not been conclusively linked to bleeding problems.

❗ NURSING PRIORITY Frequently used in combination with OTC medications. Teach client to read labels to prevent toxicity and overdose.

Appendix 3.3 SAFE CLIENT HANDLING – PREVENTION OF INJURY—cont'd

MEDICATIONS	SIDE EFFECTS	NURSING IMPLICATIONS
Piroxicam: PO Sulindac: PO Ketorolac: PO, IM, IV, intranasal	Dyspepsia, nausea, dizziness, diarrhea, nephrotoxicity	1. Piroxicam and sulindac are medications primarily indicated for clients who have rheumatoid and osteoarthritis. 2. Ketorolac: oral doses must be preceded by parenteral administration; give deep IM may cause pain at injection site; combined oral and parenteral treatment should not exceed 5 days.
COX-2 inhibitor Celecoxib: PO	Less upper GI bleeding, dyspepsia, abdominal pain, cardiovascular events, impaired kidney function	1. Short-term use is preferred to reduce side effects. 2. Monitor kidney function.

Preoperative Medications

MEDICATIONS	SIDE EFFECTS	NURSING IMPLICATIONS
Benzodiazepines **Decrease anxiety and promote amnesia before or during surgery.** *Antidote: Flumazenil (Romazicon®)*		
▲ Midazolam hydrochloride: PO, IM, IV	Respiratory depression; pain at IM or IV site; nausea, vomiting	1. Commonly used for conscious sedation and amnesia before procedures. 2. Continuous cardiac and respiratory monitoring during parenteral administration.
Lorazepam: PO, IM, IV	Drowsiness, ataxia, confusion, fatigue May produce paradoxical effects in elderly	1. Decrease stimuli in the room after administration. 2. Offer emotional support to the anxious client. 3. Maintain bed rest after administration to reduce effects of hypotension. 4. A schedule IV drug.
Diazepam: PO, IM, IV	Same as for Ativan	
Histamine (H2 Receptor Antagonists) **Decrease gastric acid secretion by blocking the H2 receptors on parietal cells, increase gastric pH, and reduce gastric volume.**		
Cimetidine Famotidine Ranitidine	See Appendix 13.2	See Appendix 13.2
Anticholinergic **Prevent bradycardia, decrease secretions.**		
Atropine: PO, IM, IV, subQ Scopolamine: PO, subQ, transdermal Glycopyrrolate: PO, IM, IV	Flushed face Dilated pupils Tachycardia Urinary retention Reduce emesis and motion sickness (Scopolamine)	1. Children and older adult clients are at increased risk for side effects. 2. Advise clients regarding atropine flush. 3. Administer with caution to clients with asthma; contraindicated for clients with glaucoma, urinary obstruction, MI, or heart failure. 4. Postural hypotension may result if client ambulates after administration. 5. Advise clients to place scopolamine transdermal batch behind the ears. 6. Monitor for urinary retention and decreased bowel sounds.

▲High-alert medication
CDC, Centers for Disease Control and Prevention; *CNS*, central nervous system; *GI*, gastrointestinal; *IM*, intramuscular; *IV*, intravenous; *MI*, myocardial infarction; *PCA*, patient-controlled analgesia; *PO*, by mouth (orally); *OTC*, over the counter; *subQ*, subcutaneous.

11. The client returns to the clinic in 2 weeks following a laparoscopic cholecystectomy.

For each assessment finding, listed below, use an X to specify whether the finding indicates whether the interventions were Effective (helped to meet expected outcomes), Ineffective (did not help meet expected outcomes) or Unrelated (not related to the expected outcome).

ASSESSMENT FINDING	EFFECTIVE	INEFFECTIVE	UNRELATED
Puncture sites are closed and healed			
Reports abdominal pain on a 5 out of 10 scale			
Has burning and frequency during urination			
Tolerates regular diet with limited fat			
Has returned to work			
Reports constipation and abdominal distention			
Shoulder pain has disappeared			

⚡Answers to Practice & Next Generation NCLEX (NGN) Questions

1. 4
Client Needs: Physiological Integrity/Basic Care and Comfort
Clinical Judgment/Cognitive Skill: Generate Solutions
Item Type: Multiple Choice
Rationale & Test-Taking Strategy: Understanding the progression of the diet for postoperative clients is essential to answering this test item. Clear liquids are usually offered first to the postoperative client. Plain gelatin, popsicles, and apple juice are clear and contain no residue. The other answers include a milk product that causes residue and are included in the next progressive step of the diet, which is full liquids.

2. 2
Client Needs: Physiological Integrity/Basic Care and Comfort
Clinical Judgment/Cognitive Skill: Prioritize Hypotheses
Item Type: Multiple Choice
Rationale & Test-Taking Strategy: Note the **key** word "best" nursing action to help the client who has vomited. This is a priority nursing care question. If the client is nauseated and vomiting, the client should not be offered any further fluids by mouth until the cause of the vomiting has been identified or the nausea has subsided. The client should be placed in either semi-Fowler position or on his or her side to prevent aspiration, and the *RN should be notified.*

3. 1
Client Needs: Psychosocial Integrity
Clinical Judgment/Cognitive Skill: Prioritize Hypotheses
Item Type: Multiple Choice
Rationale & Test-Taking Strategy: Note the **key** word, "best." This is a priority nursing care question. In many cultures, lack of

eye contact is common with the nurse or an authority figure. It does not mean that the person is not paying attention or is showing disrespect but is showing respect. It would not be appropriate to confront the son about the lack of eye contact or to ignore the son during the communication exchange.

4. 4
Client Needs: Physiological Integrity/Basic Care and Comfort
Clinical Judgment/Cognitive Skill: Generate Solutions
Item Type: Multiple Choice
Rationale & Test-Taking Strategy: To answer this test item, you will need to understand the difference between a dehiscence and an evisceration and how they are related. If an incision is dehisced or open, there is an increased risk of an evisceration, or protrusion of organs through the dehisced wound opening. Placing the client on bedrest will help to prevent further pressure on the incision. *The RN should be notified immediately of a dehiscence or evisceration.*

5. 1, 5
Client Needs: Physiological Integrity/Reduction of Risk Potential
Clinical Judgment/Cognitive Skill: Take Action
Item Type: Select All That Apply
Rationale & Test-Taking Strategy: The focus of the test item is nursing actions to prevent atelectasis and pneumonia, which are respiratory problems. The primary purpose of turn, cough, and deep breathe is to prevent respiratory complications. Use of the incentive spirometer promotes lung and alveolar expansion, which prevents atelectasis. While the other options are included in the plan of care for the postoperative client, they are not specific to reducing the risk of developing pulmonary complications.

Note: Questions 6–11 pertain to this unfolding case scenario.

6. The following is the health history of a client who is admitted to the surgical unit for a laparoscopic cholecystectomy.

Health History	Nurses' Notes	Provider Orders	Laboratory Results

A 45-year-old client who is morbidly obese with type 2 diabetes has been treated previously for acute cholecystitis. The client has a history of cholelithiasis and has been treated for the past 6 months with ursodiol to dissolve the gallstones. A recent gallbladder ultrasound reveals numerous biliary stones. Client reports pain of 6 on a 10-point scale in the upper right abdominal quadrant, along with indigestion and flatulence. Vital signs: temperature 99.0°F (37.2°C), BP 156/96 mmHg, pulse 95 and regular, respirations 20. Laboratory results: fasting blood sugar 116 mg/dL, WBC 12,900 mm^3, hemoglobin 14.4 mg/dL, hematocrit 42%.

Drag and drop the clinical findings from the choices below to fill in the blanks in the following sentence.

The assessment findings that require immediate follow up include *white blood cell count (WBC) 12,900 mm³, right upper quadrant pain, temperature 99.0°F (37.2°C),* **and** *BP 156/96 mmHg.*

CLINICAL FINDINGS
Obesity
BP 156/96 mmHg
Right upper quadrant pain
Pulse 95 and regular
Temperature 99.0°F (37.2°C)
Hemoglobin 14.4 mg/dL, hematocrit 42%
WBC 12,900 mm³

Client Needs: Physiological Integrity/Physiological Adaptation
Clinical Judgment/Cognitive Skill: Recognize Cues
Item Type: Drag and Drop Cloze
Rationale & Test-Taking Strategy: Clients with a diagnosis of chronic cholecystitis often have milder symptoms between acute attacks. Symptoms include indigestion after eating fatty foods, flatulence, nausea after eating, and some discomfort in the right upper quadrant. Low grade fever is often present. The symptom most often present in an acute flare-up of chronic cholecystitis is unbearable right upper quadrant (RUQ) pain (biliary colic). With the client scheduled for surgery, it is important for the nurse to report to the surgeon the elevated WBC, BP, and temperature. Continued presence or worsening of RUQ pain can indicate rupture of the gall bladder or obstruction of the biliary duct. Liver function tests are used to diagnose gallbladder and biliary tract disease. Alanine aminotransferase (ALT) and aspartate aminotransferase (AST) will be slightly elevated.

7. The nurse is preparing the client for laparoscopic cholecystectomy surgery and is reviewing the preoperative checklist.

   Complete the following sentences by choosing the most likely options for the missing information from the drop-down lists of options provided.

The priority for the nurse is to check and determine that the *informed consent* is present on the chart and signed by the *surgeon*, *client*, and *witness*. The nurse should verify if the client has *voided* and has signed the *informed consent* prior to administering the *preoperative medication*.

Client Needs: Safe and Effective Care Environment/Coordinated Care
Clinical Judgment/Cognitive Skill: Analyze Cues
Item Type: Drop-Down Cloze
Rationale & Test-Taking Strategy: The informed consent for surgery is a priority that must be signed and in the chart, along with laboratory work and notation of any allergies, before the client leaves the unit to go to surgery. Before any preoperative medication is given, the client needs to sign the informed consent and the nurse needs to determine if the client has voided.

CHAPTER FOUR

Coordinated Care

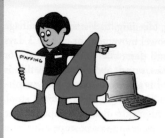

DISASTER PLANNING

A disaster is any event that causes a level of destruction, death, or injury that affects the abilities of the community to respond to the incident using available resources. A mass casualty event is one in which 100 or more individuals are involved.

Types of Disasters

A. Natural disasters.
1. Types – five most common are:
   a. Hurricane.
   b. Influenza (flu) or pandemic.
   c. Earthquake.
   d. Flooding.
   e. Tornado.
B. Man-made disasters.
1. Unconventional warfare (e.g., nuclear, chemical).
2. Transportation accidents (e.g., airplane crash, train derailment).
3. Structural building, bridge collapse.
4. Explosions/bombing, riots.
5. Active shooter events.
6. Arson, fires.
7. Hazardous materials incident.
8. Terrorism (chemical, biologic, radiologic, nuclear, explosives).
C. Agencies involved during disasters that provide relief to communities and individuals.
1. Federal Emergency Management Agency (FEMA) (Box 4.1).
2. American Red Cross.

> ⚠ **TEST ALERT** Identify nursing and assistive personnel roles during disasters. Participate in preparation for disasters (e.g., fire or natural disaster). Contribute to selection of client to recommend for discharge in a disaster situation.

Nursing Role During a Disaster

A. Disaster management stages (FEMA).
1. Prevention or mitigation stage – heightened inspections; improved surveillance and security, testing, immunizations, isolation, or quarantine; and halting chemical, biologic, radiologic, nuclear, and explosive (CBRNE) threats.

Box 4.1 FEDERAL EMERGENCY MANAGEMENT AGENCY (FEMA) LEVELS OF DISASTER

Level I Disaster – in these small-scale disasters (e.g., car accident, house fire), the nurse works in cooperation with local emergency medical systems and the community to provide medical support.

Level II Disaster – these larger disasters (e.g., airplane crash, building collapse, tornado) require the nurse to respond in a greater capacity using larger casualty practices in coordination with regional response agencies, such as state health and emergency management agencies.

Level III Disaster – these large-scale disasters (e.g., earthquakes, pandemics, hurricanes) consume local, state, and federal resources to the fullest extent and require an extended response time of nurses that can last weeks and even months.

2. Preparedness and planning stage.
   a. Personal: availability of emergency supplies; plans for family, pets, and own needs; disaster kits (Box 4.2).
   b. Professional: understanding and competence at using personal protective equipment (PPE), involvement in National Disaster Medical System (NDMS), Disaster Medical Assistance Team (DMAT), and other opportunities with the American Red Cross, etc.
   c. What nurses need to know and do to be prepared for a disaster (Box 4.3).
   d. Community preparedness.
3. Response stage – mobilization at local level of "first responders," then assessment of the scope of the disaster.
4. Recovery: returning to a "new normal" for the community.
B. *Emergency response plan* is a plan of action for coordinating services, agencies, and personnel to provide the earliest possible response in the event of a disaster or an emergency in a health care agency or community.
C. *Triage* is a standardized system of sorting clients according to medical need when resources are unavailable for all persons to be treated.
1. The overall goal of triage is to determine whether a client is appropriate for a given level of care and to ensure hospital resources are used effectively (Box 4.4).

Box 4.2   RECOMMENDED DISASTER PREPAREDNESS KIT

Recommended Items to Include in a Basic Emergency Supply Kit

- Water
  - One gallon of water per person per day for drinking and sanitation
  - Children, nursing mothers, and sick people may need more water
  - If you live in a warm climate, more water may be necessary
  - Store water tightly in clean plastic containers such as soft drink bottles
  - Keep at least a 3-day supply of water per person
- Food – at least a 3-day supply of nonperishable food
- Battery-powered or hand-crank radio and an NOAA (National Oceanic and Atmospheric Administration) weather radio with tone alert and extra batteries for both
- Flashlight and extra batteries
- First aid kit
- Whistle to signal for help
- Dust mask, to help filter contaminated air, and plastic sheeting and duct tape to shelter in place
- Moist towelettes, garbage bags, and plastic ties for personal sanitation
- Wrench or pliers to turn off utilities
- Can opener for food (if kit contains canned food)
- Local maps

Additional Items to Consider Adding to an Emergency Supply Kit

- Prescription medications and glasses
- Infant formula and diapers
- Pet food and extra water for your pet
- Important family documents such as copies of insurance policies, identification, and bank account records in a waterproof, portable container
- Cash or traveler's checks and change
- Emergency reference material such as a first aid book or information from https://www.ready.gov/
- Sleeping bag or warm blanket for each person; consider additional bedding if you live in a cold climate
- Complete change of clothing, including a long-sleeved shirt, long pants, and sturdy shoes; consider additional clothing if you live in a cold climate
- Household chlorine bleach and medicine dropper (A solution of 9 parts water to 1 part bleach can be used as a disinfectant. Or, in an emergency, you can treat water by adding 16 drops of household liquid bleach per gallon of water. Do not use scented or "color-safe" bleaches or bleaches with added cleaners.)
- Fire extinguisher
- Matches in a waterproof container
- Feminine supplies and personal hygiene items
- Mess kits, paper cups, paper plates, plastic utensils, paper towels
- Paper and pencil
- Books, games, puzzles, or other activities for children

From Zerwekh, T., Zerwekh, J. (2023). Emergency preparedness. In J. Zerwekh, A. Garneau (Eds.), *Nursing today: Transition and trends* (11th ed.). Elsevier/Saunders.
Courtesy Department of Homeland Security (www.ready.gov).

Box 4.3   THINK OF THE HELPFUL MNEMONIC IDME FOR USING THE START TRIAGE SYSTEM

Immediate – red
- Victim must be helped by immediate transport and intervention.

Delayed – yellow
- Victim's transport can be delayed.

Minimal or Minor – green
- Victim has relatively minor injuries.

Expectant – black
- Victim unlikely to survive due to severity of injuries.

For mass casualty incidents (MCIs), clients are sorted into groups – remember the mnemonic **MASS**.

Move
Assess
Sort
Send

Box 4.4   WHAT NURSES NEED TO KNOW AND DO TO BE PREPARED

- Specific types of disasters that can threaten their community
- Types of injuries to expect from different disaster situations
- Evacuation routes for agencies and the community
- Locations of shelters
- Understanding of warning systems (radio, television, and emergency apps on phones for weather, etc.)
- Information to educate others about disasters and how to prepare for and respond to them
- Maintain competency in lifesaving measures (e.g., basic first aid, cardiopulmonary resuscitation [CPR], and use of automated external defibrillators [AEDs])

! TEST ALERT The nurse needs to understand the process of implementing emergency response plans in both internal (hospital/agency) and external (hurricane, bioterrorism event) disasters and how to participate in an agency's security plan (e.g., bomb threats, newborn nursery security) and in disaster planning activities and drills.

2. Triage scoring (color) levels used during a mass casualty incident (MCI) (Table 4.1).
D. Fire.
   1. Immediately return to your unit if a fire code is called.
   2. If the fire is localized (in one room or area), remove clients from the immediate area.
   3. If clients on your unit are not in immediate danger, close all of the doors to the clients' rooms and to the unit.
   4. If you need to evacuate your unit because of an immediate danger to staff and clients, evacuate clients in this order to provide for the most rapid removal of the most clients in a short period of time:
      a. First: Ambulatory clients are first, because they can move the quickest and you can remove more clients quickly.

Legal Considerations

A. Negligence: Unintentional harm to another that occurs through failure to act in a reasonable and prudent manner.

B. Malpractice: Unprofessional nursing practice that fails to meet the minimum standard of care.

C. Invasion of privacy: Lack of protection of the constitutional right to be free from undesired publicity and exposure to public view.

1. Proper covering of the physical body.
2. Medical records.
   a. Release with signed client consent form.
   b. Release for medical "need to know," limited to caregivers only.
3. Belongings must be protected and may not be searched without specific authorization. A client's list of belongings should be explained to and signed by the client.
4. Conversations are confidential; in some states, they are protected by a specific statute.
5. Photographs and viewing procedures require consent of the client.
6. Control of visitor access to the client and client information.
7. Reporting laws are an exception – some information is required by law to be reported.

❗ TEST ALERT Follow regulation/policy for reporting specific issues (abuse/neglect, gunshot wound, or communicable disease, etc.).

   a. Communicable diseases.
   b. Injuries or deaths that are, or could be, caused by physical violence (gunshot and knife wounds).
   c. Client abuse – children and older adults.
   d. Others defined by state statute.
8. Rights may be waived by the client but never by medical personnel.
9. Nurses are obligated to maintain confidentiality of a client's health information in accordance with the Health Insurance Portability and Accountability Act (HIPAA) of 1996. (Box 4.6).

D. Informed consent (Box 4.7).

❗ TEST ALERT Obtain client's signature on the consent form. The signed informed consent form provides evidence the consent process has occurred. The nurse should verify with the client that the health care provider has discussed the risks and benefits of the procedure/surgery and that the client understands his or her rights.

E. Orders: prescriber/primary health care provider.

❗ TEST ALERT Evaluate the appropriateness of an order.

1. Question any order that is not clearly written and understood.

Box 4.6   HIPAA PRIVACY RULE

Who must follow the law?

- **Health Plans**, including health insurance companies, health maintenance organizations (HMOs), company health plans, and certain government programs that pay for health care, such as Medicare and Medicaid
- **Most Health Care Providers (HCP)** – those that conduct certain business electronically, such as electronically billing your health insurance – including most doctors, clinics, hospitals, psychologists, chiropractors, nursing homes, pharmacies, and dentists
- **Health Care Clearinghouses** – entities that process nonstandard health information they receive from another entity into a standard (i.e., standard electronic format or data content), or vice versa

What information is protected?

- Information doctors, nurses, and other health care providers put in a patient's medical record
- Conversations physicians or health care providers have about care or treatment with nurses and others
- Information about the patient's health insurer's computer system
- Billing information about the patient
- Most other health information about the patient held by those who must follow these laws

How is this information protected?

- Safeguards must be in place to protect a patient's health information.
- HCP must reasonably limit uses and disclosures to the minimum necessary to accomplish their intended purpose.
- There must be contracts in place with their contractors and others ensuring they use and disclose a patient's health information properly and safeguard it appropriately.
- There must be procedures in place to limit who can view and access a patient's health information. Groups who must follow the law need to implement training programs for employees regarding how to protect a patient's health information.

What rights does the privacy rule give patients over their health information?

Health insurers and providers must comply with the patient's rights to:

- Ask to see and get a copy of health records
- Have corrections added to health information
- Receive a notice that tells the patient how health information may be used and shared

Who can look at and receive patient health information?

The privacy rule sets limits on who can look at and receive patient health information.

The HIPAA Privacy Rule provides federal protections for personal health information held by covered entities and gives patients an array of rights with respect to that information.

Understanding HIPAA Privacy. (n.d.). U.S. Department of Health & Human Services. http://www.hhs.gov/ocr/privacy/hipaa/understanding/index.html.

2. Each medication order should contain the client's name, correct medication name, the route of administration, the dosage amount, and the time of administration.
3. Single-dose orders are for a medication to be given one time.

Box 4.7 INFORMED CONSENT

Informed consent is the process whereby the client is informed of the risks, benefits, and alternatives of certain procedures and gives consent for a procedure to be done.

What It Includes
- The nature of the proposed care, treatment, services, medications, interventions, or procedures
- The potential benefits, risks, or side effects, including potential problems related to recuperation
- The likelihood of achieving care, treatment, and service goals
- Reasonable alternatives and their respective risks and benefits, including alternatives to refusing all interventions

Nursing Considerations
- Nurses witness signatures to determine client competency, validate the signature, and ensure that the consent is voluntary.
- Witnessed signature: Do not witness unless you know the client has all information needed to make an informed decision.
- The procedure is specified in terms the client can understand.
- Client appreciates the benefits and consequences of the procedure.
- Client understands alternatives to the procedure.
- Client is informed of the health care provider performing the procedure.
- The consent form is signed while the client is free from mind-altering drugs or conditions.
- Consents are legal documents.

Withdrawal of Consent
- Can be written or verbal
- Can occur at any time, even after the procedure has begun

Exceptions
- Life-threatening emergencies or urgent situations
- Minors: For clients up to age 18, a parent's signature is generally required for consent.
- Emancipated minor: Definition may vary, but usually this is a minor who is self-supporting and living away from home.
- Mentally incapacitated individual: Consent is required from legal guardian or person specified as medical power of attorney.

Treatments Needing Informed Consent
- Admission agreements to a health care agency
- Most surgeries, even when they are not done in the hospital
- Advanced or complex medical tests and invasive procedures, such as an endoscopy and needle biopsy of the liver
- Radiation or chemotherapy to treat cancer
- Most vaccinations
- Blood transfusions
- Some blood tests, such as HIV testing (need for written consent varies by state)
- Research consents for client participating in a research study
- Special consents (use of restraints, photographing the client, disposal of body parts during surgery, donating organs after death, performing an autopsy)

4. "Stat" orders: the procedure or medication should be given/carried out immediately; new orders should be scanned initially to determine whether any "stat" orders are present.
5. The nurse is responsible for questioning any medication order if the order is not clear.

Protective Procedures

A. Documentation: written record of events surrounding a client's hospital stay.
  1. Protects client by promoting good communication among health care providers.
  2. Provides evidence in court of care given.
     a. Courts will not assume care is given unless it is recorded.
     b. Demonstrates meeting standard of care.
B. Documentation guidelines (Box 4.8).
  1. Use the agency format correctly.
  2. Complete all portions of the format.
     a. Document only factual data.
     b. Complete an honest record of events.
        (1) Do not alter the record at any time.
        (2) Record all events, even unusual events, factually.
        (3) Give all appropriate information about each note (e.g., status of incision: presence of and type of drainage, inflammation of area, foul odor, and type of dressing, if any).
        (4) Explain omissions in care.
  3. Time, date, and sign all entries.
  4. Do not skip lines; do not leave any blank spaces for other people to chart (paper charts).
  5. Correct errors properly.
     a. Draw a straight line through an error; date and initial.
        (1) No white-out on errors.
        (2) No obliteration or erasure of errors.
        (3) No recopying of a page to omit a note.
     b. Add omitted information by an "addendum" or "late entry"; give date and time of original note and date and time of the addendum.
  6. Use meaningful, specific language; do not use words you do not understand or unacceptable abbreviations.
  7. Computer documentation and the electronic health record (EHR).
     a. Do not give your username or password to anyone, because it is your legal electronic signature.
     b. Always use your own username and password when logging into the computer terminal.
     c. Review notes for accuracy before selecting "confirm" or "save."
     d. Never walk away from the computer terminal without logging off.
     e. Frequently change the log-in password to maintain security within the EHR.
     f. Shred any printout from the computer at the end of the shift.

! TEST ALERT Enter computer or electronic documentation accurately, completely, and in a timely manner.

B. Nursing interventions.
1. Provide palliative pain management – the prevention or relief of pain when a cure for the client's illness is not feasible.

> **!** **TEST ALERT** Provide care and resources for end-of-life issues and choices. Identify client's end-of-life needs (e.g., financial concerns, fear, loss of control, role changes). Identify client's ability to cope with end-of-life interventions. Provide care or support for client/family at the end of life. Assist client in resolving end-of-life issues.

   a. Pain medication is frequently administered on an around-the-clock schedule to maintain therapeutic levels of medication; do not delay or deny pain relief measures to a dying client.
   b. Moderate-to-large amounts of opioids may be required to maintain the client's comfort.
   c. Administer analgesics based on client's level of pain; medication is increased as client's pain increases.
   d. Adjuvant medications to increase effectiveness of analgesics – antiemetics, antidepressants, corticosteroids.
   e. A nurse's or family's fear that the client will become dependent on, addicted to, or tolerant to the pain medication is inappropriate in the provision of pain control in palliative care.
   f. Fear that opioids will hasten death is unsubstantiated, even in clients at the very end of life. It is important that nurses provide adequate pain relief for the terminally ill client.
2. Dehydration: maintain oral hygiene; do not force the client to eat or drink. The option to withhold artificial nutrition or hydration should be made by the client in the advance directive or by the person designated in the advance directive.
3. Respiratory distress: elevate the head of the bed, offer oxygen, and provide medications to decrease apprehension.
4. Elimination.
   a. Use incontinence pads, prevent skin irritation, and follow facility protocol for indwelling catheters.
   b. Monitor bowel function, assess for impaction, and promote normal function within client limitations.
5. Anorexia, nausea, and vomiting.
   a. Assess for precipitating cause and administer medications to decrease nausea.
   b. Offer small, frequent meals, but do not focus on the client's need to eat.
6. Determine the client's personal preferences and cultural implications regarding death. Provide family care regarding cultural needs.

Postmortem Care

> **!** **TEST ALERT** Provide postmortem care.

A. Determine whether there are any tissues or organs to be donated.

B. Perform postmortem care as soon as possible.
1. Unless the client is to have an autopsy, remove all equipment according to facility policy.
2. Cleanse the body and cover with a clean sheet. Place a pillow under the head, and leave the arms on the outside of the sheet. Deodorize the room if necessary.
3. Offer the family an opportunity to be with the client. Provide privacy in an unrushed atmosphere.
4. Return all personal belongings to the family. Document what items were taken and by whom.
5. Attach identification to the body and to the shroud. Shroud the body according to facility policy.

MANAGEMENT CONCEPTS

Management of Health Care Workers

A. RN implements the nursing process, completes the admission assessment, develops the nursing care plan, implements the teaching plan, and plans for client discharge.

> **!** **NURSING PRIORITY** Initial client assessment, provision of care to unstable clients requiring nursing judgment, discharge planning, and planning for client education are responsibilities of the RN. The PN participates in the process of providing client care.

B. Delegation is transferring to a competent individual the authority to perform a selected nursing task in a selected situation (the process for doing the work). *The nurse retains accountability for the delegation; most often, delegation is the role of the RN.*
C. Assignment describes the distribution of work that each staff member is to accomplish in a given time. To assign is to direct an individual to perform activities within an authorized scope of practice.
D. Supervision is the provision of guidance or direction, oversight, evaluation, and follow-up by the licensed nurse for the accomplishment of a nursing task delegated to nursing assistive personnel (NCSBN, 2006).
E. Role of the LPN/LVN in supervision.
1. The LPN/LVN should ensure unlicensed assistive personnel (UAP) understand the assigned task, and the UAP should acknowledge to the LPN/LVN that they understand the directions.
2. The LPN/LVN should make periodic checks to determine that the UAP are performing the tasks as directed.
3. If the UAP do not carry out the tasks correctly, the LPN/LVN should correct the action in a timely professional manner. *If the problem is not resolved, the RN should be notified.*
4. The LPN/LVN should assign tasks to the UAP that are clearly defined, within the expected expertise of the UAP, have very specific guidelines, and are non-invasive interventions: for example, bathing, ambulating, client hygiene, skin care, and range of motion.
5. The LPN/LVN can perform some invasive tasks, such as dressing changes, suctioning, urinary

catheterization, medication administration (oral, subcutaneous, intramuscular, and selected intravenous piggyback medications), and can reinforce teaching from the plan the RN has developed according to the education and job description of the LPN/LVN.

> **! TEST ALERT** Assign client care and/or related tasks (e.g., assistive personnel or LPN/LVN).

Prioritizing Client Care Assignments

A. Identify the most ill or unstable client of your assigned clients – evaluate and care for that client first.

B. Physiologic needs are the priority – education and communication needs can usually wait until the physiologic needs are met.

C. Initially, review the assigned client list – consider the report received on each client. Determine which client needs immediate physical assistance to maintain safety. (Review establishing nursing priorities in Chapter 1.)

D. Time management strategies.
   1. Get organized before the change-of-shift report.
      a. Develop a flow sheet to write down information needed to coordinate care for the client assignment.
   2. Prioritize care.
      a. Remember airway, breathing, circulation (ABCs) and Maslow's hierarchy of needs.
   3. Organize work by client.
      a. Bundle nursing care measures to accomplish several objectives in one visit to the client's room.
   4. Managing others.
      a. Use assertive communication techniques.
      b. Delegate tasks to assistive personnel.

> **! TEST ALERT** Organize and prioritize care of assigned group of clients and use effective time management skills.

Interprofessional Health Care Team Members

A. Involves health care professionals across disciplines working together to provide client care.

B. Roles and responsibilities of health care team members.
   1. Advanced practice registered nurse (APRN) – e.g., family nurse practitioner (FNP), adult-gerontology primary care nurse practitioner (AGPCNP).
   2. Dietician.
   3. Occupational therapist (OT).
   4. Pastoral care (minister, priest, rabbi).
   5. Pharmacist (PharmD, RPh).
   6. Physical therapist (PT).
   7. Physician assistant (PA).
   8. Physician (medical doctor [MD], doctor of osteopathy [DO]).
   9. Respiratory therapist (CRT, RRT).
   10. Social worker (MSW).
   11. Speech and language pathologist (speech therapist).
   12. Unlicensed assistive personnel (UAP): nursing assistant (NA), patient care associate (PCA), nursing technician, clinical assistant, orderly, health aide, nurse aide, nurse extender.

Conflict Management

A. Conflict is an active disagreement between people with opposing opinions or principles and is inevitable where there are people with differing backgrounds, needs, values, and priorities.
   1. Nurses need to become accustomed to resolving conflicts.
   2. Common employee problem areas that lead to conflict.
      a. Poor quality of work.
      b. Work schedules and assignments.
      c. Excessive tardiness or absenteeism.
      d. Personality clashes.
      e. Substance abuse.
      f. Culture-based dissension.

B. Conflict resolution.
   1. Competition: win-lose situation.
      a. Used to resolve conflict when one person has more power in a situation than the other.
      b. *Example: the charge nurse refuses your request for Christmas vacation, explaining that the staff members with more seniority have priority for vacation at Christmas time over a recent graduate nurse.*
   2. Avoidance: lose-lose situation.
      a. Unassertive and uncooperative; conflict not resolved.
      b. *Example: the nurse would not have approached the charge nurse with the Christmas schedule issue. Usually, both people involved feel frustrated and angry.*
      c. There are some situations in which avoiding the issue might be appropriate, such as when tempers are flaring or when strong anger is present. However, this is only a short-term strategy.
   3. Accommodation: lose-win situation.
      a. One person accommodates the other at his or her own expense but often ends up feeling resentful and angry.
      b. *Example: the charge nurse would put her own concern aside and let the new graduate have the vacation during Christmas, possibly even working for the new graduate during the scheduled slot. The charge nurse loses and the graduate nurse wins in this situation, which may set up conflict among staff and other recent graduates.*
   4. Compromise: no-lose-no-win situation.
      a. Bargaining is the strategy that recognizes the importance of both the resolution of the problem and the relationship between the two people.
      b. A moderately assertive and cooperative step in the right direction, in which one creates a modified win-lose outcome.

c. *Example: the charge nurse compromises with the new graduate by allowing them to have Christmas Eve off with their family but not the entire week.*
5. Collaboration: win-win situation.
   a. Deals with confrontation and problem solving when the needs, feelings, and desires of both parties are taken into consideration and reexamined while searching for proper ways to agree on goals.
   b. Is fully assertive and cooperative.
   c. *Example: the new graduate and the charge nurse discuss the week of Christmas vacation and the staffing needs and agree that the new graduate will work the first 3 days of that week and the charge nurse will work the second half of that week. The new graduate also agrees to be there the first part of the week to complete the audit on the charts from the previous week for the charge nurse. In this situation, both people are satisfied, and there is no compromising what is most important to each person. That is, the charge nurse gets her audit completed, and the recent graduate is able to spend half of the Christmas week with their family.*

! TEST ALERT Recognize and report staff conflict.

Evidence-Based Practice

A. Evidence-based practice is the use of the current best practice research, client values and preferences, and clinical expertise in the decision-making process for client care.
B. Evidence-based practice is one strategy to reduce the amount of time required to integrate new health care findings into practice.
C. Nurses should follow evidence-based practice protocols and question approaches and rationales as needed.

D. Nurses use information technology such as online resources, including research publications, to incorporate current research findings into nursing practice.

Quality improvement

A. Quality improvement (QI) is also known as performance improvement and is the framework (i.e., audit, improvement activities) in health care that systematically evaluates services provided and the results achieved compared with accepted standards to improve the ways care is delivered to clients.
B. QI processes are similar to the nursing process and involve the interprofessional team. The goal of QI is to improve client outcomes, including safety, the effectiveness of care, and the experience of health care.
C. Methods of monitoring nursing care.
   1. Nursing audit: examination of the client's records, either retrospectively (after discharge) or concurrently (while client is receiving care).
   2. Peer review: practicing nurses evaluate peer performance based on standards and criteria.
   3. Benchmarking: nurse quality indicator results are compared against the results of similar local and international institutions.
   4. Client satisfaction: a questionnaire is given to clients to determine satisfaction regarding perceptions of the care they received.
D. Participating in a QI activity such as data collection or serving on a QI committee is within the scope of PN practice and involves the following:
   1. Identify indicators to monitor the quality and effectiveness of care delivered.
   2. Gather and evaluate data to monitor the effectiveness of care.
   3. Recommend ways to improve care.
   4. Implement activities to improve care.

⚡ Practice & Next Generation NCLEX (NGN) Questions
Coordinated Care

More questions on
ℯvolve

1. While having lunch at a table with other nursing staff, a nurse asks a nurse from another unit about a friend's husband, wanting to know how he is progressing. What should the nurse from the unit do?
   1. Write the information on a piece of paper so that others at the table will not know.
   2. Inform the inquiring nurse to visit the unit and talk to the client.
   3. Ask the inquiring nurse to meet with her outside of the cafeteria to talk in a more private setting.
   4. Ask the inquiring nurse to phone the unit and ask the nurse caring for the client.

2. The nurse enters the client's room and discovers the client on the floor beside the bed. The side rails are up, and the client is confused and disoriented. What information would be included in the nurse's documentation in the occurrence or incident report?
   1. Upon entering the room, I discovered the client on the floor at the side of the bed; the side rails were up.
   2. The client fell out of the bed after the nursing assistant had explained to him the importance of not getting up.
   3. The client was confused and apparently tried to climb out over the side rails of the bed.
   4. Evidently the previous nurse did not check on the client to see that the client was confused, and then the client fell out of bed.

3. An unlicensed assistive personnel (UAP) employee is involved in a legal situation and is being held negligent. Which of the following delegations to the nursing assistant in the care of an older adult with Parkinson disease would be considered out of the scope of care for the nursing assistant?
   1. Feeding the client.
   2. Medication administration.
   3. Ambulation assistance with a walker.
   4. Obtaining a set of vital signs.

4. The nurse stopped on the highway to aid at the scene of an accident with multiple fatalities to provide assistance. Immediately after the incident, the family members were appreciative of the help the nurse provided. They offered to replace the nurse's soiled clothes. If the nurse accepts, which rights were in violation?
   1. American Nurses Association (ANA) Code of Ethics.
   2. HIPAA.
   3. Patient Self-Determination Act.
   4. Good Samaritan Act.

5. The nurse is recording a hand-off (end-of-shift) report for a client. Which information needs to be included? **Select all that apply**.
   1. Status of IVs and amount of fluid left to infuse.
   2. PRN medications given during the shift.
   3. Any abnormal vital signs.
   4. Status of all the laboratory tests since the client's admission.
   5. Routine medications given during the shift.
   6. Status of client's pain level.

6. In a mass fatality event, the nurse encounters a client with the following vital signs: walking, minor scrapes and bruises, pulse of 90 beats/min, respirations at 25 breaths/min, alert, and oriented. What triage tag designation should the client get?
   1. Green.
   2. Yellow.
   3. Red.
   4. Black.

7. A hospital has a fire on one of the units. The charge nurse is determining the acuity of clients to identify which clients can or cannot be discharged. Which client should **not** be discharged?
   1. An adult with an uncomplicated case of pneumonia who was admitted 4 days ago.
   2. An adolescent with an overdose of acetaminophen and opioids.
   3. An older adult with peripheral vascular disease and a venous leg ulcer.
   4. A young adult with a new diagnosis of Crohn disease.

8. The nurse is working with an unlicensed assistive personnel (UAP) employee to provide care to a group of assigned clients. The nurse has worked with the UAP employee and knows they are competent. What activity can the nurse delegate to the UAP employee?
   1. Giving a bed bath and turning an unconscious client.
   2. Completing the admission interview for a new client.
   3. Ambulating a cardiac client for the first time after admission.
   4. Administering an oral (PO) medication the nurse has prepared.

9. A staff nurse is beginning the evening shift. The day nurse has advised her that the suction equipment in the room of a client who has had surgery is not working properly. What is a **priority** nursing action?
   1. Troubleshoot and fix the machine.
   2. Continue to use the machine.
   3. Evaluate the function of the suction equipment.
   4. Replace the equipment.

10. Which actions by the nurse would be most effective in ensuring client confidentiality when documenting in the electronic health record (EHR)? **Select all that apply**.
    1. Allow a new nurse employee to use your username and password until they receive their own.
    2. Ask the charge nurse to provide you with another username at the beginning of each shift.
    3. Frequently change the log-in password for entering data in the EHR.
    4. Log out of the EHR when leaving the computer terminal.
    5. Always use your own username and password when logging into the computer terminal.
    6. Shred any printouts from the computer at the end of the shift.

11. The nurse is assigned to provide care for the following clients.

    Client #1: A 65-year-old man who had an open reduction and internal fixation of the right humerus 3 hours ago and reports severe pain in the operative site on a scale of 9 out of 10 and numbness of the fingers.

    Client #2: A 77-year-old woman who has Parkinson disease, mild dementia, and urinary incontinence and needs to go to the bathroom.

    Client #3: A 60-year-old female who is newly diagnosed with type 2 diabetes that has a fasting blood sugar of 150 mg/dL who is hungry and wants a snack.

    Client #4: A 40-year-old client who had a vaginal hysterectomy 4 hours ago and has noticed increased vaginal bleeding.

    Client #5: A 33-year-old client who had a flare-up of ulcerative colitis with electrolyte depletion and is being discharged tomorrow.

Complete the following sentences by choosing the most likely options for the missing information from the lists of options provided.

The nurse should assess first _____1_____ because this client is at risk for _____2_____. After attending to the priority client's needs, the second client the nurse would assess is _____1_____ because the client is at risk for _____2_____.

OPTIONS FOR 1	OPTIONS FOR 2
Client #1	Hyperglycemia
Client #2	Compartment syndrome
Client #3	Falling
Client #4	Hemorrhage
Client #5	Electrolyte imbalance

12. The clinic nurse is seeing a client who lost her home following a hurricane. **Highlight next to the Nurses' Notes the assessment findings that require follow-up by the nurse.**

Health History	Nurses' Notes	Vital Signs	Laboratory Results

A 52-year-old client reports that she is staying with her daughter at her apartment. Her daughter has 3 young children under the age of 5. The client reports feeling unwelcome by her daughter's husband and is waiting for the financial resources to move out to her own place. The client is worried that her son-in-law will make her leave and stay in a motel. Client reports difficulty sleeping, loss of appetite, and feelings of depression. Her place of employment has been supportive and has allowed her to work remotely from her daughter's home. The client starts to cry and states that she just doesn't know what to do.

⚡ Answers to Practice & Next Generation NCLEX (NGN) Questions

1. 2
Client Needs: Safe and Effective Care Environment/Coordinated Care
Clinical Judgment/Cognitive Skill: Take Action
Item Type: Multiple Choice
Rationale & Test-Taking Strategy: Ask yourself, "Is this type of behavior professional? Does it provide for client confidentiality?" The only answer that does not violate the client's right to privacy is to have the inquiring person talk directly to the client. The lunchroom is not an appropriate place to converse about how clients are doing, even if they are friends. This would be in violation of the HIPAA standards.

2. 1
Client Needs: Safe and Effective Care Environment/ Safety and Infection Control
Clinical Judgment/Cognitive Skill: Take Action
Item Type: Multiple Choice
Rationale & Test-Taking Strategy: This is the best descriptor of the event without including opinions. The nurse does not know that the client fell out of bed; the client was on the floor at the side of the bed. It is important to not place blame regarding the incident.

3. 2
Client Needs: Safe and Effective Care Environment/Coordinated Care
Clinical Judgment/Cognitive Skill: Analyze Cues
Item Type: Multiple Choice
Rationale & Test-Taking Strategy: Medication administration is to be performed by a licensed registered nurse (RN) or licensed practical/vocational nurse (LPN/LVN). Unlicensed assistive personnel (UAP) working in long-term care (LTC) are typically involved in restorative programs and may assist the client with ambulation with a walker. The UAP feeds and bathes the client and collects vital-sign data; the nurse reviews and assesses this documentation.

4. 4
Client Needs: Safe and Effective Care Environment/Coordinated Care
Clinical Judgment/Cognitive Skill: Analyze Cues
Item Type: Multiple Choice
Rationale & Test-Taking Strategy: The nurse would be in violation of the Good Samaritan Act. Allowing the family to replace the soiled clothes was a form of compensation, which is in direct violation of the Good Samaritan Act. None of the other choices

are applicable to the situation. The ANA Code of Ethics provides principles to facilitate ethical problem solving. HIPAA is a law providing confidentiality for the client to protect written and verbal communication about the client. The Patient Self-Determination Act requires that hospitalized patients indicate whether they have an advanced directive.

5. **1, 2, 3, 6**
Client Needs: Safe and Effective Care Environment/Coordinated Care
Clinical Judgment/Cognitive Skill: Take Action
Item Type: Select All That Apply
Rationale & Test-Taking Strategy: When the nurse is providing a hand-off (end-of-shift) report, the information should be pertinent to the status of the client's condition during the last shift. The nurse should include any recent changes in vital signs, pain level, new laboratory test results, or recent treatments and the client's response. Any PRN or as-needed medications given during the shift, along with the remaining amount of IV fluid to infuse, should be included in the hand-off report. It is not important to provide information about the client's routine medications or all the laboratory results since admission.

6. **1**
Client Needs: Safe and Effective Care Environment/ Safety and Infection Control
Clinical Judgment/Cognitive Skill: Analyze Cues
Item Type: Multiple Choice
Rationale & Test-Taking Strategy: Based on symptom presentation, this client is categorized as green (minimal) or "walking wounded." Green triage designation indicates the casualty requires medical attention when all higher-priority clients have been evacuated and may not require stabilization or monitoring. Yellow triage designation requires medical attention within 6 hrs. Injuries are potentially life-threatening but can wait until the red casualties are stabilized and evacuated. Red triage designation requires immediate medical attention and will not survive if not seen soon. Any compromise to the casualty's respiration, hemorrhage control, or shock control could be fatal. Black triage designation indicates the casualty is expected not to reach higher medical support alive without compromising the treatment of higher-priority clients.

7. **2**
Client Needs: Safe and Effective Care Environment/Coordinated Care
Clinical Judgment/Cognitive Skill: Prioritize Hypotheses
Item Type: Multiple Choice
Rationale & Test-Taking Strategy: The nurse should consider that the most medically stable clients may be discharged based on their acuity, including clients who are admitted for observation and diagnostic tests and are not bedridden (Crohn disease), clients who are scheduled soon to be discharged or who could be cared for at home with support from family or home health care services (PVD and venous leg ulcer), clients with no critical change in condition for the past 3 days (pneumonia), and clients who could be cared for in a rehabilitation or long-term care facility. The adolescent with an overdose needs acute care.

8. **1**
Client Needs: Safe and Effective Care Environment/Coordinated Care
Clinical Judgment/Cognitive Skill: Take Action
Item Type: Multiple Choice

Rationale & Test-Taking Strategy: The bed bath and turning of an unconscious client would be within the expected tasks for a UAP to competently perform. The admitting interview is the RN's responsibility. It would be necessary for the RN to ambulate for the first time the cardiac client to determine toleration of the activity. The nurse should never ask anyone else to administer a medication that has already been prepared.

9. **3**
Client Needs: Safe and Effective Care Environment/ Safety and Infection Control
Clinical Judgment/Cognitive Skill: Take Action
Item Type: Multiple Choice
Rationale & Test-Taking Strategy: Note the **key** word, "priority." This test item focuses on the priority nursing intervention when equipment does not function properly. The nurse should evaluate the function of the equipment based on the day nurse's comment. After evaluating the function, the nurse is responsible for replacing the equipment if it is not functioning correctly.

10. **3, 4, 5, 6**
Client Needs: Safe and Effective Care Environment/Coordinated Care
Clinical Judgment/Cognitive Skill: Take Action
Item Type: Select All That Apply
Rationale & Test-Taking Strategy: When documenting in an EHR, it is important to ensure that client information is secure and confidential. Within a hospital system, computer records and the EHR are protected by usernames, passwords, and a firewall. The nurse should never allow another nurse or user to access the EHR or computer system using their unique username and password. Each user who has access to a client record must have a secure password, which must be changed regularly to maintain security. In addition, the nurse understands that when reports or the client's chart are transmitted outside the hospital to other agencies, encryption and authentication software is used. When the nurse completes the entries in the computer terminal, the nurse needs to log off the system. Any type of paper documentation from the computer terminal (i.e., flow sheets, ISBAR-R communication sheets) that has identifiable client information must be shredded at the end of the shift.

11. The nurse is assigned to provide care for the following clients.
Client #1: A 65-year-old client who had an open reduction and internal fixation of the right humerus 3 hrs ago and reports severe pain at the operative site as a 9 on a scale of 10 and numbness of the fingers.
Client #2: A 77-year-old client who has Parkinson disease, mild dementia, and urinary incontinence and needs to go to the bathroom.
Client #3: A 60-year-old client newly diagnosed with type 2 diabetes who has a fasting blood sugar of 150 mg/dL, is hungry, and wants a snack.
Client #4: A 40-year-old client who had a vaginal hysterectomy 4 hrs ago and has noticed increased vaginal bleeding.
Client #5: A 33-year-old client who had a flare-up of ulcerative colitis with electrolyte depletion and is being discharged tomorrow.

Complete the following sentences by choosing the most likely options for the missing information from the list of options provided.

The nurse should **first** assess *client #1*, because this client is at risk for *compartment syndrome*. After attending to the priority client's needs, the second client the nurse would assess is *client #4*, because the client is at risk for *hemorrhage*.

Client Needs: Safe and Effective Care Environment/Coordinated Care
Clinical Judgment/Cognitive Skill: Prioritize Hypotheses
Item Type: Drop-Down Cloze
Rationale & Test-Taking Strategy: Client #1 should be seen first. The main sign of compartment syndrome is severe, unrelenting pain that is out of proportion to the injury and not relieved by narcotics. When the client also reports decreased sensation, numbness, and tingling, the nurse needs to immediately notify the surgeon to prevent permanent loss of function of the arm, as compartment syndrome is a serious postoperative complication that should be urgently addressed. Client #4 should be seen next because of the risk of hemorrhage following a vaginal hysterectomy. The client who has an elevated fasting blood sugar is not in acute distress. The client with Parkinson disease and dementia has a chronic illness along with incontinence, and the nurse can send the nurse's aide to assist the client to the bathroom. This client needs to be monitored for risk of falls and impaired skin integrity due to the incontinence. The client who is going to be discharged is not who the nurse would see as a priority client to assess.

---

12. The clinic nurse is seeing a client who lost her home following a hurricane. **Highlight next to the Nurses' Notes the assessment findings that require follow-up by the nurse.**

Health History	Nurses' Notes	Vital Signs	Laboratory Results

1120 A 52-year-old client reports she is staying with her daughter at her apartment. Her daughter has three young children under the age of 5. The client reports feeling unwelcome by her daughter's husband and is waiting for the financial resources to move out to her own place. The client is worried that her son-in-law will make her leave and stay in a motel. Client reports difficulty sleeping, loss of appetite, and feelings of depression. Her place of employment has been supportive and has allowed her to work remotely from her daughter's home. The client starts to cry and states that she just doesn't know what to do.

Client Needs: Physiological Integrity
Clinical Judgment/Cognitive Skill: Recognize Cues
Item Type: Highlight in Text
Rationale & Test-Taking Strategy: A traumatic event, such as a hurricane destroying a home, can cause moderate-to-severe stress reactions in individuals. Often, the person may develop depression, experience grief and anger, turn to alcohol or drugs, and even think about hurting themselves or others. Individuals react to the same disaster in different ways depending on their age, cultural background, health status, social support structure, and general ability to adapt to crisis. Typical symptoms often present when a person seeks health care assistance are excessive worry; crying frequently; excessive irritability; episodes of anger, frustration, and frequent arguing; wanting to be alone most of the time and isolate self from others; feeling anxious or fearful; feeling overwhelmed by sadness; feeling confused; having trouble thinking clearly and concentrating and/or difficulty making decisions; an increase in the amount of alcohol intake and/or substance use; increased physical (aches, pains) complaints such as headaches, neck pain, trouble with their "nerves," and loss of appetite.

CHAPTER FIVE

Pharmacology and Medication Administration

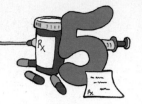

GENERAL CONCEPTS

No medication has a single action; all medications have the potential to alter more than one body function.

> **⚠ NURSING PRIORITY** Many medications have several desirable actions. Carefully evaluate the question as to what the desired response of the medication is for the specific client situation. Example: Acetylsalicylic acid (ASA) is used to prevent platelet aggregation to prevent stroke and cardiac disease, but it is also used as an antipyretic and for pain control in arthritis.

A. Drug names: The Drug Amendments of 1962 made it mandatory that each medication have one official name.
 1. Generic name (nonproprietary): the official designated name under which the medication is listed in official publications (e.g., acetaminophen).
 2. Chemical name: designates the specific chemical composition of the medication; usually quite long and complicated to pronounce and spell (e.g., N-acetyl-para-aminophenol).
 3. Trade name (proprietary, brand name): the name designated and registered by a specific manufacturer (e.g., Tylenol).

> **⚠ NURSING PRIORITY** The medications on the NCLEX-PN® examination will be identified by generic names—for example, diazepam, the generic name for Valium, will be used on the NCLEX-PN® examination. You may still encounter the trade names in the clinical setting.

B. Abuse potential: The Controlled Substances Act of 1970 defines rules for the manufacture and distribution of drugs that are considered to have a potential for abuse.
 1. Defines drugs in five categories—Schedules I, II, III, IV, V: potential for abuse becomes lower with each subsequent category; thus the higher the schedule number, the lower the potential for abuse.
 2. Schedule I drugs are highly addictive (e.g., heroin) and are not used for medicinal purposes in the United States. Schedule V drugs (e.g., diphenoxylate hydrochloride [Lomotil]) pose the lowest risk for abuse and represent the lowest level of pharmacokinetics.
C. Pharmacokinetic process: consists of four phases acting together to determine the concentration of a drug at its site of action. Use the acronym **ADME** to remember these processes.

1. **A**bsorption: movement of the drug from site of administration to the systemic circulation.
 a. Drug action may be increased or decreased by alterations in the gastric emptying time, presence of food, changes in gastric or plasma pH, or the drug form (e.g., tablets or capsules).
 b. Method of administration affects absorption (e.g., intravenous [IV] vs. oral).
2. **D**istribution: movement of the drug by the systemic circulation throughout the body.
 a. Based on blood flow of drug to tissue, ability of the drug to leave the vascular system, and ability of the drug to enter the tissue cells.
 b. Degree of binding to plasma proteins or other substances in the body. Albumin (protein) always remains in the bloodstream; drugs that are protein-bound restrict the drug distribution.
3. **M**etabolism: the enzymatic alteration of the drug structure; most drug metabolism occurs in the liver.
 a. Most important action of drug metabolism is promoting the renal excretion of the drug.
 b. Converts drugs to inactive compounds; also increases or decreases toxicity.
 c. Rates can be influenced by genetic factor, aging, drug interactions, and coexisting pathologies (chronic liver disease).
4. **E**xcretion: the removal of drugs from the body.
 a. Kidney is the most important organ for excretion of a drug; in renal failure, the duration and the intensity of drug action may increase.
 b. Kidney of a newborn is not fully developed; infants have a limited ability to excrete drugs.
 c. Aging can affect drug excretion (e.g., at the age of 80, renal clearance rate typically decreases half of what it was at age 30).
 d. Drugs are also excreted in breast milk, bile, and the lungs.

> **⚠ OLDER ADULT PRIORITY** Creatinine clearance, not serum creatinine levels, should be monitored to evaluate kidney function, as it is a more effective indicator of kidney function, especially in older adults.

Drug Actions

A. **Desired action**: the desired, predictable response for which the medication is administered.
B. **Adverse drug reactions (ADRs)**: any noxious, unintended, and undesired effect that occurs with normal drug doses.

> **! OLDER ADULT PRIORITY** ADRs are seven times more common in older adults than in young adults.

1. *Side effects*: undesirable drug effects, ranging from mild untoward effects to severe responses that occur at normal drug dosages.
2. *Toxicity*: drug reactions that primarily occur because of receiving an excessive dose (e.g., medication error, poisoning). However, toxicity also may result in severe reactions (anaphylaxis) that occur regardless of the dose.
3. *Allergic reactions*: drug reactions that occur as a result of prior sensitization and result in an immune response. Intensity can range from very mild to very severe.
4. *Idiosyncratic effect*: an uncommon drug response.

> **! TEST ALERT** Evaluate client response to medication (e.g., adverse reactions, interactions, therapeutic effects).

C. **Tolerance**: increased dose required to maintain expected drug response (e.g., when a client with chronic pain requires higher doses of a strong opioid agonist [morphine sulfate] to achieve pain relief).
D. **Dependence**: an expected response to repeated use of a drug, resulting in physical signs and symptoms of withdrawal when the serum drug level decreases suddenly (e.g., when a client abruptly stops taking a strong opioid agonist [methadone] and develops irritability, nausea, vomiting, muscle spasm, and musculoskeletal pain).
E. **Addiction**: the continued use of a psychoactive substance regardless of physical, psychological, or social harm.

Drug Interactions

A. **Synergistic or potentiation effect**: if two or more drugs are given together and this increases the therapeutic effects, it is beneficial; if it increases adverse effects, it may be detrimental.
   Example: A desirable potentiation effect occurs when a diuretic and a beta-blocker are given for hypertension. An undesirable effect can occur when warfarin and aspirin (both anticoagulants) are given together because this increases the risk for spontaneous bleeding.
B. Antagonistic or inhibitory effect: if two or more drugs are given together, one may inhibit the effect of the other; this may be beneficial or detrimental.
   Example: When you administer an adrenergic beta-blocker propranolol with an adrenergic beta stimulant isoproterenol, the action of each drug is canceled. However, the use

of naloxone to suppress the effects of morphine results in a desirable inhibitory effect.

C. Unique response effect: this occurs when two drugs are given together, and the effect creates a new response not seen when each drug is used alone.
   Example: When you administer disulfiram and the client has ingested alcohol or is using products containing alcohol, the effects are undesirable.
D. Drug incompatibility: a chemical or physical reaction that occurs when two or more drugs are combined in vitro (outside the body).
E. Drug-food interactions.

Drug Therapy Considerations Across the Life Span

A. Pediatric implications.
   1. Younger clients are more sensitive to drugs than adult clients due to organ system immaturity.
   2. Children metabolize drugs faster than adults.
B. Older adult implications (Box 5.1).
C. Food and Drug Administration (FDA) pregnancy risk categories (Table 5.1).

Herbal Supplements

A. Biologically based therapies.
   1. Dietary supplements—vitamins, minerals, herbs, and other botanical products.
   2. Herbal medicines—use of herbs to treat illness.
      a. Herbal medicine can be defined as the use of plant-derived products to promote health and relieve symptoms of disease.
      b. Herbal medicine is the most common form of alternative medicine, which can be defined as treatment practices that are not widely accepted or practiced by mainstream clinicians in a given culture.

> **Box 5.1 MEDICATION IMPLICATIONS FOR OLDER ADULT CLIENTS**
>
> **Avoiding adverse drug reactions**
> - Obtain a complete drug history that includes over-the-counter drugs and herbs.
> - Monitor client responses and drug levels.
> - Keep dosing regimen as simple as possible; use daily dosing, when possible, rather than twice a day.
> - Emphasize to clients the importance of disposing of medications they are no longer taking.
>
> **Promoting compliance**
> - Intentional underdosing (by clients) is the most common reason for nonadherence to drug regimen.
> - Provide written instructions to clients regarding medication administration, as well as why they are taking the medication.
> - Ask the pharmacist to label drug containers with large type.
> - Provide drug containers that can be opened easily.
> - Encourage clients to use a system to record or track their drug doses (calendar, pill organizer).
> - Determine whether clients can afford their medications.

Table 5.1 FDA PREGNANCY AND LACTATION LABELING RULE (PLLR) REQUIREMENTS

Sections	Subsections	Headings and/or Content

Pregnancy	1. Pregnancy Exposure Registry
	2. Risk Summary
	3. Clinical Considerations
	4. Data
		1. There is a pregnancy exposure registry that monitors pregnancy outcomes in women exposed to (name of drug) during pregnancy.
		2. Risk summaries are statements that summarize outcomes for the following content relative to drug dosage, length of time drug was taken, and weeks of gestation when the drug was taken, as well as known pharmacologic mechanisms of action.
		3. Information is provided for the following five headings:
		  a. Disease-associated maternal and/or embryo/fetal risk
		  b. Dose adjustments during pregnancy and the postpartum period
		  c. Maternal adverse reactions
		  d. Fetal/neonatal adverse reactions
		  e. Labor or delivery
		4. This section describes research that served as a source of data for Risk Summaries (e.g., human data, animal data).

Lactation	1. Risk Summary
	2. Clinical Considerations
	3. Data
		1. Risk summaries are statements that summarize outcomes for the following content:
		  a. Presence of drug in human milk
		  b. Effects of drug on the breast-fed child
		  c. Effects of drug on milk production/excretion
		  d. Risk and benefit statement
		2. Information is provided for the following headings:
		  a. Minimizing exposure
		  b. Monitoring for adverse reactions
		3. This section expands on the Risk Summary and Clinical Considerations subsections.

Females and males of reproductive potential	No defined subsections	The following headings are included to address the need for pregnancy testing or contraception and adverse effects associated with preimplantation loss or adverse effects on fertility:
		  a. Pregnancy testing
		  b. Contraception
		  c. Infertility

Adapted from Burcham, J.R., Rosenthal, L.D. (2022). FDA Pregnancy and Lactation Labeling Rule (PLLR) Requirements in *Lehne's pharmacology for nursing care* (11cd.). Elsevier (Table 11.2, page 94).

    c. The word *natural* is not synonymous with safe! Remember, poison ivy and tobacco are natural, too.
    d. All herbal products must be labeled as "dietary supplements."
    e. The product label must state that it is not intended to diagnose, treat, cure, or prevent any disease and that it has not been evaluated by the FDA.
  3. Probiotics—live microorganisms (e.g., "good" bacteria) ingested that have similar function to beneficial organisms.

! NURSING PRIORITY Clients need to be advised that herbal therapy may need to be discontinued 2 to 3 weeks prior to surgery.

B. Some commonly used medicinal herbs are identified in Table 5.2.

! NURSING PRIORITY Unlike conventional drugs, herbal and other dietary supplements can be marketed without any proof of safety or efficacy. Dietary supplements are not regulated by the FDA.

MEDICATION ADMINISTRATION

! NURSING PRIORITY The nurse's responsibility in administering medication is influenced by three primary factors: nursing guidelines for safe medication administration, pharmacologic implications of the medication, and the legal aspects of medication administration.

Nursing Responsibilities in Medication Administration

A. Follow the "Six Rights" of medication administration (Fig. 5.1).

! TEST ALERT Administer medications according to the Six Rights of Medication Administration.

B. Nurses should administer *only* those medications that they have prepared.
C. Be familiar with the medication.
  1. General purpose for which the client is receiving the medication.

Table 5.2   COMMONLY USED MEDICINAL HERBS

Medicinal Herb	Drug Interactions
• **Aloe** is used for topical skin ailments with little or no topical side effects. Oral aloe is used for constipation and can cause severe diarrhea. Fresh aloe is more effective than stored product.	None noted with topical therapy.
• **Black cohosh** is a popular treatment for acute symptoms of menopause and premenstrual syndrome. Minor side effect of upset stomach may occur.	May potentiate hypotensive effects of antihypertensive drugs, as well as hypoglycemic action of insulin and oral hypoglycemics.
• **Dehydroepiandrosterone (DHEA)** may increase levels of testosterone and estrogen; has antiaging effects and antidepressant effects.	Carries a risk, especially because it can raise male and female hormone levels.
• **Echinacea** is used orally to stimulate the immune functions and suppress inflammation; has antiviral properties. Side effects include unpleasant taste, fever, nausea, and vomiting.	May oppose effects of immunosuppressant drugs.
• **Feverfew** is used for treatment of migraine and fever; it stimulates menstruation and suppresses inflammation.	May suppress platelet aggregation and increase risk for bleeding in clients on anticoagulant medications (aspirin, warfarin, heparin).
• **Flaxseed** treats constipation and dyslipidemias.	May reduce the absorption of conventional medications.
• **Garlic** reduces levels of triglycerides and LDLs and raises HDLs.	Suppresses platelet aggregation and can increase the risk for bleeding.
• **Ginger root** is used for nausea and vomiting caused by motion sickness and perhaps nausea caused by chemotherapy.	Suppresses platelet aggregation and can increase risk of bleeding; lowers blood glucose.
• **Ginkgo biloba** is used for increased circulation (peripheral vasodilator effects), memory, clear thinking, and impotence. It may cause stomach upset and dose-related headache.	May suppress coagulation and may promote seizures.
• **Goldenseal** is used for bacterial, fungal, and protozoal infections of mucous membranes in the respiratory, gastrointestinal, and genitourinary tracts. It is also used to treat inflammation of the gallbladder. It is generally well tolerated but can be toxic in high doses.	Contraindicated in pregnancy.
• **Glucosamine** is used to treat osteoarthritis symptoms.	May increase the risk of bleeding.
• **Melatonin** regulates sleep; treats insomnia and "jet lag."	Large doses can cause hangover, headache, nightmares.
• **Milk thistle** has antiinflammatory and antioxidant effects; treats liver and gall bladder disorders.	May mimic the effects of estrogen.
• **St. John's wort** is used for depression. Potential interactions with other drugs are possible.	May interfere with oral contraceptives; reduced anticoagulation in clients taking warfarin; decreased effectiveness of cyclosporine; caution in use with antidepressants.
• **Saw palmetto** is used to relieve urinary symptoms related to BPH and is well tolerated. May cause a false-negative result on PSA test.	Should not use with finasteride (Proscar) in treatment of BPH; has antiplatelet effect.
• **Valerian** is a sedative to promote sleep and reduce restlessness.	Can potentiate the actions of other drugs with CNS-depressant actions; may cause daytime drowsiness. With high doses and long-term use, headache, nervousness, or cardiac abnormalities can occur.

BPH, Benign prostatic hypertrophy; *CNS*, central nervous system; HDL, high-density lipoprotein; LDL, low-density lipoprotein; *MAO*, monoamine oxidase; *PMS*, premenstrual syndrome; *PSA*, prostate-specific antigen.

2. Common side effects.
3. Average dose or range of safe dosage.
4. Any specific safety precautions that apply before administration (e.g., digoxin: check apical pulse; heparin: check clotting times).

D. Check the medication against the health care provider's orders and document according to policy.
E. Evaluate client's overall condition and assess for changes that may indicate the medication is contraindicated (e.g., morphine would be contraindicated in a client who has increased intracranial pressure).

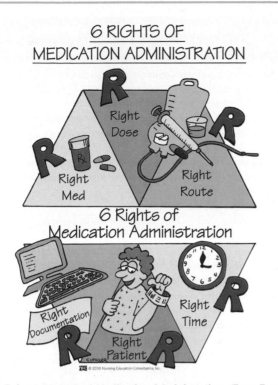

FIG. 5.1 **"6 Rights" of Medication Administration.** (From Zerwekh, J., Garneau, A., & Miller, C. J. [2017]. *Digital collection of the memory notebooks of nursing images* [4th ed]. Chandler, AZ: Nursing Education Consultants, Inc.)

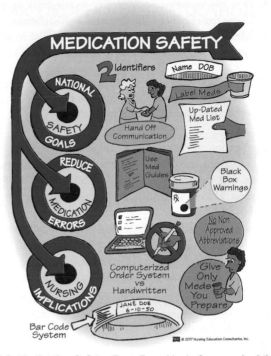

FIG. 5.2 **Medication Safety.** (From Zerwekh, J., Garneau, A., & Miller, C. J. [2017]. *Digital collection of the memory notebooks of nursing images* [4th ed]. Chandler, AZ: Nursing Education Consultants, Inc.)

common prefixes and suffixes of medications (Appendix 5.1, 5.2, and 5.3).

Nurse's Legal Responsibilities in Administration of Medication

A. The nurse administers a medication only by order of a physician or health care provider and according to provisions of the specific institution.

B. The nurse should not automatically carry out an order if the dosage is outside the normal range or if the route of administration is not appropriate; the nurse should consult the physician.

C. The nurse is legally responsible for the medication administered, even when the medication is administered according to a physician's order.

D. The nurse is responsible for evaluating the client before and after the administration of an as-needed (PRN) medication.

E. The medication should be charted as soon as possible after administration.

F. When taking oral orders on the phone, the nurse should carefully repeat all the orders (read-back) to verify they are correct.
   Example of a read-back:
   Doctor: "Give 25 mg diphenhydramine PO."
   Nurse: "Give 25 mg diphenhydramine PO."
   Doctor: "That's correct."

G. Medication errors (Fig. 5.2).
   1. If an error is found in a drug order, it is the nurse's responsibility to question the order.
   2. Always report medication errors to the appropriate health care provider immediately.

Box 5.2 FACTORS INFLUENCING DOSE-RESPONSE RELATIONSHIPS

- Age: Infants and older adults are generally more sensitive to medications.
- Presence of disease process, specifically kidney and liver problems.
- Method of administration—IV is much more rapid than PO.
- Adequate cardiac output.
- Emotional factors: Clients are more likely to respond to a medication in a positive manner if they have confidence in their treatment and anticipate the therapeutic effects.

F. Evaluate compatibility with other medications the client is receiving.

G. Use appropriate aseptic technique when preparing and administering medication.

H. Do not leave medications at the client's bedside without a doctor's order to do so.

I. If client is to self-administer medication, review the correct method of administration (e.g., eyedrops) with the client.

J. Before procedures, label medications that are not labeled, for example, medications in syringes, cups, or basins, and do the labeling in the area where medications and supplies are set up.

K. Factors affecting dose-response relationships (Box 5.2).

L. Understand conversions, common abbreviations and symbols, the list of "do not use" abbreviations, and

TRANSDERMAL MEDICATION ADMINISTRATION

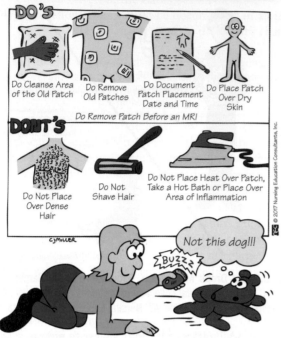

FIG. 5.4 Transdermal Medication Administration. (From Zerwekh, J., Garneau, A., & Miller, C. J. [2017]. *Digital collection of the memory notebooks of nursing images* [4th ed]. Chandler, AZ: Nursing Education Consultants, Inc.)

ADMINISTRATION OF MEDICATIONS BY INHALATION

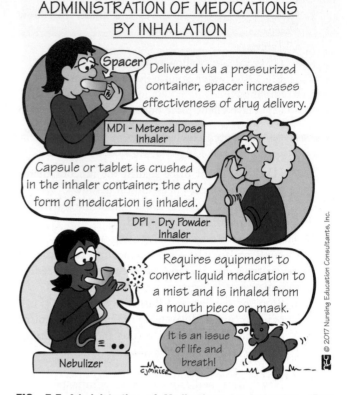

FIG. 5.5 Administration of Medications by Inhalation. (From Zerwekh, J., Garneau, A., & Miller, C. J. [2017]. *Digital collection of the memory notebooks of nursing images* [4th ed]. Chandler, AZ: Nursing Education Consultants, Inc.)

INJECTION ROUTES

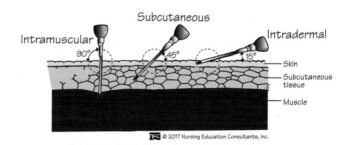

FIG. 5.6 Injection Routes. Needle insertion angles for intramuscular, subcutaneous, and intradermal injections. (From Zerwekh, J., Garneau, A., & Miller, C. J. [2017]. *Digital collection of the memory notebooks of nursing images* [4th ed]. Chandler, AZ: Nursing Education Consultants, Inc.)

5. Patch must come in contact with skin; excessive body hair may need to be removed. Do not shave the area; use scissors to clip hair from area.

E. Inhalation medication: medication is in an aerosol or powder form and is inhaled and absorbed throughout the respiratory tract (Fig. 5.5).
1. Place client in semi-Fowler position.
2. Check instructions for use of inhaler and make sure client understands.
   a. Shake the metered-dose inhaler (MDI) vigorously (3–5 seconds) to mix the medication.
   b. Insert the MDI mouthpiece into the spacer and place into the mouth.
   c. Press down once while inhaling slowly through the mouth.
   d. Hold breath for 10 seconds.
   e. Remove the inhaler from the mouth and exhale slowly through pursed lips.
   f. Repeat, if ordered. (Wait 1 minute between inhalation of bronchodilators to allow medication to take effect.)
   g. Rinse mouth with water and spit it out. (Removes remaining medication and reduces risk of infection and irritation.)

F. Parenteral medications: administration of medications by some method of injection.
1. Injection routes (Fig. 5.6).
2. Selection of a syringe: Select a syringe and type of needle that are appropriate for the type of parenteral medication to be administered.

3. Intradermal injection: administered just below the skin surface.
   a. Use a syringe with appropriate calibrations because amount is small in volume (0.01–0.1 mL).
   b. Use a tuberculin or 1-mL syringe with a small-gauge (25- or 27-gauge) needle, ⅜ to ⅝ inch long.
   c. Select area where skin is thin (e.g., inner surface of forearm, middle of back).
   d. Insert needle bevel edge up at a 5- to 15-degree angle.

e. Frequently used for tuberculin testing, administration of local anesthetic, allergy testing.

4. Subcutaneous injection: medication is injected into fatty tissue, just below the dermis.

   a. Medication should be small in volume (0.5–1 mL) and nonirritating.

   b. Areas on outer surface of upper arm, anterior surface of the thigh, and the abdomen are frequent sites.

   c. Use a 25-gauge needle that is ⅝ inches long and insert at a 45-degree angle or a 25-gauge needle that is ½ inch long and insert at a 90-degree angle.

DELTOID MUSCLE INJECTION SITE in the UPPER ARM

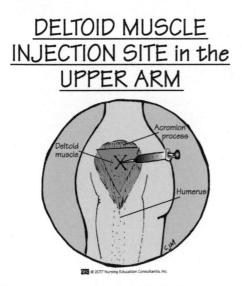

FIG. 5.7 Deltoid Muscle Injection Site in the Upper Arm. (From Zerwekh, J., Garneau, A., & Miller, C. J. [2017]. *Digital collection of the memory notebooks of nursing images* [4th ed]. Chandler, AZ: Nursing Education Consultants, Inc.)

5. Intramuscular (IM) injection: injection of medication into the muscle.

   a. The amount of medication is usually 0.5 to 3 mL.

   b. Appropriate sites.
      (1) Deltoid (Fig. 5.7).
      (2) Ventrogluteal (Fig. 5.8) and vastus lateralis muscles (Fig. 5.9).

   c. Use a 1-inch to 1½-inch needle; gauge of needle depends on viscosity of medication; insert needle at 90-degree angle.
      (1) For oil-based or viscous medications, use an 18- to 22-gauge needle.
      (2) For less viscous medications, use a 20- to 22-gauge needle.

   d. Aspirate when needle is in place (make sure the needle is not in a vein or artery); if no blood returns, administer medication at a rate of 1 mL every 10 seconds. According to the Centers for Disease Control and Prevention, there is no longer any need to aspirate after the needle is injected when *administering vaccines*.

   e. Z-track technique is used to prevent medication from leaking back through the needle track and irritating or staining subcutaneous tissue.
      (1) After medication is drawn up, change the needle.
      (2) Pull skin over to one side at the injection site.
      (3) Inject medication into taut skin at site selected.
      (4) Remove the needle and release the skin. As the stretched skin returns to its original position, the needle track is sealed.
      (5) The preferable site is the ventrogluteal area.

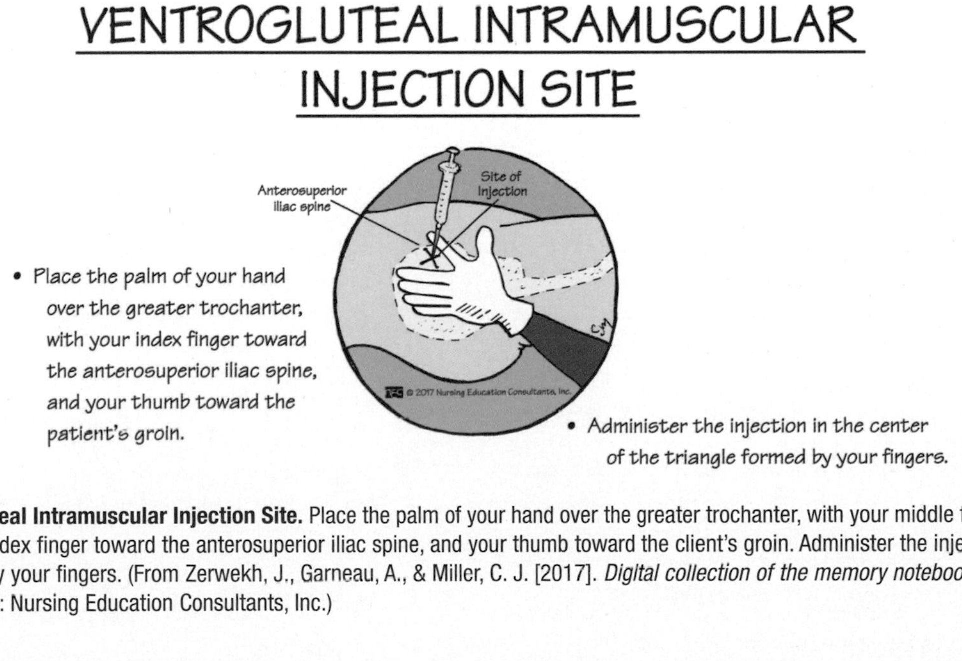

VENTROGLUTEAL INTRAMUSCULAR INJECTION SITE

- Place the palm of your hand over the greater trochanter, with your index finger toward the anterosuperior iliac spine, and your thumb toward the patient's groin.

- Administer the injection in the center of the triangle formed by your fingers.

FIG. 5.8 Ventrogluteal Intramuscular Injection Site. Place the palm of your hand over the greater trochanter, with your middle finger pointed toward the iliac crest, your index finger toward the anterosuperior iliac spine, and your thumb toward the client's groin. Administer the injection in the center of the triangle formed by your fingers. (From Zerwekh, J., Garneau, A., & Miller, C. J. [2017]. *Digital collection of the memory notebooks of nursing images* [4th ed]. Chandler, AZ: Nursing Education Consultants, Inc.)

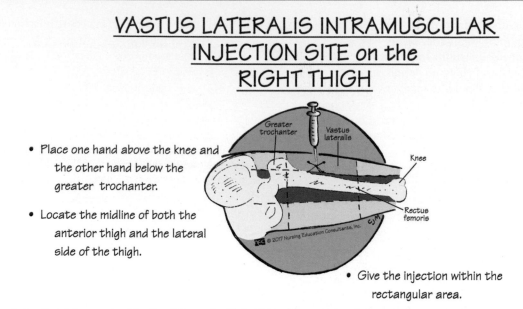

VASTUS LATERALIS INTRAMUSCULAR INJECTION SITE on the RIGHT THIGH

- Place one hand above the knee and the other hand below the greater trochanter.

- Locate the midline of both the anterior thigh and the lateral side of the thigh.

- Give the injection within the rectangular area.

FIG. 5.9 Vastus Lateralis Intramuscular Injection Site on the Right Thigh. Place one hand above the knee and the other hand below the greater trochanter. Locate the midline of both the anterior thigh and the lateral side of the thigh. Give the injection within the rectangular area. (From Zerwekh, J., Garneau, A., & Miller, C. J. [2017]. *Digital collection of the memory notebooks of nursing images* [4th ed]. Chandler, AZ: Nursing Education Consultants, Inc.)

f. Intramuscular injections in children.
   (1) Vastus lateralis muscle is a common site in infants (see Fig. 5.9).
   (2) Ventrogluteal site is the preferred site in children.
   (3) A 22-gauge, 1-inch needle is appropriate for an IM injection in most children.

> **❗ NURSING PRIORITY** Subcutaneous, intramuscular, and intradermal routes are avoided in clients with bleeding tendencies.

6. IV administration: injection of medication into the blood (Table 5.3).
   a. Administration of large volumes of liquid by infusion.
   b. Administration of irritating medications by piggyback method.
      (1) Dilute medication according to directions, usually 25 to 250 mL of a compatible intravenous fluid like normal saline (NS).
      (2) Assess patency of primary infusion.
      (3) Connect medication and adjust flow rate for the time designated, usually 30 to 45 minutes.
      (4) Administration of medications through IV piggyback method enhances the action of the medication.
      (5) *Always follow facility and state guidelines regarding parenteral nutrition (PN) administration of IV piggyback medication.*
      (6) *IV push or bolus is administered by the registered nurse.*

> **❗ TEST ALERT** Calculate and monitor intravenous flow rate. Administer intravenous piggyback (secondary) medications.

c. Vascular access device (VAD) or central IV therapy: placed in a central bold vessel such as the superior vena cava (SVC). Multiple types are available, depending on the purpose, the duration of the therapy being administered, and the availability of insertion sites.
   (1) Peripherally inserted central catheter (PICC).
   (2) Nontunneled percutaneous central catheter.
   (3) Tunneled central catheter.
   (4) Implanted port.
d. Epidural catheter: inserted in the epidural space allowing for the administration of bolus or continuous infusion. Analgesia administered into the epidural space can reach the systemic circulation in significant amounts, which could cause respiratory depression.

Forms of Medication Preparations

A. Solids.
   1. Capsule: medication is placed in cylindrical gelatin container.
   2. Pills, tablets: medication is pressed into solid form in various shapes and colors.
      a. Enteric-coated: prevents medication from being released in stomach; dissolves in intestine. Do not crush enteric-coated, extended-release (ER), or sustained-release (SR) tablets.
      b. Lozenge: flavored tablet is held in the mouth for slow release of medication.
   3. Suppositories: keep these in cool area; will melt at body temperature; may produce local or systemic effects.
      a. Rectal.
      b. Vaginal.

Table 5.3 INTRAVENOUS MEDICATION ADMINISTRATION

Method	Injection Rate	Nursing Implications
IV push or bolus	Rate of administration is determined by the amount of medication that can be given each minute based on each drug's protocol.	1. Drug is not diluted and is injected directly into the client's venous system. 2. Access is most often through an existing IV infusion. Use the access port closest to the client. 3. It has a rapid effect on the CNS and cardiopulmonary systems. 4. IV push or bolus is the most dangerous delivery method. Extreme care should be taken in following the drug protocol. If in doubt, do not deliver the bolus.
Intermittent infusion or piggyback (IVPB)	Medication is diluted in 25–250 mL and infused over 15–60 minutes.	1. Drug is diluted to decrease toxicity and hypertonicity of the solution. 2. It is the method of choice for multiple daily doses, especially antibiotics. 3. Concentrated medications require higher dilution and longer infusion time.
Constant and variable-rate infusion	Pump is set to deliver constant rate of infusion based on dose and dilution of medication.	1. This method is used for medications that need to be highly diluted (chemotherapeutic drugs). 2. It provides for continuous medication infusion.
Intermittent venous access or saline or heparin lock	IV catheter is capped off on the end with a small chamber covered by a rubber diaphragm or specially designed cap.	1. Increased mobility, safety, and comfort for the client. 2. Access must be flushed after medication is administered; generally normal saline is used; some agencies use heparin, which needs flushed before as well as after the medication.

CNS, Central nervous system; *IV*, intravenous.
Note: Always follow agency and nurse practice act guidelines for IV administration of medications by the licensed practical nurse/licensed vocational nurse.

4. Ointments: used for external application.
5. Powders: finely ground medications that are stable only in dry form; frequently mixed with solution before administration.
B. Solutions.
   1. Syrups: medication prepared in an aqueous sugar solution.
   2. Elixirs: solutions containing alcohol, sugar, and water.
   3. Suspensions: finely ground particles of medication dispersed in a liquid; shake all suspensions well before preparing dose (antacids).
   4. Emulsions: medication is dispersed in an oil or fat solution; shake all emulsions well before preparing dose.
   5. Liniments, lotions: medication dispersed in a mixture of oil, soap, alcohol, or water; used for external application.

Calculation of Medication Dosages

Occasionally, the health care provider orders medications in amounts not supplied by the pharmacy. In these situations, the nurse must calculate the correct dosage. Another important area of calculation is in the administration of IV solutions. Thus it is essential that the nurse have a good working knowledge of the fundamental principles of mathematics to calculate medication dosages correctly.

Oral Medication Calculations

Dose desired ÷ Dose on hand = Amount to give

Example: Order reads to give cephalexin 500 mg. Dose on hand is 250 mg capsules.

$$500 \div 250 = 2 \text{ capsules}$$

Dose desired ÷ Dose on hand × Quantity = Amount to give

Example: Order reads to give ampicillin 350 mg. Dose on hand is 250 mg in 5 mL.

$$350 \div 250 \times 5 = x$$
$$350 \div 250 = 1.4$$
$$1.4 \times 5\,\text{mL} = 7\,\text{mL}$$

The problem also can be set up as an algebraic proportion:

$$350/x = 250/5\,\text{mL}$$
$$250x = 1750\,\text{mL}$$
$$x = 7\,\text{mL}$$

Parenteral Medication Calculations

Dose desired ÷ Dose on hand × Quantity of solution = Amount to give

Example: Order reads gentamicin 60 mg IM. Dose on hand is 80 mg in 1 mL.

$$60\,mg \div 80\,mg \times 1\,mL = x$$
$$60 \div 80 = 0.75$$
$$0.75 \times 1\,mL = 3/4\,mL\,or\,0.75\,mL$$

Set up as an algebraic proportion, the equation reads:

$$60\,mg\,/\,x = 80\,mg\,/\,1\,mL$$
$$80x = 60$$
$$x = 0.75\,mL\,or\,3/4\,mL$$

Intravenous Medication Calculations

- To determine how long an infusion will run, divide the total number of milliliters to infuse by the hourly infusion rate.

$$\text{Amount to infuse} \div \text{Hourly rate} = \text{Number of hours}$$

Example: Order reads 1000 mL at 125 mL/hr. How long will it take the 1000 mL to infuse?

$$1000 \div 125 = x$$
$$1000 \div 125 = 8\,hours$$

- To determine the rate in milliliters per hour at which an infusion will run, divide the total number of milliliters to infuse by the infusion time.

$$\text{Amount to infuse} \div \text{Total infusion time} = \text{Rate}(mL/hr)$$

Example: Order reads 1000 mL to run every 8 hours. At what rate in milliliters per hour will the medication be infused?

$$1000\,mL \div 8\,hr = 125\,mL/hr$$

- Calculating drop factors: Check the IV equipment to determine how many drops are delivered in 1 mL. For example, a drop factor of 10 gtt per 1 mL is used. The following are two formulas with which to calculate this factor.

$$\text{Total mL/Time in min} = mL\,/\,min \times \text{Drop factor}$$
$$= gtt\,/\,min$$

Example: 1000 mL is ordered to infuse in 8 hours. Set drop factor is 10 gtt/mL.

$$1000\,mL \div 480\,min = 2.08\,mL/min$$
$$2.08 \times 10 = 20.8\,or\,21\,gtt/min$$

Example: 500 mL is ordered to infuse in 2 hours (250 mL/hr to infuse). Set drop factor is 10 gtt/mL.

$$500\,mL \div 120\,min = 4.16 \times 10 = 41.6\,or\,42\,gtt/min$$

- Determine the number of milliliters per hour and divide by 60 (60 minutes in 1 hour). This equals the number of milliliters per minute. Multiply by set drop factor calibration of number of drops per milliliter.

$$\text{Number of milliliters per hour} \div 60 = mL\,/\,min$$
$$\text{Rate}(mL/min) \times \text{Set calibration} = gtt\,/\,min$$

Example: 500 mL is ordered to infuse in 2 hours. Set drop factor is 10 gtt/mL (250 mL/hr to infuse).

$$250\,mL \div 60 = 4.16\,mL/min$$
$$4.16\,mL \times 10 = 41.6\,or\,42\,gtt/min$$

Note: *There may be a difference of 2 to 4 gtt when different formulas are used.*

Appendix 5.1 CONVERSIONS

CELSIUS AND FAHRENHEIT	POUNDS AND GRAMS
Fahrenheit reading = 9/5 × Celsius reading + 32	1 pound = 454 gm
Example: Temperature is 50°C	To convert pounds to grams, multiply the number of pounds by 454.
Fahrenheit = 9/5 × 50 + 32	7.5 × 454 = 3405 gm
90 + 32 = 122°F	To convert grams to pounds, divide the number of grams by 454.
	Example: An infant weighs 3405 gm
	3405/454 = 7.5 lb, or 7 lb 8 oz

Appendix 5.2 COMMON ABBREVIATIONS AND SYMBOLS

Ac	before meals
ad lib	as desired
bid	twice daily
c	with
Ca	calcium
CBC	complete blood count
Cl	chloride
gm	gram
gtt	drops
H2O	water
H2O2	hydrogen peroxide
K	potassium
L	liter
Mg	magnesium
mcg	micrograms
mL	milliliter
N	nitrogen
Na	sodium
NPO	nothing by mouth
OOB	out of bed
pc	after meals
po	by mouth
PRN	as needed
qid	four times a day
q2h	every 2 hours
q3h	every 3 hours
S	without
Stat	immediately
tab	tablet
tid	three times a day

Appendix 5.3 UNDERSTANDING MEDICAL TERMINOLOGY: PREFIXES AND SUFFIXES

Prefixes

cef-	antibiotic (cephalosporin)
ceph-	antibiotic (cephalosporin)
nitr-	vasodilator
sulf-	antibiotic (sulfonamide)

Suffixes

-actone	potassium-sparing diuretic
-ane	general anesthetic
-arin, -aban, - rudin	anticoagulant

Continued

Appendix 5.3 UNDERSTANDING MEDICAL TERMINOLOGY: PREFIXES AND SUFFIXES—cont'd

R̲x̲

-ase	thrombolytic
-azine	antiemetic
-azole	antifungal
-azosin	alpha blocker
-barbital	barbiturate (sedative-hypnotic)
-caine	local anesthetic
-cillin	antibiotic (penicillin)
-coxib	COX-2 inhibitors
-cycline	antibiotic (tetracycline)
-dipine	calcium-channel blocker
-done	opioid analgesics
-dronate	bisphosphonates
-floxacin	antibiotic (fluoroquinolone)
-gliptin	oral hypoglycemic (DPP-4 inhibitor)
-glitazone	oral hypoglycemic (glitazone)
-grel	antiplatelet
-ide	oral hypoglycemic and loop diuretic
-kinase	thrombolytic
-lam	antianxiety agent; benzodiazepines
-mycin (micin)	antibiotic (aminoglycosides, macrolides)
-mide	diuretics
-nium	neuromuscular blocking agents
-olol	beta-blockers
-oxin	cardiac glycoside
-pam	antianxiety agent
-phylline	bronchodilator
-prazole	proton pump inhibitor (PPI)
-pril	angiotensin-converting enzyme (ACE) inhibitor
-profen	nonsteroidal antiinflammatory drug (NSAID)
-ridone	atypical antipsychotic
-sartan	angiotensin II blocker
-sone	steroid
-statin	antihyperlipidemic; HMG-CoA reductase inhibitor
-stigmine	cholinergic
-stine	antineoplastic
-tidine	H2 receptor antagonist (antiulcer)
-triptan	antimigraine
-vir	antiviral (protease inhibitors)
-zepam, -zolam	benzodiazepine
-zide	thiazide diuretic
-zine	phenothiazine
-zole	antifungal (azoles)
-zone	oral hypoglycemic (glitazone)

Use these helpful prefixes and suffixes to assist in identifying medication generic names (Fig. 5.10).

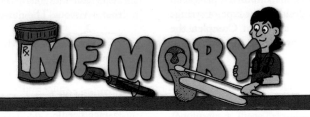

FIG. 5.10 Memory. (From Zerwekh, J., & Miller, C. J. [2020]. *NCLEX review course.* Chandler, AZ: Nursing Education Consultants, Inc.)

⚡ Practice & Next Generation NCLEX (NGN) Questions

More questions on

Pharmacology and Medication Administration

1. The health care provider orders an IV piggyback of cefotetan 1 gm in 100 mL D5W to run over 30 minutes. The drop factor for the tubing is 10 gtt/mL. At what rate in drops per minute would you run the IV? **Fill in the blank**.
   Answer: _____ gtt/min

2. A client has an order for fluoxetine 20 mg in the a.m. and at noon; 10-mg tablets are available. How many tablets will the client receive each day? **Fill in the blank**.
   Answer: _____ tablets

3. A client is prescribed heparin 5000 units subcutaneously, every 12 hours. The medication vial reads heparin 10,000 units/mL. The nurse prepares how many mL to administer one dose? **Fill in the blank**.
   Answer: _____ mL

4. The health care provider has indicated that ampicillin and gentamicin are to be given piggyback in the same hour, every 6 hours (2400-0600-1200-1800). How would the nurse administer these drugs?
   1. Give both drugs together IV push.
   2. Give each drug separately, flushing between drugs.
   3. Retrograde both drugs into the tubing.
   4. Give one drug every 4 hours and one every 6 hours.

5. What should the nurse take into consideration when planning to give medication to an older adult client?
   1. Multiple simultaneous drugs can be dangerous.
   2. The older client metabolizes and excretes medications differently from younger clients.
   3. Medications affect the older client during the early hours of the morning.
   4. Medications have an effect on the respiratory system of the older adult.

6. Which of the following is correct regarding the administration of an intradermal injection?
   1. It forms a bleb in the epidermis area of the skin.
   2. The injection is given at a 40-degree angle.
   3. The injection site is pressed and rubbed in a circular motion.
   4. A 16-gauge needle is used.

7. What is the correct method for administering eyedrops to an older adult client?
   1. Drop the medication directly on the cornea.
   2. Instruct the client to rapidly open and close their eye to distribute the medication.
   3. Place the applicator tip on the lower conjunctival sac and instill the drops.
   4. Instill the drops in the lower conjunctival sac.

8. At the shift handoff report, a nurse is told that one of their clients is becoming tolerant to pain medication. What nursing observation would agree with this conclusion?
   1. The current medication order, which has previously been effective, is no longer providing adequate pain relief.
   2. The client becomes irritable and confused before the next scheduled dose of medication.
   3. Pain medication is being administered every 3 to 4 hours around the clock for adequate pain relief.
   4. The client is sleeping, arouses with physical and verbal stimulation, but is very lethargic.

9. The nurse is preparing to administer an intramuscular injection to an infant who is 8 months old. Which muscle would be the most appropriate injection site?
   1. Deltoid.
   2. Dorsogluteal.
   3. Vastus lateralis.
   4. Ventrogluteal.

10. A client is postoperative thyroidectomy and is experiencing some dysphagia following surgery. The nurse is to administer the client's oral medications. What is an appropriate nursing intervention?
   1. Crush only enteric-coated medications.
   2. Crush each medication and administer separately.
   3. Mix all crushed medications together and dilute with water for ease of administration.
   4. Obtain only sustained-release preparations of the medications so the capsules can be opened.

12. An adult client is being scheduled for outpatient surgery for repair of a deviated nasal septum. The surgery is scheduled for the following week. **Highlight information in the client's health history that require further action and follow-up by the nurse prior to the scheduled surgery.**

Health History	Nurses' Notes	Provider Orders	Laboratory Results

1400 Client has a history of difficulty breathing through the nose for the past 2 years and has been diagnosed with a deviated nasal septum. Client denies nosebleeds, sneezing, headaches, or buzzing in the ears, but has difficulty smelling. A septoplasty and rhinoplasty procedure is scheduled. Client reports taking several herbal remedies for various conditions, including saw palmetto, ginkgo biloba, and garlic.

Other findings noted on the assessment include:

- Bruised, ecchymosis area on forehead
- Random blood sugar 89 mg/dL at 1000
- Temperature: 100°F (37.9°C)
- BP: 124/78 mmHg
- Heart rate: 68 bpm and regular
- Respirations: 18 breaths/min
- SpO$_2$: 98% on room air

Client Needs: Physiological Integrity/Pharmacological Therapies
Clinical Judgment/Cognitive Skill: Recognize Cues
Item Type: Highlight in Text
Rationale & Test-Taking Strategy: Difficulty breathing through the nose and loss of smell are associated with a deviated nasal septum. The health care provider must know of all medications – including nonprescription drugs, supplements, and herbs that the client is taking. Before surgery, the client should stop taking drugs like aspirin, ibuprofen, naproxen, and certain herbal supplements, as many herbal remedies can affect coagulation; they should be stopped at least a week before surgery. Garlic suppresses plate aggregation and can increase the risk of bleeding. Ginkgo biloba may suppress coagulation and promote seizures. Saw palmetto has an antiplatelet effect. The temperature elevation should be followed up. Blood sugar is within normal limits for a random specimen. The bruised area on the forehead could be a symptom related to taking the herbal medications.

CHAPTER SIX

Homeostasis and Immune Concepts

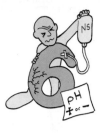

FLUID AND ELECTROLYTES

Physiology

A. Basic concepts of body fluid.

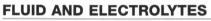

1. Water is the primary component of body fluid. It is used to transport nutrients, electrolytes, and oxygen to the cells and to remove waste products.
2. Intracellular fluid: provides the cell with internal fluid necessary for cellular function.
   a. Approximately 40 to 50% of body weight (two-thirds of total body water).
   b. Electrolytes: potassium (primary), magnesium, phosphate.
3. Extracellular (intravascular and interstitial) fluids: transport system for cellular waste, oxygen, electrolytes, and nutrients; help regulate body temperature; lubricate and cushion joints.
   a. Approximately 20 to 30% of body weight (one-third of total body water).
   b. An infant maintains a larger percentage of extracellular fluids than does an older child or adult.
   c. Vascular: circulating plasma volume.
   d. Interstitial: fluid surrounding tissue cells.
   e. Electrolytes: sodium (primary), chloride, bicarbonate.

B. Dynamic transport of fluid and electrolytes.
1. Diffusion: movement of molecules from an area of high concentration to an area of low concentration.
2. Osmosis: movement of water through a semipermeable membrane from an area of low electrolyte concentration to an area of high concentration; osmotic pressure is the term used to describe osmosis (water goes where the salt is).
3. Filtration: movement of water and electrolytes through a semipermeable membrane from an area of high pressure to an area of low pressure.
4. Hydrostatic pressure: term used to describe the force of filtration exerted by the pumping action of the heart.
5. Osmolality refers to the concentration of the dissolved particles in a solution; osmolality controls the movement of fluid in each of the compartments.
   a. Hyperosmolar (hypertonic): fluids in which the concentration of solutes is higher than in the cells.
   b. Hypo-osmolar (hypotonic): fluids in which the concentration of solutes is less than in the cells.
   c. Iso-osmolar (isotonic): fluids with the same osmolality as the cells; normal distribution of solutes and water in body fluid.

C. Fluid shifts.
1. Plasma to interstitial fluid shift (edema).
   a. Edema: accumulation of fluid in interstitial spaces.
   b. Hypovolemia may occur as a result of excessive fluid shift into the interstitial spaces, resulting in circulatory collapse (client with burns).
2. Interstitial to plasma fluid shift: movement of fluid back into the circulatory volume, as in a client with mobilization of burn edema or in the case of excessive administration of hypertonic solution; client may demonstrate symptoms of circulatory overload.
3. Fluid spacing.
   a. First spacing: normal distribution of fluids.
   b. Second spacing: abnormal accumulation of interstitial fluid—edema.
   c. Third spacing: fluid that is trapped and cannot easily move back into extracellular fluid (ECF) (e.g., edema associated with burns and ascites).

TEST ALERT Identify signs and symptoms of client fluid and/or electrolyte imbalances and provide interventions to restore client fluid and/or electrolyte balance.

Fluid Imbalances

Assessment: Recognize Cues

A. *Fluid deficit*: extracellular fluid volume deficit hypovolemia results from vascular fluid volume loss.
1. Sensible fluid loss: fluid loss of which an individual is aware, as in urine.
2. Insensible fluid loss: fluid loss of which an individual is not aware (approximately 600–900 mL of fluid is lost every 24 hours through the skin and lungs in a healthy adult).
3. Causes of fluid deficit (all result from loss of both water and sodium).
   a. Decreased fluid intake.
   b. Loss of fluid through the gastrointestinal (GI) tract, as in vomiting, nasogastric suctioning, diarrhea, colostomy, and/or ileostomy drainage.
   c. Excessive excretion due to kidney disease.
   d. Loss due to overuse of diuretics or inadequate replacement of fluid loss.
   e. Increased insensible fluid loss through skin and lungs due to febrile state, increased respiratory rates.

policy) unless complications (inflammation, irritation, or fluid extravasation) occur at the site.

B. Carefully monitor the infusion rate: control with either a roller clamp or an infusion pump.

C. Discontinue intravenous infusion.
1. Perform hand hygiene and apply clean gloves (Box 6.1).
2. Turn off infusion rate.
3. Remove IV site dressing and any tape securing catheter (do not use scissors).
4. Hold catheter hub and clean site with antiseptic swab and allow to dry.
5. Place sterile gauze over venipuncture site and apply light pressure while withdrawing catheter using a slow, steady motion. Keep hub parallel to skin, that is, do not raise or lift catheter before it is completely out of vein.
6. Inspect end of catheter, being sure it is intact after removal.
7. Document removal in client chart.

> **! NURSING PRIORITY** Check the IV fluid for expiration date, color, and clarity. Always monitor the rate of infusion by evaluating the amount of fluid that has actually been infused and by checking the pump or IV control settings.

Indications for Use of Infusion Pumps

A. To deliver a medication that requires a precise rate of administration (vasopressor agents, patient-controlled analgesia).

B. To deliver fluids that would precipitate adverse effects if administered too rapidly (total parenteral nutrition).

♣ C. To deliver fluids in controlled amounts to clients very sensitive to volume administered (infants, children younger than 10 years of age, older adult clients, clients with pulmonary edema, cardiac problems, hypertension, and with decreased kidney function).

> **TEST ALERT** Operate and monitor the use of an infusion pump.

COMPLICATIONS OF PERIPHERAL INTRAVENOUS THERAPY (FIG. 6.3)

> **TEST ALERT** Identify and treat a client IV line infiltration.

Infiltration

Assessment: Recognize Cues

A. Common causes: dislodging of the needle/catheter by client movement or obstruction of fluid flow.

B. Signs and symptoms: edema, *blanching of skin*, discomfort at site, fluid that is flowing slowly or has stopped, *cooler skin temperature*.

Nursing Intervention: Take Action

A. Preventive nursing management: use the smallest gauge of catheter possible; use an arm board to stabilize

> **Box 6.1 GUIDELINES TO DECREASE INFECTION RELATED TO INTRAVENOUS THERAPY**
>
> - Use a >0.5% chlorhexidine skin preparation with alcohol for antisepsis.
> - Avoid routine replacement of central venous catheters.
> - Select catheters on the basis of intended duration of use, known infectious and noninfectious complications, and experience of individual catheter operators.
> - Use a midline catheter or PICC instead of a short peripheral catheter when the duration of IV therapy will likely exceed 6 days.
> - Remove peripheral venous catheters if the client develops signs of phlebitis, infection, or a malfunctioning catheter.
> - When adherence to aseptic technique cannot be ensured, replace the catheter as soon as possible.
> - Perform hand hygiene by washing hands with conventional soap and water or with alcohol-based hand rubs. Hand hygiene should be performed before and after palpating, inserting, replacing, accessing, repairing, or dressing an intravascular catheter site.
> - Use either sterile gauze or sterile, transparent, semipermeable dressing to cover the catheter site.
> - Replace catheter site dressing if the dressing becomes damp, loosened, or visibly soiled.
> - Do not use topical antibiotic ointment on insertion sites.
> - Replace gauze dressings every 2 days and transparent dressings every 7 days.
> - Use a sutureless securement device to reduce the risk of infection for IV catheters.
> - Replace tubing used for blood, blood products, or fat emulsions within 24 hr of initiating the infusion.
> - Replace tubing used to administer propofol infusions every 6 to 12 hr.
>
> *IV*, Intravenous; *PICC*, peripherally inserted central catheter.
> From Centers for Disease Control and Prevention (CDC). 2011 *Guidelines for the prevention of intravascular catheter-related infections.* Updated February 15, 2017. https://www.cdc.gov/infectioncontrol/guidelines/BSI/index.html

catheter, especially for restless, confused clients or those with catheters placed in the antecubital fossa area; check frequently for coolness of skin around site; avoid looping tubing below bed level; check IV flow rate at least every 1 to 2 hours.

B. Discontinue IV solution and remove catheter.

C. Apply warm, moist heat for 20 minutes to increase fluid absorption (if not contraindicated); may reapply warm, moist heat three to four times throughout the day; raise affected extremity to increase venous return and reduce swelling.

D. *If infiltrated solution contains an irritating medication (chemotherapy, vasoconstrictive fluids), notify the registered nurse (RN) immediately. Do not remove IV catheter as an antidote will be administered directly to the site by the RN.*

E. *Anticipate the RN will insert an IV at another site.*

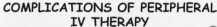
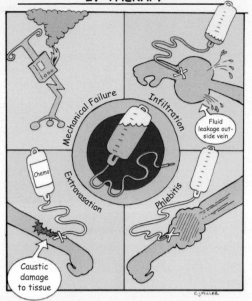

FIG. 6.3 Complications of Peripheral IV Therapy. (From Zerwekh, J. [2023]. *Mosby's fluids and electrolytes memory notecards: Visual, mnemonic, and memory aids for nurses* [3rd ed.]. Mosby.)

Phlebitis

Assessment: Recognize Cues

A. Common causes: overuse of a vein; irritating infusion solutions or medications; catheter left in vein for too long; use of large-gauge catheters.

B. Signs and symptoms: tenderness, pain along the course of the vein, edema, *redness at insertion site*, red streak along course of vein, *extremity with IV feels warmer than other extremity.*

Nursing Intervention: Take Action

A. Change IV site every 72 to 96 hours or per policy.

B. Use large veins to administer irritating solutions.

C. Stabilize cannula.

D. Dilute medications adequately and infuse at prescribed rates.

E. Choose the smallest-gauge catheter possible to administer solutions.

F. Apply warm, moist compresses to stimulate circulation and promote absorption.

TEST ALERT Evaluate client response to parenteral fluid therapy.

ACID-BASE BALANCE

Basic Concepts of Acid-Base Balance

A. Terms used to describe acid-base balance.
 1. pH: the chemical abbreviation for negative logarithm of hydrogen ion concentration.

Table 6.1 BLOOD GAS VALUES

Component	Normal Values
pH	7.4 (7.35–7.45)
PaO_2	80–100 mm Hg
$PaCo_2$	35–45 mm Hg
HCO_3^-	22–26 mEq/L(mmol/L)

Acid-Base Mnemonic (ROME)

Remember **ROME**—the acid-base mnemonic to interpret blood gas values!

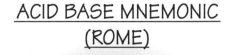
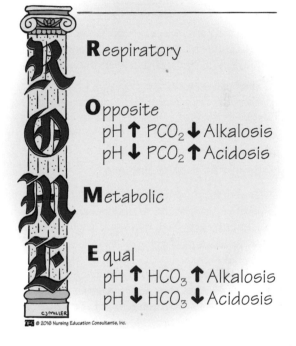

2. CO_2: carbon dioxide.
3. $PaCo_2$: pressure of dissolved CO_2 gas in the blood.
4. O_2: oxygen.
5. PaO_2: pressure of dissolved O_2 gas in the blood.
6. HCO_3^-: bicarbonate.
7. mm Hg: millimeters of mercury.
8. H^+: hydrogen ion concentration.

B. Normal blood gas values (Table 6.1).
 1. pH 7.4 (7.35–7.45).
 2. PaO_2: 80 to 100 mm Hg.
 3. $PaCo_2$: 35 to 45 mm Hg.
 4. HCO_3^-: 22 to 26 milliequivalents (mEq/L).

C. The H^+ concentration determines the acidity or alkalinity of a solution (pH); increased pH has fewer H^+ ions and is more alkaline; decreased pH has more H^+ ions and is more acidic (Fig. 6.4).

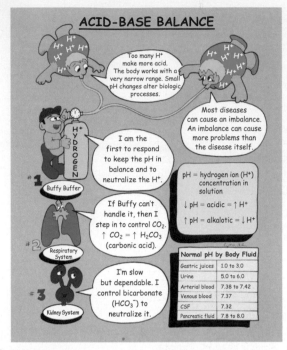

FIG. 6.4 Acid-Base Balance. (From Zerwekh, J. [2023]. *Mosby's fluids and electrolytes memory notecards: Visual, mnemonic, and memory aids for nurses* [3rd ed.]. Mosby.)

Regulation of Acid-Base Balance

A. Buffer system: continuously regulates acid-base balance.

B. Respiratory system: the second most rapid response in regulating the acid-base balance. Carbonic acid is transported to the lungs, where it is converted to CO_2 and water, then excreted.

> ❗ **NURSING PRIORITY** Hyperventilation is associated with an increase in pH or a decrease in P_{CO2} ($CO2$ is lost). Hypoventilation is associated with a decrease in pH or an increase in P_{CO2} ($CO2$ is retained).

C. Kidney system: the slowest, but very effective, mechanism of acid-base regulation.

Alterations in Acid-Base Balance

> **TEST ALERT** Identify laboratory values for arterial blood gases (ABGs).

A. **Respiratory acidosis**: characterized by excessive retention of CO_2 due to hypoventilation; therefore an increased carbonic acid concentration produces an increase in H^+ ions and a decrease in pH (decreases below 7.35).

Assessment: Recognize Cues

1. Causes: conditions that cause decreased respiratory function.
   a. Head injuries.
   b. Oversedation with sedatives and/or narcotics.
   c. Asthma, bronchitis, emphysema, cystic fibrosis.
   d. Pneumonia, atelectasis.
   e. Thoracic trauma: flail chest.
   f. Guillain-Barré syndrome, myasthenia gravis, polio.
   g. Mechanical hypoventilation.
2. Clinical manifestations.
   a. Rapid, shallow respirations (hypoventilation).
   b. Disorientation, decreased level of consciousness.
   c. Decreased blood pressure.
   d. Ventricular irritability related to hyperkalemia.
   e. Hypoxemia secondary to respiratory depression.
3. Blood gas values.
   a. pH decreases below 7.35.
   b. $PaCO_2$ increases above 45 mm Hg.
   c. HCO_3^- remains normal, unless compensating, then increases.

Nursing Intervention: Take Action

1. Preventive management.
   a. Have client turn, cough, and deep-breathe every 2 hours after surgery.
   b. Use narcotics carefully in the immediate postoperative period.
   c. Maintain adequate hydration.
2. Use semi-Fowler position to facilitate deep breathing.
3. Thoroughly assess client's pulmonary function.
4. Perform postural drainage and percussion, followed by suction, to remove excessive pulmonary secretions.
5. Anticipate the need for mechanical ventilation if client does not respond to pulmonary hygiene.
6. Anticipate use of bronchodilator.
7. Administer O_2 with caution because it may precipitate CO_2 narcosis.
8. Monitor for hyperkalemia.
9. *Report any changes in the client's respiratory status to the RN.*

> **TEST ALERT** Identify changes in respiratory status; provide pulmonary hygiene. The concept of respiratory acidosis may be tested in a variety of situations, especially if the condition causes obstruction of the airway or depresses the respiratory system.

B. **Respiratory alkalosis:** characterized by a low $PaCO_2$ due to hyperventilation. An excessive amount of CO_2 is exhaled, resulting in a decrease in H^+ concentration and an increase in pH (above 7.45).

Assessment: Recognize Cues

1. Causes of respiratory alkalosis.
   a. Primary stimulation of central nervous system (CNS): hyperventilation.
      (1) Emotional origin (anxiety, fear, apprehension).
      (2) CNS infection (encephalitis).
      (3) Salicylate poisoning.
   b. Hypoxia stimulates hyperventilation (heart failure, pneumonia, pulmonary emboli).
   c. Fever.
   d. Mechanical hyperventilation, resulting in "overbreathing."

2. Clinical manifestations.
   a. Deep, rapid breathing (hyperventilation).
   b. CNS stimulation, resulting in confusion, lethargy, seizures.
   c. Hypokalemia.
   d. Hyperreflexia, muscle weakness, tingling of extremities.
3. Blood gas values.
   a. pH increases above 7.45.
   b. $PaCo_2$ decreases below 35 mm Hg.
   c. HCO_3^- remains normal, unless compensating, then decreases.
4. Compensation/correction.
   a. Compensation: kidney system will compensate by increasing HCO_3^- excretion and retaining H^+ ions, thus returning pH to a more normal level.
   b. Correction: prevent loss of CO_2 from respiratory systems.

Nursing Intervention: Take Action

1. Identify and eliminate (if possible) causative factor.
2. Evaluate need for sedation.
3. Use rebreathing mask or techniques (paper bag, cupped hands) to increase CO_2 levels.
4. Remain with client to decrease anxiety levels.

C. **Metabolic acidosis**: characterized by a decrease in HCO_3^- level in the serum, leading to an increase in H^+ concentration and a decrease in pH (below 7.35).

Assessment: Recognize Cues

1. Causes.
   a. Diabetic ketoacidosis.
   b. Starvation.
   c. Shock, resulting in lactic acidosis.
   d. Deep, prolonged vomiting may cause excessive loss of base products.
   e. Severe diarrhea and loss of pancreatic secretions.
   f. Renal insufficiency and failure.
   g. Salicylate poisoning due to accumulation of ketone bodies produced as a result of the increased metabolic rate.
2. Clinical manifestations.
   a. Drowsiness, confusion, headache, disorientation.
   b. Deep, rapid respirations (Kussmaul) compensatory action by the lungs.
   c. GI problems: nausea, vomiting, diarrhea.
   d. Dysrhythmias related to hyperkalemia.
   e. Decreased blood pressure.
3. Blood gas values.
   a. pH decreases below 7.35.
   b. $PaCo_2$ remains normal.
   c. HCO_3^- decreases below 22 mEq/L (mmol/L).

Nursing Intervention: Take Action

1. Assist in identification of underlying problem.
2. In severe acidosis, HCO_3^- may be given intravenously to neutralize acid and return pH to normal.
3. In clients with diabetes, evaluate for ketoacidosis and administer insulin accordingly.

4. Assess kidney function and hydration status.
5. Maintain accurate intake and output records.
6. Evaluate laboratory values for hyperkalemia.
7. Support respiratory system to promote compensation.

D. **Metabolic alkalosis**: characterized by an increase in the HCO_3^- levels in the serum, leading to a decrease in the H^+ concentration and an increase in pH (increase above 7.45).

Assessment: Recognize Cues

1. Causes.
   a. Diuretic therapy.
   b. Excessive loss of H^+ ions.
      (1) Prolonged nasogastric suctioning without adequate electrolyte replacement.
      (2) Excessive vomiting, resulting in loss of hydrochloric acid and K^+.
   c. Prolonged steroid therapy.
   d. Excessive intake of bicarbonate (baking soda).
   e. Hypokalemia.
2. Clinical manifestations.
   a. Nausea, vomiting.
   b. Increased irritability, disorientation, restlessness.
   c. Muscle cramping, tremors, seizures.
   d. Shallow, slow respirations (hypoventilation).
   e. Dysrhythmias (tachycardia) related to hypokalemia.
3. Blood gas values.
   a. pH increases above 7.45.
   b. $PaCo_2$ remains normal.
   c. HCO_3^- increases above 26 mEq/L (28 mmol/L).

Nursing Intervention: Take Action

1. Preventive.
   a. Provide foods high in potassium and chloride for client receiving diuretics.
   b. Administer potassium supplement to client receiving long-term diuretic therapy.
   c. Administer IV solution with replacement electrolytes.
2. Maintain accurate intake and output records.
3. Evaluate the laboratory values for a decrease in serum potassium levels.

INFLAMMATION

Inflammation is the tissue response to localized injury or trauma. It is an expected response to tissue injury.

Basic Concepts of Inflammation

A. Acute.
   1. Occurs rapidly.
   2. Neutrophils (white blood cells) arrive first and are usually the predominant cell.
   3. Essential for normal tissue repair.
   4. Examples: skin infection, tonsillitis.
B. Chronic.
   1. Characterized by pain, redness, and swelling.
   2. Persists longer than 2 weeks; has a damaging course that lasts for weeks, months, or even years.

Box 6.3 OLDER ADULT CARE FOCUS

Infections

- Infection may be manifested by changes in behavior: confusion, disorientation.
- Client may not exhibit fever or pain.
- Closely monitor client response to antibiotics, especially with regard to kidney function.
- Maintain adequate hydration.
- Monitor GI function; diarrhea is common with antibiotics.

Box 6.4 SIGNS OF INFECTION

Generalized
- Fever, chills, increased pulse, increased respiratory rate, localized inflammation, joint pain, fatigue, and increased white blood cells

Gastrointestinal Tract
- Diarrhea, nausea, and vomiting

Respiratory Tract
- Purulent sputum, sore throat, chest pain, and congestion

Urinary Tract
- Urgency and frequency, hematuria, purulent discharge, dysuria, and flank pain

---

G. Identify clients at increased risk for infections.
  1. Older adults (Box 6.3).
  2. Immunocompromised clients.
  3. Clients compromised by chronic health care problems.
  4. Poorly nourished clients.
  5. Client with high-risk lifestyle (IV drug use, unprotected sex).

Goal: To promote healing.

A. Encourage high fluid intake when client has a fever: 2000 to 3000 mL daily for adults.
B. Encourage a diet high in protein, carbohydrates, and vitamins—specifically vitamins A, C, and B complex.
C. Immobilize an injured extremity with a cast, splint, or bandage.
D. Administer antipyretic medications (see Appendix 3.2).
E. Identify early signs of infection to facilitate treatment (Box 6.4).

Goal: To decrease pain.

A. Cold packs applied after initial trauma may help decrease swelling and pain.
B. Heat may be used later to promote healing and to localize the inflammatory agents.
C. Elevate the injured area to decrease edema and promote venous return.

TEST ALERT Use correct hand hygiene techniques—soap and water or an antimicrobial cleanser.

Goal: To prevent complications.

A. Identify clients with compromised immune response; they are at high risk for opportunistic infection.
B. Increase surveillance for clients with leukopenia or impaired circulation, clients receiving steroids or drugs that depress bone marrow, and clients exposed to a communicable disease.
C. Protect healing wounds from injury that could be caused by pulling or stretching.

TEST ALERT Protect immunocompromised clients from exposure to infectious diseases and organisms.

Antibiotic-Resistant Infections

Assessment: Recognize Cues

A. Common antibiotic-resistant organisms.
  1. Methicillin-resistant *Staphylococcus aureus*: wound, skin and soft tissue, pneumonia, and bloodstream infections.
  2. Methicillin-resistant *Staphylococcus epidermidis*: skin and mucosa, common with catheter and implants.
  3. Aminoglycoside-resistant *Enterococcus faecalis* and *faecium:* oral root canals and urinary tract infections.
  4. Penicillin-resistant *Streptococcus pneumoniae:* pneumonia.
  5. Cephalosporin-resistant *Klebsiella pneumoniae:* pneumonia.
  6. Cephalosporin-resistant *Neisseria gonorrhoeae:* sexually transmitted infections.
B. Transmission.
  1. Most common mode of transmission is from person to person, including from health care workers to hospitalized clients.
  2. HAIs.
C. Clients at increased risk.
  1. Treatment with multiple antibiotics.
  2. Multiple hospitalizations.
  3. Older adults with chronic conditions.
  4. Clients with compromised immune function.

Analyze Cues and Prioritize Hypotheses

The most important problem is fever as a result of the pathogen and the potential for sepsis and septic shock.

Generate Solutions

Treatment

Culture and sensitivity followed by administration of antibiotics sensitive to identified organism.

Nursing Intervention: Take Action

Goal: To decrease spread of infection.

A. Routine cultures of health care workers in some settings.
B. Identification of clients at increased risk.
C. Add contact precautions to the standard precautions.
  1. Private room, gown, and gloves.
  2. Masks are not necessary unless the client has a respiratory tract infection.
  3. Teach family the importance of gloves and gowns.

Sepsis

Sepsis causes a systemic inflammatory response to infection.

A. Gram-negative and gram-positive bacteria are primary organisms.

B. Increased risk in clients with urinary catheters, respiratory infections, invasive procedures (arterial lines, central venous pressure [CVP], any indwelling line).

C. At-risk clients: older adults, clients with chronic health problems or immunosuppression or who are malnourished.

Assessment: Recognize Cues

A. Clinical manifestations.
   1. Hypo- or hyperthermia.
   2. Compromised respiratory function.
      a. Initially, hyperventilation occurs as a compensating mechanism.
      b. Hypoventilation and respiratory acidosis occur.
      c. Respiratory failure and development of adult respiratory distress syndrome (ARDS).
   3. Compromised cardiac function—tachycardia, hypotension.
   4. Altered mental status.
   5. Significant edema.
   6. Oliguria.

Analyze Cues and Prioritize Hypotheses

The most important problems are widespread infection, potential for clotting issues, and poor gas exchange due to organ dysfunction.

Generate Solutions

Treatment

A. Prevention of infection.

B. Aggressive treatment of infections as soon as blood cultures are obtained.

C. Aggressive pulmonary support.

D. Fluid resuscitation.

E. Vasopressor—administration to maintain blood pressure.

Nursing Intervention: Take Action

See care of a client in shock (see Chapter 12).

A. Functions of the immune system (Fig. 6.6).
   1. Defense—protect against invading microorganisms.
   2. Homeostasis—removal of damaged cellular substances.
   3. Surveillance—recognition and destruction of foreign cells.

B. Body recognizes foreign proteins, called *antigens*, which will elicit a response from the immune system—the production of antibodies, which attack and destroy the invading antigens.

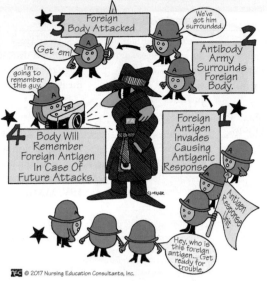

FIG. 6.6 **Immune System Response.** (From Zerwekh, J., Garneau, A., & Miller, C. J. [2017]. *Digital collection of the memory notebooks of nursing* [4th ed.]. Nursing Education Consultants.)

   1. Antigens are foreign to the body and are frequently associated with bacteria, viruses, or other pathogens; antigens react with antibodies or antigen receptors on B and T cells.
   2. Allergens are antigens that produce an allergic response.

Immunologic Responses

A. Properties of the immunologic response.
   1. *Specificity:* the formation of a specific antibody for each antigen; antibodies produced against one pathogen will not protect the body from other pathogens.
      Example: Antibodies against chickenpox will not protect the body against measles.
   2. *Memory:* both responses are capable of "remembering" the antigen and responding more rapidly if exposed to same antigen again.
      Example: The body remembers how to make the antibody against the chickenpox virus.
   3. *Self-recognition:* the immune system has the ability to distinguish self or self-antigens from nonself or foreign antigens; the self-antigens do not illicit the immune response.
      Example: When the body does not recognize its own cells, the condition is called autoimmunity and can lead to autoimmune diseases or disorders.

B. Types of specific immunity.
   1. Innate immunity: present at birth; is not antigen specific and involves a nonspecific response; first line of defense.
   2. Acquired immunity: develops either actively or passively (Table 6.3).

B. If hypersensitivity is suspected, a localized skin test may be done before the administration of substance.

C. Prevention is the priority.

Goal: To maintain adequate ventilation.

> **⚠ NURSING PRIORITY** Airway positioning and mouth-to-mouth resuscitation will not provide adequate ventilation when client has airway edema. An emergency tracheotomy or intubation may be indicated.

A. Maintain bed rest; place client in low-Fowler position with the legs elevated.

B. High oxygen concentrations if airway is compromised.

C. Anticipate use of airway adjuncts (tracheostomy, endotracheal intubation).

D. Administration of medications to reverse bronchospasm (albuterol, corticosteroid, epinephrine).

Goal: To restore adequate circulation.

A. Administer IV fluids (normal saline or lactated Ringer solution) to correct loss of fluid to third-space shifts and vasodilation.

B. Carefully titrate fluid replacement with vital signs.

> **⚠ NURSING PRIORITY** Monitor the client's fluid status closely; as fluid begins to shift back into the vascular compartment, it is easy to cause fluid overload.

C. Vasopressors and volume expanders may be used to increase blood pressure if fluid replacement is not effective.

Goal: Client will verbalize actions to prevent recurrence.

A. Once causative agent is identified, instruct client accordingly.

B. Advise client to wear identification tag or medic-alert bracelet.

C. Explain to client that if any level of allergic reaction had occurred previously, the next exposure could be worse (penicillin, insect stings, etc.).

📋 Systemic Lupus Erythematosus

SLE is a multisystem inflammatory autoimmune disorder; the disease affects multiple organs. SLE is characterized by a diffuse production of autoantibodies that attack and cause damage to body organs and tissue.

A. Tissue injury in SLE results from deposition of the immune complexes throughout the body (kidneys, heart, skin, brain, and joints); this activates the inflammatory response.

B. The severity of symptoms varies greatly throughout the course of the disease; periods of exacerbation and remission occur.

Assessment: Recognize Cues

A. Risk factors.
  1. More common in women, 20 to 40 years of age.
  2. Familial tendencies.

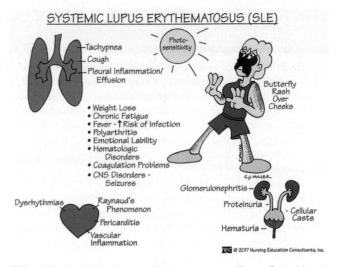

FIG. 6.8 Systemic Lupus Erythematosus. (From Zerwekh, J., Garneau, A., & Miller, C. J. [2017]. *Digital collection of the memory notebooks of nursing* [4th ed.]. Nursing Education Consultants.)

  3. More prevalent in African Americans, Asian Americans, Hispanics, and Native Americans than Caucasians.
  4. May be triggered by environmental stimulus, infections, and medications; sun exposure most common.

B. Clinical manifestations (Fig. 6.8).

C. Diagnostics
  1. No specific test is diagnostic; assess configuration of symptoms.
  2. Presence of antinuclear antibody (ANA), high levels of anti-DNA, and presence of anti-Smith (Sm) are most suggestive of a diagnosis of SLE.
  3. C-reactive protein (CRP), ESR—monitor progress of inflammation and therapy effectiveness.

Analyze Cues and Prioritize Hypotheses

The most important problems are persistent pain, chronic inflammation, fatigue, potential loss of tissue integrity, and decreased self-esteem due to body image.

Generate Solutions

Treatment

SLE has no known cure.

A. Nonsteroidal antiinflammatory drugs (NSAIDs).

B. Corticosteroids for exacerbations of polyarthritis.

C. Immunosuppressants; methotrexate.

D. Antimalarial agents (e.g., hydroxychloroquine).

Nursing Interventions: Take Action

Goal: To prevent exacerbations.

A. Maintain good nutritional status; eat a low-cholesterol diet.

B. Avoid exposure to infections.

C. Teach client about skin problems: discoid lesions, loss of hair, dry scaly scalp.

D. Teach client personal hygiene to prevent urinary tract infections.

E. Make sure client understands how to take medications.

F. Avoid exposure to sunlight; use a sunscreen with a minimum SPF 30 when exposure is unavoidable.

G. Contact health care provider before participating in any immunization procedures.

H. Counseling regarding pregnancy.

Goal: To maintain adequate tissue perfusion.

A. Assess for indications of impaired peripheral perfusion—numbness, tingling, and weakness of hands and feet.

B. Prevent injury to extremities—especially fingers.

C. Carefully evaluate fluid status with regard to cardiac status, fluid retention, and weight gain.

Goal: To promote effective pain control.

A. Establish schedule to conserve energy, but still maintain physical activity.

B. NSAIDs to control arthritic pain.

C. Nonpharmacologic therapies to supplement analgesics (see Chapter 3).

D. Evaluate response of pain to decreased inflammation from corticosteroids.

Goal: To maintain kidney function.

A. Monitor for peripheral edema, hypertension, hematuria, and decreased output.

B. Monitor blood urea nitrogen and creatinine levels.

C. Monitor for urinary tract infections (glomerulonephritis).

D. Assess for peripheral edema and excess fluid volume.

Goal: To assist client to maintain psychological equilibrium.

A. Observe for behavioral changes that may indicate CNS involvement: headaches, inappropriate speech, difficulty concentrating.

B. Encourage client to participate in support groups and to seek counseling to deal with stress.

Human Immunodeficiency Virus Infection

A. Human immunodeficiency virus (HIV) infection is caused by a retrovirus that causes immunosuppression.

B. The person infected with HIV is more susceptible to infection due to the diminished response of the immune system.

Assessment: Recognize Cues

Transmission of Human Immunodeficiency Virus

A. Blood transmission.

1. Needlesticks that occur when the client has a high viral load carry a higher risk than those that occur when client is at a low viral load.

2. Exposure to an infected client's blood via open wounds or mucous membranes carries a lower risk than does a needlestick.

3. Transmission via blood transfusions has been greatly reduced with the screening of donated blood.

   a. A risk remains when the blood is donated within the first few months of infection and the screening blood test does not identify the donor as being HIV-positive.

B. Sexual transmission—most common mode of transmission.

1. Sexual practices, not preferences, place people at increased risk.

2. Risk for infection is greater for the partner who receives the semen during oral, vaginal, or anal sex.

3. Any sexual activity that involves direct contact with vaginal secretions and semen may transmit HIV.

C. Perinatal transmission.

1. Exposure can occur during pregnancy, at the time of delivery, or during the postpartum period through breast milk.

2. Twenty-five percent of infants born to untreated HIV-positive mothers are infected.

3. Prophylactic antiretroviral medications (zidovudine, AZT) during pregnancy can reduce rate of transmission to less than 2%.

4. Decreased incidence occurs with cesarean delivery of HIV-positive mothers.

D. How HIV *cannot* be transmitted (Fig. 6.9).

E. The level of CD4+ T cells is used to monitor the stages and progression of the virus; normal CD4+ T-cell count is at least 800 cells/µL (0.80×10^9/L) of blood.

F. The viral load in the semen, blood, vaginal secretions, or breast milk is an important variable in the transmission. The higher the viral load, the greater the risk of transmission.

> ⚠ **NURSING PRIORITY** As a nurse, it is essential for you to know the modes of transmission of HIV; activities that do *not* transmit the virus; and the nursing care to protect yourself, your clients with acquired immunodeficiency syndrome (AIDS), and other clients you are caring for.

Clinical Manifestations

A. Acute HIV infection.

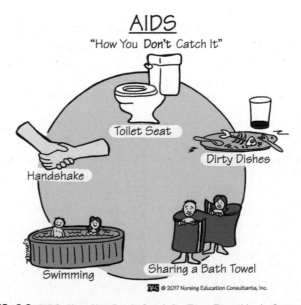

FIG. 6.9 AIDS: How You Don't Catch It. (From Zerwekh, J., Garneau, A., & Miller, C. J. [2017]. *Digital collection of the memory notebooks of nursing* [4th ed.]. Nursing Education Consultants.)

1. Intense viral replication and dissemination of HIV throughout the body.
2. Symptoms are mild, ranging from no symptoms to flulike symptoms (fever, swollen lymph glands, muscle and joint pain, diarrhea, sore throat, headache).
3. Window of seroconversion: time period from when the person is infected with the virus until HIV antibodies can be detected.
4. Average time for seroconversion to occur is 1 to 3 weeks.
5. A client may have vague, nonspecific symptoms for years.
6. During this period, there is a high viral load and the CD4+ T-cell count falls, but only temporarily.

B. Chronic HIV infection.
1. Asymptomatic infection—CD4+ T-cell count greater than 500 cells/μL (0.50 × 10⁹/L) and low viral load.
   a. Viral replication has reached a steady state.
   b. Considered asymptomatic phase; however, chronic vague symptoms persist (fatigue, fever, headache, night sweats).
   c. Persistent generalized lymphadenopathy.
2. Symptomatic infection—CD4+ T-cell count between 200 and 500 cells/μL (0.02 and 0.50 × 10⁹/L) and increased viral load.
   a. Exacerbation of symptoms.
   b. Client begins to experience localized infections, increased lymphadenopathy, and neurologic manifestations.
   c. *Candida* is a common problem—persistent oropharyngeal or vulvovaginal candidiasis.
   d. Hairy oral leukoplakia, which may also be indication of progression of disease.
   e. Shingles, oral or genital herpes lesions.
   f. Kaposi sarcoma.
      (1) A cutaneous skin lesion that looks like a bruise; later will turn dark violet or black.
      (2) Invades body organs, extremities, skin, and torso.
      (3) May become painful.
3. AIDS—CD4+ T-cell count less than 200 cells/μL (0.20 × 10⁹/L) and viral load increases. *A diagnosis of AIDS is made when the HIV-positive client develops at least one of the following disease processes.*
   a. CD4+ T-cell count below 200 cells/μL (0.20 × 10⁹/L).
   b. AIDS dementia complex.
   c. Wasting syndrome caused by HIV.
   d. At least one opportunistic cancer—invasive cervical cancer, Kaposi sarcoma, Burkitt lymphoma, immunoblastic lymphoma, primary lymphoma of the brain.
   e. At least one opportunistic infection—viral (cytomegalovirus), fungal (PCP, coccidioidomycosis), bacterial, or protozoal infection.

Opportunistic Diseases

A. Diseases and infections that occur in clients with AIDS are called *opportunistic* because they take advantage of the suppressed immune system.
1. The type of infection and its extent varies with each client, depending on the extent of immunosuppression.
2. Single opportunistic infections are rare; a client usually has multiple infections.

B. Infections may be delayed or prevented by antiretroviral therapy, vaccines (hepatitis B, influenza, and pneumococcal), and disease-specific prevention.

C. *Coccidioides jiroveci* pneumonia, *Pneumocystis jiroveci* pneumonia (previously called *Pneumocystis carinii* and abbreviated as PJP or PCP).
1. May be caused by a pathogen in the body that is dormant.
2. Is not common in healthy individuals; immune system must be compromised for the infection to occur.
3. Symptoms: fever, night sweats, nonproductive cough, progressive dyspnea.

D. Tuberculosis.

E. Fungal infections: histoplasmosis (pneumonia, meningitis), coccidioidomycosis (pneumonia).

F. Kaposi sarcoma: a bruised, dry-appearing skin lesion; may be present internally as well.

G. Candidiasis of the esophagus, mouth, vagina.

H. Viral infections: cytomegalovirus (CMV), CMV retinitis, herpes simplex with chronic ulcers or bronchitis, esophagitis, or pneumonitis.

Diagnostics

> **!** **NURSING PRIORITY** A positive test result means the person has HIV—it does not predict the course of the disease. A negative test result means that HIV antibodies were not detected; however, this can occur during the window period of seroconversion.

A. HIV antibody/antigen testing (fourth-generation testing): highly sensitive test that detects antibodies and antigens associated with HIV.
1. Fourth-generation testing algorithm includes confirmatory testing with HIV viral load testing for any indeterminate results.
2. If the client has a negative fourth-generation test but reports risky behavior, encourage retesting in 4 to 6 weeks.
3. If results are positive, assist in finding follow-up HIV primary care.

B. Rapid HIV tests—ready within 20 minutes, but results are preliminary and must be confirmed.
1. Client needs to return for a standard HIV assay if the results are positive.
2. In-home testing kits are available that use an oral fluid sample (saliva).

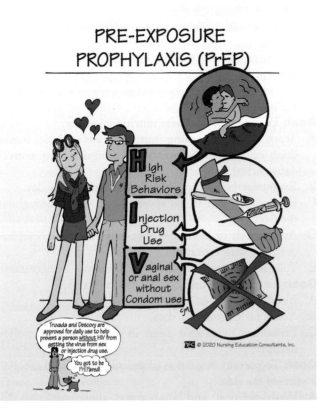

FIG. 6.10 Preexposure Prophylaxis (PrEP). (From Zerwekh, J., & Garneau, A. [2021]. *Mosby's pharmacology memory notecards: Visual, mnemonic, and memory aids for nurses* [6th ed.]. Elsevier.)

C. CD4$^+$ T cell (receptor cell on the T4 helper cell) count: below 200 cells/µL (0.20×10^9/L) in an HIV-positive client indicates progression to acute HIV infection.
D. Serum monitoring after diagnosis.
   1. CD4$^+$ T-cell counts and plasma assays (HIV RNA viral load).
   2. Evaluation for drug resistance.

Analyze Cues and Prioritize Hypotheses

The most important problems are potential for infection, inadequate gas exchange and nutrition, pain, diarrhea, and reduced tissue integrity.

Generate Solutions

Treatment

A. Medications: antiretroviral therapy (ART) (see Appendix 6.1).
   1. Prescribed according to the viral load and the CD4$^+$ T-cell counts.
   2. Combination of at least three or more ART drugs.
   3. Women should begin ART even if they are pregnant, except for Sustiva, which can cause fetal anomalies.
   4. Combination drug therapy attacks virus at different stages of replication.

B. Medications do not cure the client but decrease the viral replication and slow disease process.
C. Adherence to drug schedules is critical; nonadherence to drug regimen can lead to mutations of the virus and increased virus resistance.

> **! NURSING PRIORITY** Frequently, the treatment for the client with AIDS causes problems in other areas: the high-dose antibiotics may increase the level of leukopenia and the chemotherapy medications will further decrease the bone marrow functions. The client with AIDS receiving chemotherapy will be even further immunosuppressed.

D. PrEP (**Pr**e-**E**xposure **P**rophylaxis) is medication for people at risk for HIV who take daily medicine to prevent HIV. PrEP is highly effective for preventing HIV from sex or injection drug use (Fig. 6.10).

Nursing Interventions: Take Action

See Nursing Interventions for immunocompromised clients.
Goal: To provide and promote client and public education regarding transmission of HIV.
A. Safe sex.
   1. Maintain monogamous relationships.
   2. Sex with female or male prostitutes is a high-risk activity.
   3. Avoid all direct contact with a partner's mouth, penis, vagina, or rectum if the HIV status of the partner is not known.
   4. Avoid all sexual activities that cause cuts or tears in the vagina, on the penis, or in the rectum.
   5. Males should wear a condom if multiple partners are involved.
   6. If the HIV status of a sexual partner is not known, a condom should always be used during intercourse.
   7. Anyone who has been involved in any high-risk sexual activities or who has injected IV recreational drugs should have a blood test to determine presence of HIV.
B. Needles should not be recapped or shared. Dispose of them in an impenetrable sealed container.

> **! NURSING PRIORITY** Public and client teaching regarding the transmission of HIV is vital in the control of this disease. The period of time from when the client is infected until the condition is diagnosed is when the majority of new infections are transmitted.

Home Care

A. An employee in a health care setting should advise employer of HIV-positive status.
B. Kitchen and bathroom facilities may be shared, provided that normal sanitary practices are observed.
C. Clean up spills of body fluids or waste immediately with a solution of 1 part bleach to 10 parts water. A bleach solution can be used to disinfect kitchen and bathroom floors, showers, sinks, and toilet bowls.

Appendix 6.1   POTASSIUM, SODIUM, AND CALCIUM IMBALANCES AND CORRECTING MEDICATIONS—cont'd   ℞

Electrolyte Imbalances: Sodium

CAUSES	SYMPTOMS	NURSING IMPLICATIONS
Normal serum sodium (Na) levels: 135–145 mEq/L (mmol/L)		
Hyponatremia: Serum Na⁺ below 135 mEq/L (mmol/L) (loss of sodium or water excess)		
Inadequate Na⁺ intake (rare) Loss of sodium-rich fluids Cystic fibrosis Fluid gain, overhydration (dilutional) Increased kidney excretion: • Thiazide diuretics • Adrenal insufficiency—Addison disease • Increased ADH or SIADH Edema Excessive administration of D₅W GI losses Massive tissue injury: • Burns • Trauma	**Solution deficit (Na⁺ loss):** CNS problems: changes in level of consciousness, confusion, seizures Weakness, restlessness Oliguria Abdominal cramps Postural hypotension Cold and clammy skin **Dilutional hyponatremia (water excess):** CNS problems: confusion, headache, seizures Hypertension Muscle twitching, cramping Increased urine Weight gain	1. Identify source of depletion. 2. Maintain accurate I&O records and determine weight daily (best measurement of fluid status). 3. Irrigate nasogastric tubes with normal saline solution. 4. Seizure precautions. 5. Monitor blood pressure. 6. Restrict fluid intake if client has fluid excess.

> ❗ **NURSING PRIORITY** Older adult clients and infants are at higher risk because of variations in total body water; carefully monitor clients receiving fluid replacement with D5W.

Hypernatremia: Serum Na+ above 145 mEq/L (mmol/L) (sodium retention or water loss)		
Decreased fluid intake Excessive salt intake Excessive water loss: • Diarrhea • Febrile state Increased kidney retention Cushing syndrome	**Fluid excess (Na⁺ retention):** • Pitting edema • Weight gain • Flushed skin • Lethargic • Hypertension • Decreased hematocrit **Fluid deficit (hemoconcentration of Na, water loss):** • Concentrated urine • Dry mucous membranes • Flushed skin, tachycardia, increased temperature, weight loss, decreased CVP	1. Identify origin of increase. 2. Maintain accurate I&O records and determine weight daily. 3. Administer D₅W IV if fluid is normal or there is a fluid deficit. 4. Administer diuretics to remove excess Na⁺ 5. Restrict fluid intake if client has fluid excess. 6. Assess for cerebral edema— lethargy, headache, nausea, vomiting, increased BP.

Medications to Correct Sodium Imbalance

MEDICATION	NURSING IMPLICATIONS
Sodium Supplements Sodium chloride (NaCl, table salt) Saline solutions: 3%, 0.9%, and 0.45% saline solution for infusion ▲ High-alert medication	1. Administer with caution to clients with HF, kidney problems, edema, or hypertension. 2. Determine weight daily; maintain accurate I&O records to evaluate fluid retention. 3. Evaluate serum Na⁺ levels. 4. Do not store containers of sodium chloride above a concentration of 0.9% (normal saline) on the nursing unit.

Electrolyte Imbalances: Calcium

CAUSES	SYMPTOMS	NURSING IMPLICATIONS
Normal serum calcium (Ca²⁺) levels: 9–11 mg/dL (2.25–2.75 mmol/L)		
Hypocalcemia: Serum Ca²⁺ below 8.6 mg/dL (1.7 mmol/L) or below 3.5 mEq/L (.875 mmol/L) in infants		

Note: A reciprocal relationship exists between phosphorus and calcium; when one is increased the other is decreased.

Appendix 6.1 POTASSIUM, SODIUM, AND CALCIUM IMBALANCES AND CORRECTING MEDICATIONS—cont'd ℞

Electrolyte Imbalances: Calcium

CAUSES	SYMPTOMS	NURSING IMPLICATIONS
Acute pancreatitis Laxative abuse Dietary lack of Ca^2+ and vitamin D Hypoparathyroidism Hyperphosphatemia Excessive blood transfusions Excessive IV fluids Alkalosis	Tetany: + Chvostek sign; + Trousseau sign (see Chapter 9) Neuromuscular irritability Numbness and tingling in extremities or around mouth Laryngeal stridor Seizures Abdominal cramping and distention Hyperreflexia Dysrhythmias	1. Identify origin of deficiency. 2. Keep Ca^{2+} replacement medications easily accessible for clients who have had thyroid or parathyroid surgically removed. 3. Assess for tetany. 4. Reduce environmental stimuli for both adults and infants. 5. Institute seizure precautions. 6. Provide client education regarding Ca^{2+} intake.

Hypercalcemia: Serum Ca^{2+} above 10.2 mg/dL (2.55 mmol/L)

CAUSES	SYMPTOMS	NURSING IMPLICATIONS
Metastatic malignancy Hyperparathyroidism Thiazide diuretics Prolonged immobilization Vitamin D overdose	Anorexia, nausea, constipation CNS depression Decreasing muscle tone, coordination Pathologic fractures Dysrhythmias—increases sensitivity to digitalis preparations Kidney stones	1. Identify origin of increase. 2. Administer loop diuretics to facilitate removal of serum Ca^+, normal saline fluid replacement. 3. Increase client's fluid intake 3000–4000 mL/24 hr. 4. Decrease Ca^{2+} intake. 5. Encourage client mobility. 6. Provide client education regarding supplemental vitamins. 7. Increase fiber intake. 8. Assess client taking digitalis for symptoms of toxicity.

Medications to Correct Calcium Imbalance

MEDICATION	ACTION	NURSING IMPLICATIONS
Calcium Salts Calcium citrate: PO Calcium gluconate: IV, PO Calcium carbonate: PO Loop diuretics may be used to enhance excretion of calcium in treatment of hypercalcemia.	Necessary for cardiac muscle function IV infusion for treatment of hypocalcemic tetany	1. May be given in conjunction with vitamin D to enhance absorption. 2. PO supplements are more effective if taken ½–1 hr after meals. 3. Prevent IV infiltration; Ca^{2+} solutions cause tissue hypoxia and sloughing. 4. Do not add Ca^{2+} preparations to solutions containing carbonates or phosphates. 5. Use with caution for client receiving digitalis. 6. Monitor infusion rate carefully; sudden increase in serum Ca^{2+} level may precipitate severe cardiac dysrhythmias. 7. Corticosteroids decrease Ca^{2+} absorption. Administer several hours apart.

Electrolyte Imbalances: Phosphorus

CAUSES	SYMPTOMS	NURSING IMPLICATIONS

Normal serum phosphorus (PO4) levels: 2.4–4.4 mg/dL (0.78–1.42 mmol/L)

Hypophosphatemia: Serum phosphorus below 2.4 mg/dL (0.78 mmol/L)

Note: A reciprocal relationship exists between phosphorus and calcium; when one is increased the other is decreased.

Continued

Appendix 6.1 POTASSIUM, SODIUM, AND CALCIUM IMBALANCES AND CORRECTING MEDICATIONS—cont'd ℞

Electrolyte Imbalances: Phosphorus

CAUSES	SYMPTOMS	NURSING IMPLICATIONS
Malabsorption Chronic diarrhea Malnutrition, vitamin D deficiency Parenteral nutrition Chronic alcoholism Phosphate-binding antacids Diabetic ketoacidosis Hyperparathyroidism Refeeding syndrome Respiratory alkalosis	CNS depression (confusion, coma) Muscle weakness, including respiratory muscle weakness Polyneuropathy, seizures Cardiac problems (dysrhythmias, heart failure) Osteomalacia, rickets Rhabdomyolysis	1. Identify origin of deficiency. 2. Increase oral intake of foods high in phosphate and/or administer a supplement (e.g., dairy). 3. Monitor for hypocalcemia, hyperkalemia, hypotension, and dysrhythmias during IV administration.

Hyperphosphatemia: Serum phosphorus above 4.4 mg/dL (1.42 mmol/L)

Kidney failure Phosphate enemas (e.g., Fleet enema) Excessive ingestion (e.g., phosphate-containing laxatives) Rhabdomyolysis Tumor lysis syndrome Thyrotoxicosis Hypoparathyroidism Sickle cell anemia, hemolytic anemia Hyperthermia	Hypocalcemia Numbness and tingling in extremities and region around mouth Hyperreflexia, muscle cramps Tetany, seizures Calcium-phosphate precipitates in skin, soft tissue, cornea, viscera, blood vessels	1. Identify origin of increase and treat underlying cause. 2. Administer oral phosphate-binding agents (e.g., calcium carbonate) to facilitate removal of excess. 3. Restrict foods high in phosphate (e.g., dairy products). 4. Increase client's fluid intake 3000–4000 mL/24 hr. 5. Volume expansion and forced diuresis with a loop diuretic may facilitate phosphorus excretion. 6. Hemodialysis may be required with severe cases.

Medications to Correct Phosphorus Imbalance

MEDICATION	ACTION	NURSING IMPLICATIONS
Inorganic Phosphates Calcium-based phosphate binders: • Calcium carbonate: PO • Calcium acetate: PO Calcium-free phosphate binders: • Sevelamer carbonate: PO • Lanthanum: PO	Both groups of binders have GI effects Calcium-based phosphate binders promote hypercalcemia	1. Medication taken daily with meals. 2. Monitor calcium levels with calcium-based phosphate binders. 3. Calcium-free phosphate binders are more expensive but do not promote hypercalcemia or metabolic acidosis.

Electrolyte Imbalances: Magnesium

CAUSES	SYMPTOMS	NURSING IMPLICATIONS
Normal serum magnesium (Mg+) levels: 1.5–2.5 mg/dL (0.75–1.25 mmol/L)		

Hypomagnesemia: Serum Mg+ below 1.5 mg/dL (0.75 mmol/L)

GI tract fluid losses (e.g., diarrhea, NG suction) Chronic alcoholism Malabsorption syndromes Prolonged malnutrition Increased urine output Hyperglycemia Proton pump inhibitor therapy	*Symptoms similar to hypocalcemia:* • Confusion • Muscle cramps • Tremors, seizures • Vertigo Hyperactive deep tendon reflexes Chvostek and Trousseau signs Increased pulse, increased BP, dysrhythmias Associated with digitalis toxicity	1. Identify origin of deficiency. 2. Administer oral magnesium supplements and encourage foods high in magnesium (e.g., dark chocolate, avocados, nuts, legumes, tofu, leafy greens). 3. Assess for tetany. 4. Reduce environmental stimuli for both adults and infants. 5. Institute seizure precautions.

Hypermagnesemia: Serum Mg+ above 2.5 mg/dL (1.25 mmol/L)

Appendix 6.1   POTASSIUM, SODIUM, AND CALCIUM IMBALANCES AND CORRECTING MEDICATIONS—cont'd   ℞

Electrolyte Imbalances: Magnesium

CAUSES	SYMPTOMS	NURSING IMPLICATIONS
Kidney failure	Lethargy, drowsiness	1. Identify origin of increase.
IV administration of magnesium, especially for treatment of eclampsia	Muscle weakness	2. Limit dietary intake of foods high in magnesium (e.g., dark chocolate, avocados, nuts, legumes, tofu, leafy greens).
	Urinary retention	
	Nausea, vomiting	
Tumor lysis syndrome	Diminished deep tendon reflexes	3. Administer diuretics if client's kidney function is adequate to promote urinary excretion of magnesium.
Hypothyroidism	Flushed, warm skin, especially facial	
Metastatic bone disease	Increased pulse, increased BP	
Adrenal insufficiency		4. Increase client's fluid intake 3000–4000 mL/24 hr.
Antacids, laxatives		5. Calcium gluconate is the antidote for magnesium overdose.

Medications to Correct Magnesium Imbalance

MEDICATION	ACTION	NURSING IMPLICATIONS
Magnesium oxide: PO	Excessive levels of magnesium cause neuromuscular blockade—leads to respiratory depression	1. IV administration preferred treatment for severe deficiency.
Magnesium sulfate: IV		2. Calcium gluconate can reverse excess effects.
	Excessive oral doses may cause diarrhea	3. See Appendix 21.2 for obstetric implications of magnesium administration.

▲High-alert medication

ACE, angiotensin-converting enzyme; *ADH*, antidiuretic hormone; *BP*, blood pressure; *BUN*, blood urea nitrogen; *CHF*, congestive heart failure; *CNS*, central nervous system; *CVP*, central venous pressure; *D5W*, 5% dextrose in water; *ECG*, electrocardiogram; *GI*, gastrointestinal; *HF*, heart failure; *I&O*, intake and output; *IM*, intramuscular; *IV*, intravenous; *NG*, nasogastric; *NPO*, nothing by mouth; *PO*, by mouth (orally); *PVC*, premature ventricular contraction; *SIADH*, syndrome of inappropriate antidiuretic hormone secretion.

Appendix 6.2   MEDICATIONS: ANTI-INFLAMMATORY, ANTIBIOTIC, ANTIRETROVIRAL   ℞

Anti-inflammatory Medications

General Nursing Implications
- Give oral medications with or after meals to decrease GI irritation and side effects.
- After therapy, withdrawal from steroids *must be done* gradually.
- For clients on long-term therapy, increased amounts of corticosteroids will be required during periods of stress such as surgery.
- Decrease client's ability to respond to and fight infection.
- Closely evaluate the client on digitalis preparations and thiazide diuretics for the development of hypokalemia.
- Use with NSAIDs increases risk for intestinal irritation and perforation (see Appendix 3.2).
- Uses: inflammatory conditions—respiratory, GI, joint inflammation, and skin conditions. Adrenocortical hormone replacement is necessary if adrenal glands are insufficient or have been removed. Suppress rejection of transplanted organs.

MEDICATIONS	SIDE EFFECTS	NURSING IMPLICATIONS
Adrenocortical Hormones (corticosteroids, glucocorticoids): *Antiinflammatory action:* Suppress the inflammatory response. Suppress infiltration of area by phagocytes and suppress production of lymphocytes, further reducing the immune response and inflammation. Used as immunosuppressant for delaying organ rejection. Long-term use will suppress the function of the adrenal glands.		
Hydrocortisone base: PO	Increased susceptibility to infections (body-wide)	1. Administer medication before 0900 to decrease adrenal cortical suppression.
Hydrocortisone sodium succinate: IV, IM	GI upset, gastric irritation	2. Monitor for psychological changes.
	Osteoporosis	

Continued

Appendix 6.2 MEDICATIONS: ANTIINFLAMMATORY, ANTIBIOTIC, ANTIRETROVIRAL—cont'd

MEDICATIONS	SIDE EFFECTS	NURSING IMPLICATIONS
Tetracyclines: Bacteriostatic: Broad-spectrum; interfere with protein synthesis of infectious organism and thus diminish its growth and reproduction		
Tetracycline: PO, IV, IM Doxycycline: PO, IV Demeclocycline: PO Minocycline: PO, IV Oxytetracycline: PO Tigecycline: IV	PO may cause GI irritation (loose stools, diarrhea), sore throat, photosensitivity Diarrhea may indicate severe superinfection (pseudomembranous colitis) in bowel Discoloration of teeth in children up to 8 years old Can cause staining of developing teeth in the fetus if taken after fourth month of gestation and in children before permanent teeth have come in Photosensitivity	1. Administer on empty stomach; withhold antacids, dairy foods, and foods high in calcium at least 2 hr after PO administration; do not administer with milk. 2. Can give doxycycline and minocycline with food. 3. Do not give at the same time as iron preparations. Give them as far apart as possible (e.g., 2–3 hr). 4. Advise client to avoid direct or artificial sunlight. 5. If diarrhea occurs, important to determine cause. 6. Observe for development of superinfections.
Monobactams: Bactericidal: Synthetic beta-lactam		
Aztreonam: IM, IV	Rash, nausea, vomiting, and diarrhea	1. Often combined with other antibiotics for treatment of intraabdominal and gynecologic infections.
Sulfonamides: Bacteriostatic: Suppress bacterial growth by inhibiting synthesis of folic acid		
Sulfisoxazole: PO, IV, IM Trimethoprim sulfamethoxazole (also referred to as TMP-SMZ): PO, IV	Blood dyscrasias—hemolytic anemia Hypersensitivity—rash, "drug fever," photosensitivity Kidney dysfunction—crystalluria (irritation and obstruction) Stevens-Johnson syndrome	1. Encourage 8–10 glasses of water per day to prevent crystalluria. 2. Contraindicated during pregnancy and for nursing mothers and infants under 2 months of age. 3. Avoid prolonged exposure to sun.
Macrolides: Bacteriostatic: Inhibit protein synthesis		
Erythromycin base: PO Azithromycin: PO, IV Clarithromycin: PO	Nausea, vomiting, abdominal distress, diarrhea Cholestatic hepatitis: abnormal liver function studies, jaundice, fever	1. Administer with a full glass of water.
Fluoroquinolones: Bactericidal: Inhibit bacterial DNA		
Ciprofloxacin: PO, IV Levofloxacin: PO, IV Norfloxacin: PO Moxifloxacin: PO, IV Gemifloxacin: PO	GI: Nausea, vomiting, abdominal distress, diarrhea CNS: dizziness, headache, confusion Superinfections, hypersensitivity Tendon rupture with Cipro	1. Absorption is reduced by milk products, antacids. 2. Administer IV infusions over 60 min. 3. Instruct client to report joint pain promptly.
Other Antibiotics		
Metronidazole: PO, IV	Nausea, dry mouth, headache Disulfiram reaction when taken with alcohol: nausea, copious vomiting, flushing, palpitations, headache; may last 30 min to an hour	1. Classified as an antiprotozoal antibiotic; is effective against anaerobic microorganisms. 2. Avoid concurrent use with alcohol or products containing alcohol. Will cause a disulfiram (Antabuse) reaction.
Clindamycin: PO, IV, topical	Mild nausea, vomiting, or stomach pain and joint pain Vaginal itching or discharge Monitor for diarrhea—risk of pseudomembranous colitis	1. Bactericidal or bacteriostatic, depends on the concentration of drug. 2. Contraindicated in those with ulcerative colitis or enteritis. 3. High risk for pseudomembranous colitis development.

Appendix 6.2 MEDICATIONS: ANTIINFLAMMATORY, ANTIBIOTIC, ANTIRETROVIRAL—cont'd

MEDICATIONS	SIDE EFFECTS	NURSING IMPLICATIONS
Vancomycin: PO, IV	Ototoxicity, thrombophlebitis at site Red man syndrome: flushing, rash, pruritus, tachycardia, and hypotension	1. Acts by inhibiting cell wall synthesis; used only for serious infections. 2. IV infusions over at least 60 min to prevent adverse effects. 3. Serum peak and trough levels are monitored. 4. Used to treat MRSA.
Linezolid: PO, IV	GI: diarrhea, nausea Myelosuppression—anemia, leukopenia, thrombocytopenia	1. New class of antibiotics—oxazolidinones. 2. Monitor for blood dyscrasias. 3. Reserved for treatment of infections from MDROs, especially VRE.

Antifungal

Nystatin: PO, topical Amphotericin B: IV Fluconazole: PO, IV	GI: diarrhea, nausea, vomiting, stomach pain Amphotericin B: hypokalemia, cardiac dysrhythmias, neurotoxicity, kidney toxicity and infusion-related fever, chills, headaches, malaise, hypotension, anemia	1. Used for treatment of candidiasis (mouth, esophagus, vagina). 2. Oral treatment—encourage client to hold medication in the mouth and "swish" around to provide good contact with all affected areas.

Antiretroviral Therapy

General Nursing Implications

- Highly active antiretroviral therapy (ART) is used for treatment of clients with HIV infection and AIDS.
- Report any sore throat, white patches on tongue or throat, fever, or other signs of infection to the health care provider.
- It is important to administer the medication at the same time each day to maintain consistent blood levels and to decrease drug resistance.
- No vaccines or immunity-conferring agents should be administered while client is immunosuppressed.
- Maintain standard precautions; use contact, droplet, and airborne precautions as indicated.
- Medications do not cure AIDS or reduce the risk for transmission.

MEDICATIONS	SIDE EFFECTS	NURSING IMPLICATIONS

Nonnucleoside Reverse Transcriptase Inhibitors (NNRTIs): All bind directly to the HIV transcriptase and inhibit the enzyme.

Efavirenz: PO	CNS symptoms, rash, hepatotoxic, teratogenic	Monitor LFTs; avoid getting pregnant; avoid taking with St. John's wort.
Etravirine: PO	Hypersensitivity reactions, rash, malaise, blisters, facial edema, nausea	Take after meals.
Nevirapine: PO	Rash (may be severe—blistering, joint pain, oral lesions), hepatotoxic, hepatitis	Monitor LFTs; rash may be so severe that drug is discontinued; resistance may occur if drug is used alone; therefore administer concurrently with another antiretroviral drug.
Rilpivirine: PO	Depression, insomnia, headache	Take medication with food.

Nucleoside/Nucleotide Reverse Transcriptase Inhibitors (NRTIs): All NTRIs suppress the synthesis of viral DNA by reverse transcriptase. Medications are given with other antiretroviral agents; they are not used alone because of rapid development of resistance. *Adverse effects of all NRTIs:* Potentially fatal lactic acidosis with hepatic steatosis can occur. Avoid NRTIs during pregnancy because of increased risk of lactic acidosis and hepatic steatosis.

Zidovudine: PO, IV Known as ZDV or AZT	Bone marrow suppression, anemia, neutropenia	Maintain upright position to decrease esophageal irritation; monitor levels of anemia and neutropenia.
Didanosine: PO	Nausea, diarrhea, peripheral neuropathy, liver damage, pancreatitis	Food decreases absorption; give on empty stomach 30 min before eating or 2 hr after. Avoid alcohol.
Stavudine: PO	Pancreatitis, lactic acidosis, diarrhea, peripheral neuropathy	Report peripheral neuropathy. Monitor serum amylase and triglyceride levels.
Tenofovir: PO, powder	Kidney toxicity, decreases bone mineralization	Powder may be mixed with food, but it is bitter. Will not dissolve in water.

Continued

8. Place contaminated linens in a leak-proof bag; handle contaminated linens in a manner that prevents contamination and transfer of microorganisms.

9. Discard all sharps in puncture-resistant container. Do not bend, break, reinsert them into their original sheaths, or handle them unnecessarily. Discard them intact immediately after use.

10. Place clients who pose a risk for transmission to others in a private room. This includes clients who cannot contain secretions/excretions or wound drainage and infants with respiratory or intestinal infections.

11. Practice good hand hygiene.

Respiratory Hygiene and Cough Etiquette

1. Educate health care personnel regarding measures to contain their own respiratory secretions.

2. Post signs in strategic places regarding covering the mouth and nose with a tissue when coughing or sneezing; provide no-touch receptacles for disposal of tissue.

3. Teach client importance of hand hygiene.

Safe Injection Practices

1. Use single-dose vials for parenteral administration when possible.

2. If multidose vials must be used, the needle or cannula and the syringe used to access the vial must be sterile.

3. Do not use the same syringe to administer medications to multiple clients, even if the needle is changed.

4. Do not keep multidose vials in the immediate client treatment area.

Airborne Precautions (droplets smaller than 5 micrometers)

1. Place client in airborne isolation infection room (AIIR) as soon as possible.

2. Personal protection equipment (PPE):
   - Wear respiratory protection (N95 respirator mask approved by the National Institute for Occupational Safety and Health [NIOSH]) when entering the room).
   - Wear gloves and gown when entering the room; remove before leaving room.

3. Limit client transport and client movement out of the room. Health care personnel who are not immune are restricted from entering the client's room.

4. Conditions requiring use of airborne precautions include pulmonary or laryngeal tuberculosis, varicella, rubella, and smallpox.

Droplet Precautions (droplets larger than 5 micrometers)

1. Applicable to clients known to be, or suspected of being, infected with pathogens that are transmitted via respiratory droplets (sneezing, coughing, talking).

2. Place the client in a private room whenever possible; may place two clients in the same room if they are infected with the same pathogen.

3. PPE:
   - Wear a mask when entering the client room or examination area.
   - No recommendation regarding routine use of eye protection.

4. Place a mask on the client if transporting in the health care setting.

5. Instruct client and family regarding respiratory hygiene/cough etiquette.

6. Limit movement of the client from the room; if the client must leave the room, have them wear a surgical mask.

Contact Precautions

1. Applicable to clients with diseases easily transmitted by direct contact such as GI, respiratory tract, skin, or wound infections and clients colonized with multiple drug-resistant bacteria.

2. Place the client in a private room if condition (e.g., uncontrolled drainage, incontinence) may facilitate transmission. Two clients infected with same pathogen may be placed in the same room.

3. PPE:
   - Wear a gown when entering the client's room; remove gown before leaving the room.
   - Wear gloves when entering the client's room. Always change gloves after contact with infected material. Remove gloves before leaving the client's room and perform hand hygiene; do not touch anything in the room as you are leaving.
   - Wear gloves when touching the client's intact skin and surfaces and articles in close proximity to the client.

4. Dedicate use of noncritical client care equipment to the single client; if common equipment use is unavoidable, the equipment must be disinfected before use on another client.

5. Limit the transport or movement of the client outside the room; if it is necessary to move the client, ensure that infected or colonized areas of the client's body are contained and covered.

6. Evidence shows that MDROs can be carried from one person to another via the hands of health care personnel.

Protective Environment Precautions

1. Precautions may be used for clients who are severely immunosuppressed—clients with stem cell transplants, clients with organ transplant, AIDS clients.

2. Place the client in a private room that has positive-pressure air flow and high-efficiency particulate air (HEPA) filtration for incoming air.

3. Wear respiratory protection (N95 respirator mask), gloves, and gown when entering the room.

4. Limit client transport and client movement out of the room.

5. No fresh flowers, fresh fruits/vegetables, or potted plants are allowed in room.

TEST ALERT Use critical thinking to ensure standard transmission-based precautions are implemented; prevent environmental spread of infectious diseases.

From Centers for Disease Control and Prevention (CDC). *2007 Guideline for isolation precautions: Preventing transmission of infectious agents in healthcare settings.* https://www.cdc.gov/hicpac/pdf/isolation/isolation2007.pdf

Appendix 6.4 VASCULAR ACCESS DEVICES

Peripheral intravenous therapy: Most common vascular access device (VAD) is the *short peripheral catheter* placed in the veins of the arm. A *midline catheter* is another type of VAD that is used for peripheral IV therapy and is usually inserted into the median antecubital vein when IV therapy is given longer than 6 days and up to 14 days.

Central intravenous therapy: A VAD (central line) is inserted into the venous system within the superior vena cava near its junction with the right atrium. A chest x-ray is performed to confirm placement.

1. Peripherally inserted central catheter (PICC).
   • May be single, dual, or triple lumen.
   • Insertion methods use guidewires and ultrasound devices.
   • May be in place for several months.
2. Nontunneled percutaneous central venous catheters (CVCs).
   • Inserted by a health care provider, physician assistant, or nurse practitioner through the subclavian vein in the upper chest or the internal jugular veins in the neck using sterile technique.
   • Client is placed in the Trendelenburg position, usually with a rolled towel between the shoulder blades and catheter inserted using ultrasound guidance.
3. Tunneled central venous catheters.
   • Requires surgical placement; has an external port. The distal tip lies in the superior vena cava just above the right atrium.
   • Not used to obtain CVP readings.
   • Examples are Hickman, Broviac, Leonard.

Implanted ports: A vascular access line port is implanted under the skin; activities are not restricted and is used most often for chemotherapy.

Hemodialysis catheters: Used for hemodialysis procedures or pheresis procedures.

Arterial lines: Used to obtain arterial blood sample for ABGs, monitor hemodynamic pressures, infuse chemotherapy or fibrolytics.

⚡ Practice & Next Generation NCLEX (NGN) Questions

Homeostasis and Immune Concepts

More questions on
Ꭼvolve

1. A client is being started on prednisone. What is important to teach the client regarding his medication?
   1. Increase fluid intake.
   2. Increase dose as needed.
   3. Do not discontinue medication abruptly.
   4. Do not take medication with food.

2. The nurse is evaluating an older adult client for adequacy of hydration. What would the nurse observe if the client has a fluid volume deficit?
   1. Peripheral edema
   2. Weight gain of 2 pounds in 24 hours.
   3. Dizziness when standing at bedside.
   4. Light-color urine in increased amounts.

3. Which client would the nurse identify as being at the greatest risk for having a significant fluid imbalance if their fluid intake was significantly reduced?
   1. 46-year-old diabetic adult
   2. 3-week-old infant
   3. 12-year-old underweight teenager
   4. 25-year-old obese adult

4. What is important for the nurse to teach the HIV-positive client regarding transmission of the human immunodeficiency virus? It is most frequently transmitted: **Select all that apply**.
   1. via sexual contact with an infected individual
   2. through contact with the HIV-positive client's sweat
   3. from the HIV-positive mother via the placenta at birth
   4. by sharing a bathroom with an infected individual
   5. by drinking after someone using the same glass

5. A client is prescribed amikacin for a severe bacterial infection of a surgical wound. What is important for the nurse to monitor while the client is receiving this medication? **Select all that apply**.
   1. Polyuria
   2. Malaise
   3. Dizziness
   4. Tinnitus
   5. Muscle and joint pain

6. The nurse is evaluating the fluid balance on an older adult client. What is the **most** accurate measurement to determine changes in a client's fluid balance?
   1. Adequacy of skin turgor
   2. Daily body weight
   3. Measure intake and output
   4. Measure circumference of the legs

7. The nurse is performing a dressing change on a client who has a *Staphylococcus aureus* infection in an abdominal incision. What infection control precautions will the nurse implement? **Select all that apply**.
   1. Put on a face shield.
   2. Wear sterile clean gloves to remove the soiled dressing.
   3. Remove extra dressings and supplies from the room.
   4. Dispose of the gown and mask in container outside client's door.
   5. Wear personal protective equipment.
   6. Cleanse the stethoscope and scissors that came in contact with the client before removing from the room.

8. Trimethoprim-sulfamethoxazole (TMP-SMZ) is prescribed for a client. The nurse would instruct the client to report which symptom if it developed while taking this medication therapy? **Select all that apply**.
   1. Sore throat
   2. Diarrhea
   3. Constipation
   4. Rash
   5. Nausea and vomiting

9. A client is beginning long-term medication therapy with methylprednisolone. What is important to teach the client regarding the medication?
   1. The medication will decrease the client's inflammatory response and ability to fight infections.
   2. The client should return to have anticoagulant blood studies drawn every 3 months.
   3. The client should carry a dose of epinephrine autoinjector in case of an allergic reaction.
   4. It will be important for the client to maintain a high fluid intake with supplemental potassium.

10. The nurse is caring for a client who is admitted with a diagnosis of fever of unknown origin. The client's temperature is 103.6 °F (39.8 °C). The health care provider has ordered a broad-spectrum antibiotic and acetaminophen for the fever. Which nursing intervention is the **priority**?
    1. Administer the antibiotic and acetaminophen ASAP due to the high temperature.
    2. Wait to administer the antibiotic until the blood culture results are reported.
    3. Obtain a blood culture before the first dose of the antibiotic is administered.
    4. Administer the antipyretic as soon as possible.

11. The charge nurse is teaching a group of student nurses the importance of understanding the signs and symptoms of electrolyte imbalance. **For each client finding, use an X to specify whether the finding is consistent with the electrolyte** imbalance of hyperkalemia, hypercalcemia, or hyponatremia. **Each finding may support more than one electrolyte imbalance.**

CLIENT FINDING	HYPERKALEMIA	HYPERCALCEMIA	HYPONATREMIA
Pathologic fractures			
Muscle weakness			
Tetany			
Frequent bowel movements			
Paresthesias in hands and feet			
Confusion			
Decreased deep tendon reflexes			

12. An adult client has a nosocomial or health care–associated infection (HAI). The client has been diagnosed with a methicillin-resistant *Staphylococcus aureus* (MRSA) surgical site infection and has been receiving several IV antibiotics to treat the infection. Recently the client has had severe diarrhea most likely due to *Clostridium difficile*. The nursing staff is working on measures to decrease infection, including improving hand hygiene by all nursing staff members.

    For each nursing action listed below regarding hand hygiene measures, use an X to specify whether the action would be Indicated (appropriate or necessary), Non-Essential (makes no difference or not necessary), or Contraindicated (could be harmful) for the client's care at this time.

NURSING ACTIONS	INDICATED	NON-ESSENTIAL	CONTRA-INDICATED
Take client's temperature q2h.			
Monitor for signs of electrolyte imbalance.			
Perform hand hygiene with an alcohol-based antiseptic cleanser.			
Wash hands under warm water for 20 seconds.			
Wash hands before client care and following client care.			
Have client wash hands after urination and defecation.			
Use antibacterial soap, allow to lather, and wash hands using friction around hands and fingers.			
Use warm water for the washing and cool water to rinse hands.			

⚡ Answers to Practice & Next Generation NCLEX (NGN) Questions

1. 3
Client Needs: Physiological Integrity/Pharmacological Therapies
Clinical Judgment/Cognitive Skill: Take Action
Rationale & Test-Taking Strategy: Think about what type of medication the prednisone is and what its side effects are. When two options have similar wording, "Do not..." often is the correct answer. When a client is taking any corticosteroid, it is important for the client to continue the medication schedule, and the medication should be taken with food. The body is dependent on the level of steroid intake to maintain homeostasis and discontinuing the medication could have very serious side effects. A side effect is fluid retention; therefore, the client needs to watch his fluid intake. Corticosteroids must be taken exactly as prescribed; the client should never increase the dose as needed. To decrease gastrointestinal upset, the client should take the medication with a glass of milk or food.

2. 3
Client Needs: Physiological Integrity/Physiological Adaptation
Clinical Judgment/Cognitive Skill: Recognize Cues
Item Type: Multiple Choice
Rationale & Test-Taking Strategy: How are fluid volume deficit and dehydration related? Dehydration frequently precedes the development of fluid deficit. Orthostatic hypotension is an early sign of problems with fluid deficit. Peripheral edema and weight gain are indications of fluid retention. Dilute urine in normal amounts indicates adequate fluid balance. When fluid deficit occurs, hypovolemia may develop and there is an increased risk of the client developing low blood pressure and consequences of poor cardiac output.

3. 2
Client Needs: Physiological Integrity/Physiological Adaptation
Clinical Judgment/Cognitive Skill: Prioritize Hypotheses
Item Type: Multiple Choice
Rationale & Test-Taking Strategy: Think about what age groups are most often affected by fluid imbalance. The very young and older adults (over 65 years) are more susceptible to fluid changes. These two client groups frequently do not have adequate compensatory mechanisms to deal with sudden changes in fluid balance. The older adult client frequently has chronic conditions that affect the ability to compensate for sudden changes in fluid status. An infant's body is comprised of over 75% water; for this reason, any small change in fluid volume can disrupt their fluid balance.

4. 1, 3
Client Needs: Safe and Effective Care Environment/ Safety and Infection Control
Clinical Judgment/Cognitive Skill: Analyze Cues
Item Type: Select All That Apply
Rationale & Test-Taking Strategy: Go through each of the options and decide whether the statement is true or false. HIV is transmitted via unprotected sexual contact, maternal transmission to an infant from vaginal delivery or through breast milk, and through receiving an organ transplant from a person with HIV, blood transfusion from a person with HIV, or exposure through an open-bore needle stick with an HIV-contaminated needle. HIV is not transmitted through sweat or by sharing a bathroom with a person who is HIV positive.

5. 3, 4
Client Needs: Physiological Integrity/Pharmacological Therapies
Clinical Judgment/Cognitive Skill: Recognize Cues
Item Type: Select All That Apply
Rationale & Test-Taking Strategy: First, determine to which antibiotic classification amikacin belongs. Clients who receive aminoglycosides such as amikacin need to be monitored for two serious side effects – ototoxicity and nephrotoxicity. Ototoxicity signs include dizziness, tinnitus, and progressive hearing loss. Nephrotoxicity is assessed by monitoring the blood urea nitrogen (BUN), creatinine, decreasing urine output and specific gravity, and blood in the urine. Malaise, muscle aches, and joint pain are not associated with use of this medication. It is not necessary to immediately contact the primary health care provider nausea occurs.

6. 2
Client Needs: Physiological Integrity/Physiological Adaptation
Clinical Judgment/Cognitive Skill: Prioritize Hypotheses
Item Type: Multiple Choice
Rationale & Test-Taking Strategy: Look at the **key** word, "most." This is a priority question. The best way to determine the adequacy of body fluids is to measure the daily weight at the same time each day. Sudden increase or loss of body weight is most often due to fluid loss or retention. Assessment of skin turgor will not provide a reliable indicator of fluid volume status in an older adult client due to the skin being inelastic. Measuring intake and output and leg circumference do not adequately account for fluid volume shifts that may occur in the client's body.

7. 5
Client Needs: Safe and Effective Care Environment/ Safety and Infection Control
Clinical Judgment/Cognitive Skill: Take Action
Item Type: Select All That Apply
Rationale & Test-Taking Strategy: Contact precautions require the nurse to wear personal protective equipment (PPE):
- Wear a gown when entering the client's room; remove gown before leaving the room.
- Wear gloves when entering the client's room. Always change gloves after contact with infected material. Remove gloves before leaving the client's room and perform hand hygiene; do not touch anything in the room as you are leaving.
- Wear gloves when touching the client's intact skin and surfaces and articles in close proximity to the client.
- Dedicate use of noncritical client care equipment to the single client, i.e., blood pressure cuff, stethoscope, scissors, etc.

Removing soiled dressings does not require sterile gloves. A face shield is not necessary unless splattering of fluids is anticipated. The gown and mask should be disposed of in the client's room; they should not be removed from the room. The nurse needs to leave all extra dressing supplies in the room. The stethoscope and scissors should not be taken into the client's room.
(Note: This is a "select all that apply" question that has only one correct answer. Remember the correct answer could be only one of the options, any number of the options, or all of the options.)

8. 1, 4
Client Needs: Physiological Integrity/Pharmacological Therapies
Clinical Judgment/Cognitive Skill: Take Action
Item Type: Select All That Apply

Rationale & Test-Taking Strategy: Think about the serious side effects of drugs that belong to the antibiotic classification of sulfonamides. Clients taking trimethoprim-sulfamethoxazole need to be informed about adverse effects, which include hypersensitivity reactions, blood dyscrasias (disorders), and crystalluria. The most severe hypersensitivity reaction is Stevens-Johnson syndrome, which is characterized by a skin rash, lesions of the mucous membranes, fever, malaise, and toxemia. Early signs of blood disorders include sore throat, fever, and pallor. At any appearance of a rash, the client should be taught to immediately stop taking TMP-SMX, and the health care provider should be notified of the sore-throat symptom.

9. 1
Client Needs: Physiological Integrity/Pharmacological Therapies
Clinical Judgment/Cognitive Skill: Take Action
Item Type: Multiple Choice
Rationale & Test-Taking Strategy: All corticosteroids are antiinflammatory medications. These medications decrease the body's ability to fight infection. The nursing priority would be to teach the client how to avoid infections – hand washing, avoiding crowds of people. There is no need for anticoagulant studies or epinephrine.

While the client may require supplemental potassium to prevent hypokalemia associated with corticosteroid use, clients are generally on decreased fluids because steroids increase fluid retention.

10. 3
Client Needs: Physiological Integrity/Physiological Adaptation
Clinical Judgment/Cognitive Skill: Prioritize Hypotheses
Item Type: Multiple Choice
Rationale & Test-Taking Strategy: Notice the **key** word, "priority." The priority nursing intervention is to obtain any cultures (i.e., blood, wound, etc.) prior to administering the first dose of the antibiotic. If the antibiotic is administered first, the blood culture results may not be as effective in identifying the microorganism causing the infection. Acetaminophen, an antipyretic, is indicated for the fever, but the priority is obtaining specimens for culture. Most often, the antibiotic treatment will be initiated before the blood culture test results are available. This is called empiric antibiotic treatment, which means the antibiotic ordered is based on experience and an educated guess as to what will treat the infection and is typically a broad-spectrum antibiotic.

11. The charge nurse is teaching a group of student nurses the importance of understanding the signs and symptoms of electrolyte imbalance. **For each client finding, use an X to specify whether the finding is consistent with the electrolyte imbalance of hyperkalemia, hypercalcemia, or hyponatremia. Each finding may support more than one electrolyte imbalance.**

CLIENT FINDING	HYPERKALEMIA	HYPERCALCEMIA	HYPONATREMIA
Pathologic fractures		X	
Muscle weakness	X	X	X
Tetany			
Frequent bowel movements	X		X
Paresthesias in hands and feet	X		
Confusion		X	X
Decreased deep tendon reflexes	X		X

Client Needs: Physiological Integrity/Physiological Adaptation
Clinical Judgment/Cognitive Skill: Analyze Cues
Item Type: Matrix Multiple Response
Rationale & Test-Taking Strategy: Review in your mind the signs and symptoms of the electrolyte imbalances listed. Two of them are "hyper" conditions (too much electrolyte) and one is a "hypo" condition (too little electrolyte). The client experiencing hyperkalemia (potassium greater than 5.0 mEq/L) would have cardiovascular problems, such as bradycardia and hypotension. Bowel movements are frequent and watery. Muscles twitch in the early stages of hyperkalemia, and the client may report tingling and burning sensations, followed by numbness in the hands and feet and around the mouth (paresthesia). As hyperkalemia worsens, muscle weakness occurs with decreased reflexes, followed by flaccid paralysis. Hyperkalemia is rare in clients with normal kidney function. Clients at greatest risk are those who are chronically ill or debilitated, older adults, and those taking potassium-sparing

diuretics. Cardiovascular changes are the most serious and lifethreatening problems associated with hypercalcemia. Initially, there is increased heart rate and blood pressure, later progressing to bradycardia and other dysrhythmias, and cardiac arrest. The characteristic findings with hypercalcemia (calcium greater than 11 mg/dL) include confusion, anorexia, nausea, abdominal pain, constipation, muscle weakness, oliguria, renal calculi, and pathologic fractures. Cerebral changes are the most prominent signs and symptoms of hyponatremia (sodium below 135 mEq/L) due to cerebral edema and increased intracranial pressure, along with general muscle weakness, diminished deep tendon reflexes (DTRs), hyperactive bowel sounds, and frequent watery bowel movements. Tetany is associated with hypocalcemia. Paralytic ileus is associated with severe hypokalemia. *Notice that muscle weakness is a common finding with all three electrolyte imbalances and is also found with hypokalemia and hypernatremia.*

12. An adult client has a nosocomial or health-care associated infection (HAI). The client has been diagnosed with a methicillin-resistant *Staphylococcus aureus* (MRSA) surgical site infection and has been receiving several IV antibiotics to treat the infection. Recently, the client has had severe diarrhea, most likely due to *Clostridium difficile*. The nursing staff is working on measures to decrease infection, including improving hand hygiene by all nursing staff members.

For each nursing action listed below regarding hand hygiene measures, use an X to specify whether the action would be indicated (appropriate or necessary), nonessential (makes no difference or not necessary), or contraindicated (could be harmful) for the client's care at this time.

NURSING ACTIONS	INDICATED	NON-ESSENTIAL	CONTRA-INDICATED
Take client's temperature q2h.		X	
Monitor for signs of electrolyte imbalance.		X	
Perform hand hygiene with an alcohol-based antiseptic cleanser.			X
Wash hands under warm water for 20 sec.	X		
Wash hands before and after client care.	X		
Have client wash hands after urination and defecation.	X		
Use antibacterial soap, allow to lather, and wash using friction around hands and fingers.	X		
Use warm water for the washing and cool water to rinse hands.			X

Client Needs: Safe and Effective Care Environment/Safety and Infection Control
Clinical Judgment/Cognitive Skill: Take Action
Item Type: Matrix Multiple Choice
Rationale & Test-Taking Strategy: The focus of this question is on hand hygiene practices. Hand hygiene is considered of utmost importance when practicing standard precautions and is the single most effective measure in preventing the spread of infection. The hands should be washed for at least 20 sec with a facility-approved soap, running hands under a flow of warm water (not cool or too hot). Hands should be washed thoroughly with a firm, circular motion using friction on the back of hands, palms, and wrists. The nurse should wash each finger individually, paying special attention to areas between the fingers and knuckles by interlacing fingers and thumbs and moving hands back and forth, causing friction. Hands are to be washed before client care and after touching blood, body fluids, secretions, excretions, and contaminated items, regardless of whether gloves are worn. Perform hand hygiene immediately after gloves are removed, between client contacts, and when otherwise indicated to prevent the transfer of microorganisms to other clients or environments. The nurse should wash hands between tasks and procedures on the same client to prevent cross-contamination of different body sites. The nurse should encourage the client to wash their hands after urination and defecation. It is strongly recommended in taking care of clients with diarrhea that soap and water for hand hygiene be used in place of alcohol-based hand cleansers, because the spores of *Clostridium difficile* are not killed by alcohol. Although monitoring vital signs and signs of electrolyte imbalance are important nursing actions for this client, they do not relate to measures to reduce infection, specifically, effective hand hygiene.

CHAPTER SEVEN

Psychosocial Nursing Care

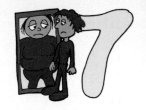

SELF-CONCEPT

A. *Self-concept*: all beliefs, convictions, and ideas that constitute an individual's knowledge of themselves and influence their relationships with others.

B. *Self-esteem*: an individual's personal judgment of their own worth obtained by analyzing how well their behavior conforms to their self-ideal.

> **! NURSING PRIORITY** A healthy self-concept (i.e., positive self-esteem) is essential to psychological wellbeing; it is universal.

Assessment: Recognize Cues

A. Factors affecting self-esteem.
   1. Parental rejection in early childhood experiences.
   2. Lack of recognition and appreciation by parents as child grows older.
   3. Overpossessiveness, overpermissiveness, and control by one or both parents.
   4. Unrealistic self-ideals or goals.

> **! OLDER ADULT PRIORITY** The use of wheelchairs, canes, walkers, hearing aids, adaptive devices, or any combination of these will affect the self-esteem of the older client.

B. Behaviors associated with low self-esteem.
   1. Self-derision and criticism: describes self as stupid, no good, or a loser.
   2. Self-diminution: minimizes one's ability.
   3. Guilt and worrying.
   4. Postponing decisions and denying pleasure.
   5. Disturbed interpersonal relationships.
   6. Self-destructiveness and boredom.
   7. Conflicted view of life.

> **! TEST ALERT** Promoting a positive self-concept is basic to all psychotherapeutic interventions. Look for options that focus on this concept; acknowledging the client as a person is an example.

Nursing Interventions: Take Action

A. Expand self-awareness.
   1. Promote an open, trusting therapeutic relationship.
   2. Maximize the client's participation in the therapeutic relationship.

B. Self-exploration.
   1. Encourage the client to accept their own feelings and thoughts.
   2. Help the client clarify their concept of self and relationship with others through appropriate self-disclosure.
   3. Explore false assumptions with the client such as:
      a. Catastrophizing: thinking that the worst will happen.
      b. Minimizing and maximizing: tendency to minimize the positive and maximize the negative.
      c. All-or-nothing thinking: tendency to look at situations in extremes; no middle ground.
      d. Overgeneralization: thinking that if something happens once, it will happen again.
      e. Filtering: selectively taking certain details out of context while neglecting to look at more positive facts.
   4. Communicate empathically, not sympathetically, and remind client that they have the power to change themself.

C. Self-evaluation.
   1. Encourage client to define and identify problem.
   2. Identify irrational beliefs such as:
      a. "I must be loved by everyone."
      b. "I must be competent and never make mistakes."
      c. "My whole life is a disaster if it doesn't turn out exactly as planned."
   3. Identify areas of strength by exploring, for example, the client's hobbies, skills, work, school, character traits, personal abilities.

> **♣ ! PEDIATRIC NURSING PRIORITY** If parents help children identify and accomplish goals that are important to them, children begin to develop a sense of personal competence and independence.

   4. Explore client's adaptive and maladaptive coping responses.
      a. Determine "pay-offs" for maintaining self-defeating behaviors such as:
         (1) Procrastination.
         (2) Avoiding risks and commitments.
         (3) Retreating from the present situation.
         (4) Not accepting responsibility for one's actions.
      b. Identify the disadvantages of the maladaptive coping responses.

BODY IMAGE

Evaluation of Body-Image Alteration

A. Types of body-image disturbances.
 1. Changes in body size, shape, or appearance (rapid weight gain or loss, plastic surgery, pregnancy, burns, hair loss, hirsutism).
 2. Pathologic processes causing changes in structure or function of one's body (e.g., Parkinson disease, cancer, heart disease).
 3. Failure of a body part to function properly (paraplegia or stroke).
 4. Physical changes associated with normal growth and development (puberty, aging process).
 5. Threatening medical or nursing procedures (fecal or urinary diversion[s], radiation therapy, organ transplantation).
 6. Gender dysphoria creating marked incongruence between one's experience/expressed gender and assigned gender.
B. Principles.
 1. Body characteristics that have been present from birth or acquired early in life seem to have less emotional significance than those arising later.
 2. Body-image changes, handicaps, or changes in body function that occur abruptly are far more traumatic than ones that develop gradually.
 3. The location of a disease or injury greatly affects the emotional response to it; internal diseases are generally less threatening than external changes (trauma, disfigurement).
 4. Changes in genitals or breasts are perceived as a great threat and reawaken fears about sexuality and virility.

SPECIFIC SITUATIONS OF ALTERED BODY IMAGE AND NURSING INTERVENTIONS

> ❗ **TEST ALERT** Provide support to client with changes in body image.

Obesity

Assessment: Recognize Cues

A. Body weight exceeds 20% above the normal range for age, sex, and height.
B. Feeding behavior is gauged according to external environmental cues (i.e., odors, stress, availability of food), rather than hunger (increased gastrointestinal motility).
C. Increased incidence of diabetes, cardiovascular disease, cancer, and delayed wound healing.
D. Obese client often has symptoms of depression, fatigue, dyspnea, tachycardia, and hypertension.

Nursing Interventions: Take Action

A. Encourage behavior modification programs.
B. Promote activities and interests not related to food or eating.
C. Identify client's need to eat and relate the need to preceding events or situations.
D. Decrease guilt and anxiety related to being obese.
E. Provide long-range nutritional counseling.
F. Encourage an exercise program.
G. Assess for complications (hypertension, cardiovascular disease).
H. Provide pre- and postoperative care for client undergoing bariatric surgery.

Stroke

Assessment: Recognize Cues

A. Change of body function resulting from loss of bowel and bladder control, speech, and cognitive skills.
B. Disordered orientations in relationship to body and position sense in space; body-image boundaries disrupted.

Nursing Interventions: Take Action

A. Decrease frustration related to speech problems by encouraging speech effort, speaking slowly, and clarifying statements.
B. Promote reintegration of altered body image caused by paralyzed body part by means of tactile stimulation and verbal reminders of the existing body part.

Amputation

Assessment: Recognize Cues

A. Feelings of loss, lowered self-esteem, guilt, helplessness.
B. Depression, passivity, and increased emotional vulnerability.
C. Phantom limb pain occurs in most clients: increased experience if amputation occurs after 4 years of age; almost universal experience after 8 years of age.

Nursing Interventions: Take Action

A. Anticipatory guidance and therapeutic preparation of a client who is to undergo amputation.
B. Discussion of phantom limb phenomenon and exploration of client's fears regarding amputation.
C. Assist family members to work through their feelings and to accept client as a whole person.
D. Acknowledge phantom limb pain; reassure client that this is a normal process.
E. Provide pain medication as needed.
F. Educate client and family members on proper fitting of prosthesis (if applicable.)

Pregnancy

Assessment: Recognize Cues

A. Produces marked changes in a woman's body, resulting in major alterations in body configuration within a short period of time.
B. Second trimester: woman becomes aware that her body is widening and requires more space.
C. Third trimester: woman is very much aware of increased size; may feel ambivalent about the changes in her body.

D. Woman perceives her body as vulnerable, yet also as a protective space for the unborn.

E. Significant other experiences change body image and sympathetic symptoms during a woman's pregnancy.

Nursing Interventions: Take Action

A. Explain and offer reassurance about the normal physiologic changes that are occurring.

B. Provide discussions of alterations in body image for both mates.

C. Encourage verbalization of feelings relating to changed body image.

Cancer

Assessment: Recognize Cues

A. Clients with cancer may experience many changes in body image.

B. Side effects of chemotherapy, radiation, and surgery may affect body image.

C. Removal of sex organs (breasts, uterus) has a significant effect on a client's perception of sexuality.

D. Disfiguring head-and-neck surgery has a devastating effect on body image because the face is one of the primary means by which people communicate.

E. Symptoms of depersonalization, loss of self-esteem, and depression may occur.

Nursing Interventions: Take Action

A. Assess client for depression.

B. Provide anticipatory guidance to help client cope with crisis of changed body image.

C. Set long-term goals to help client with cancer adjust to physiologic and psychological changes.

Enterostomal Surgery

Assessment: Recognize Cues

A. Client is often shocked at initial sight of ostomy.

B. Client may experience lowered self-esteem, fear of fecal or urine spillage, alteration in sexual functioning, and feelings of disfigurement and rejection.

Nursing Interventions: Take Action

A. Preoperative explanation by use of drawings, models, or pictures of how stoma will appear.

B. Reassurance that reddish appearance of stoma and large size will diminish in time.

C. Encourage discussion and recognize importance of client talking with a successful ostomate.

D. Educate client on performing ostomy care (pouching ostomy, emptying drainage bag/reservoir, observing peristomal skin).

HUMAN SEXUALITY

Key Nursing Concepts

A. Principles.

1. Sexual role identity may be altered during the illness process.

2. Cultural variables influence one's expression of sexuality.

3. Sexual problems are addressed through short-term, behavior-oriented treatment; the goal is to decrease fear of performance and to facilitate communication.

4. Nursing plays a key role in sex-health education; nurses need to be aware of their own attitudes toward sex to respond helpfully to clients.

B. Effect of illness and injury on sexuality.

1. Depressive episodes often precipitate a decrease in libido.

2. Sexual preoccupations and overtones may be experienced by the client with psychosis.

3. Certain medications contribute to sexual dysfunction, failure to reach orgasm in women, and impotence or failure to ejaculate in men (e.g., antipsychotic agents, reserpine, phenothiazine, and estrogen use in men decreases libido; androgen use in women increases libido).

4. Clients with spinal cord injuries may lose sexual functioning.

5. Trauma and disfigurement may precipitate an alteration in sexuality.

C. Effect of the aging process on sexuality.

1. Physiologic changes in women are frequently caused by decreasing estrogen supply, which results in decreased vaginal lubrication, shrinkage, and loss of elasticity in vaginal canal and decrease in breast size.

2. Physiologic changes in men include a decrease in testosterone, decrease in spermatogenesis, longer length of time to achieve erection, and decrease in the firmness of erection.

3. Prolonged abstinence from sexual activity can lead to disuse syndrome in which the physiologic changes are experienced to a greater degree.

CONCEPT OF LOSS

> ⚠ **TEST ALERT** Provide care or support to client and family at end of life. Assist with coping related to grief or loss.

Definition

1. Loss includes both biologic and physiologic aspects; loss of function.

2. Components of loss include death, dying, grief, and mourning.

   a. Grief: the sequence of subjective states that follow loss and accompany mourning.

   b. Anticipatory grief: grief that occurs before the actual loss (e.g., diagnosis of a terminal illness, client receiving hospice care).

   c. Maladaptive grief: loss that is not associated with normal grieving (e.g., disenfranchised grief, chronic grief, delayed grief, exaggerated grief, masked grief).

Assessment: Recognize Cues

A. Characteristic stages.
   1. Death and dying (Kübler-Ross, 1969).
      a. Denial and isolation.
      b. Anger.
      c. Bargaining.
      d. Depression.
      e. Acceptance.
   2. Grief.
      a. Shock and disbelief.
      b. Developing awareness.
      c. Restitution or resolution of the loss.

Coping and Reactions to Death Throughout the Life Cycle

♣ A. Infant-toddler (ages 1-3).
   1. No specific concept of death.
   2. Reacts more to pain and discomfort of illness and immobilization; separation anxiety; intrusive procedures; change in ritualistic routine.

> ❗ **NURSING PRIORITY** Parents of a dying child may have feelings of guilt and may need to talk out these feelings before being able to help each other and their child.

♣ B. Preschooler (ages 3-5).
   1. Death is viewed as a departure, a kind of sleep.
   2. Life and death can change places with one another.
   3. If a pet dies, may request a funeral, burial, or some other type of ceremony to symbolize the loss.

> ❗ **PEDIATRIC NURSING PRIORITY** A young child's fear of death is often a fear of aloneness, of being away from their parents. It is important for parents to interact with the nurse in the child's presence so that the nurse can be identified as a trustworthy substitute caretaker.

♣ C. School-age child (ages 5-12).
   1. Death is personified; fantasies of a separate person or distinct personality (e.g., skeleton-man, devil, ghost, or death-man).
   2. Fear of mutilation and punishment is often associated with death; anxiety is released by nightmares and superstitions.
♣ D. Adolescent (ages 12-18).
   1. Has a mature understanding of death.
   2. Concerned more with the here and now (i.e., the present).
   3. May have strong emotions about death (anger, frustration, despair); silent, withdrawn.
   4. Often worries about physical changes in relationship to terminal illness.
E. Adult.
   1. Concerned about death as a disruption in lifestyle and its effect on significant others.

   2. Adults tend to think about loss in terms of unmet goals and/or an impediment to future plans; often experience delayed grief and threat to emotional integrity.
F. Older adult.
   1. Aware of death as inevitable; life is over.
   2. Emphasis on religious belief for comfort; a time of reflection, rest, and peace.

Nursing Interventions: Take Action

Goal: To acknowledge the pain of loss
A. Assist the griever in recognizing that they must yield to the painful process of grief.
B. Explain how grief affects all areas of one's life.
C. Try to view the loss from the griever's perspective.

Goal: To assist the grieving and/or dying client to accept the reality of loss and/or death
A. Encourage expression and verbalization of feelings without interruption (i.e., crying, talking).
B. Listen nonjudgmentally and with acceptance.
C. Reach out and make contact with client and family; let genuine concern and caring show.

Goal: To provide for spiritual needs of the grieving and/or dying client
A. Ask clergy to visit.
B. Pray with client and family (if requested to do so), read inspirational literature, play music.
C. Encourage the griever to allow self-respite times from the grieving process.

Goal: To promote adjustment to life and living after the experience of loss
A. Encourage reinvesting energies into new undertakings and relationships.
B. Promote letting go and moving on.

PSYCHOSOCIAL

Assessment: Recognize Cues

Complete assessment includes descriptions of the intellectual functions, behavioral reactions, emotional reactions, and dynamic issues of the client relative to adaptive functioning and response to present situations.

> ❗ **TEST ALERT** Collect data regarding client's psychosocial functioning.

📋 Psychiatric History

Purpose: A psychiatric history is used to obtain data from multiple sources (e.g., client, family, friends, police, mental health personnel) as a means of identifying patterns of functioning that are healthy and patterns that create problems in the client's everyday life.

> ❗ **OLDER ADULT PRIORITY** Allow ample time to gather psychosocial data from older clients (Box 7.1).

Box 7.1 OLDER ADULT CARE FOCUS: AGING AND MENTAL HEALTH

- Sensory losses (hearing and vision) can have behavioral changes that can be mistaken for disorientation.
- Financial and physical changes of aging can lead to social isolation.
- Exaggerated personal characteristics occur as a person ages.
- Anxiety, fear, and depression can occur from experiencing multiple losses (death, job changes, relocation from home, loss of independence) and grief, especially if they occur quickly.
- Alcoholism is often found in the older adult.
- Behaviors commonly seen are hopelessness and helplessness, which can lead to suicide.
- To assist coping with life circumstances, encourage reminiscence and life review.

A. General history of a client.
   1. Demographic information, such as address, age, religious affiliation, occupation, and insurance company.
   2. Pertinent personal history, such as birth, growth and development, illness, and marital history.
   3. Previous mental health hospitalizations or treatment.
B. Components of psychiatric history.
   1. Chief complaint: main reason client is seeking psychiatric help.
   2. Presenting symptoms: onset and development of symptoms or problems.
   3. Family history: Have any of client's family members sought psychiatric treatment?
   4. Personality profile: client's interests, feelings, mood, and usual leisure activities or hobbies; how they handle stress, overall mood, social relationships.

Mental Status Examination

The *mental status examination* differs from the psychiatric history in that it is used to identify an individual's present mental status and behavior.

NURSING PRIORITY First, assess client's level of consciousness, vision, and hearing (e.g., alert, lethargic, stuporous, obtunded, or comatose) and ability to comprehend the interview.

Assessment: Recognize Cues

A. Components of a mental status exam.
   1. Appearance and general behavior.
   2. Speech and motor activity.
   3. Mood and affect.
   4. Thought process, thought content, and perception.
   5. Cognitive abilities: attention, language, memory, abstract reasoning, intelligence.
   6. Insight, attitude, judgment.

Nursing Interventions: Take Action.

A. Collect data on client's mental status and participate in the psychosocial assessment process.
B. *Report any changes in the client's mental status to the RN, especially if there are active suicidal thoughts.*

Coping Mechanisms

Specific defense processes are used by individuals to relieve or decrease anxieties caused by uncomfortable situations that threaten self-esteem.

Assessment: Recognize Cues

A. Related principles.
   1. The primary functions of coping mechanisms are to decrease emotional conflicts, provide relief from stress, protect from feelings of inadequacy and worthlessness, prevent awareness of anxiety, and maintain an individual's self-esteem.
   2. Everyone uses defense mechanisms to a certain extent. If used to an extreme degree, defense mechanisms distort reality, interfere with interpersonal relationships, limit one's ability to work productively, and may lead to pathologic symptoms.
B. Types of coping mechanisms (Box 7.2).

Nursing management: Take Action

A. Accept coping mechanisms.
B. Discuss alternative coping mechanisms and problem-solving situations.
C. Assist the client in learning new or alternative coping patterns for healthier adaptation.
D. Use techniques to decrease anxiety.

THERAPEUTIC NURSING PROCESS

A therapeutic interpersonal relationship is the interaction between two persons: the nurse promotes goal-directed activities that help alleviate the discomfort of the client by promoting growth and satisfying interpersonal relationships.

Assessment: Recognize Cues
Characteristics

A. Goal-directed.
B. Empathetic understanding.
C. Honest, open communication.
D. Concreteness; avoids vagueness and ambiguity.
E. Acceptance; nonjudgmental attitude.
F. Involves nurse's understanding of self and personal motives and needs.

Phases

A. Preorientation phase: Goal is to *obtain* relevant client data.
   1. During this phase, the nurse obtains relevant information from another caregiver regarding the client's care.
   2. The nurse locates a comfortable setting for interviewing the client.
B. Orientation phase: goal is to *build trust*.
   1. Explore the client's perceptions, thoughts, feelings, and actions.
   2. Identify the purpose of the meeting and the client's problem.
   3. Assess levels of anxiety of self and client.
   4. Mutually define specific goals to pursue.

Box 7.2 TYPES OF COPING MECHANISMS

Compensation: Attempting to make up for or offset deficiencies, either real or imagined, by concentrating on or developing other abilities.

Conversion: Symbolic expression of intrapsychic conflict expressed in physical symptoms.

Denial: Blocking out or disowning painful thoughts or feelings.

Displacement: Feelings are transferred, redirected, or discharged from the appropriate person or object to a less threatening person or object.

Dissociation: Separating and detaching an idea, situation, or relationship from its emotional significance; helps the individual put aside painful feelings and often leads to a temporary alteration of consciousness or identity.

Identification: Attempting to pattern or resemble the personality of an admired, idealized person.

Intellectualization: Attempt to avoid emotional conflict by focusing on concrete, logical events.

Introjection: Acceptance of another's values and opinions as one's own.

Projection: Attributing one's own unacceptable feelings and thoughts to others.

Rationalization: Attempting to justify or modify unacceptable needs and feelings to the ego, in an effort to maintain self-respect and prevent guilt feelings.

Reaction formation: Assuming attitudes and behaviors that one consciously rejects.

Regression: Retreating to an earlier, more comfortable level of adjustment.

Repression: An involuntary, automatic submerging of painful, unpleasant thoughts and feelings into the *unconscious.*

Sublimation: Diversion of unacceptable instinctual drives into personally and socially acceptable areas to help channel forbidden impulses into constructive activities.

Suppression: Intentional exclusion of forbidden ideas and anxiety-producing situations from the conscious level; a voluntary forgetting and postponing mechanism.

Undoing: Actually or symbolically attempting to erase a previous consciously intolerable experience or action; an attempt to repair feelings and actions that have created guilt and anxiety.

C. Working phase: goal is *behavioral change.*
   1. Encourage client participation.
   2. Focus on problem-solving techniques; choose between alternate courses of action and practice skills.
   3. Explore thoughts, feelings, and emotions.
   4. Develop constructive coping mechanisms.
   5. Increase independence and self-responsibility.
D. Termination phase: goal is to *evaluate goals* set forth and terminate relationship.
   1. Plan for termination early in formation of relationship (in orientation phase).
   2. Discuss client's feelings about termination.
   3. Evaluate client's progress and goal attainment.

❗ NURSING PRIORITY To effectively interview a client, be sure to start with a broad, empathetic statement; explore normal behaviors before discussing maladaptive behaviors; phrase inquiries or questions sensitively to decrease the client's anxiety; ask the client to clarify vague statements; refocus on pressing problems when the client begins to ramble; interrupt nonstop talking by the client as tactfully as possible; express empathy toward the client while they are expressing feelings.

Nursing Interventons: Take Action
Therapeutic Nurse-Client Communication Techniques

A. Planning and goals.
   1. Demonstrate active listening; use face-to-face communication.
   2. Demonstrate unconditional positive regard, interest, congruence, respect.
   3. Develop trusting relationship; accept client's behavior and display nonjudgmental, objective attitude.
   4. Be supportive, honest, authentic, genuine.

   5. Focus on emotional needs and emotionally charged area.
   6. Focus on here-and-now behavior and expression of feelings.
   7. Attempt to understand the client's point of view.
   8. Develop an awareness of the client's likes and dislikes.
   9. Encourage expression of both positive and negative feelings.
   10. Use broad openings and ask open-ended questions; avoid questions that can be answered by yes or no.
   11. Use reflections of feelings, attitudes, and words.
   12. Explore alternatives rather than answers or solutions.
   13. Focus feedback on *what* is said rather than *why* it is said.
   14. Paraphrase to assist in clarifying client's statements.
   15. Promote sharing of feelings, information, and ideas instead of giving advice.
B. Examples of therapeutic communication responses (Table 7.1).
C. Examples of nontherapeutic communication responses (Table 7.2 and Box 7.3).

❗ TEST ALERT Listen to the client's concerns and use therapeutic interventions to increase client's understanding of their behavior.

INTERVENTION MODALITIES

📋 Crisis Intervention

A crisis is a self-limiting situation in which usual problem-solving or decision-making methods are not adequate.

Table 7.1	THERAPEUTIC COMMUNICATION
Response	**Example**
1. Exploring	"What seems to be the problem?" "Tell me more about . . . ."
2. Reflecting	Client: "I am really mad at my mother for grounding me." Nurse: "You sound angry."
3. Focusing	"Give an example of what you mean." "Let's look at this more closely."
4. Clarifying	"I'm not sure that I understand what you're saying." "Do you mean . . . . ?"
5. Using general leads	"Go on . . . ." "Talk more about . . . ."
6. Broad opening leads	"Where would you like to begin?" "Talk more about . . . ."
7. Validating	"Did I understand you to say . . . .?"
8. Informing	"The time is . . . ." "My name is . . . ."
9. Accepting	"Yes." "Okay." Nodding, "Uh hmm."
10. Sharing observations	"You appear anxious. I noticed that you haven't been coming to lunch with the group."
11. Presenting reality	"I do not hear a noise or see the lights blinking." "I am not Cleopatra; I am your nurse."
12. Summarizing	"During the past hour we talked about . . . ."
13. Using silence	Nurse remains silent to allow time for client to gather thoughts and begin speaking.

Table 7.2	NONTHERAPEUTIC COMMUNICATION
Response	**Example**
1. False reassurance	"Don't worry; you will be better in a few weeks." "Don't worry. I had an operation just like it; it was a snap."
2. Giving advice	"What you should do is . . . ." "If I were you, I would do . . . ."
3. Rejecting	"I don't like it when you . . . ." "Please, don't ever talk about . . . ."
4. Belittling	"Everybody feels that way." "Why? You shouldn't feel that way."
5. Probing	"Tell me more about your relationships with other men."
6. Excessive questioning	"Hi, I am JoAnn, your student nurse. How old are you? What brought you to the hospital? How many children do you have? Do you want to fill out your menu right now?"
7. Asking "why" questions	"Why are you crying?"
8. Clichés	"Gee, the weather is beautiful outside." "Did you watch that new TV show last night? Everybody's talking about it."

Box 7.3 INEFFECTIVE COMMUNICATION RESPONSES AND NURSE BEHAVIORS

- Not listening; talking too much
- Looking too busy
- Seeming uncomfortable with silence
- Avoiding sensitive topics
- Changing the subject
- Laughing nervously; smiling inappropriately
- Showing a closed body posture
- Focusing on personal issues of the nurse
- Making flippant comments
- Being defensive or making excuses

A. A crisis offers opportunities for growth and renewal.

B. Crisis intervention strategies view people as capable of personal growth and able to control their own lives.

C. Types of crisis intervention strategies.
  1. Individual crisis counseling.
  2. Crisis groups.
  3. Telephone counseling.

D. Crisis intervention requires support, protection, and enhancement of the client's self-image.

E. Goals of crisis intervention are to promote client safety and reduce client's anxiety by providing anxiety reduction techniques.

Group Therapy

Group therapy **is a structured or semistructured process in which individuals (7-12 members is an ideal size) are interrelated and interdependent and may share common purposes and norms.**

A. Emphasis on clear communication to promote effective interaction.

B. Disturbed perceptions can be corrected through consensual validation.

C. Socially ineffective behaviors can be modified through peer pressure.

Family Therapy

Family therapy **is a treatment modality designed to bring about a change in communication and interactive patterns between and among family members.**

A. A family can be viewed as a system that is dynamic. A change or movement in any part of the family system affects all other parts of the system.

B. A family seeks to maintain a balance or "homeostasis" among various forces that operate within and on it.

C. Emotional symptoms or problems of an individual may be an expression of the emotional symptoms or problems in the family.

D. Therapeutic approaches involve helping family members look at themselves in the here and now and recognize the influence of past models on their behavior and expectations.

Milieu

> ⚠ **TEST ALERT** Maintain a therapeutic milieu/environment that is safe and supportive for the client.

Milieu **is a scientifically planned, purposeful manipulation in the environment aimed at causing changes in the behavior and personality of the client.**

A. Nurse is viewed as a facilitator and a helper to clients rather than as a therapist.

B. The *therapeutic community* is a special kind of milieu therapy in which the total social structure of the treatment unit is involved as part of the helping process.

C. Emphasis is placed on open communication, both within and between staff and client groups.

Complementary and Alternative Medicine Therapies

These *alternative therapies* **are different from traditional Western medicine and are often influenced by traditional Chinese medicine, which focuses on maintaining unity with nature and balancing our energy systems.**

A. Energy therapies – healing touch, therapeutic touch, Reiki therapy.

B. Body-based or manipulative therapies – acupressure, chiropractic medicine, massage.

C. Mind-body therapies – biofeedback, guided imagery, music therapy, transcendental meditation, tai chi, yoga, Pilates.

D. Whole medical systems – ayurvedic medicine, homeopathic medicine, naturopathic medicine, traditional Chinese medicine.

> ⚠ **TEST ALERT** Assess client's use of alternative/complementary practices; evaluate client's response to alternative therapy. Use alternative/complementary therapy in providing client care (e.g., music therapy).

Electroconvulsive Therapy

Electroconvulsive therapy **(ECT) is an electric shock delivered to the brain through electrodes that are placed on the head. The shock artificially induces a seizure.**

Assessment: Recognize Cues

Indications.

1. Severe depression; when other treatment modalities are ineffective.
2. Suicide risk/starvation.
3. Number of treatments: usually given in a series that varies according to the client's presenting problem and response to therapy; two to three treatments per week for a period of 2 to 6 weeks.

Nursing Interventions: Take Action.

A. Assess client's record for routine preoperative-type checklist for information (informed consent).

B. NPO for 6 hrs before treatment.

C. Remove dentures, hairpins, contact lenses, and hearing aids.

D. Administer preprocedure medication after electrodes are applied and before convulsion occurs.

E. Provide for safety and observe progress of seizure.

F. Care immediately after treatment.
1. Provide orientation to time.
2. Temporary memory loss is usually confusing; explain that this is a common occurrence.
3. Assess vital signs for 30 min to 1 hr after treatment.
4. Deemphasize preoccupation with ECT; promote involvement in regularly scheduled activities.

Other Therapies

A. Restraints (Box 7.4).
1. Must consider client's civil liberties.
2. Mechanical restraints include camisoles, wrist and ankle restraints, and sheet restraints.

Box 7.4 USE OF RESTRAINTS

- Obtain an order or a consent to apply restraints.
- Selecting a restraint: it should restrict movement as little as possible, be obscure to others, not interfere with the client's treatment, be readily changeable, and be safe for the age of the client (to keep an active child in bed, use a jacket restraint as opposed to a wrist restraint).
- Secure restraint: check for adequate blood circulation to extremities.
- Pad bony prominences (wrists and ankles) before applying restraint.
- Always tie limb restraint with a knot (e.g., clove hitch) that will not tighten when pulled.
- Never tie ends of restraint to a side rail or to part of fixed bed frame if the bed position is going to be changed.
- Assess restraint every 30 min and document.
- Release all restraints every 2 hrs and provide range of motion (ROM) and skin care, offer fluids, and assist to bathroom; stay with client when restraint is removed and document.
- Keep in mind the principle of least restriction: restrain the client to the extent necessary to accomplish the restraint's purpose.

TEST ALERT Implement least restrictive restraints or seclusion.

3. Chemical restraints include the use of medications – antianxiety or antipsychotic.

❗ NURSING PRIORITY Legally, the nurse must have a health care provider's order to apply restraints and must provide for client's biologic needs (e.g., hygiene, elimination, nutrition, and ability to communicate) by following a protocol for timed client monitoring (e.g., safety checks).

B. Seclusion.
1. Confinement to a room that may be locked. Often, the room is without a mattress or linens, and the client is wearing a hospital gown.
2. There is limited opportunity for communication.
C. Activities therapy: a number of vital programs belong in this category, such as pet therapy, music therapy, occupational therapy, art therapy, recreational therapy, ropes course therapy or course, dance or movement therapy, etc.

STRESS AND ADAPTATION

Stress is a state produced by a change in the environment that is perceived as challenging, threatening, or damaging to the individual's equilibrium.

Adaptation is a constant, ongoing process that occurs along the time continuum, beginning with birth and ending with death.

📋 Stressors

A. Physiologic stressors.
1. Chemical agents: drugs, poisons, alcohol.
2. Physical agents: heat, cold, radiation, electrical shock, trauma.
3. Infectious agents: viruses, bacteria, fungi.
4. Environment: noise, air pollution.
5. Faulty immune mechanisms.
6. Genetic disorders.
7. Nutritional imbalance.
8. Hypoxia.
B. Psychosocial stressors.
1. Accidents and the survivors (e.g., airplane crash, hurricane, earthquake survivors).
2. Death of a close friend; neighbor being robbed and/or beaten.
3. Horrors of history: Auschwitz, Hiroshima, Chernobyl, etc.
4. Fear of aggression, mutilation, and destruction.
5. Events of history brought into our living rooms through various media.
6. Life crises: situational, developmental, role.
7. Inherent conflicts in social relations.

❗ TEST ALERT Identify stressors that may affect recovery or health maintenance (e.g., lifestyle, body changes, environmental). Assist client to cope/adapt to stressful events and changes in health status.

Stress Response

❗ NURSING PRIORITY Understanding of the stress response is basic to many nursing interventions.

A. Sympathetic: fight-or-flight response.
1. Increased pulse, blood glucose level, and coagulability of blood.
2. Pupils dilated.
3. Mental activity enhanced.
4. Cold, clammy skin.
5. Respirations rapid and shallow.
B. Stress reduction methods.
1. Proper nutrition, regular exercise, physical activity, and recreation; meditation, breathing exercises, guided imagery, mindfulness.
2. Biofeedback, progressive muscle relaxation, journaling.
3. Group process and social support.
4. Thought-stopping, self-hypnosis, refuting irrational self-talk, cognitive reframing.

COMMON BEHAVIORAL PATTERNS

❗ TEST ALERT Identify inappropriate behavior, use client behavior modification techniques, and use therapeutic interventions to increase client's understanding of their behavior. Reinforce education to caregivers/family on ways to manage client with behavioral disorders.

📋 Interpersonal Withdrawal

Interpersonal withdrawal is behavior characterized by avoidance of interpersonal contact and a sense of unreality.

Assessment: Recognize Cues

A. Physical withdrawal: client sits or stands apart from others; may hide, assume a catatonic posture, or (in extreme form) attempt suicide.
B. Verbal withdrawal: avoidance through silence or (in extreme form) mutism; silence may indicate resistance, a pensive moment, or the indication that nothing more is to be said.

Nursing Interventions: Take Action

A. Avoid punishment of client.
B. Decrease isolation.
C. Invite the client to speak.
D. State the amount of time you are willing to stay with the client, whether they choose to speak or not.
E. Change the context of the contact (e.g., go for a walk together).
F. Encourage the client to share responsibility for the continuance of the relationship.

Regression

Regression is a selective, defensive operation in which the individual resorts to earlier, childish, or less complex patterns of behavior that once brought the client attention or pleasure.

Nursing Interventions: Take Action

A. Avoid fostering dependency and childlike attitudes.
B. Be patient and understanding.
C. Confront client directly about their plan.
D. Compliment client when they do something unusually well or assumes more responsibility.
E. Promote problem solving, reality orientation, and involvement in social activities.
F. Avoid punishment after periods of regression; instead, explore the meaning of the regressive behavior.
G. Remember that regression is a normal occurrence in young children who are hospitalized.

Anger

Anger is an unconscious process used to obtain relief from anxiety that is produced by a sense of danger; it involves a sense of powerlessness. Fear of expressing anger is related to fear of rejection.

Nursing Interventions: Take Action

A. Have client acknowledge or name feelings.
B. Explore source of personal fear or perceived threat (e.g., illness, disability, disfigurement, or emotional crisis).
C. Encourage verbalization of anxiety.
D. Explore appropriate external expression of feelings.
E. Avoid arguing with client.
F. Acting-out behavior is often an indirect expression of anger; it attracts attention and often represents the feelings the person is experiencing.

> **⚠ NURSING PRIORITY** Nontherapeutic responses to a client's anger include defensiveness, retaliation, condescension, and avoidance.

Hostility/Aggressiveness

Hostility is an antagonistic feeling; the client wishes to hurt or humiliate others; the result may be a feeling of inadequacy or self-rejection resulting from a loss of self-esteem.

Nursing Interventions: Take Action

A. Prevent aggressive contact by early recognition of increased anxiety.
B. Maintain client contact rather than avoiding it.
C. Reduce environmental stimuli.
D. Avoid reinforcement behavior (e.g., joking, laughing, teasing, and competitive games).
E. Use distraction or remove the client from the immediate environment to reestablish self-control.

F. Set limits on unacceptable behavior.
G. Protect other clients.

> **⚠ NURSING PRIORITY** When two clients are arguing, engage the dominant client first by using distraction or removing the client from the setting to allow time for de-escalation and processing of the situation.

Violence

Violence is behavior that is physically assaultive and risks injury to the self, others, and the environment.

Nursing Interventions: Take Action

> **⚠ NURSING PRIORITY** Immediate intervention should focus on control and safety, followed by discussion to alleviate guilt and identify alternative behaviors to help prevent future episodes of violence.

A. Establish eye contact.
 1. Conveys attention and concern.
 2. Elicits more information.
 3. Ask the person to look at you.

> **⚠ OLDER ADULT PRIORITY** Expect some older clients to have vision problems; they may not know who you are. Hearing problems occur often with older adults; do not shout or talk rapidly.

B. Avoid asking, "Why?" Instead ask, "What's bothering you?"
 1. *Why* questions are threatening and decrease self-esteem.
 2. Open-ended questions seek to identify the problem, convey concern, and elicit more information.
C. Speak to the client softly, slowly, and with assurance.
D. Give directions clearly and concisely. Tell the client what you want them to do.
E. Encourage client to verbalize feelings.
 1. Give the client an outlet for the physical tension – "Walk with me. Tell me what happened."
 2. Keep the conversation slow; pace yourself – "Wait, I can't follow that. Tell me what you said."
 3. Listen more than talk.
 4. Let the client walk or move around or provide something for the client to safely "pound" on to release the tension before you talk.
F. Self-protection and protection of other clients are primary concerns.
 1. Position yourself near the door for safety purposes.
  a. Do not block the door.
  b. Do not box the client into a corner.
 2. Never remain alone with a potentially violent client; call security or other personnel.
 3. Keep a comfortable distance from client; do not intrude on their personal space.
  a. With a client experiencing mild or moderate anxiety: sit near, about 2 ft away.

    b. With a client experiencing severe anxiety or panic: stay 4 to 6 ft away (or farther).

   4. Be prepared to move quickly; violent clients act quickly and unpredictably.

   5. Determine that the client has no weapons before approaching them.

   6. Be supportive and intervene to increase client's self-esteem.

   7. Be honest; tell the client you are concerned that they are out of control, but you are not going to let anyone get hurt.

   8. Stay with the client but do not touch them until you have asked permission and it has been given to you.

G. Once the client is in control of their behavior, review and process the situation to alleviate the client's guilt and to discuss alternatives in case the client becomes anxious or angry in the future.

Manipulation/Acting Out

Manipulation or acting out **is a type of controlling behavior in which an individual uses others to meet their own needs or to achieve specific goals; often disguises underlying feelings of inadequacy, inferiority, and unworthiness; an attempt to protect against failure or frustration and to gain power over another.**

Nursing Interventions: Take Action

A. Be consistent and firm in the expectations of behavior.

B. Allow some freedom within set limits.

C. Consistently enforce previously set limits.

D. Be alert to client's attempt to intimidate; allow verbal anger.

E. Avoid involvement and intellectualization.

F. Watch carefully for client's use of manipulative patterns; be alert to the many guises in which it may be manifested.

G. Keep staff united, firm, and consistent.

H. Encourage open communication about real needs and feelings.

I. Maintain a sense of authority.

J. Do not accept gifts, favors, flattery, or other forms of manipulation.

Dependence

Dependence **is a behavior pattern characterized by adopting a helpless, powerless stance; a reliance on other people to meet a basic need.**

Nursing Interventions: Take Action

A. Assess client's abilities and capacities.

B. Set firm and consistent limits on behavior.

C. Provide only help needed.

D. Encourage problem-solving and decision-making skills; emphasize accountability.

E. Avoid making decisions for client or assuming responsibility for client's ability to make decisions.

F. Maintain an attitude of firmness and confidence in client's ability to make decisions.

G. Discourage reliance beyond actual needs.

H. Give positive reinforcements for development of independent, growth-facilitating behavior.

I. Encourage successful participation in social relationships.

Shame

Shame **is the inner sense of being completely diminished or insufficient as a person (e.g., feeling "less than").**

Nursing Interventions: Take Action

A. Assist client to begin to externalize rather than internalize feelings of shame.

B. Encourage client to share feelings honestly with individuals they feel "safe" with.

C. Involve client in "debriefing," which is writing and talking about past shame experiences.

D. Encourage client to make positive self-affirmations and involve themself in creative visualization activities to improve self-concept.

Detachment

Detachment **is characterized by aloofness, superficiality, denial, and intellectualization in interpersonal contact.**

Nursing Interventions: Take Action

A. Establish awareness of the process of detachment.

B. Explore fears and fantasies inhibiting emotional expression.

C. Encourage verbalization from global generalities to specific personal comments.

D. Provide clarification of client's unclear responses.

E. Emphasize awareness and exploration of feelings.

ABUSE

Abuse is difficult to define because the term has been politicized and is not a clinical or scientific term.

> **⚠ TEST ALERT** Recognize risk factors for domestic, child, and/or elder abuse/neglect and sexual abuse. Follow regulation/policy for reporting abuse. Provide safe environment and emotional support for abused/neglected client. (see Box 7.5)

Types of Abuse

A. **Physical abuse**: nonaccidental, intentional physical injury inflicted on another person.

B. **Physical neglect**: willing deprivation of essential care needed to sustain basic human needs and to promote growth and development.

C. **Emotional abuse**: use of threats, verbal insults, or other acts of degradation that are intended to be injurious or damaging to another's self-esteem.

Box 7.5 DOCUMENTATION FOR SUSPECTED ABUSE

Procedure

1. Obtain the client's or parent's permission before photographing the victim.
2. Do not make assumptions about the identity of the perpetrator.
3. Chart the exact words used by the client/child to describe the abuser.
4. Record information objectively; do not record your feelings, assumptions, or opinions of the incident or how it occurred.

History

1. Specify the time, date, and location as described by the client.
2. Report the sequence of events before the abuse/attack.
3. Identify and explain the period of time between the abuse/attack and initiation of medical attention.
4. List other people/children in the immediate vicinity of the abuse/attack.
5. Include quotations from the client.
6. Use objective, specific documentation when recording observations of the client and the person who brought the client to the emergency department.
7. Observe and record the interaction of the child and the parents and the older adult client with their family.
8. Do conduct the interview in private.

Physical examination

1. Be specific in describing the location, size, and shape of bruises and lacerations. If possible, photograph the client to demonstrate the extent of the injuries.
2. If possible, describe the location and extent of injuries on an anatomic diagram.
3. Identify the presence of other injuries.
4. Describe the victim's reaction to pain, level of pain, and location of pain.

D. **Emotional neglect**: absence of a warm, interpersonal atmosphere that is necessary for psychosocial growth, development, and the promotion of positive feelings of self-worth and self-esteem.

E. **Economic abuse**: failing to provide financial support to an individual, even though funds are available (e.g., not paying utility bills and water/electricity being shut off to home).

F. **Sexual abuse**: lack of comprehension and consent on the part of the individual involved in sexual activities that are either exploitative or physically intimate in nature (e.g., rape, fondling, oral or genital contact, masturbation, unclothing, etc.).

G. **Incest**: sexual activity performed between members of a family group.

Family Violence

Patterns of dysfunctional, violent families can frequently be traced back for several generations. Adult behavior and role models for parenting are influenced by the childhood experiences within the family system.

> **! TEST ALERT** Assess dynamics of family interactions; identify risk factors; plan interventions to assist the client and family to cope.

Assessment: Recognize Cues

A. The incorporation of violence within the family teaches children that the use of violence is appropriate. When the children grow up and form their own families, they tend to recreate the same parent-child, husband-wife relationships experienced in their original family.

B. Frequently, the abuser has inappropriate expectations of family members; the abuser may expect perfection and may be obsessed with discipline and control.

C. Family members are confused regarding their roles in the family; parents may be unable to assume adult roles in the family. Adult family members who feel inadequate in their roles may use violence in an attempt to prove themselves and to maintain superiority.

D. Family is usually isolated, both physically and emotionally. The family tends to have few friends and is frequently isolated from the extended family. Family members are ashamed of what is occurring and tend to withdraw from social contacts in fear that the family activities might become known to others.

E. The *hostage response* is when victims assume responsibility for the violence inflicted on them.

Characteristics of Abuse: The Perpetrator

A. The person who abuses – the perpetrator.
   1. Perpetrator has an inability to control impulses; explosive temper; low tolerance for frustration.
   2. Possesses greater physical strength than the victim.
   3. Has low self-esteem and depression; feels they are a victim.
   4. Tends to project shortcomings and inadequacies onto others.
   5. Emotional immaturity; decreased capacity to delay satisfaction.
   6. Suspicious of everyone; fear of being exposed; tends to isolate self from family.
   7. High incidence of drug and alcohol abuse.
   8. Often has experienced abuse as a child; has a greater tendency to demonstrate violence in their adult relationships.

B. Common similarities between person who abuses and victim.
   1. Poor self-concept and feelings of insecurity.
   2. Feelings of helplessness, powerlessness, and dependence.
   3. Difficulty in handling or inability to handle anger.

Older Adult Abuse

Assessment: Recognize Cues

A. Types of older adult abuse (Box 7.6).
B. Typical victim.
   1. Woman of advanced age with few social contacts.

Box 7.6   OLDER ADULT CARE FOCUS

Older Adult Abuse

Types of older adult abuse

- Physical: willful infliction of injury
- Neglect: withholding goods or services (such as food or attention) to the detriment of the older adult's physical or mental health
- Emotional: withholding affection or imposing social isolation
- Exploitation: dishonest or inappropriate use of the older person's property, money, or other resources

Neglect indicators

- Poor hygiene, nutrition, and skin integrity
- Contractures
- Urine burns/excoriation
- Pressure ulcers
- Dehydration
- Bruises in various stages of healing
- Outdated medications
- No access to assistive devices if used by older adult (i.e., cane, wheelchair, hearing aid)

---

2. At least one physical or mental impairment, limiting the person's ability to perform activities of daily living.

C. Symptoms: contusions, abrasions, sprains, burns, bruising, human bite marks, sexual molestation, untreated or previously treated conditions, erratic hair loss from hair pulling, fractures, dislocations, head and face injuries (especially orbital fractures, black eyes, and broken teeth).

D. Behavior: clinging to the abuser, extreme guardedness in the presence of the abuser, wariness of strangers, expression of ambivalence toward family/caregivers, depression, social or physical isolation, denial of abuse for fear of retaliation.

Nursing Interventions: Take Action

Goal: To assess for older adult abuse

A. Use a private, separate setting for interviewing victim and perpetrator.

B. The interview must be unbiased, accurate, and appropriately documented.

C. Avoid signs of disapproval that might evoke shame or anger in the older client; be nonjudgmental.

Goal: To establish a safe environment

A. It is important for the nurse to be knowledgeable of the legal responsibilities in regard to state practice acts and reporting of abuse.

B. Client and family teaching in the areas of nutrition, general physical care, etc.

Spousal or Intimate Partner Abuse

Assessment: Recognize Cues

A. Most often, the spouse abused is the wife; frequently, the violence is a pattern in the woman's life. The violence in the family is frequently associated with alcohol; often,

there is a history of the woman's parents having a violent relationship.

B. It is not uncommon for the husband or abuser to have been exposed to violent family dynamics during childhood.

Nursing Interventions: Take Action

Goal: To establish a safe environment

A. Emergency treatment, counseling, and work that goes on in shelters toward rehabilitating and providing long-term support to victims of abuse.

> **! NURSING PRIORITY** When working with an abused victim, avoid anything that sounds like blaming the individual for their situation.

RAPE

A. Legal definition of rape (varies from state to state): forced, violent sexual attack on an individual without their consent. Includes sex acts other than forced intercourse as rape; some states do not recognize rape by the husband.

B. Sexual assault is not a means of sexual gratification; it is a violent physical and emotional attack. Men attack women in an attempt to demonstrate their power and dominance; it is an attempt to control, terrify, and degrade the woman.

C. Majority of rapes are not sudden and impulsive; they are well planned.

D. Most women know the rapist; most rape assaults occur between people of the same race.

E. Rape-trauma syndrome: variant of posttraumatic stress disorder; has two phases, an acute phase and a long-term reorganization phase.

Assessment: Recognize Cues

A. Woman may experience a wide range of emotional responses: fear, shock, disbelief, anger, denial, guilt, embarrassment, physical trauma, skeletal muscle tension, gastrointestinal and genitourinary symptoms/discomfort.

B. Advise the woman to not "clean up" after a rape, because the physical evidence may be destroyed; advise the woman to come immediately to the emergency department.

C. Assist with complete physical assessment.

Nursing Interventions: Take Action

Goal: To assist the client after the rape experience

A. Encourage the client to verbalize her feelings regarding the attack.

B. Ensure that written consent is obtained for the examination, photographs, laboratory tests, release of information, and laboratory samples.

C. Respond to the client in a warm, respectful, accepting manner; protect the client from becoming overwhelmed

Table 7.3 STAGES OF ALZHEIMER'S DISEASE

Stage	Hallmarks
Mild Alzheimer's disease (early-stage)	May function independently, but notices memory lapses. Friends, family, or neighbors start to notice memory or concentration difficulties. Difficulty choosing the right word or name and remembering names when introduced to new people. Greater difficulty noticed when performing tasks in social or work settings. Forgetting material that one has just read. Losing or misplacing a valuable object. Increasing trouble with planning or organizing.
Moderate Alzheimer's disease (middle-stage)	Longest stage that can last for many years. Forgetfulness of events or about one's own personal history. Feeling moody or withdrawn, especially in socially or mentally challenging situations. Being unable to recall their own address or telephone number or the high school or college from which they graduated. Confusion about where they are or what day it is. May refuse to bathe and needs help choosing proper clothing for the season or the occasion. Trouble controlling bladder and bowels in some individuals. Changes in sleep patterns, such as sleeping during the day and becoming restless at night. An increased risk of wandering and becoming lost. Personality and behavioral changes, including suspiciousness and delusions or compulsive, repetitive behavior like handwringing or tissue shredding.
Severe Alzheimer's disease (late-stage)	Person requires full-time, around-the-clock assistance with daily personal care. Lose awareness of recent experiences and of their surroundings. Require high levels of assistance with activities of daily living (ADLs). Experience changes in physical abilities, including the ability to walk, sit, and eventually, swallow. Have increasing difficulty communicating. Become vulnerable to infections, especially pneumonia.

Used with permission and adapted from Alzheimer's Association. (2019). *Stages of Alzheimer's.* https://www.alz.org/alzheimers-dementia/stages?type=alzfooter.

Box 7.7 TEN WARNING SIGNS OF ALZHEIMER DISEASE

1. Memory loss that disrupts daily life
   - Most common sign – especially forgetting recently learned information. Others include forgetting important dates or events; asking for the same information over and over; increasingly needing to rely on memory aides (e.g., reminder notes or electronic devices) or family members for things they used to handle on their own.
   What's a typical age-related change?
   Sometimes forgetting names or appointments but remembering them later.
2. Challenges in planning or solving problems
   - Experience changes in their ability to develop and follow a plan or work with numbers; trouble following a familiar recipe or keeping track of monthly bills; difficulty concentrating and take much longer to do things than they did before.
   What's a typical age-related change?
   Making occasional errors when balancing a checkbook.
3. Difficulty completing familiar tasks at home, at work, or at leisure
   - Hard to complete daily tasks: trouble driving to a familiar location, managing a budget at work, or remembering the rules of a favorite game.
   What's a typical age-related change?
   Occasionally needing help use the settings on a microwave or to record a television show.
4. Confusion with time or place
   - Lose track of dates, seasons, and the passage of time; trouble understanding something if it is not happening immediately; forget where they are or how they got there.
   What's a typical age-related change?
   Getting confused about the day of the week but figuring it out later.
5. Trouble understanding visual images and spatial relationship
   - Vision problems: difficulty reading, judging distance, and determining color or contrast, which may cause problems with driving.
   What's a typical age-related change?
   Vision changes related to cataracts.
6. New problems with words in speaking or writing
   - Trouble following or joining a conversation; may stop in the middle of a conversation and have no idea how to continue or they may repeat themself; struggle with vocabulary; have problems finding the right word; or call things by the wrong name (e.g., calling a "watch" a "hand-clock").
   What's a typical age-related change?
   Sometimes having trouble finding the right word.
7. Misplacing things and losing the ability to retrace steps
   - May put things in unusual places; lose things and be unable to go back over their steps to find them again; accuse others of stealing – this may occur more frequently over time.

Box 7.7 TEN WARNING SIGNS OF ALZHEIMER DISEASE—cont'd

What's a typical age-related change?
Misplacing things from time to time and retracing steps to find them.

8. Decreased or poor judgment
   - Experience changes in judgment or decision-making; poor judgment when dealing with money; giving large amounts to telemarketers; pay less attention to grooming or keeping themself clean.
   What's a typical age-related change?
   Making a bad decision once in a while.
9. Withdrawal from work or social activities
   - Starts to remove themself from hobbies, social activities, work projects, or sports; trouble keeping up with a favorite sports team or remembering how to complete a

favorite hobby; avoids being social because of the changes they have experienced.
What's a typical age-related change?
Sometimes feeling weary of work, family, and social obligations.

10. Changes in mood and personality
    - Mood and personalities can change; become confused, suspicious, depressed, fearful, or anxious; may be easily upset at home, at work, with friends, or in places where they are out of their comfort zone.
    What's a typical age-related change?
    Developing very specific ways of doing things and becoming irritable when a routine is disrupted.

Reprinted with permission from Alzheimer's Association. (2022) *Ten Warning Signs of Alzheimer's Disease*. https://www.alz.org/alzheimers-dementia/10_signs#signs.

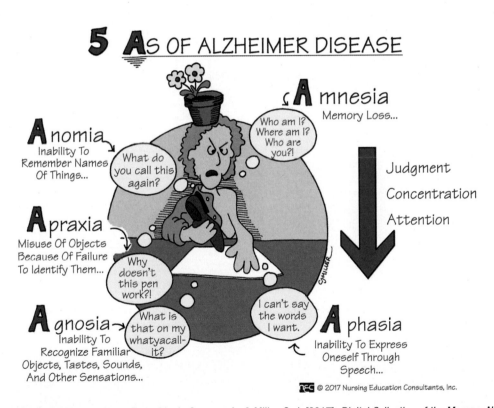

FIG. 7.2 Five As of Alzheimer Disease. (From Zerwekh, J., Garneau, A., & Miller, C. J. [2017]. *Digital Collection of the Memory Notebooks of Nursing* [4th ed.]. Chandler, AZ: Nursing Education Consultants, Inc.)

Goal: To administer medication to slow the dementia disease process (Appendix 7.1).

Goal: To provide a quiet, structured environment to increase consistency and promote feelings of security

A. Avoid dependency.

B. Establish routine for activities of daily living.
C. Meet client's physical needs.
D. Do not isolate client from others in the unit.
E. Provide handrails, walkers, and wheelchairs.
F. Do not change schedules suddenly.

SUNDOWNING SYNDROME

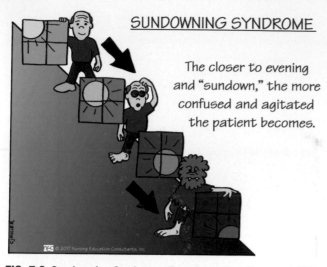

The closer to evening and "sundown," the more confused and agitated the patient becomes.

FIG. 7.3 Sundowning Syndrome. (From Zerwekh J, Garneau A, Miller CJ. [2017]. *Digital Collection of the Memory Notebooks of Nursing* [4th ed.]. Chandler, AZ: Nursing Education Consultants, Inc.)

> ❗ **NURSING PRIORITY** The 3 Rs – **routine, reinforcement,** and **repetition** – are key aspects of care, not only for the intellectually disabled, but for the older adult client with dementia as well.

G. Check for hazards in the environment (e.g., rugs on floor); make sure environment is well lighted.
H. Prevent client from wandering away from care area.

> ❗ **TEST ALERT** Orient the client to reality and monitor activities of the confused client. (Knowledge about providing care for the older client, especially the client with Alzheimer disease, is often tested.) Participate in reminiscence therapy and validation therapy.

Goal: To promote contact with reality
A. Make brief and frequent contact.
B. Give feedback.
C. Supply stimulation to motivate client to engage in activities.
D. Use concrete ideas in communication.
E. Maintain reality orientation by encouraging client to reminisce *(reminiscence therapy)* – encourage client to remember events, places, and people from their past.
F. Use *validation therapy* with older adults who misperceive their setting or life situation by communicating respect and acknowledgment of the older adults' feelings.
G. Orient client frequently to reality and surroundings.
   1. Allow client to have familiar objects around them.
   2. Use other items such as clocks, calendars, and daily schedules.
H. Use simple explanations and face-to-face interaction.
I. Do not shout message into client's ear.
J. Allow sufficient time for client to complete projects.

Table 7.4   ASSESSMENT OF ANXIETY

Physiologic	*Psychological*
Sympathetic Responses	**Behavioral Responses**
Tachycardia	Restlessness
Elevated blood pressure	Agitation
Increased perspiration	Tremors (fine to gross shaking of the body)
Dilated pupils	Startle reaction
Hyperventilation with difficulty breathing	Rapid speech
Cold, clammy skin	Lack of coordination
Dry mouth	Withdrawal
Constipation	
Parasympathetic Responses	**Cognitive Responses**
Urinary frequency	Impaired attention
Diarrhea	Poor concentration
	Forgetfulness
	Blocking of thought
	Decreased perceptual field
	Decreased productivity
	Confusion
Related Responses	**Affective Responses**
Headaches	Tension
Nausea or vomiting	Jittery feeling
Sleep disturbances	Worried
Muscular tension	Apprehension, nervousness
	Irritability
	Dread
	Fear
	Panic
	Fear of impending doom

K. Reinforce reality-oriented comments and orientation to time, place, and date.

> ❗ **NURSING PRIORITY** Speaking slowly and in a face-to-face position is most effective when communicating with an older adult experiencing hearing loss. Visual cues facilitate understanding. Shouting causes distortion of high-pitched sounds, and in some instances, creates a feeling of discomfort for the client.

Goal: To provide diversion activities that enhance self-esteem
A. Name sign and picture on door identifying client's room.
B. Identifying sign on outside of dining room door.
C. Large clock, with oversized numbers and hands, appropriately placed.

Table 7.5 NURSING MANAGEMENT OF ANXIETY

Level of Anxiety	Data Collection	Goal	Nursing Management
Mild	Increased alertness, motivation, and attentiveness	To assist client to tolerate some anxiety	1. Help the client identify and describe feelings. 2. Help the client develop the capacity to tolerate mild anxiety and use it consciously and constructively.
Moderate	Perception narrowed, selective inattention, poor concentration, physical discomforts	To reduce anxiety; directed toward helping client understand cause of anxiety and new ways of controlling it	1. Provide an outlet for tension, such as walking; crying; or working at simple, concrete tasks.
Severe	Behavior becomes automatic; connections between details are not seen; senses are drastically reduced	To assist in channeling anxiety	1. Recognize own level of anxiety. 2. Link the client's behavior with feelings. 3. Protect defenses and coping mechanisms. 4. Identify and modify anxiety-provoking situations.
Panic	Overwhelmed; inability to function or communicate; potential for bodily harm to self and others; loss of rational thought; hallucinations or delusions may be present	To be supportive and protective	1. Provide a nonstimulating, structured environment. 2. Avoid touching. 3. Stay with the client. 4. Medicate the client with tranquilizers if necessary.

! NURSING PRIORITY Decreasing stimuli in the environment by providing a calm, quiet atmosphere is a priority nursing action for the client experiencing anxiety.

D. Large calendar, indicating 1 day at a time, with month, day, and year identified in bold print.

! OLDER ADULT PRIORITY The 4 Ps for clients with dementia: Protecting dignity, Preserving function, Providing a safe environment, and Promoting quality of life.

ANXIETY

Anxiety is an emotion, a subjective experience; a feeling state that is experienced as vague uneasiness, tension, or apprehension; it occurs when the ego is threatened, is provoked by the unknown, and precedes all new experiences.
A. Assessment: Recognize Cues (Table 7.4).
B. Nursing Interventions: Take Action (Table 7.5).

! TEST ALERT Assist client in using behavioral strategies to decrease anxiety.

Anxiety Disorders

Anxiety can be a predominant disturbance (panic and generalized anxiety), or anxiety can be experienced as a person attempts to confront a dreaded situation (phobic disorder) or resist the obsessions and compulsions of an obsessive-compulsive disorder. In general, these are common responses to emotional problems that are seldom treated in a psychiatric setting because the person does not have a great defect in reality testing and does not demonstrate severe antisocial behavior (Table 7.6).

Somatic Symptom Disorders

Somatic symptom disorders are disorders in which the person has physical symptoms suggesting a physiologic etiology; however, after in-depth assessment and diagnostic testing, no organic disease or physiologic abnormalities are found.

Assessment: Recognize Cues

A. Conversion disorder is a loss of, or alteration in, voluntary and/or sensory functioning that suggests a neurologic disorder but is related to expression of a psychological conflict or need; person appears calm while experiencing symptoms.
  1. Development of one or more voluntary and/or sensory impairments (e.g., blindness, deafness, loss of sensation), suggesting a neurologic disorder.
  2. Symptoms are not under voluntary control.
  3. *La belle indifference*: an attitude toward the symptoms in which there is a lack of concern.

Table 7.7 PERSONALITY DISORDERS

Paranoid Personality	Antisocial Personality	Avoidant Personality
Suspicious and mistrustful of people	Violates rights of others	Fear of criticism or disapproval
Secretive	Lacks responsibility	Hypersensitive to potential rejection
Questions loyalty of others	Manipulative	Views self as socially inept, personally unappealing, and inferior to others
Jealous	Unable to sustain a job; frequent job changes and lengthy periods of unemployment	Inhibited in interpersonal relationships
Overly concerned with hidden motives and special meanings	Financial dependency	Reluctant to take personal risks
Hypersensitive and alert	Common behaviors observed – lying, stealing, truancy	Unwilling to get involved with people unless certain of being liked
Exaggerates	Excessive drinking and drug use	
Unable to relax	Criminality	
Takes offense quickly	Vagrancy	
Impaired affect	Lack of remorse	
Unemotional and cold		
No sense of humor		
Absence of soft, tender, sentimental feelings		
Distorts reality		
Uses projection		

Schizoid Personality	Borderline Personality	Dependent Personality
Unable to form social relationships	Unstable interpersonal relationships and moods; splitting behavior (admires then devalues a person)	Submissive; clinging behavior
Cold and aloof; flat affect		Fear of separation
Indifferent to praise or criticism	Impulsiveness and unpredictability that may be self-damaging (e.g., spending, sex, reckless driving, drug use)	Difficulty making everyday decisions
Has little or no desire for social involvement	Identity disturbance	Needs others to assume responsibility
Appears reserved, withdrawn, and seclusive; emotionally detached from others	Recurrent suicidal behavior, gestures, or threats	Wants others to take care and nurture
	Self-mutilating behavior	Feels uncomfortable or helpless when left alone
	Inappropriate, intense anger; lack of anger control; shifts in mood	Difficulty initiating projects independently
	Chronic feelings of emptiness	

Schizotypal Personality	Histrionic Personality	Obsessive-Compulsive Personality
Magical thinking (e.g., telepathy, superstition)	Excessive emotionality and attention-seeking behavior	Preoccupation with rules, lists, organization, schedules
Ideas of reference	Uncomfortable when not center of attention	Perfectionistic
Social isolation	Uses physical appearance to draw attention to self	Excessive devotion to work
Recurrent illusion	Self-dramatization, theatrical, and exaggerated expression of emotion	Overly conscientious and inflexible
Oddities of thought, perception, speech, and behavior	Easily suggestible	Reluctant to delegate tasks
Inappropriate affect		Hoards money; frugal
Excessive social anxiety		Rigid and stubborn in thoughts

	Narcissistic Personality	
	Grandiose self-importance	
	Preoccupation with fantasies of success	
	Belief that they are "special or unique"	
	Need for excessive amount of admiration	
	Unrealistic sense of entitlement	
	Interpersonal exploitation	
	Lack of empathy	
	Arrogant and haughty	
	Fears rejection by others	

D. Anticipate and deal with depression in a client who gradually acquires enough insight to realize and accept responsibility for their behavior.

E. Common sources of frustration for nurses.
1. Client's immature behavior.
2. Poor communication skills.

Goal: To minimize manipulation and "acting-out" behaviors and encourage verbal communication

A. Set firm, consistent limits without being punitive.

B. Be aware of how client may manipulate other staff members (e.g., playing one against the other or splitting).

C. Promote expression of feelings versus acting out.

D. Promote client's acceptance of responsibility for their own actions and a social responsibility to others.

Goal: To set realistic limits

A. Break the health-attention-avoidance cycle that usually exists in relating to this type of client.

B. Support the client who is gradually making more decisions on their own.

C. Offer assistance only when needed.

SUBSTANCE-RELATED AND ADDICTIVE DISORDERS

Substance use disorders are characterized by behavior changes, regular use of a substance (alcohol or another drug) that affects the central nervous system (CNS), and withdrawal symptoms when the substance is not taken. The term "addiction" is defined as a chronic disease of brain reward related to drug dependence or compulsive use and involves loss of control with respect to use of the drug or alcohol.

Polydrug dependence involves the regular use of three or more psychoactive substances over a period of at least 6 months.

A. Substance abuse.
1. A pattern of pathologic use.
   a. Intoxication during the day.
   b. Inability to cut down or stop drinking.
   c. Daily need of the substance to function.
   d. Blackouts and medical complications from use.
   e. Impairment of social or occupational functioning.
2. Tolerance.
   a. Increased amounts of the substance are required to achieve the desired effect.
   b. Markedly diminished effect with regular use of the same dose.
3. Withdrawal: a specific syndrome of symptoms that develops when the person abruptly stops ingesting the substance.

B. Psychological dependence.
1. Habituation: the need to take the substance.
2. Physiologic dependence is not necessary.
3. No physiologic symptoms on withdrawal.

Alcohol Dependence (Alcoholism)

A chronic pattern of pathologic alcohol use is characterized by impairment in social or occupational functioning, along with tolerance or withdrawal symptoms.

General Concepts

A. Incidence.
1. Alcohol abuse is more common among men than women.
2. Only 25% of individuals with alcohol dependence seek treatment.

B. Effects of use.
1. Central nervous system (CNS) depressant drug.
2. Measured in the bloodstream by the blood alcohol level (BAL).
3. A BAL of 8% to 10% (0.08 mg to 0.10 mg) or more is considered the legal level of intoxication in most states.

Assessment: Recognize Cues

A. Risk factors.
1. History of alcoholism in family.
2. History of total abstinence.
3. Broken or disrupted home.
4. Last or near-last child in a large family.
5. Heavy smoking.
6. Cultural groups: Irish, Eskimo, Scandinavian, Native American.

B. General personality characteristics of alcoholics.
1. Dependent behavior along with resentment of authority.
2. Demanding and domineering with a low tolerance for frustration.
3. Dissatisfied with life; tendency toward self-destructive acts, including suicide.
4. Low self-esteem and poor self-concept.

C. Signs and symptoms of possible alcohol abuse.
1. Sprains, bruises, and injuries of questionable origin.
2. Diarrhea and early morning vomiting.
3. Chronic cough, palpitations, and infections.
4. Frequent Monday morning illnesses; blackouts (inability to recall events or actions while intoxicated).

D. Alcohol withdrawal syndrome. The withdrawal syndrome develops in heavy drinkers who have increased, decreased, or interrupted the intake of alcohol.
1. Alcohol withdrawal.
   a. Anorexia, irritability, nausea, tremulousness.
   b. Insomnia, nightmares, irritability, hyper-alertness.
   c. Tachycardia, increased blood pressure, diaphoresis.
   d. Onset within several hrs after cessation of drinking (usually 48-72 hrs); clears up within 5 to 7 days.
2. Alcohol withdrawal delirium (Fig. 7.4).
   a. Autonomic hyperactivity: tachycardia, sweating, increased blood pressure.

ALCOHOL WITHDRAWAL DELIRIUM
"Delirium Tremens (DTs)"

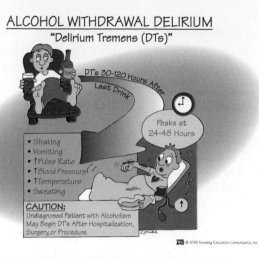

FIG. 7.4 Alcohol Withdrawal Delirium. (From Zerwekh J, Garneau A, Miller CJ. [2017]. *Digital Collection of the Memory Notebooks of Nursing* [4th ed.]. Chandler, AZ: Nursing Education Consultants, Inc.)

    b. Vivid hallucinations, delusions, confusion.
    c. Coarse, irregular tremor is almost always seen; fever may occur.
    d. Onset within 24 to 72 hrs after the last ingestion of alcohol; usually lasts 2 to 3 days.
    e. Convulsions/seizures may occur.

❗ NURSING PRIORITY Alcohol withdrawal delirium is a medical emergency!

E. Wernicke encephalopathy.
  1. An acute, reversible neurologic disorder.
  2. Triad of symptoms: global confusion, ataxia, and eye movement abnormality (nystagmus).
  3. Occurs primarily in clients with chronic alcoholism; may develop in illnesses that interfere with thiamine (vitamin B_1) absorption (e.g., gastric cancer, malabsorption syndrome, regional enteritis).
  4. Treatment: thiamine 100 mg, given intravenously (IV) initially, then followed by 50 to 100 mg/day intramuscularly (IM) or IV, usually reverses nystagmus within 2 to 3 hrs of treatment.
F. Korsakoff syndrome (alcohol amnesiac disorder).
  1. A chronic, *irreversible* disorder, often following Wernicke encephalopathy.
  2. Triad of symptoms: memory loss, learning deficit, confabulation (filling in of memory gaps with plausible stories).
G. Other disorders associated with chronic alcoholism: pneumonitis, esophageal varices, cirrhosis, pancreatitis, diabetes (these are addressed in the appropriate chapter discussing the system).

Nursing Interventions: Take Action

Goal: To assess for alcoholism in a client through careful questioning
A. Frequently used acronym – *CAGE-AID* – suggests asking the following questions. An answer of "yes" to any question can indicate a problem.

  1. Have you ever felt the need to:
     Cut down on your drinking?
  2. Have you ever felt:
     Annoyed by criticism of your drinking?
  3. Have you had:
     Guilty feelings about drinking?
  4. Do you ever take a morning:
     Eye-opener?
  5. **AID** – **A**dapt questions to **I**nclude **D**rugs.
B. Identify the alcoholic client in the preoperative period.
  1. Often, alcoholics are undiagnosed at the time of surgery and may go into withdrawal or alcohol withdrawal delirium after the NPO (nothing by mouth) period.
  2. Preoperative medication doses need to be adjusted; usually, if tolerant of alcohol, clients are also tolerant of other medications, including anesthetics.
  3. Client usually takes longer to be fully responsive during postoperative period; client is susceptible to severe respiratory complications; client has more difficulty with healing because of poor nutritional state.

Goal: To assist in the medical treatment of alcohol withdrawal
A. Benzodiazepines for agitation (Appendix 12.2).
B. Thiamine (vitamin B_1) to prevent Wernicke encephalopathy.
C. Magnesium sulfate is used to increase effectiveness of vitamin B_1, because it helps reduce post withdrawal seizures.
D. Anticonvulsant (phenytoin or carbamazepine), if necessary, for seizure control.
E. Encourage use of multivitamins, especially folic acid, B_{12}, and vitamin C.
F. Antipsychotic agents (chlorpromazine or haloperidol) for alcohol withdrawal delirium.
G. Beta-adrenergic blockers (atenolol, propranolol) to improve vital signs; encourage intake of fluids, but do not force.

Goal: To provide for the basic needs of rest, comfort, safety, and nutrition
A. Safety measures, such as bed rest and use of bed rails, may be necessary.
B. *If client is experiencing delirium tremens, stay with them and notify RN.*
C. Have room adequately lit to help reduce confusion and avoid shadows and unclear objects.
D. Monitor vital signs every 1 to 4 hrs.
E. Encourage a soft, high-carbohydrate diet.

Goal: To recognize complications of alcohol use
A. Obstetric implications.
  1. Use of alcohol during pregnancy may lead to fetal alcohol syndrome.
  2. Chronic alcoholism can lead to maternal malnutrition, especially folic acid deficiency, bone marrow suppression, infections, and liver disease.
  3. Alcohol withdrawal syndrome may occur in the intrapartum period as early as 12 to 48 hrs after the last drink.

4. Alcohol withdrawal delirium may occur in the post-partum period.

♣ B. Neonatal implications (fetal alcohol syndrome).
1. Teratogenic effects may be seen along with growth and developmental delay.
2. Increased risk for anomalies of the heart, head, face, and extremities.
3. Withdrawal symptoms can occur shortly after birth and are characterized by tremors, agitation, sweating, and seizure activity.
4. Maintain seizure precautions.

C. Medical complications of alcohol abuse.
1. Trauma related to falls, burns, hematomas.
2. Liver disease: cirrhosis, esophageal varices, hepatic coma.
3. Gastrointestinal disease: gastritis, bleeding ulcers, pancreatitis.
4. Nutritional disease: malnutrition, anemia caused by iron or vitamin B_{12} deficiency, thiamine deficiency.
5. Infections, especially pneumonia.
6. Neurologic disease: polyneuropathy and dementia.

Goal: To assist in the long-term rehabilitation of the client
A. Avoid sympathy, because clients tend to rationalize and use dependent, manipulative behavior to seek privileges.
B. Maintain a nonjudgmental attitude.
C. Set behavior limits in a firm but kind manner.
D. Place responsibility for sobriety on client; do not give advice or punish or reprimand client for failures.
E. Provide opportunities to decrease social isolation by encouraging participation in social groups and activities.
F. Encourage client to develop coping mechanisms other than alcohol to deal with stress.
G. Refer clients and family to available community resources.
1. Alcoholics Anonymous (AA): a self-help group focusing on education, guidance, and the sharing of problems and experiences unique to the individual.
2. Al-Anon: a self-help support group for the spouses and significant others of the alcoholic.
3. Alateen: the support group for teenagers with an alcoholic parent.
4. Adult Children of Alcoholics (ACOA): support group for ACOA and dysfunctional individuals.
5. Families Anonymous: support group for the families whose lives have been affected by the addicted client's behavior.
6. Codependents Anonymous: support group for code-pendents who may be alcoholics or drug addicts and for persons who are close to an addict.
H. Promote adherence to prescribed therapeutic regimens.
1. Disulfiram: a drug that produces intense side effects after ingestion of alcohol or application of lotions/mouthwashes that contain alcohol (severe nausea, vomiting, flushed face, hypotension, blurred vision).
2. Naltrexone: opioid antagonist that decreases the craving for alcohol.
3. Acamprosate: a drug that helps clients abstain from alcohol.

Polydrug Dependence

Polydrug dependence is the regular use of three or more psychoactive substances over a period of at least 6 months.

General Concepts

A. Effects of use.
1. Relieves anxiety.
2. Overdose can occur.
B. General personality characteristics.
1. Inability to cope with stress, frustration, or anxiety.
2. Rebellious, immature, desire for immediate gratification.
3. Passivity and low self-esteem.
4. Difficulty forming warm, personal relationships.
5. Uses coping mechanisms: denial, rationalization, intellectualization.

Assessment: Recognize Cues

A. General data collection.
1. Determine the pattern of drug use.
   a. Which drugs are being used by the client?
   b. When was the last use?
   c. How much does the client use and how often?
   d. How long has the client been using drugs?
   e. What combination of drugs is being used?
2. Determine whether there are any physical changes present (e.g., needle tracks, swollen nasal mucous membranes, reddened conjunctivae).
B. Narcotic dependence.
   Examples of narcotics and street names: opium, heroin, morphine, codeine, fentanyl, methadone, oxycodone; horse, junk, smack (heroin); black poppy (opium); M (morphine); dollies (methadone); terp (terpin hydrate or cough syrup with codeine).
1. Administration.
   a. Heroin: sniffed, smoked, injected intravenously (mainlining), injected subcutaneously (skin popping).
   b. Other narcotics are usually taken orally or by injection.
2. Symptoms of use.
   a. Drowsiness and decreased blood pressure, pulse, and respiratory rate.
   b. Pinpoint pupils, needle tracks, scarring.
   c. Overdose effects: slow, shallow breathing, clammy skin, convulsions, coma, pulmonary edema, possible death.
3. Withdrawal symptoms.
   a. Onset of symptoms approximately 8 to 12 hrs after the last dose.
   b. Lacrimation, sweating, sneezing, yawning.
   c. Gooseflesh (piloerection), tremor, irritability, anorexia.
   d. Dilated pupils, abdominal cramps, vomiting, involuntary muscle spasms.
   e. Symptoms generally subside within 7 to 10 days.

C. Sedative-hypnotic dependence.

Examples of sedative-hypnotics and street names: barbiturates (pentobarbital, secobarbital) and the benzodiazepines (chlordiazepoxide, diazepam); green and whites, roaches (chlordiazepoxide); red birds, red devils (secobarbital); blue birds (amobarbital capsules); yellow birds (pentobarbital); downers, rainbow, 7145 (barbiturates; tranquilizers).

1. Administration: oral or injected.
2. Symptoms of use.
   a. Alterations in mood, thought, behavior.
   b. Impairment in coordination, judgment.
   c. Signs of intoxication: slurred speech, unsteady gait, decreased attention span or memory.
   d. Barbiturate use: often violent, disruptive, irresponsible behavior.
3. Withdrawal symptoms.
   a. Insomnia, anxiety, profuse sweating, weakness.
   b. Severe reactions of delirium, grand mal seizures, cardiovascular collapse.

> **! NURSING PRIORITY** Abrupt withdrawal of CNS depressants may lead to death. Client must be tapered off drug slowly.

D. Cocaine abuse.

Examples and street names: coke, toot, nose candy, snow, C, powder, lady, blow, bump, Charlie, flake, rock.

1. Administration: intranasal ("snorting") or by intravenous or subcutaneous injection; also smoked in pipe (freebasing).
2. Symptoms of use.
   a. Euphoria, grandiosity, and a sense of well-being.
   b. Amphetamine-like or stimulant-like effects such as increased blood pressure, dilated pupils, racing of the heart, paranoia, anxiety.
   c. Used regularly, cocaine may disrupt eating and sleeping habits, leading to irritability and decreased concentration.

> **! NURSING PRIORITY** Crack (rock) has been labeled the most addictive drug. It is a potent form of cocaine hydrochloride mixed with baking soda and water, heated (cooked), allowed to harden, and then broken or "cracked" into little pieces and smoked in cigarettes or glass water pipes. Cardiac dysrhythmias, respiratory paralysis, and seizures are some of the dangers associated with crack use.

3. Withdrawal symptoms.
   a. Severe craving.
   b. Coming down from a "high" often leads to a severe "letdown," depressed feeling.
   c. Psychological dependence often leads to cocaine becoming a total obsession.

E. Methamphetamine dependence.

Example and street names: dextroamphetamine; meth, crystal, crank, bennies, wakeups, uppers, chalk, dunk, gak, ice, pootie, quartz, scooby, speed or trash (amphetamines).

1. Administration: inhalation, oral, or injected.
2. Symptoms of use.
   a. Elation, agitation, hyperactivity, irritability, visual and auditory hallucinations, paranoia, and profound dental caries – "meth mouth."
   b. Increased pulse, respiration, and blood pressure.
   c. Fine tremor, muscle twitching, and mydriasis (pupillary dilation).
   d. Large doses: convulsions, cardiovascular collapse, respiratory depression, coma, death.
3. Withdrawal symptoms.
   a. Appear within 2 to 4 days after the last dose.
   b. Depression, overwhelming fatigue, suicide attempts.

F. PCP (phencyclidine hydrochloride) abuse.

Examples and street names: peace pill, hog, super pill, elephant tranquilizer, angel dust, rocket fuel, primo, sherms, embalming fluid (PCP), zoom (PCP mixed with marijuana).

1. Administration: snorted, smoked, or orally ingested; usually smoked along with marijuana.
2. Symptoms of use.
   a. Euphoria, feeling of numbness, mood changes.
   b. Diaphoresis, eye movement changes (nystagmus), hypertension, catatonic-like stupor with eyes open.
   c. Seizures, shivering, decerebrate posturing, possible death.
   d. Synesthesia: experiencing one sense when another is actually being stimulated (e.g., seeing colors when a loud sound occurs).
3. Overdose symptoms ("bad trip"): psychosis, possible death.
   a. User may become violent, destructive, and confused.
   b. Users have been known to go berserk; users may harm themselves and others.
   c. Intoxicating symptoms lighten and worsen over a period of 48 hrs.

G. Hallucinogen abuse.

Examples and street names: LSD (lysergic acid diethylamide), psilocybin ("magic mushroom"), mescaline (peyote), DMT, MDA; acid, blotter, boomers, cid, golden dragon, looney tunes, Lucy Mae, microdust, tabs, yellow sunshine.

1. Administration: usually oral, but LSD and mescaline can be injected.
2. Symptoms of use.
   a. Pupillary dilation, tachycardia, sweating.
   b. Visual hallucinations, depersonalization, impaired judgment and mood.
   c. Flashbacks and "bad trips."
   d. Usually no signs of withdrawal symptoms after use has been discontinued.

H. Marijuana dependence.

Examples and street names: marijuana, hashish, tetrahydrocannabinol (THC); joints, reefers, pot, grass, shit, dope blunt, doobie, ganja, herb, skunk, smoke, stinkweed, trees, hemp, boom, Mary Jane and sinsemilla (marijuana), hash and gangster (hashish).

1. Administration: oral, sniffed, and smoked.
2. Symptoms of use.
   a. Euphoria, relaxation, tachycardia, and conjunctival congestion.

b. Paranoid ideation; impaired judgment.

c. Rarely, panic reactions and psychoses.

d. Heavy use leads to apathy and general deterioration in all aspects of living.

e. Overdose effects: flashbacks, bronchitis, personality changes.

3. Withdrawal symptoms.

a. Anxiety, sleeplessness, sweating.

b. Lack of appetite, nausea, general malaise.

I. Designer drugs.

Examples and street names: ecstasy, Adam, rolls, skittles, sweets, beans, candy, E-bomb, thizz, love drug, Molly (MDMA [methylenedioxy-methamphetamine]), China white (MTPT).

1. Called *analog drugs* because they retain the properties of controlled drugs (e.g., MTPT is an analog of meperidine).

2. Symptoms of use and side effects are similar to those associated with the controlled substance from which they are derived.

Nursing Interventions: Take Action

Goal: To assess the drug use pattern

Goal: To assist in medical treatment during detoxification or withdrawal.

A. Narcotics.

1. Narcotic antagonists, such as naloxone, nalorphine, or levallorphan, are administered intravenously for narcotic overdose.

2. Withdrawal is managed with methadone tapering and naltrexone chloride. Substitution therapy with buprenorphine may be instituted to decrease withdrawal symptoms for longer effects.

B. Opiates.

1. Substitution therapy with methadone hydrochloride may be instituted to decrease withdrawal symptoms.

2. Some health care providers prescribe buprenorphine as needed for objective symptoms, gradually decreasing the dosage until the drug is discontinued.

C. Stimulants.

1. Treatment of overdose is geared toward stabilization of vital signs.

2. IV antihypertensives may be used, along with IV diazepam, to control seizures.

3. Chlordiazepoxide may be administered orally for the first few days while client is "crashing."

4. Withdrawal symptoms are managed with tricyclic antidepressants, such as desipramine, and dopamine agonists, such as bromocriptine.

D. Hallucinogens and marijuana.

1. Medications are normally not prescribed for withdrawal from these substances.

2. In the event of overdose, diazepam or chlordiazepoxide may be given as needed to decrease agitation.

E. Be aware that gradual withdrawal, detoxification, or dechemicalization is necessary for the client addicted to barbiturates, narcotics, or tranquilizers.

F. Abrupt withdrawal, or quitting "cold turkey," is often dangerous and can be fatal.

G. Maintain a patent airway; have oxygen available.

H. Provide a safe, quiet environment (i.e., remove harmful objects, place bed in low position).

Goal: To decrease problem behaviors of manipulation and "acting out."

A. Set firm, consistent limits.

B. Confront client with manipulative behaviors.

Goal: To promote alternative coping methods

A. Encourage responsibility for own behavior.

B. Encourage the use of hobbies, exercise, or alternative therapies as a means to deal with frustration and anxiety.

Goal: To recognize complications of substance abuse

A. Obstetric implications.

1. Narcotic addiction.

a. Increased risk for pregnancy-induced hypertension, malpresentation, and third-trimester bleeding.

b. Provide methadone maintenance therapy for the duration of the pregnancy – withdrawal is not advisable because of the risk to the fetus.

2. Use of other drugs causes increased risk to mother and fetus.

B. Neonatal complications.

1. Withdrawal symptoms depend on type of drug mother used.

2. Restlessness, jitteriness, hyperactive reflexes, high-pitched shrill cry; feeds poorly.

3. Maintain seizure precautions.

4. Administer antiepileptics to treat withdrawal and prevent seizures.

5. Swaddle infant in snug-fitting blanket.

6. Increased risk for congenital malformations and prematurity.

C. Medical implications.

1. Increased risk for hepatitis, malnutrition, and infections in general.

Goal: To assist in the long-term process of drug rehabilitation

A. Refer client to drug rehabilitation programs.

B. Promote self-help residential programs that foster self-support systems and use ex-addicts as rehabilitation counselors.

C. Methadone maintenance programs.

1. Must be 18 years old and addicted for more than 2 years with a history of detoxification treatments.

2. Methadone is a synthetic narcotic that appeases desire for opiates.

a. Controlled substance; given only under urinary surveillance.

b. Administered orally; prevents opiate withdrawal symptoms.

D. 12-step self-help groups.

1. Narcotics Anonymous: support group for clients who are addicted to narcotics and other drugs.

2. Nar-Anon: support group for relatives and friends of narcotic addicts.

3. Families Anonymous.

Gambling Disorder

Gambling is a compulsive activity that causes economic problems and significant disturbances in personal, social, or occupational functioning. Individuals with this disorder are preoccupied with the behavior, experience an increasing desire to gamble, and lie to conceal the extent of the problem.

Assessment: Recognize Cues

A. Disrupts, damages, or compromises family, personal, and vocational pursuits.
B. Evidence of forgery, fraud, embezzlement.
C. Unable to pay debts or meet other financial obligations.
D. Borrows money, either legally or illegally.
E. Loss of work because of frequent absenteeism.

Nursing Interventions: Take Action

Goal: To encourage client to develop alternative ways of dealing with stress
A. Refer client to self-help groups: Gamblers Anonymous (GAM-ANON).
B. Assist client in determining when anxiety and tension are increasing and provide a plan of action to prevent acts of stealing, setting fires, or destroying property.

MOOD DISORDERS

The bipolar disorders and major depressive disorder are characterized by disturbances of mood.

General Concepts

A. Incidence.
   1. More prevalent among family members when there is a positive family history.
   2. Major depression is seen more often in women.
   3. More common in higher socioeconomic groups.

Assessment: Recognize Cues

A. Bipolar disorder (Fig. 7.5). There are currently three types of bipolar disorder ranging from mild to severe forms and they include: bipolar I disorder (most severe), bipolar II disorder (low-level severity), and cyclothymic disorder (low-level severity; more common in children).
   a. Bipolar I disorder exhibits features of mania for at least 1 week with psychotic features (hallucinations, delusions) and is the most severe.
   b. Bipolar II disorder exhibits features of low-level mania (hypomania) followed by profound depression.
   c. Cyclothymic disorder resembles similar manifestations of bipolar II disorder with more irritable hypomanic episodes; some experience rapid cycling (4 mood episodes in a 12-month period); usually begins in adolescence or early adulthood.
   1. Mania.
      a. Onset before the age of 30 years.
      b. Mood: elevated, expansive, or irritable.

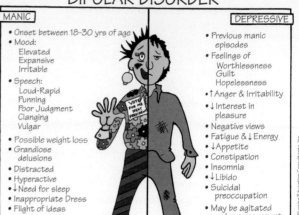

FIG. 7.5 Bipolar Affective Disorder. (From Zerwekh J, Garneau A, Miller CJ. [2017]. *Digital Collection of the Memory Notebooks of Nursing* [4th ed.]. Chandler, AZ: Nursing Education Consultants, Inc.)

   c. Speech: loud, rapid, difficult to interpret, punning, rhyming, clanging (using words that sound like the meaning rather than the actual word).
   d. Cognitive skills: flight of ideas, grandiose delusions, easily distracted.
   e. Psychomotor activity: hyperactive, decreased need for sleep, exhibitionistic, vulgar, profane, may make inappropriate sexual advances and be obscene.
   f. Course of manic episode: begins suddenly, rapidly escalates over a few days, and ends more abruptly than major depressive episodes.
   2. Hypomania (depressive).
      a. Has had one or more manic episodes.
      b. Mood: dysphoric, depressive, despairing, loss of interest or pleasure in most usual activities.
      c. Cognitive process: negative view of self, world, and of the future; poverty of ideas; crying; suicidal preoccupation.
      d. Psychomotor: may have either agitation or retardation in movements, feelings of fatigue, lack of appetite, constipation, sleeping disturbances (insomnia or early morning wakefulness), decrease in libido.
A. Major depressive disorder.
   1. May occur at any age.
   2. Differentiated as either a single episode or a recurring type.
   3. Severity and type of depression vary with the ability to test reality.
      a. Diagnosis is made when five or more of the following symptoms identified are present nearly every day over a 2-week period:
         (1) Depressed mood most of day.
         (2) Inability to feel pleasure.
         (3) Insomnia or hypersomnia.
         (4) Weight loss or weight gain.
         (5) Increased or decreased psychomotor activity.

(6) Suicidal thoughts or plan to harm self.

(7) Loss of energy or fatigue every day.

(8) Feelings of worthlessness or guilt.

(9) Poor concentration; unable to make decisions.

b. Delusional thoughts or hallucinations present with psychotic major depression.

Nursing Interventions: Take Action (manic episode)

Goal: To provide for basic human needs of safety and rest/activity

A. Reduce outside stimuli and provide a nonstimulating environment.

B. Monitor food intake: provide a high-calorie, high-vitamin, high-fiber diet with finger foods to be eaten as the client moves about.

> **! NURSING PRIORITY** Physiologic needs are the first priority in providing client care.

C. Encourage noncompetitive solitary activities such as walking, swimming, or painting.

D. Assist with personal hygiene.

> **! NURSING PRIORITY** During the manic phase, the client's physical safety is at risk because the hyperactivity may lead to exhaustion, and ultimately, cardiac failure.

Goal: To establish a therapeutic nurse-client relationship

A. Use firm, consistent, honest approach.

B. Assess client's abilities and involve client in their own care planning.

C. Promote problem-solving abilities; recognize that a false sense of independence is often demonstrated by loud, boisterous behavior.

D. Do not focus on or discuss grandiose ideas.

Goal: To set limits on behavior

A. Instructions should be clear and concise.

B. Initiate regularly scheduled contacts to demonstrate acceptance.

C. Maintain some distance between self and client to allow freedom of movement and to prevent feelings of being overpowered.

D. Maintain neutrality and objectivity: realize that client can be easily provoked by harmless remarks and may demonstrate a furious reaction but calm down quickly.

E. Use measures to prevent overt aggression (e.g., distraction, recognition of behaviors of increased excitement).

Goal: To promote adaptive coping with constructive use of energy

A. Do not hurry client; this leads to anxiety and hostile behavior.

> **! NURSING PRIORITY** In a hyperactive state, the client is extremely distractible, and responses to even the slightest stimuli are exaggerated.

B. Provide activities and constructive tasks that channel the agitated behavior (e.g., cleaning game room, going for a walk, gardening, playing catch).

Goal: To assist in the medical treatment

A. Administer lithium carbonate (Appendix 7.1).

B. Risperidone is a first-line treatment for severe mania.

C. Lamotrigine is a first-line treatment for acute manic episodes and maintenance therapy.

1. Clients taking lamotrigine need to be instructed to seek immediate medical attention if a skin rash appears, because this drug can cause a severe and potentially life-threatening rash.

Nursing Interventions: Take Action (depressive episode)

> **! NURSING PRIORITY** Depression and suicidal behaviors may be viewed as anger turned inward on the self. If this anger can be verbalized in a nonthreatening environment, the client may be able to resolve these feelings, regardless of the discomfort involved.

Goal: To assess for suicide potential

A. Recognition of suicidal intent.

1. Self-destructive behaviors are viewed as attempts to escape unbearable life situations.

2. Anxiety and hostility are overwhelmingly present.

3. There is the presence of ambivalence; living versus self-destructive impulses.

4. Depression, low self-esteem, and feelings of hopelessness are critical to evaluate, because suicide attempts are often made when the client feels like giving up.

5. Assess for *indirect* self-destructive behavior: any activity that is detrimental to the physical well-being of the client in which the potential outcome is death.

   a. Eating disorders: anorexia nervosa, bulimia, obesity, and overeating.

   b. Noncompliance with medical treatment (e.g., diabetic who does not take insulin).

   c. Cigarette smoking, gambling, criminal and/or socially deviant activities.

   d. Alcohol and drug abuse.

   e. Participation in high-risk sports (e.g., automobile racing; skydiving).

B. Suicide danger signs.

1. The presence of a suicide plan: specifics relating to method, its lethality, and likelihood for rescue.

2. Change in established patterns in routines (e.g., giving away personal items, making a will, saying good-bye).

3. Anticipation of failure: loss of a job, preoccupation with physical disease, actual or anticipated loss of a significant other.

4. Change in behavior, presence of panic, agitation, or calmness; often, as depression lifts, client has enough energy to act on suicidal feelings.

5. Hopelessness: feelings of impending doom, futility, and entrapment.

6. Withdrawal and rejection of help.

B. Negative symptoms – the absence of something that should be present.
   1. Loss of pleasure, blunted affect, loss of motivation, "avolition."
   2. Rigidity and mutism; poverty of thought.
C. Cognitive symptoms – symptoms associated with cognition, thinking.
   1. Difficulty concentrating.
   2. Problems with decision making.
   3. Impaired judgment, memory impairment.
D. Affective symptoms – symptoms that involve emotions and expression of emotion.
   1. Suicidal ideation.
   2. Hopelessness.
   3. Dysphoria.
E. Four *A*s: Eugen Bleuler's classic symptoms.
   1. *Associative looseness*: lack of logical thought progression, resulting in disorganized and chaotic thinking.
   2. *Affect*: emotion or feeling tone is one of indifference or is flat, blunted, exaggerated, or socially inappropriate.
   3. *Ambivalence*: conflicting, strong feelings (e.g., love and hate) that neutralize each other, leading to psychic immobilization, and difficulty in expressing other emotions.
   4. *Autism*: extreme retreat from reality characterized by fantasies, preoccupation with daydreams, and psychotic thought processes of delusion and hallucination.
      a. Hallucinations: false sensory perceptions with no basis in reality; may be auditory, olfactory, tactile, visual, gustatory; most common is auditory.
      b. Delusions: fixed, false beliefs not corrected by logic; develop as a defense against intolerable feelings or ideas that cause anxiety.
         (1) Delusions of grandeur: related to feelings of power, fame, splendor, magnificence.
         (2) Delusions of persecution: belief that others are out to harm, injure, or destroy.
      c. Ideas of reference: belief that actions and speech of others have reference to oneself; ideas symbolize feelings of guilt, insecurity, and alienation.
      d. Depersonalization: feeling alienated from oneself; difficulty distinguishing self from others; loss of boundaries between self and environment.
F. Additional characteristics.
   1. Regression: extreme withdrawal and social isolation.
   2. Negativism: doing the opposite of what is asked; typical behavior is to speak to no one and answer no one; used to cover feelings of unworthiness and inadequacy.
   3. Religiosity: excessive religious preoccupation.
   4. Impulsivity: unable to resist impulses.
   5. Motor retardation: slowed movement.
   6. Motor agitation: pacing or running; constantly on the move.

Nursing Interventions: Take Action
Goal: To build trust

TEST ALERT Building trust is the primary goal when working with the client with schizophrenia. Identify needs and assist in the care of a client experiencing sensory/perceptual alterations.

A. Encourage free expression of feelings (either negative or positive) without fear of rejection, ridicule, or retaliation.
B. Use nonverbal level of communication to demonstrate warmth, concern, and empathy, because client often distrusts words.
C. Consistency, reliability, acceptance, and persistence build trust.
D. Allow client to set pace; proceed slowly in planning social contacts.
Goal: To provide a safe and secure environment
A. Maintain familiar routines. Make sure persons who come in contact with the client are recognizable to the client.
B. Avoid stressful situations or increasing anxiety.
Goal: To clarify and reinforce reality
A. Involve client in reality-oriented activities.
B. Help client find satisfaction in the external environment and ways of relating to others.
C. Focus on clear communication and the immediate situation.
Goal: To promote and build self-esteem
A. Encourage simple activities with limited concentration and *no* competition.
B. Provide successful experiences with short-range goals realistic for client's level of functioning.
C. Relieve client of decision making until they are ready.
D. Avoid making demands.
Goal: To encourage independent behavior
A. Anticipate and accept negativism.
B. Avoid fostering dependency.
C. Encourage client to make their own decisions, using positive reinforcement.
Goal: To provide care to meet basic human needs
A. Determine client's ability to meet responsibilities of daily living.
B. Attend to nutrition, elimination, exercise, hygiene, and signs of physical illness.
Goal: To assist in medical treatment
A. Administer antipsychotic medications (Appendix 7.1).

NURSING PRIORITY As the client's symptoms lessen, they will often discontinue therapy and medication, which can lead to recurrence of symptoms.

Goal: To deal effectively with withdrawn behavior
A. Establish a therapeutic one-to-one relationship.
   1. Initiate interaction by seeking out client at every opportunity.
   2. Maintain a nonjudgmental, accepting manner in what is said and done.

3. Attempt to draw client into a conversation without demanding a response.
B. Promote social skills by helping client feel more secure with other people.
   1. Accept one-sided conversations.
   2. Accept client's negativism without comments.
C. Attend to physical needs of client as necessary.
D. Have client focus on reality.
E. Protect and restrain client from potential destructiveness to self and others.

Goal: To deal effectively with hallucinations
A. Clarify and reinforce reality.
   1. Help client recognize hallucination as a manifestation of anxiety.
   2. Provide a safe, secure environment.
   3. Avoid denying or arguing with client when they are experiencing hallucinations.

4. Acknowledge client's experience but point out that *you* do not share the same experience.
5. Do not give attention to content of hallucinations.
6. Direct client's attention to real situations, such as singing along with music.
7. Protect client from injury to self or others when they are prompted by "voices" or "visions."
B. Encourage social interaction to help client find satisfactory ways of relating with others.
   1. Increase interaction gradually.
   2. Respond verbally to anything real that client talks about.

Appendix 7.1   MEDICATIONS: ALZHEIMER'S, ANTIANXIETY, ANTIMANIC, ANTIDEPRESSANT, AND ANTIPSYCHOTIC

Alzheimer Medications

General Nursing Implications

- Drugs do not cure and do not stop disease progression, but they may slow down the progression by a few months.

MEDICATIONS	SIDE EFFECTS	NURSING IMPLICATIONS
Cholinesterase Inhibitors		
Donepezil: PO Galantamine: PO Rivastigmine: PO, transdermal	GI symptoms: nausea, vomiting, dyspepsia, diarrhea dizziness and headache bradycardia, syncope	1. Abrupt withdrawal of medication can lead to a rapid progression of symptoms. 2. Monitor for side effects, because the drug is typically given in high doses to produce the greatest benefit. 3. Donepezil is better tolerated.
N-methyl-D-aspartate (NMDA) Receptor Antagonists		
Memantine: PO	Dizziness, headache, confusion, constipation	1. Used for moderate-to-severe cases. 2. Better tolerated than cholinesterase inhibitors. 3. Monitor kidney function; contraindicated in clients with severe kidney impairment.

Antianxiety Agents

General Nursing Implications

- Withhold or omit one or more doses if excessive drowsiness occurs.
- Assess for symptoms associated with a withdrawal syndrome in hospitalized clients: anxiety, insomnia, vomiting, tremors, palpitations, confusion, and hallucinations.
- When discontinuing, the drug dosage should be gradually decreased over a period of months, depending on the dose and length of time the client has been taking the medication.
- Scheduled IV drug requires documentation.
- Promote safety with the use of side rails and assistance with ambulation as necessary.
- Teach the client and family not to drink alcohol while taking an antianxiety agent and not to stop taking the medication abruptly.

Continued

Appendix 7.1   MEDICATIONS: ALZHEIMER'S, ANTIANXIETY, ANTIMANIC, ANTIDEPRESSANT, AND ANTIPSYCHOTIC—cont'd

MEDICATIONS	SIDE EFFECTS	NURSING IMPLICATIONS

Benzodiazepines: Reduce anxiety and promote anticonvulsant activity and skeletal muscle relaxation.

MEDICATIONS	SIDE EFFECTS	NURSING IMPLICATIONS
Alprazolam: PO Chlordiazepoxide: PO, IM, IV Diazepam: PO, IM, IV Clonazepam: PO Clorazepate: PO Lorazepam: PO, IV Midazolam: IM, IV	CNS depression, drowsiness (decreases with use), ataxia, dizziness, headaches, dry mouth *Adverse effects:* tolerance commonly develops, physical dependency	1. May cause paradoxical effects and should not be taken by mothers who are breastfeeding. 2. Assess for symptoms of leukopenia, such as sore throat, fever, and weakness. 3. Encourage the client to rise slowly from a supine position and to dangle feet before standing. 4. Chlordiazepoxide: Do not inject or add IV chlordiazepoxide to an existing IV infusion; inject directly into a large vein over a 1-min period. 5. Do not mix chlordiazepoxide or diazepam with any other drug in a syringe or add to existing IV fluids. 6. Midazolam is commonly used for induction of anesthesia and sedation before diagnostic tests and endoscopic examinations. 7. Flumazenil is approved for the treatment of benzodiazepine overdose; it has an adverse effect of precipitating convulsions, especially in clients with a history of epilepsy. *Uses:* anxiety and tension, muscle spasm, preoperative medication, acute alcohol withdrawal, and to induce sleep

Nonbenzodiazepine Agents: Decrease anxiety; lack muscle-relaxant and anticonvulsant effects; do not cause sedation or physical or psychological dependence; do not increase CNS depression caused by alcohol or other drugs.

MEDICATIONS	SIDE EFFECTS	NURSING IMPLICATIONS
Buspirone: PO	Dizziness, drowsiness, headache, nausea, fatigue, insomnia	1. Not a controlled substance. 2. Some improvement can be noted in 7-10 days; however, it usually takes 3-4 weeks to achieve effectiveness. 3. Better tolerated than benzodiazepines. *Uses:* short-term relief of anxiety and anxiety disorders

Mood Stabilizers: Antimanic medications.

MEDICATIONS	SIDE EFFECTS	NURSING IMPLICATIONS

Lithium Carbonate: Believed to affect electrical conductivity in neurons; blocks binding of serotonin to its receptors. *Uses:* bipolar disorder (manic episode).

MEDICATIONS	SIDE EFFECTS	NURSING IMPLICATIONS

Lithium: PO	*High incidence:* increased thirst, increased urination (polyuria)
	Frequent: 1.5 mEq/L (1.5 mmol/L) levels or less – nausea, vomiting, slurred speech, dry mouth, lethargy, fatigue, muscle weakness, headache, GI disturbances, fine hand tremors
	Adverse effects: 1.5-2.0 mEq/L (1.5-2.0 mmol/L) may produce confusion, persistent GI disturbances, ECG changes, drowsiness, incoordination, coarse hand tremors, muscle twitching 2.0-2.5 mEq/L (2.0-2.5 mmol/L) may result in ataxia, tinnitus, seizures, clonic movements, high output of dilute urine, blurred vision, severe hypotension
		1. Monitor lithium blood levels: blood samples are obtained 12 hrs after dose was given.
		2. Teach client the following:
		  • Symptoms of lithium toxicity.
		  • Importance of frequent blood tests (every 2-3 days) to check lithium levels at the beginning of treatment (maintenance blood levels done every 1-3 months).
		  • Importance of taking dose at same time each day, preferably with meals or milk to reduce GI symptoms.
		  • Encourage a diet containing normal amounts of salt and a fluid intake of 3 L per day; avoid caffeine because of its diuretic effect.
		  • Report polyuria, prolonged vomiting, diarrhea, or fever to health care provider (may need to temporarily reduce dosage or discontinue use).
		  • Do not crush, chew, or break the extended-release or film-coated tablets.

MEDICATIONS	SIDE EFFECTS	NURSING IMPLICATIONS
	Acute toxicity greater than 2.5 mEq/L (2.5 mmol/L): generalized convulsions, oliguria, coma, death	3. Assess clients at high risk for developing toxicity: postoperative, dehydrated, hyperthyroidism, those with renal disease, or those taking diuretics. 4. Blood levels: • Extremely narrow therapeutic range: 0.5-1.5 mEq/L (0.5-1.5 mmol/L) • Toxic serum lithium level: greater than 2 mEq/L (2 mmol/L) • Acute mania: 0.8-1.4 mEq/L (0.8-1.4 mmol/L) • Long-term maintenance levels: 0.4-1.0 mEq/L (0.4-1.0 mmol/L) 5. Management of lithium toxicity: possible hemodialysis. 6. Long-term use may cause goiter; may be associated with hypothyroidism.

Other Agents: Both of the following medications were originally developed and used for seizure disorders. Both have mood-stabilizing effects.

MEDICATIONS	SIDE EFFECTS	NURSING IMPLICATIONS
Carbamazepine: PO	Drowsiness, dizziness, visual problems (spots before eyes, difficulty focusing, blurred vision), dry mouth *Toxic reactions:* blood dyscrasias	1. Used primarily for clients who have not responded to lithium or who cannot tolerate the side effects. 2. Avoid tasks that require alertness and motor skills until response to drug is established. 3. Monitor CBC frequently during initiation of therapy and at monthly intervals thereafter.
Valproic acid: PO	Nausea, GI upset, drowsiness, may cause pancreatitis, hepatotoxicity	1. Monitor liver function studies. 2. Administer with food to avoid GI upset.

Antidepressant Medications

General Nursing Implications
- Selective serotonin reuptake inhibitors (SSRIs) are overtaking tricyclic antidepressants (TCAs) as drugs of choice for depression.
- Serotonin/norepinephrine reuptake inhibitors (SNRIs) are indicated for major depression, generalized anxiety disorder, and chronic pain disorder.
- Because of the potential interactions with other drugs and certain foods, monoamine oxidase inhibitors (MAOIs) are used as second-line drugs for the treatment of depression.
- The therapeutic effect has a delayed onset of 7 to 21 days; however, SSRIs may take as long as 4 to 6 weeks to become effective.
- These drugs can potentially produce cardiotoxicity, sedation, seizures, and anticholinergic effects and may induce mania in clients with bipolar disorder (SSRIs are less likely to cause these problems).
- Drugs are usually discontinued before surgery (10 days for MAOIs; 2-3 days for TCAs) because of adverse interactions with anesthetic agents.

MEDICATIONS	SIDE EFFECTS	NURSING IMPLICATIONS

Tricyclic Antidepressants (TCAs): Prevent the reuptake of norepinephrine or serotonin, which results in increased concentrations of these neurotransmitters.

MEDICATIONS	SIDE EFFECTS	NURSING IMPLICATIONS
Imipramine hydrochloride: PO, IM Nortriptyline hydrochloride: PO Doxepin hydrochloride: PO Amitriptyline hydrochloride: PO, IM	Drowsiness, dry mouth, blurred vision, constipation, weight gain, and orthostatic hypotension *Adverse reactions:* cardiac dysrhythmias, nystagmus, tremor, hypotension, restlessness	1. TCAs should not be given at the same time as an MAOI; a time lag of 14 days is necessary when changing from one drug group to the other. 2. Because of marked sedation, client should avoid activities requiring mental alertness (driving or operating machinery). 3. Instruct client to move gradually from lying to sitting and standing positions to prevent postural hypotension.

Continued

Appendix 7.1	MEDICATIONS: ALZHEIMER'S, ANTIANXIETY, ANTIMANIC, ANTIDEPRESSANT, AND ANTIPSYCHOTIC—cont'd	R̶x

MEDICATIONS	SIDE EFFECTS	NURSING IMPLICATIONS
		4. Doxepin is better tolerated by older adults and has less effect on cardiac status; dilute the concentrate with orange juice.
		5. TCAs are contraindicated in clients with epilepsy, glaucoma, and cardiovascular disease.
		6. TCAs are usually given once daily at bedtime.
		Uses: depression; imipramine is also used to treat enuresis in children.

Selective Serotonin Reuptake Inhibitors (SSRIs): Cause selective inhibition of serotonin uptake and produce CNS excitation rather than sedation; have no effect on dopamine or norepinephrine.

MEDICATIONS	SIDE EFFECTS	NURSING IMPLICATIONS
Fluoxetine: PO Sertraline: PO Paroxetine: PO Citalopram: PO Escitalopram: PO Fluvoxamine: PO	Nausea, headache, anxiety, nervousness, insomnia, weight gain, skin rash, sexual dysfunction *Adverse reactions (serotonin syndrome):* tachycardia, delirium, restlessness, fever, seizures	1. Medication is usually given once a day. 2. Interacts with St. John's wort and MAOI; may cause serotonin syndrome. 3. Discontinue SSRI 5 weeks before starting MAOI. *Uses:* depression, obsessive-compulsive disorder, bulimia

Serotonin/Norepinephrine Reuptake Inhibitors (SNRIs): Block reuptake of serotonin and norepinephrine, and effects are similar to those of the SSRIs.

MEDICATIONS	SIDE EFFECTS	NURSING IMPLICATIONS
Duloxetine: PO Venlafaxine: PO	Nausea, dizziness, nervousness, insomnia, hypertension, sexual dysfunction	1. Monitor blood pressure. 2. May be administered with food, preferably in the morning. 3. May cause serotonin syndrome. *Uses:* generalized anxiety disorder, depression, chronic pain disorder

Monoamine Oxidase Inhibitors (MAOIs): Inhibit the enzyme monoamine oxidase, which breaks down norepinephrine and serotonin, increasing the concentration of these neurotransmitters.

MEDICATIONS	SIDE EFFECTS	NURSING IMPLICATIONS
Isocarboxazid: PO Phenelzine sulfate: PO Tranylcypromine: PO	Drowsiness, insomnia, dry mouth, urinary retention, hypotension *Adverse reactions:* Serotonin syndrome, tachycardia, tachypnea, agitation, tremors, seizures, heart block, hypotension	1. Potentiate many drug actions: narcotics, barbiturates, sedatives, and atropine-like medications. 2. Have a long duration of action; therefore 2-3 weeks must go by before another drug is administered while a client is taking an MAOI. 3. MAOIs interact with specific foods and drugs (ones containing tyramine or sympathomimetic drugs) and may cause a severe hypertensive crisis characterized by marked elevation of blood pressure, increased temperature, tremors, and tachycardia. Foods and drugs to avoid: coffee, tea, cola beverages, aged cheeses, beer and wine, pickled foods, avocados, and figs and many over-the-counter cold preparations, hay fever medications, and nasal decongestants. 4. Monitor for bladder distention by checking urinary output. 5. Tranylcypromine: most likely to cause hypertensive crisis; onset of action is more rapid. *Uses:* primarily psychotic depression and depressive episode of bipolar affective disorder.

MEDICATIONS	SIDE EFFECTS	NURSING IMPLICATIONS
Miscellaneous Antidepressants		
Trazodone: PO	Sedation, orthostatic hypotension, nausea, vomiting, can cause priapism (prolonged, painful erection of the penis)	See *General Nursing Implications.* *Uses:* depression, insomnia

Appendix 7.1 MEDICATIONS: ALZHEIMER'S, ANTIANXIETY, ANTIMANIC, ANTIDEPRESSANT, AND ANTIPSYCHOTIC—cont'd

MEDICATIONS	SIDE EFFECTS	NURSING IMPLICATIONS
Bupropion: PO	Weight loss, dry mouth, dizziness, agitation	See *General Nursing Implications*. *Uses:* depression, smoking cessation

Antipsychotic (Neuroleptic) Medications

General Nursing Implications

- Use cautiously in older adults.
- These drugs should make the client feel better and experience fewer psychotic episodes.
- Maintain a regular schedule; usually take daily dose 1 to 2 hrs before bedtime.
- Explain to client and family the importance of compliance with medication regimen.
- Medications are not addictive.
- Discuss side effects and importance of notifying primary care provider if client experiences undesired side effects.
- When mixing for parenteral use, do not mix with other drugs.
- Inject deep IM; client should stay in reclined position 30 to 60 mins after dose administration.

MEDICATIONS	SIDE EFFECTS	NURSING IMPLICATIONS
Phenothiazines: Block dopamine receptors and also thought to depress various portions of the reticular activating system; have peripherally exerting anticholinergic properties (atropine-like symptoms: dry mouth, stuffy nose, constipation, blurred vision). Classified by chemical type (aliphatic, piperazine, piperidine types) and potency.		
Aliphatic type: Conventional/ First generation: Chlorpromazine hydrochloride **(low potency):** PO, IM, IV suppository *Piperidine type:* Conventional/First generation: Fluphenazine hydrochloride **(high potency):** PO, IM Conventional/ First generation: Trifluoperazine (high potency): PO, IM *Piperidine type:* Conventional/First generation: Thioridazine (low potency): PO	**Extrapyramidal effects (movement disorder):** occur early in therapy and are usually managed with other drugs *Acute dystonia* – painful spasm of muscles of tongue, face, neck, or back; oculogyric crisis (upward deviation of the eyes); opisthotonus (spasm of the back muscles causing trunk to arch forward and limbs to move backward) *Parkinsonism* – muscle tremors, rigidity, spasms, shuffling gait, stooped posture, cogwheel rigidity *Akathisia* – motor restlessness, pacing **Tardive dyskinesia:** occurs late in therapy; symptoms are often irreversible – earliest symptom is slow, wormlike movements of the tongue; later symptoms include fine twisting, writhing movements of the tongue and face, grimacing; lip smacking; involuntary movements of the limbs, toes, fingers, and trunk **Neuroleptic malignant syndrome:** rare problem, fever (105°F [41°C]), "lead pipe" muscle rigidity, agitation, confusion, delirium, respiratory and acute renal failure *Endocrine* – amenorrhea, increased libido in women, decreased libido in men, delayed ejaculation, increased appetite, weight gain, hypoglycemia, and edema *Dermatologic* – photosensitivity *Hypersensitivity reaction* – jaundice, agranulocytosis	1. Check blood pressure before administration; to avoid postural hypotension, encourage client to rise slowly from sitting or lying position. 2. Be aware of the antiemetic effect of the phenothiazines; may mask other pathology such as drug overdose, brain lesions, or intestinal obstruction. 3. Client teaching: protect skin from sunlight – wear long-sleeved shirts, hats, and sunscreen lotion when out in the sunlight. 4. Explain importance of reporting any signs of sore throat, fever, or symptoms of infection. 5. Encourage periodic liver function studies to be done. 6. Teach that drug may turn urine pink or reddish brown. 7. Extrapyramidal symptoms treated with anticholinergics (e.g., benztropine). 8. Long-term use of phenothiazines requires assessment of involuntary movement screening (AIMS). *Uses:* severe psychoses, schizophrenia, manic phase of bipolar affective disorder, personality disorders, and severe agitation and anxiety

Other Antipsychotic Drugs

First generation/ Conventional: Haloperidol: PO, IM	High potency antipsychotic agent Significant extrapyramidal effects; low incidence of sedation, orthostatic hypotension; does not elicit photosensitivity reaction	1. May reduce prothrombin time. 2. Often used as the initial drug for treatment of psychotic disorders.
Second generation/Atypical: Risperidone: PO	Anxiety, somnolence, extrapyramidal symptoms, dizziness, constipation, GI upset, rhinitis	1. *Uses:* tics, vocal disturbances, and psychotic schizophrenia. 2. Risperidone is the most frequently prescribed antipsychotic because of less serious side effects.

Continued

Appendix 7.1   MEDICATIONS: ALZHEIMER'S, ANTIANXIETY, ANTIMANIC, ANTIDEPRESSANT, AND ANTIPSYCHOTIC—cont'd

MEDICATIONS	SIDE EFFECTS	NURSING IMPLICATIONS
Second generation/Atypical: Clozapine: PO	Blood dyscrasias (agranulocytosis), sedation, weight gain, orthostatic hypotension, seizures, diabetes	1. Used with caution in clients with diabetes and those with history of seizures. 2. Mandatory monitoring of WBC and absolute neutrophil count (ANC) – weekly for first 6 months, then every 2 weeks for the next 6 months, then monthly after 1 year of treatment.
Third generation (dopamine system stabilizer): Aripiprazole: PO	Very low extrapyramidal effects and tardive dyskinesia, headache, nervousness, insomnia, dizziness	1. Only medication in this category.

⚡ Practice & Next Generation NCLEX (NGN) Questions

Psychosocial nursing care

More questions on
ⓔvolve

1. A client taking lithium carbonate reports increased thirst, frequent urination, nausea, vomiting, abdominal bloating, and dry mouth. The client has been newly prescribed this medication and is having the lithium level checked as a part of the routine follow-up. The lithium level is 0.8 mEq/L (0.8 mmol/L). What does this level **most likely** indicate?
   1. Toxic.
   2. Slightly elevated.
   3. Desired level.
   4. Nontherapeutic.

2. The nurse is admitting an older adult client to an extended care facility. The client is confused, malnourished, and has contusions with bruises and welts over the trunk. What would be the most important nursing intervention at this time?
   1. Perform a physical assessment.
   2. Notify the nursing supervisor regarding client's condition.
   3. Establish communication and rapport with the client.
   4. Notify authorities regarding suspected elderly abuse.

3. A client is suspicious about their surroundings and is paranoid toward the nursing staff. What therapeutic approach should be implemented by the nurse?
   1. Maintain silence and do not attempt to explain circumstances.
   2. Make sure you have the client's attention and maintain direct eye contact.
   3. Accept the need for the client to be suspicious and be direct and honest in responses.
   4. Sit with the client and console through touch and being very open and friendly.

4. The nurse is monitoring a client who has been prescribed an antipsychotic medication for extrapyramidal symptoms. Which clinical finding indicates the client is experiencing extrapyramidal symptoms from this medication? **Select all that apply**.
   1. Blood pressure of 92/58 mm Hg.
   2. Dyspnea, respiratory rate 26.
   3. Muscle cramps and spasms in the neck.
   4. Dry mouth and anorexia.
   5. Tremor.
   6. Slowness of movement.

5. A client is diagnosed with schizophrenia and is started on risperidone. What would be important to teach the client to report to the health care provider?
   1. Weight loss.
   2. Strange dreams.
   3. Difficulty falling asleep.
   4. Dizziness.

6. The nurse is concerned a client is becoming depressed. What nursing observations would support the development of depression?
   1. Insomnia, loss of libido, restlessness.
   2. Overwhelming sadness, fatigue, poor grooming.
   3. Hypervigilance, overeating, poor grooming.
   4. Flight of ideas, weight loss, lack of interest.

7. A client is experiencing auditory hallucinations. What would the nurse be **most** concerned about?
   1. Feelings of depression when the voices stop.
   2. How the voices are telling them to hurt someone.
   3. Feelings of happiness to hear the voices.
   4. How the voices sound like a woman's voice.

8. A client has been receiving memantine for moderate Alzheimer's disease (AD). How would the nurse know that the medication is effective?
   1. The client is less forgetful.
   2. The client has normal liver function studies.
   3. The client has improved short-term memory.
   4. The client is less agitated and more cooperative.

9. The nurse is developing a teaching plan for a client receiving clozapine. What is important to reinforce in the teaching plan?
   1. Monitor white blood cell (WBC) count and differential weekly for first 6 months, then every 2 weeks.
   2. Monitor liver function studies monthly and watch for signs of jaundice.
   3. Have a monthly electroencephalogram (EEG) and polysomnography.
   4. Have a follow-up echocardiogram and adenosine stress-test.

10. A client has been prescribed disulfiram. The nurse is reinforcing what was taught about the medication. What is important for the nurse to explain to the client? **Select all that apply**.
    1. Medication needs to be taken three times a day.
    2. Avoid crushing or mixing the medication.
    3. Wait at least 12 hrs after the last alcohol drink before taking the first dose.
    4. Avoid colognes and aftershave lotions.
    5. Check labels of all foods to determine whether alcohol is present.

11. A client has been prescribed lithium for treatment of bipolar disorder. The client is being seen at the clinic for possible adverse effects of the medication. The nurse evaluates the client for these symptoms. **For each symptom, mark an X to indicate whether the finding is significant for an adverse effect associated with lithium or an unrelated finding.**

SYMPTOM	SIGNIFICANT FINDING	UNRELATED FINDING
GI disturbances		
Excessive thirst		
Polyuria		
Severe hypertension		
Speech difficulty		
Sweating		

12. A 42-year-old is admitted to the psychiatric unit for evaluation. The client's spouse is worried about her husband's preoccupation that the neighbors are spying on them using binoculars. She relates how he has withdrawn from their friends. The spouse has not noted any unusual behavior by the neighbors. The client has a history of low back pain and has a TENS unit in the lumbar area and reports that they are receiving signals from the device implanted in their body. They relate that, when they receive the signals, it tells them to pace around the room. Recently, the client was laid off from work as a result of labor dispute issues, which has led to increased stress. Client is uncommunicative and withdrawn during the interview.

The nurse is reviewing the client's assessment data to prepare the client's plan of care.

Complete the diagram by dragging from the choices below to specify what condition the client is most likely experiencing, two actions the nurse should take to address that condition, and two parameters the nurse should monitor to assess the client's progress.

Action to Take		Parameter to Monitor
Action to Take.	Condition Most Likely Experiencing	Parameter to Monitor

ACTIONS TO TAKE	POTENTIAL CONDITIONS	PARAMETERS TO MONITOR
Isolate the client from others on the unit.	Paranoid disorder	Watch for auditory hallucinations.
Set firm limits.	Phobia	Observe for any repetitive compulsive behaviors, e.g., pacing.
Maintain nonjudgmental manner.	Schizophrenia	Monitor effectiveness of medication.
Tell the client the TENS unit does not broadcast signals.	Obsessive-compulsive disorder	Remains safe and refrains from acting upon any delusion.
Clarify and reinforce reality.	Borderline personality disorder	Limit number of stressful situations.

⚡ Answers to Practice & Next Generation NCLEX (NGN) Questions

1. 3
Client Needs: Physiological Integrity/Pharmacological Therapies
Clinical Judgment/Cognitive Skill: Prioritize Hypotheses
Item Type: Multiple Choice
Rationale & Test-Taking Strategy: Recall there is an extremely narrow therapeutic range for lithium, which is 0.5 to 1.5 mEq/L. Lithium levels should range from 0.4 to 1 mEq/L. Generally, levels are desired between 0.6 and 0.8 mEq/L. Levels of 0.8 to 1 mEq/L may be more effective but carry a greater risk for adverse effects. Lithium levels must be kept below 1.5 mEq/L; levels greater than this can produce significant toxicity signs and symptoms. Remember, the mnemonic – 2.0 mEq/L is too much! Early adverse effects include nausea, diarrhea, abdominal bloating, and anorexia, which are quite common but transient. There is a high incidence of polyuria and thirst at desired blood levels.

2. 1
Client Needs: Physiological Integrity/Physiological Adaptation
Clinical Judgment/Cognitive Skill: Generate Solutions
Item Type: Multiple Choice
Rationale & Test-Taking Strategy: Note the **key** word, "most." This is a nursing priority question. While it is important to establish rapport and trust with the client, physiologic needs must be taken care of first; it is important to determine the extent of client injuries, check vital signs, and establish if the client is stable or unstable. The client is exhibiting symptoms of elder abuse, but assessment data must be obtained before further action can be taken.

3. 3
Client Needs: Physiological Integrity
Clinical Judgment/Cognitive Skill: Take Action
Item Type: Multiple Choice
Rationale & Test-Taking Strategy: It is important to be direct and honest but not overly friendly with a paranoid client. Touching should be avoided because it may be misinterpreted as a threat (delusion of persecution). It is important to make contact with the paranoid client; being silent and making direct eye contact may escalate the client's paranoid behavior.

4. 3, 5, 6
Client Needs: Physiological Integrity/Pharmacological Therapies
Clinical Judgment/Cognitive Skill: Recognize Cues
Item Type: Select All That Apply
Rationale & Test-Taking Strategy: Recall the symptoms associated with the complication of extrapyramidal symptoms. Extrapyramidal symptoms are movement disorders resulting from the effects of antipsychotic drugs. Symptoms include: *acute dystonia* – spasm of muscles of tongue, face, neck, and back, opisthotonos; *parkinsonism* – bradykinesia (slowness of movement), mask-like facies, tremor, rigidity, shuffling gait, drooling, cogwheeling, stooped posture; *akathisia* – compulsive, restless movement; symptoms of anxiety and agitation; *tardive dyskinesia* – oral-facial dyskinesias (sticking out tongue, lip smacking), choreoathetoid movements. Low blood pressure, elevated respiratory rate, dyspnea, dry mouth, and anorexia are not extrapyramidal symptoms.

5. 4

Client Needs: Physiological Integrity/Pharmacological Therapies
Clinical Judgment/Cognitive Skill: Take Action
Item Type: Multiple Choice
Rationale & Test-Taking Strategy: Risperidone is an antipsychotic medication. Think about the side effects of this type of medication. Are there safety issues to be concerned about? Clients should report dizziness, because orthostatic hypotension can cause potential safety issues (falls, etc.) Risperidone can cause metabolic effects, such as weight gain, diabetes, and dyslipidemia. Adverse effects that have led to drug discontinuation include agitation, dizziness, somnolence, and fatigue. Dreaming and difficulty falling asleep can occur with risperidone but are related to excessive dosages and are not associated with safety issues, such those related to orthostatic hypotension.

6. 2

Client Needs: Psychosocial Integrity
Clinical Judgment/Cognitive Skill: Recognize Cues
Item Type: Multiple Choice
Rationale & Test-Taking Strategy: Review each of the options and keep in mind that all the information in each option must be correct for it to be the right answer. During a depressive episode, there is a general slowing down of body systems and behavior (e.g., anorexia, sad affect, fatigue, anergia, psychomotor retardation, lack of social interaction, and poor grooming). The other options are manifestations associated with mania.

7. 2

Client Needs: Psychosocial Integrity
Clinical Judgment/Cognitive Skill: Prioritize Hypotheses
Item Type: Multiple Choice
Rationale & Test-Taking Strategy: Notice the **key** word, "most." This is a nursing priority question. Safety is a concern when a client experiences an auditory hallucination, as the client may hear a voice that tells them to do something harmful to themselves or others. While the other responses are important to make note of, the correct answer is most concerned with physiologic wellbeing and safety.

8. 4

Client Needs: Physiological Integrity/Pharmacological Therapies
Clinical Judgment/Cognitive Skill: Evaluate Outcomes
Item Type: Multiple Choice
Rationale & Test-Taking Strategy: When determining whether a medication is effective, you would expect to see a lessening of the troublesome symptoms. Memantine is used to treat moderate-to-severe symptoms (i.e., agitation, aggression, confusing words, behavioral problems), not the early stages of AD. Early-stage symptoms are short-term memory loss and forgetfulness, which would more likely be treated with donepezil. Memantine reduces renal clearance, and renal function studies, not liver function studies, should be monitored.

9. 1

Client Needs: Physiological Integrity/Pharmacological Therapies
Clinical Judgment/Cognitive Skill: Take Action
Item Type: Multiple Choice
Rationale & Test-Taking Strategy: Clozapine is an antipsychotic that can cause a potentially fatal blood dyscrasia characterized by agranulocytosis (i.e., decreased WBC count, specifically neutrophils). Although this adverse effect is rare, it is potentially fatal if not detected early, which is the reason for weekly monitoring of the WBC count and ANC. Adverse reactions to clozapine include sedation, dizziness, salivation, anticholinergic toxicity (gastrointestinal paralysis), seizures, myocarditis (heart muscle inflamed and weakened from the medication, causing symptoms of heart failure, which may mimic a heart attack), and neuroleptic malignant syndrome. A monthly EEG is not necessary; however, an electrocardiogram, not an echocardiogram, would be indicated if myocarditis symptoms appeared.

10. 3, 4, 5

Client Needs: Physiological Integrity/Pharmacological Therapies
Clinical Judgment/Cognitive Skill: Take Action
Item Type: Select All That Apply
Rationale & Test-Taking Strategy: Disulfiram is a medication that interferes with alcohol metabolism, which causes the client to experience intense side effects of severe nausea, throbbing headache, blurred vision, tachycardia, tachypnea, flushing, hypotension, and sweating within 5 to 15 min of alcohol consumption. The duration of the reaction is variable, from 30 to 60 min in mild cases, up to several hours in more severe cases or as long as there is alcohol remaining in the blood. Clients need to avoid all forms of alcohol, including alcohol in vinegar, sauces, and cough syrups, and alcohol applied to the skin in aftershave lotions, colognes, and liniments. Checking food labels to see if alcohol is present is important. Teach the client not to administer the first dose until at least 12 hrs after their last alcohol drink. The effects of disulfiram will persist about 2 weeks after the last dose, and alcohol must not be consumed during this time. Dosing is done once daily. Disulfiram may be crushed or mixed with liquid.

11. A client has been prescribed lithium for treatment of bipolar disorder. The client is being seen at the clinic for possible adverse effects of the medication. The nurse evaluates the client for these symptoms. **For each symptom, mark an X to indicate whether the finding is significant for an adverse effect associated with lithium or an unrelated finding.**

SYMPTOM	SIGNIFICANT FINDING	UNRELATED FINDING
GI disturbances	X	
Excessive thirst	X	
Polyuria	X	
Severe hypertension		X
Speech difficulty	X	
Sweating		X

Client Needs: Physiological Integrity/Pharmacological Therapies
Clinical Judgment/Cognitive Skill: Analyze Cues
Item Type: Matrix Multiple Choice
Rationale & Test-Taking Strategy: Review each symptom and determine if it is a significant side effect of lithium. Clients who take lithium may experience increased thirst and increased urination (polyuria). Other frequent adverse effects include nausea, vomiting, slurred speech, dry mouth, lethargy, fatigue, muscle weakness, headache, gastrointestinal (GI) disturbances, and fine hand tremors. As the level of lithium rises in the body, symptoms may include confusion, persistent GI disturbances, ECG changes, drowsiness, incoordination, coarse hand tremors, and muscle twitching. Acute toxicity can lead to generalized seizures, oliguria, coma, and death. Blood pressure should not be elevated, as it is often low. Sweating is not an adverse effect.

12. A 42-year-old is admitted to the psychiatric unit for evaluation. The client's spouse is worried about her husband's preoccupation that the neighbors are spying on them using binoculars. She relates how he has withdrawn from their friends. The spouse has not noted any unusual behavior by the neighbors. The client has a history of low back pain and has a transcutaneous electrical nerve stimulation (TENS) unit in the lumbar area and reports he is receiving signals from the device implanted in his body. He relates that when he receives the signals, they tell him to pace around the room. Recently, the client was laid off from work due to labor dispute issues, which has led to increased stress. Client is uncommunicative and withdrawn during the interview.

The nurse is reviewing the client's assessment data to prepare the plan of care.

Complete the diagram by dragging from the choices below to specify what condition the client is most likely experiencing, two actions the nurse should take to address that condition, and two parameters the nurse should monitor to assess the client's progress.

Actions to Take		Parameters to Monitor
Maintain nonjudgmental manner.		Remains safe and refrains from acting upon any delusion.

Actions to Take	Condition Most Likely Experiencing	Parameters to Monitor
Clarify and reinforce reality.	Schizophrenia	Effectiveness of the medication.

Actions to Take	Potential Conditions	Parameters to Monitor
Isolate the client from others on the unit.	Paranoid disorder	Watch for auditory hallucinations.
Set firm limits.	Phobia	Look for any repetitive compulsive behaviors, e.g., pacing.
Maintain nonjudgmental manner.	Schizophrenia	Monitor effectiveness of medication.
Tell the client the TENS unit does not broadcast signals.	Obsessive-compulsive disorder	Remains safe and refrains from acting upon any delusion.
Clarify and reinforce reality.	Borderline personality disorder	Limit number of stressful situations.

Client Needs: Psychosocial Integrity
Clinical Judgment/Cognitive Skill: Recognize Cues, Analyze Cues, Prioritize Hypotheses, Generate Solutions, Take Action
Item Type: Bowtie
Rationale & Test-Taking Strategy: With this type of test item, it is important first to determine what condition the client is most likely experiencing. The client has altered thought processes of believing that the neighbors are spying on him and that his TENS unit is sending him signals. These are delusions, which are associated with schizophrenia. TENS units are battery powered devices that deliver pulses of electrical energy for pain relief, and they are not implanted in the body. All individuals diagnosed with schizophrenia have at least one psychotic symptom, such as hallucinations, delusions, and/or disorganized speech or thought. The symptoms are severe enough to disrupt normal activities such as school, work, family and social interaction, and selfcare. Basic needs such as hygiene, nutrition, and health care are often neglected, and socialization and relationships are often disrupted (i.e., lack of communication and withdrawn behavior). It will be important for the nurse to establish trust in a nonjudgmental, accepting manner. Also, clarifying reality and maintaining a safe environment are important actions. The client's safety and response to medication therapy are parameters to monitor. Limit setting is not appropriate for this client. A person with a phobia experiences excessive, irrational fear of a specific activity, situation, or object. This fear can lead to avoidance or extreme anxiety that interferes with normal responsibilities and routines. Common phobias include fear of heights (acrophobia), spiders (arachnophobia), and enclosed spaces like elevators (claustrophobia). The main features of borderline personality disorder include marked emotional and mood instability, self-image distortion, impulsivity, and difficulty in interpersonal relationships with emotions and relationships experienced with heightened intensity. A person with obsessive-compulsive disorder (OCD) experiences an obsession, recurrent or intrusive thoughts that they cannot stop thinking about, and these thoughts create anxiety. A compulsive act is an act that the person feels compelled to perform.

CHAPTER EIGHT

Eye and Ear: Care of Adult Clients

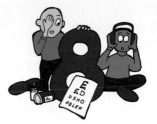

THE EYE

Physiology of the Eye

A. Eyes (Fig. 8.1).
1. Sclera: tough, protective covering of the outside of the eye; the "white" of the eye.
2. Cornea: transparent tissue that covers the front of the eye over the pupil.
3. Conjunctiva: the thin, transparent mucous membrane that covers the outer surface of the eye and lines the inner surface of the eyelid.
4. Ciliary muscle: muscular body that allows the eye to focus through contraction and relaxation.
5. Ciliary body: produces aqueous humor.
6. Iris: controls the size of the pupil in order to regulate the amount of light that enters the eye; gives the eye its characteristic color.
7. Pupil: the opening in the center of the iris; the size of the pupil determines the amount of light that enters the eye.
8. Retina: thin innermost lining (or the inside back wall) of the eye; contains millions of light-sensitive nerve cells to coordinate and transmit signals via the optic nerve to the brain; similar to film in a camera.

9. Macula: part of the retina responsible for providing optimal visual focusing.
10. Aqueous humor: fluid that fills anterior and posterior chambers; circulates through the pupil and empties into canal of Schlemm.
11. Vitreous humor: fluid that fills the cavity posterior to the lens.
12. Crystalline lens: provides for the convergence and refraction of light rays and images onto the retina; enables vision to be focused.
13. Optic nerve: exits the eye through the retina at the location of the optic disc.
B. Eyelids: protective coverings of the eye.
1. Conjunctiva: inner lining of the eyelid.
2. Lacrimal gland: excretes lacrimal fluid (tears) to lubricate, clean, and protect the outer surface of the eye.

System Assessment: Recognize Cues

A. External data collection.
1. Assess position and alignment of the eyes: both eyes should fixate on one visual field simultaneously.
2. Evaluate for presence of ptosis (drooping eyelids).
3. Inspect lids and conjunctiva for signs of inflammation, such as discharge, erythema, or edema.
4. Assess eyelids for entropion (turning inward) or ectropion (turning outward).
5. Assess color of sclera: normally, a thin white coating; may yellow with age and with jaundice.
6. Evaluate size and equality of pupils: both should be equal in size and shape.
7. Evaluate pupillary reaction to light.
   a. Direct light reflex: constriction of pupil when stimulated with light.
   b. Consensual reflex: constriction of opposite pupil when stimulated with light.
B. Evaluate visual acuity and check for refractive errors (see Appendix 8.1).
1. Myopia (nearsightedness): vision for near objects is better than vision for distant objects.
2. Hyperopia (farsightedness): vision for distant objects is better than vision for near objects.
3. Assess for any blurred or double vision.
C. Assess for presence of pain and any recent change in vision.

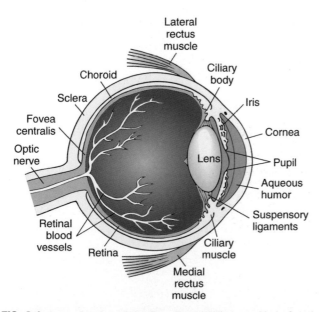

FIG. 8.1 Cross-Section of the Eye. (From Willihnganz, M. J., Guretiz, S. L., & Clayton, B. D. [2020]. *Clayton's basic pharmacology for nurses* [18th ed.]. Elsevier.)

TEST ALERT Assist client to cope with sensory impairment (e.g., hearing, sight, etc.).

DISORDERS OF THE EYE

📋 Glaucoma

Glaucoma is a group of disorders characterized by an increase in intraocular pressure, optic nerve atrophy, and progressive loss of vision. It is an acute or chronic condition and a leading cause of blindness and can be prevented with early detection/treatment.

Types

A. Primary open-angle glaucoma (POAG—chronic): most common form.
1. Flow of aqueous humor is slowed or stopped by obstruction, thus increasing intraocular pressure.
2. Characterized by a slow onset.
3. Chronic and progressive peripheral vision loss late in the disease process.
B. Primary angle-closure glaucoma (PACG—acute).
1. Rapid increase in intraocular pressure due to a reduction in the outflow of aqueous humor; may also occur in the client with prolonged pupil dilation.
2. Symptoms occur suddenly; immediate medical treatment is required because it may cause total blindness within hours to a day.
C. Secondary glaucoma: caused by trauma or optic neoplasm.

Assessment: Recognize Cues

A. Risk factors for POAG.
1. Family history.
2. Aging—occurs most often in clients more than 40 years of age.
3. Chronic diseases such as diabetes mellitus.
4. History of eye injury.
5. Cataract surgery.
B. Risk factors for PACG.
1. Anything that causes pupil dilation such as dark rooms, emotional excitement, or drug-induced mydriasis.
C. Diagnostics: intraocular pressure is greater than 22 mm Hg (see Appendix 8.1).
D. Clinical manifestations of POAG—develop slowly and frequently without symptoms (Fig. 8.2).
1. Gradual loss of peripheral vision (i.e., tunnel vision).
2. Blindness may occur if untreated.
3. Central vision is normal, even with loss of peripheral vision.
E. Clinical manifestations of PACG.
1. Sudden, severe pain in and around the eye.
2. Nausea and vomiting.
3. Blurred vision, redness of the eye.
4. Colored halos around lights.

Analyze Cues and Prioritize Hypotheses

The most important problems are impaired vision and sensory perception due to glaucoma.

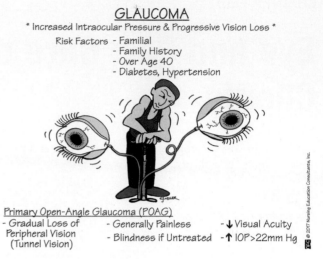

GLAUCOMA
* Increased Intraocular Pressure & Progressive Vision Loss *
Risk Factors - Familial
- Family History
- Over Age 40
- Diabetes, Hypertension

Primary Open-Angle Glaucoma (POAG)
- Gradual Loss of Peripheral Vision (Tunnel Vision)
- Generally Painless
- Blindness if Untreated
- ↓ Visual Acuity
- ↑ IOP>22mm Hg

FIG. 8.2 Glaucoma. (From Zerwekh, J., Garneau, A., & Miller, C. J. [2017]. *Digital collection of the memory notebooks of nursing* [4th ed.]. Nursing Education Consultants.)

Generate Solutions

Treatment

A. Medications (see Appendix 8.2).
1. Topical (ophthalmic) beta blockers (can have an additive effect with systemic beta blockers), carbonic anhydrase inhibitors, and alpha-adrenergic agonists decrease the amount of aqueous humor produced.
2. Cholinergics (miotics) and prostaglandin analogs increase the outflow of aqueous humor.
3. Oral glycerin preparations promote diuresis and lower intraocular pressure.
4. Medications may be used alone or in combination.
B. Surgical intervention: most often done on outpatient basis with topical anesthetic.
1. Argon laser trabeculoplasty: microscopic laser burns applied to the trabecula open the fluid channels, facilitating outflow of aqueous humor.
2. Trabeculectomy: creation of an artificial drain to bypass the trabecular meshwork, allowing outflow of aqueous humor.
3. Laser peripheral iridotomy: may be used for PACG, allowing flow of the aqueous humor to occur through a newly created opening in the iris into the normal outflow channels. Permanent change in pupil shape.

Nursing Interventions: Take Action

Goal: To prevent progression of visual impairment.

A. Teaching plan.
1. Explanation of the problem of increased intraocular pressure.
2. Visual damage cannot be corrected, but further damage can be slowed.
3. Correct use of prescribed medications; client must continue to take medication to control disease; otherwise visual problem will progress.
4. Importance of continued follow-up medical care.

5. Advise all health care providers of glaucoma condition.
6. Avoid medications that increase intraocular pressure such as atropine, antihistamines, and decongestants.
7. Wear medical alert identification.

Goal: To decrease intraocular pressure.

A. Avoid straining with defecation, lifting, or stooping.
B. Administer medications to decrease intraocular pressure.

Goal: To provide appropriate preoperative nursing measures if surgery is indicated.

A. Surgery and treatments are frequently done on an outpatient basis and with a local anesthetic. Orient the client to the surroundings and sounds that will occur during the procedure.
B. For outpatient surgery, client should wear comfortable clothes and arrange for someone to provide transportation home.
C. Postoperative instructions should be given to the client or family in writing, as well as verbally clarify any questions the client may have regarding postoperative care.

Goal: To prevent client from experiencing postoperative complications (surgery frequently done under local anesthesia).

A. Administer medications: miotics, antibiotics, and steroids.
B. Be sure medication is administered in the eye for which it is ordered; the unaffected eye may be treated with a different medication.
C. Client may eat and ambulate as desired after the initial sedative effect is gone.

Home Care

A. Emphasize the importance of follow-up care.
B. Teach the client not to rub the eyes; wear an eye shield or patch at night to prevent inadvertent rubbing of the eyes.
C. Demonstrate the correct administration of eye medication and have the client return the demonstration.
D. Advise the client to avoid activities that increase intraocular pressure.
E. Teach the client to report pain that is not relieved by prescribed analgesics.

Cataract

A *cataract* is a complete or partial opacity of the lens, which compromises the sharpness of images on the retina. It may occur at birth (congenital cataract); however, it occurs most commonly in adults past middle age (senile cataracts).

Assessment: Recognize Cues

A. Risk factors.
1. Diabetes mellitus, hypertension.
2. Corticosteroids: long-term systemic or topical use.
3. Advanced age—due to metabolic changes within the lens.

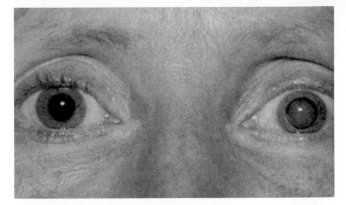

FIG. 8.3 **Cataract in Subject's Left Eye.** (From Swartz, M. H. [2002]. *Textbook of physical diagnosis* [4th ed.]. Saunders.)

4. Trauma to the eye.
5. Exposure to radioactive materials, ultraviolet (UV) radiation, x-rays.

B. Clinical manifestations.
1. Painless, with gradual decrease in visual acuity, blurry vision.
2. Pupil appears gray or yellowish brown to milky white (Fig. 8.3).
3. Red light reflex is distorted on direct ophthalmoscopic examination.
4. Poor color perception.
5. Glare due to light scatter on lens; worse at night.

C. Diagnostics – slit lamp (see Appendix 8.1).

Analyze Cues and Prioritize Hypotheses

The most important problems are impaired visual acuity due to the opacity of the lens.

Generate Solutions

Treatment

A. Nonsurgical: corrective lenses, increased lighting, adaptions in lifestyle.
B. Surgical treatment occurs when palliative measures no longer provide an acceptable level of vision; surgery is usually performed when client begins to experience problems in activities of daily living (Box 8.1). If both eyes require surgical correction, each is treated individually, about 4 to 8 weeks apart.
C. Phacoemulsification (phaco): a small incision is made on the side of the cornea, allowing a tiny probe to be inserted to emit ultrasound, which fragments the lens; cataract is then aspirated.
D. Intraocular lens (IOL) implant is inserted to restore vision.

Nursing Interventions: Take Action

Goal: To provide appropriate teaching and nursing care.

A. Orient the client to the surroundings and sounds that will occur during the procedure.
B. For outpatient surgery, client should wear comfortable clothes and arrange for someone to provide transportation home.

ASSISTING at the TABLE and LOCATING FOOD USING a CLOCK FACE

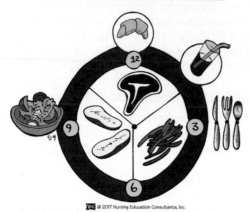

FIG. 8.5 Assisting at the Table and Locating Food Using a Clock Face. (From Zerwekh, J., Garneau, A., & Miller, C. J. [2017]. *Digital collection of the memory notebooks of nursing* [4th ed.]. Nursing Education Consultants.)

C. Promote independence in clients with decreased vision (see Box 8.1).
D. To assist with meals, arrange food on the plate according to numbers on a clock (Fig. 8.5).
E. Psychosocial support in dealing with issues such as loss of independence (e.g., inability to continue driving as visual impairment progresses).

📋 Eye Trauma

Eye trauma **may include surface injuries (e.g., burns or splash injuries), embedded or impaled objects, or orbital trauma. History is usually congruent with eye injury.**

A. Assessment and treatment are often carried out at the same time.
B. As soon as the eye injury is detected, the client should be seen by a physician (ophthalmologist).

Assessment: Recognize Cues

A. Identify eye in which trauma occurred.
B. Determine whether client has a contact lens in the affected eye.
C. Pain, inability to open the eye, photophobia, tearing.
D. Decreased visual acuity: may be unable to distinguish light and images.
E. Ecchymosis, swelling, or visible foreign body.

Analyze Cues and Prioritize Hypotheses

The most important problems are relief of pain and protecting against the potential permanent loss of vision.

Generate Solutions

Treatment

A. If there is visible trauma but no penetrating object, gently apply dressing soaked with normal saline solution to prevent drying during transport.
B. Any suspected or known corneal abrasion should be examined with fluorescein (see Appendix 8.2), followed by ocular irrigation with normal saline solution (see Appendix 8.3).
C. Nonpenetrating foreign objects may be removed by irrigation with normal saline solution.
D. Penetrating foreign bodies must be removed by a physician (ophthalmologist) as soon as possible. *Do not attempt to remove foreign objects from eye but stabilize the object and protect from movement by patching the other eye while seeking emergency care.*
E. Do not attempt to stop bleeding from the eye or the eyelid with direct pressure; do not patch the eye until type of injury is determined.
F. For chemical eye burns, before going to emergency department (ED), irrigate the eye with copious amounts of warm tap water to remove chemical for at least 15 to 20 minutes. Normal saline irrigation is used in the ED; injury may require short-acting ophthalmic anesthetic drops.

Nursing Interventions: Take Action

Goal: To prevent further eye damage.

A. Have client "rest" the eyes: provide dimly lit room; use eye patches, if necessary.
B. Irrigate eyes with normal saline solution from inner canthus to outer canthus so solution does not flow into unaffected eye.
C. Eye may remain irritated after foreign body is removed and the anesthetic drops wear off; eye patch may be necessary.
D. If penetrating eye injury is present, decrease activities that cause increased ocular pressure, such as any Valsalva maneuver, blowing nose, sneezing, bending at the waist, etc.
E. Keep client immobilized until evaluated by an ophthalmologist.

Goal: To care for a client with an enucleation (removal of the eye).

A. Immediate: obtain vital signs; monitor for bleeding.
B. Instillation of topical ointments until prosthesis is fitted.
C. A clear "conformer" may be placed in the eye socket to allow the area to heal until a permanent prosthesis can be fitted.
D. Eye prosthesis.
1. *Insertion:* notched end of prosthesis should be closest to the client's nose; lift upper eyelid (using nondominant hand) and insert saline solution–rinsed prosthesis into socket area with top edge slipping under upper lid; gently retract lower lid until bottom edge of prosthesis slips behind it.

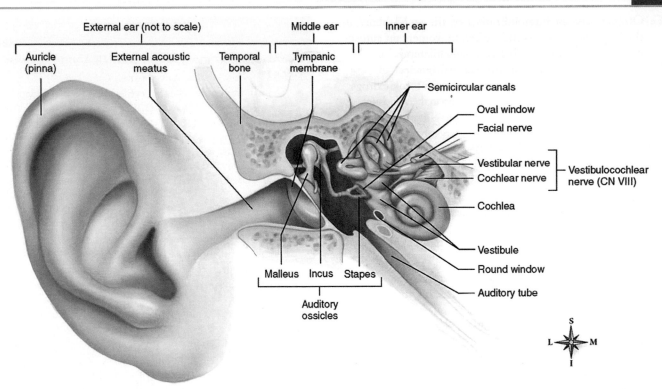

FIG. 8.6 Ear Anatomy. (From Patton, K. & Thibodeau, G. [2013]. *Anatomy & physiology* [8th ed.]. Elsevier.)

2. *Removal*: retract the lower lid and apply slight pressure just below the eye—this should release the suction holding the prosthesis in place; assess the socket for signs of infection.
3. The prosthesis is usually cleansed with normal saline.

THE EAR

Physiology of the Ear

A. External ear (Fig. 8.6).
   1. External auditory canal: function is to transmit the collected sound waves to the tympanic membrane; outer half of canal secretes cerumen, or wax, which has a protective function.
   2. Tympanic membrane: a tough membrane separating the external and middle ear; transmits vibrations from external ear to the malleus of the middle ear; normally a pearly gray color.
B. Middle ear.
   1. Middle ear is filled with air at atmospheric pressure by means of the eustachian tubes; the eustachian tubes of infants and young children are shorter, wider, straighter, and more horizontal than those of adults.
   2. The function of the external and middle ear is to transmit and magnify sound waves by air conduction.
   3. Problems in the external and middle ear cause conductive hearing loss.
C. Inner ear.
   1. Assists in maintaining equilibrium.
   2. Cochlea: contains organ of Corti, which is the receptive end organ for hearing.

3. Disease of the inner ear or nerve pathway can result in sensorineural hearing loss.

System Assessment: Recognize Cues

A. Assessment of the ear.
   1. Assess placement of the ears: low-set ears may be indicative of congenital anomalies in the newborn.
   2. Movement of the auricle should not elicit pain.
   3. Note presence of any discharge in the external canal.
   4. Note color and consistency of cerumen.
B. Assess for vertigo: ask client to close eyes and stand on one foot; have client walk with eyes closed; client may fall to one side or complain of the room spinning.

DISORDERS OF THE EAR

Hearing Loss

Hearing loss results from an impairment of the transmission of sound waves.

A. Conductive hearing loss results from mechanical dysfunction in transmission of sound from the outer or middle ear or both. Client will be able to benefit from a hearing aid. An example of conductive hearing loss is impacted cerumen, which often occurs in older adults.
B. Sensorineural (perceptive) hearing loss results from a problem in the inner ear (cochlea) or auditory nerve pathway. It often results from injury to cilia that transmit sound. Incoming sound cannot be analyzed correctly. Client may benefit from cochlear implant. An example of sensorineural hearing loss is presbycusis, which occurs in older adults.

Ophthalmic Diagnostics

The **Snellen chart** is used in screening for visual acuity problems. Client is placed 20 feet (6 m) from the chart, and visual acuity is expressed as a ratio (what the client *should* see at 20 feet [6 m] with normal vision compared with what they *can* see at 20 feet [6 m]). A ratio of 20/50 means that the client can see at 20 feet (6 m) what they should see at 50 feet (15 m). Normal visual acuity is 20/20. Legal blindness is defined as the best-corrected vision in the better eye of 20/200 or less.

Noncontact tonometer is an instrument used to measure intraocular pressure noninvasively. Normal pressure is 12 to 22 mm Hg. A puff of air is directed toward the cornea, which causes indentation and allows measurement of intraocular pressure—a screen for diagnosis of glaucoma.

Direct ophthalmoscopy is examination of the fundus or back portion of the interior of the eyeball, which provides for visual evaluation of the retina, vascular patterns, and optic disk.

Biomicroscopy (slit-lamp examination) is used to assess the anterior eye for problems of the cornea, iris, and lens and to evaluate the depth of the anterior chamber.

Fluorescein angiography provides information about flow of blood through retinal vessels and involves the IV administration of fluorescein followed by taking photographs of the retina. Yellow-orange discoloration of urine and skin may occur.

Refractive error evaluation determines what refractive errors have occurred because light is not correctly focused on the retina. Conditions that occur in refractive errors are:

- **Myopia** (nearsightedness)—sees near objects clearly; has problem seeing distant objects
- **Hyperopia** (farsightedness)—sees distant objects clearly; has problem seeing close objects
- **Presbyopia**—a decrease in the elasticity of the lens that causes poor accommodation for near vision (common in older adults); difficulty seeing objects that are close
- **Astigmatism**—an uneven curvature of the cornea; light rays do not focus on the retina at the same time

Hearing Diagnostics

Audiometry is used to measure a client's hearing by the use of various tones and intensities of sound produced by an audiometer.

Rinne test is conducted by holding a tuning fork on the mastoid bone (bone conduction). The client who hears normally will continue to hear the vibrations. This demonstrates that air conduction will last twice as long as bone conduction (2:1 ratio). When the tone is louder through air, the test result is positive and indicates normal hearing. If the bone conduction is louder than air conduction, it is indicative of a conductive loss.

Weber test is conducted by placing a vibrating tuning fork on top of the client's head or in the middle of the forehead; the sound should be heard equally well in each ear. Sound is heard better in impaired ear with conduction deafness and sound is heard only in normal ear with sensorineural hearing loss.

Otoscopy is the examination of the external ear and the tympanic membrane by the use of an otoscope.

Ophthalmic Medications

General Nursing Implications

- Only use ophthalmic preparations of medications; the container should say "for ophthalmic use only."
- To decrease systemic absorption of ophthalmic topical medications, teach the client to apply gentle pressure (punctal occlusion) to the nasolacrimal duct (tear duct) for 30 to 60 seconds immediately after instillation of drops.
- Instruct the client or family in proper administration of eyedrops or ointment (i.e., maintain sterile technique and prevent dropper contamination; clearly mark each container to indicate what eye medication is for, and do not share medication).
- Expect some blurriness from ointments; apply at bedtime, if possible, to avoid safety problems from diminished vision.
- Instruct the client to report changes in vision, blurring, difficulty breathing, or flushing.
- Teach the client to gently close eye and allow medication to distribute evenly over eye.
- If client has difficulty instilling eyedrops, provide information about adaptive equipment that positions the bottle of eyedrop medication directly over the eye.

MEDICATIONS	SIDE EFFECTS	NURSING IMPLICATIONS
Glaucoma Medications		
Alpha2-Adrenergic Agonists: Decrease the production of aqueous humor and increase outflow.		
Apraclonidine Brimonidine Dipivefrin	Dry mouth, ocular hyperemia, local burning and stinging Systemic absorption: hypotension Dipivefrin may cause hypertension and tachycardia	1. Can be absorbed into contact lens; wait 15 min after drops are instilled to replace contacts. 2. Dipivefrin is contraindicated in clients with narrow-angle glaucoma.

Appendix 8.2   OPHTHALMIC MEDICATIONS—cont'd   ℞

MEDICATIONS	SIDE EFFECTS	NURSING IMPLICATIONS
Glaucoma Medications		
Contraindicated with a history of cardiac problems, such as bradycardia, heart block, or hypertension.		
Nonselective Beta$_1$ and Beta$_2$ Blockers: Decrease the production of aqueous humor.		
Timolol maleate Carteolol	Eye irritation, dry eyes Bradycardia, AV block, bronchospasm	1. Assess for cardiac and respiratory changes with systemic absorption—can constrict airways and drop heart rate and blood pressure. 2. Contraindicated in clients with COPD or asthma.
Selective Beta$_1$ Blockers: Decrease the production of aqueous humor.		
Betaxolol	Bradycardia, AV block	1. Recommended for use in clients with history of COPD. 2. Contraindicated in clients with bradycardia or overt cardiac failure. 3. Assess for systemic absorption.
Prostaglandin Analogs: Increase the outflow of aqueous fluid from the eye.		

Bimatoprost
Latanoprost
Travoprost
	Increases pigmentation of
	    eyelid and growth of
	    eyelashes; conjunctiva
	    hyperemia
		1. Systemic effects are minimal.
		2. May cause local brown pigmentation of the iris.
		3. If only one eye is to be treated, teach the client not to place drops in the other eye to try to make the eye colors similar.

Carbonic Anhydrase Inhibitors: Inhibit the production of aqueous humor; do not affect the flow or absorption of the fluid.		
Brinzolamide Dorzolamide	Bradycardia, AV block	1. Drugs are similar to the sulfonamides; check client for allergies because an allergy is likely with these eyedrops. 2. Teach client to shake eye medication before applying because it separates. 3. Drug is absorbed by contact lenses, which will discolor and become cloudy.
Cholinergics—Direct Acting: Contract the ciliary muscle, which causes the iris to be withdrawn, permitting drainage of aqueous humor and decreased pressure within the eye.		

Carbachol
Pilocarpine
    hydrochloride
	Conjunctiva irritation,
	    transient ocular
	    discomfort
	Headache, dizziness,
	    increased saliva
		1. Cholinergics are contraindicated in clients with inflammatory eye conditions.
		2. Miotic; causes constriction of pupil.

> **❗ NURSING PRIORITY** Only use ophthalmic preparations of any clinically indicated medication (drops or ointment) that is instilled into the eye.

Other Eye Medications

MEDICATIONS	SIDE EFFECTS	NURSING IMPLICATIONS
Cycloplegic and Mydriatics: Work by blocking the response of the sphincter muscle of the iris to produce dilation of the pupil; may cause paralysis of accommodation. Used in eye examination and diagnosis. *All are contraindicated in glaucoma because dilated pupils cause an increase in intraocular pressure.*		

Atropine sulfate
Cyclopentolate HCl
Tropicamide
	Blurred vision, photophobia,
	    headache, hyperemia; systemic
	    effects: flushing, sweating, dry
	    mouth, dizziness
		1. These are contraindicated in clients with glaucoma.
		2. Dark glasses may be worn to decrease discomfort from photophobia.
		3. Use only ophthalmic preparations.

Diagnostics: Surface of eye absorbs dye, thus enhancing the visualization of corneal abrasions in eye trauma.		

Fluorescein sodium
Rose Bengal
Lissamine green
	Stinging, burning sensation,
	    nausea, vomiting, pruritus, and
	    paresthesias
		1. Cornea remains uncolored; abrasions and defects turn green.
		2. IV fluorescein is used to facilitate visualization of retinal blood vessels in evaluating diabetic retinopathy.

Continued

POTENTIAL NURSING ACTION	INDICATED	NON-ESSENTIAL	CONTRA-INDICATED
Have client sit upright in bed at all times.			X
Provide a regular diet and snacks.		X	
Maintain bedrest in a quiet, dimly lit room	X		
Avoid unnecessary nursing procedures.	X		
Minimize stimulation and sudden position changes.	X		
Rise and change positions (especially of the head) slowly.	X		
Limit number of visitors.		X	
Increase sodium in the diet to treat an acute attack.			X

Client Needs: Physiological Integrity/Physiological Adaptation
Clinical Judgment/Cognitive Skill: Generate Solutions
Item Type: Matrix Multiple Choice
Rationale & Test-Taking Strategy: The question is asking for nursing actions that promote a safe environment. Ménière disease is an inner-ear disorder characterized by recurrent episodes of vertigo, most typically associated with fluctuating progressive hearing loss and tinnitus. The primary goal in planning care for this client is to provide for client safety, along with emotional and physical support during an acute attack. Nursing interventions would include maintaining bedrest in a quiet, dimly lit room and avoiding flickering lights and television, having the client take a position of comfort (sitting up may not be helpful), avoiding unnecessary nursing procedures, and minimizing stimulation and sudden position changes. If the client is severely nauseated, administer medications via routes other than oral. Instruct client to always call before getting out of bed. Teach the client to rise and change positions (especially of the head) slowly. Clients are placed on a low-sodium diet and diuretic to reduce the inner pressure and volume.

---

12. The nurse is reviewing the admission nurses' notes on a client with bilateral cataracts.

    In the following nurses' notes, highlight the assessment findings that are prevalent in a client with impaired vision due to cataracts in both eyes.

Health History	Nurses' Notes	Vital Signs	Laboratory Results

1500 AA 75-year-old client reports being a retired nuclear engineer with a history of type 2 diabetes. Client reports progressive blurring of vision since last year's visit and relates difficulty in reading street signs while driving. Client wears bifocal glasses and has difficulty driving at night due to a glare seen on car headlights. Client denies any flashes or floaters, eye discomfort, or pain. There is no appearance of eye redness or drainage coming from either eye.

Client Needs: Physiological Integrity/Physiological Adaptation
Clinical Judgment/Cognitive Skill: Recognize Cues
Item Type: Highlight in Text
Rationale & Test-Taking Strategy: The nurses' notes indicate the client has age-related cataract formation. Think about the symptoms that a client with cataracts experiences. Cataract signs and symptoms include clouded, blurred, or dim vision; increasing difficulty with vision at night; and sensitivity to light and glare. Also, clients typically need brighter light for reading and other activities. Predisposing factors for cataracts include age; recent or past eye trauma; exposure to radioactive materials, x-rays, or ultraviolet (UV) light; diabetes mellitus; hypertension; and prolonged use of corticosteroids, chlorpromazine, beta blockers, or miotic drugs. There should not be any signs of inflammation with cataracts.

CHAPTER NINE

Endocrine: Care of Adult Clients

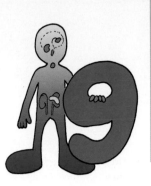

PHYSIOLOGY OF THE PITUITARY GLAND

The pituitary gland is often referred to as the "master gland" and is located deep in the brain. It secretes hormones that control hormone secretion of other endocrine glands (Fig. 9.1). It has two lobes—anterior and posterior—that secrete hormones promoting growth, water absorption by the kidney, and sexual development and function.

System Assessment: Recognize Cues

A. Assess for growth imbalance.
1. Assess for excessive or retarded growth.
   a. In adults, assess for excessive growth of small bones and soft tissue.
   b. In children, assess for excessive or retarded growth in height.
2. Evaluate excessive weight gain or loss.
B. Evaluate familial tendencies.
1. Parents who displayed slower growth patterns.
2. Compare rate of growth of siblings at age comparable to that of client.
3. Assess for specific characteristics and/or genetic traits in the adults of the immediate family.
C. Assess for secondary sexual characteristics appropriate to age and gender.
D. Onset of endocrine problems can be slow and insidious or abrupt and life-threatening depending on the endocrine gland involved.

DISORDERS OF THE PITUITARY GLAND

Hyperpituitarism: Acromegaly

Acromegaly **is most often the result of a benign slow-growing tumor (pituitary adenoma) that secretes growth hormone (GH) in adults. It occurs after the closure of epiphyses of the long bones. Pediatric GH excess is called gigantism.**

Assessment: Recognize Cues

A. Clinical manifestation.
1. Enlargement of the hands and feet and hypertrophy of the skin.
2. Peripheral neuropathy and joint pain may also be present.
3. Changes in facial features: protruding jaw, slanting forehead, thickened lips, and an increase in the size of the nose.
4. Severe enlargement of the pituitary gland may cause pressure on the optic nerve, resulting in changes in vision and headaches.
B. Diagnostics—hormone levels (see Appendix 9.1).

Analyze Cues and Prioritize Hypotheses

The most important problems are body image disturbances, sexual dysfunction, and depression.

Generate Solutions

Treatment

A. Treatment consists of surgery, radiation therapy, drug therapy, or a combination of these therapies.
B. Surgical intervention includes a hypophysectomy, which may be accomplished by the transsphenoidal approach (endoscopic transnasal).

Nursing Interventions: Take Action

Goal: To provide supportive preoperative care (see Chapter 3).
Goal: To decrease the chances of complications after hypophysectomy.
A. Elevate the head of the bed 30 degrees.
B. Assess for signs of cerebrospinal fluid leakage (client swallowing frequently or complaints of postnasal drip or headache); monitor gauze pad placed under the nose regularly for drainage. If any clear drainage is present, check for glucose and protein using a urine dipstick.
C. Discourage bending, coughing, sneezing, or straining (Valsalva maneuver) to prevent cerebrospinal fluid leak.
D. Assess for symptoms of increasing intracranial pressure (see Chapter 16).
E. Evaluate urine for excessive increase in volume (greater than 200 mL/h for 3 consecutive hours) or specific gravity less than 1.005 (i.e., development of diabetes insipidus [DI]). Replace fluids to avoid hypovolemia.
F. Do not brush teeth but use mouthwash and daily flossing.
G. Increase fiber and use laxatives to prevent constipation.
Goal: To assist client to reestablish hormone balance after hypophysectomy (adrenal insufficiency, hypothyroidism, and DI are most common complications).
A. Administer corticosteroids.

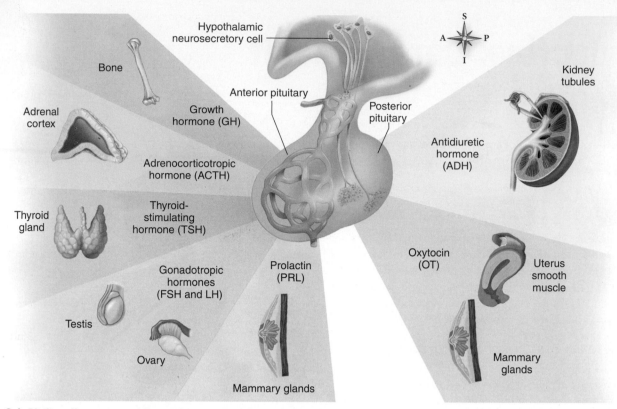

FIG. 9.1 Pituitary Hormones and Target Organs. (From Patton, K. T. & Thibodeau, G. A. [2014]. *The human body in health and disease* [6th ed.]. Elsevier/Mosby.)

B. If output becomes excessive (because of decrease in antidiuretic hormone [ADH]), anticipate administration of ADH-regulating medications; see Appendix 9.2).

C. Evaluate serum glucose levels for significant changes.

D. Monitor for problems related to hypothyroidism.

E. Cortisone and thyroid hormone replacement throughout lifetime.

Hypopituitarism

A deficiency of one or more pituitary hormones is called *hypopituitarism*. Deficiencies of adrenocorticotropic hormone (ACTH) or thyroid-stimulating hormone (TSH) can be life-threatening. In children a deficiency is usually related to GH deficiency.

Assessment: Recognize Cues

A. Clinical manifestations.
   1. Child—slow growth pattern after 1 year of age leading to short stature and other symptoms related to decreased TSH and ACTH.
   2. Adult—changes in secondary sex characteristics, headaches, diplopia, limited eye movements, reduced muscle mass, reduced exercise capacity, increased mortality from cardiovascular causes.

B. Diagnostics—measurement of anterior and posterior pituitary hormones.

Analyze Cues and Prioritize Hypotheses

The most important issue is the need for hormone replacement for improvement of overall well-being.

Generate Solutions

Treatment

A. Replacement of target hormones for deficiency problems (GH therapy administered at bedtime).

B. Identify underlying cause (surgery, irradiation of a tumor, etc.) in the adult and replace the deficient pituitary hormones.

Nursing Interventions: Take Action

Goal: To have early recognition of growth problems and other endocrine deficiencies.

A. Prepare child and family for diagnostic testing.

B. Reinforce client education regarding signs and symptoms of both hypo- and hyperfunction of the pituitary related to insufficient or excess hormone replacement.

Goal: To provide child and family support.

A. Encourage counseling to assist the child and family in setting realistic expectations regarding improvement with GH therapy.

B. Refer to community agencies—treatment is quite expensive.

DISORDERS OF THE POSTERIOR PITUITARY

Diabetes Insipidus

DI is characterized by a deficiency of ADH or the kidney's inability to respond to ADH. When it occurs, it is most often associated with neurologic conditions, brain surgery, tumors, head injury, drug therapy, or central nervous system (CNS) inflammatory problems.

Assessment: Recognize Cues

A. Clinical manifestations.
   1. Polyuria: excretion of excessive amounts urine (4–30 L/day).
   2. Polydipsia.
   3. Low urine specific gravity (less than 1.005).
   4. Severe dehydration (tachycardia, poor skin turgor, dry mucous membranes, hypotension).
   5. Hypernatremia and elevated serum osmolality (greater than 295 mOsm/kg or 295 mmol/kg).
   6. Hemoconcentration (increased hemoglobin, hematocrit, blood urea nitrogen [BUN]).
B. Diagnosis: water deprivation test; measurement of ADH level.

Analyze Cues and Prioritize Hypotheses

The most important problems are disturbances in fluid and electrolyte balance that can lead to excess water loss through polyuria and dehydration.

Generate Solutions

Treatment

A. Administration of ADH-regulating medications (desmopressin, vasopressin) (see Appendix 9.2).

Nursing Interventions: Take Action

Goal: To maintain fluid and electrolyte balances.
A. Encourage intake of fluids containing electrolytes.
B. Monitor intake and output carefully; weigh daily.
C. Evaluate urine specific gravity for changes.
D. Assess hydration status.
E. Correlate hydration status with weight gain or loss.
F. Closely monitor sodium and potassium levels with fluid shifts (hypernatremia).

> **! NURSING PRIORITY** Because the client cannot reduce urine output, they are at risk for severe dehydration if they are deprived of fluids for more than 4 hours.

Syndrome of Inappropriate Antidiuretic Hormone

The *syndrome of inappropriate antidiuretic hormone* (SIADH) is a condition in which there is continued release or high production of ADH, regardless of the level of plasma osmolarity, which may be normal or low.

Assessment: Recognize Cues

A. Clinical manifestations.
   1. Low urinary output with weight gain and no obvious edema.
   2. Decreased (dilutional hyponatremia) serum sodium level and hypochloremia.
   3. Gastrointestinal (GI) disturbances (anorexia, nausea, vomiting).
   4. Cerebral edema: altered mental status, headaches, seizures.
   5. High urine specific gravity (greater than 1.025).
   6. Fatigue and muscle aches.
B. Diagnostics—increased urine and decreased serum osmolality.

Analyze Cues and Prioritize Hypotheses

The most important problems are disturbances in fluid and electrolyte balance that can lead to water retention and fluid overload.

Generate Solutions

Treatment

A. Treat underlying cause.
   1. Fluid restriction (limit fluids to 800–1000 mL/24 hours).
   2. Monitor sodium correction carefully; correct deficit slowly.
B. Administration of vasopressin receptor antagonist medications when hyponatremia is present.

Nursing Interventions: Take Action

Goal: To maintain fluid and electrolyte balances.
A. Restrict fluids.
B. Monitor intake and output carefully; weigh daily.
C. Evaluate urine specific gravity for changes.
D. Assess hydration status.
E. Closely monitor sodium and potassium levels with fluid shifts (hyponatremia).
F. Maintain seizure and fall precautions and perform neurologic checks.

Physiology of the Thyroid Gland

The *thyroid gland* is located in the anterior portion of the neck below the Adam's apple and in front of the trachea. Primary function of thyroid hormone is to control the level of cellular metabolism by secreting thyroxin (T4) and triiodothyronine (T3).

System Assessment: Recognize Cues

A. Assess for changes in metabolism.
   1. Significant increase or decrease in weight.
   2. Diarrhea or constipation.

Generate Solutions

Treatment

A. Medical management.
1. Replacement of thyroid hormone.
2. Low-calorie diet to promote weight loss.
3. Minimize constipation; increase fiber in diet and fluids.

Complications

A. Thyroid hormone replacement will increase the workload of the heart and increase myocardial oxygen requirements.
B. Observe client for development of *myxedema coma*, which can lead to organ damage and death—reduced level of consciousness, respiratory and cardiac failure, hypoglycemia, and hypothermia.

Nursing Interventions: Take Action

Goal: To assist the client to return to hormone balance.

A. Begin thyroid replacement and evaluate client's response; advise client that it will be about 7 days before beginning to feel better.
B. Provide a warm environment.

> ❗ **NURSING PRIORITY** Administer sedatives and hypnotics with caution because of increased susceptibility. These medications tend to precipitate respiratory depression in the client with hypothyroidism.

C. Prevent and/or treat constipation.
D. Assess progress.
1. Decrease in body weight.
2. Intake and output balance.
3. Decrease in visible edema.
4. Energy level and mental alertness should increase in 7 to 14 days and continue to rise until normal.
E. Evaluate cardiovascular response to medication.

Goal: To assist client to understand implications of disease and requirements for health maintenance.

A. Need for lifelong drug therapy.
B. Client with diabetes needs to evaluate blood glucose levels more frequently; thyroid preparations may alter effects of hypoglycemic agents.
C. Continue to reinforce teaching as client begins to make progress; early in the disease, the client may not comprehend importance of information.

Physiology of the Parathyroid

Four small parathyroid glands are located near, or embedded in, the thyroid gland. The hormone secreted is parathyroid hormone (PTH), also called parathormone, which is primarily involved in the control of serum calcium levels.

System Assessment: Recognize Cues

A. History of problems of calcium metabolism and/or thyroid surgery.

B. Assess for changes in mental or emotional status.
C. Evaluate reflexes and neuromuscular response to stimuli.
D. Evaluate serum and urine calcium levels.

DISORDERS OF THE PARATHYROID

Hyperparathyroidism

Hyperparathyroidism **is characterized by excessive secretion of PTH, resulting in hypercalcemia.**

Assessment: Recognize Cues

A. Clinical manifestations.
1. Bone cysts and pathologic fractures occur because of bone decalcification.
2. Hypercalcemia.
3. Urinary calculi; azotemia.
4. Hypertension caused by chronic kidney disease.
5. Repeated urinary tract and kidney infections.
6. CNS problems of lethargy, stupor, and psychosis.
7. GI problems.
   a. Anorexia, nausea, and vomiting.
   b. Constipation; development of peptic ulcer.
B. Diagnostics.
1. Increased level of serum total calcium; decreased level of serum phosphorous; increased PTH.
2. Computed tomography (CT) scan and/or x-ray film show demineralized cystic areas in bone.
3. Increased urine calcium and phosphorous levels.

Analysis: Analyze Cues and Prioritize Hypotheses

The most important problems are related to elevated serum calcium levels due to increased PTH secretion.

Generate Solutions

Treatment

A. Decrease level of circulating calcium.
B. Parathyroidectomy.

Nursing Interventions: Take Action

Goal: To decrease the level of serum calcium.

A. High fluid intake to dilute serum calcium and urine calcium levels.
B. If IV is necessary, generally administer normal saline solution.
C. Furosemide, a loop diuretic, may be used to increase excretion of calcium.
D. Encourage mobility because immobility increases demineralization of bones.
E. Limit foods high in calcium.
F. Phosphate replacement.

Goal: To assess client's tolerance of and response to increased PTH level.

A. Assess for skeletal involvement.
B. Assess for kidney involvement.
1. Strain urine for stones.
2. Evaluate for low back pain (kidney).
3. Check for hematuria.
4. Assess intake and output carefully.

C. Assess for presence of bone pain.

D. Assess cardiac response to increased level of calcium.

Goal: To provide appropriate preoperative measures if surgery is indicated (see Chapter 3).

Goal: To prevent postoperative complications of parathyroidectomy.

A. Care of client who has undergone parathyroidectomy is same as that for client who has undergone thyroidectomy.

B. Bone pain is relieved shortly after surgery; bone lesions frequently heal; serious kidney disease may not be reversible.

Hypoparathyroidism

Hypoparathyroidism **is characterized by a decrease in the PTH level, resulting in hypocalcemia and elevated serum phosphate levels. Severe hypocalcemia results in tetany.**

Assessment: Recognize Cues

A. Insidious onset.
   1. Muscle weakness/spasms.
   2. Loss of hair; dry skin.

B. Overt/acute tetany (potentially fatal).
   1. Bronchospasm; laryngospasm.
   2. Seizures; cardiac dysrhythmias.
   3. Positive Chvostek sign (sign is positive when sharp tapping over the facial nerve elicits mouth, nose, and eye twitching).
   4. Trousseau phenomenon (present when carpopedal spasm, i.e., involutary contraction of the hand and wrist muscles, that occurs after compression of the upper arm with a blood pressure cuff).

C. Diagnostics.
   1. Decreased serum calcium levels.
   2. Increased serum phosphate levels.
   3. Low PTH levels.

Analysis: Analyze Cues and Prioritize Hypotheses

The most important problems for this rare disorder are low serum calcium levels that can lead to tetany and vitamin D deficiency.

Generate Solutions

Treatment

A. Vitamin D to enhance calcium absorption.

B. Increased calcium in the diet and supplements.

TEST ALERT Adjust food and fluid intake to improve fluid and electrolyte balances.

C. Acute.
   1. Replace calcium through slow IV infusion (calcium gluconate, calcium chloride).
   2. Sedatives, anticonvulsants.

Nursing Interventions: Take Action

Goal: To assist client to increase serum calcium levels.

A. Administer calcium preparations.

B. Evaluate for an increase in serum calcium levels and a decrease in serum phosphate levels.

C. Client will require lifelong medical care to maintain homeostasis.

Goal: To prevent complications of neuromuscular irritability.

A. Quiet environment.

B. Low lights.

C. Seizure precautions.

D. Have client breathe in and out of a breathing mask or bag (reduces serum pH, thereby increasing total calcium available in its free form).

Goal: To help client avoid complications of respiratory distress.

A. Bronchodilators.

B. Tracheotomy and suction set readily available.

C. Frequent assessment of respiratory status. *Immediately report to registered nurse (RN) any significant changes.*

Goal: To prevent complications of cardiac problems.

A. Assess client for history of cardiac problems.

B. Assess frequently for dysrhythmias.

C. Calcium will potentiate effects of digoxin; use cautiously together.

PHYSIOLOGY OF THE PANCREAS

The pancreas is located in the upper left aspect of the abdominal cavity and produces the enzymes trypsin, amylase, and lipase, along with insulin, amylin, and glucagon from the islets of Langerhans.

System Assessment: Recognize Cues

A. Evaluate changes in weight, particularly weight gain in an adult and weight loss in a child.

B. Evaluate alterations in fluid balance.

C. Evaluate changes in mental status.

D. Evaluate serum glucose and pancreatic enzyme studies.

E. Evaluate the abdomen for epigastric pain and abdominal discomfort.

DISORDERS OF THE PANCREAS

Diabetes Mellitus

Diabetes mellitus **(DM) is a complex, multisystem disease characterized by the absence of, or a severe decrease in, the secretion or utilization of insulin.**

A. Pathophysiology.
   1. The primary function of insulin is to facilitate the movement of glucose from the blood into the cell, thus decreasing the blood glucose level.
      a. Necessary for the transport of glucose into the cells of the liver, muscles, and other tissues.
      b. Regulates the rate of carbohydrate metabolism and conversion to glucose; normally insulin is decreased during fasting and increased after eating (prandial).
   2. Insulin is secreted by the beta cells in the islets of Langerhans in the pancreas.

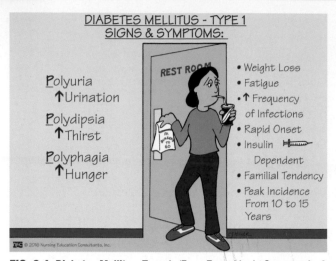

FIG. 9.4 Diabetes Mellitus, Type 1. (From Zerwekh, J., Garneau, A., & Miller, C. J. [2017]. *Digital collection of the memory notebooks of nursing* [4th ed.]. Nursing Education Consultants.)

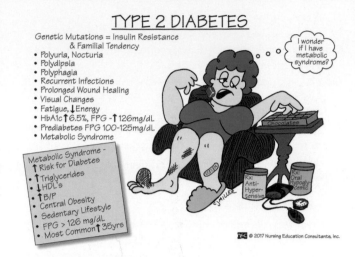

FIG. 9.5 Diabetes Mellitus, Type 2. (From Zerwekh, J., Garneau, A., & Miller, C. J. [2017]. *Digital collection of the memory notebooks of nursing* [4th ed.]. Nursing Education Consultants.)

3. Insulin allows the body to use carbohydrates more effectively for conversion of glucose for energy.
   a. Adequate intake of carbohydrates.
   b. Available insulin to facilitate the movement of glucose into cells.
   c. Adequate reserves of glucagon (released by pancreas; converts glycogen to glucose in the liver).
4. If carbohydrates are not available to be used for energy, cells will begin to oxidize the fats and protein stores.
   a. Breakdown of fat results in the production of ketone bodies.
   b. Protein is wasted during insulin deficiency. Protein is broken down and converted to glucose by the liver, thus contributing to the increase in circulating glucose.
   c. When fats are used as the primary energy source, the serum lipid level rises and contributes to the accelerated development of atherosclerosis.
5. When circulating glucose cannot be used for energy, the level of serum glucose will increase (hyperglycemia).
6. Pathophysiologic bases for symptoms.
   a. *Polyuria*: because of the increased serum osmolarity, there is more circulating volume; water is not reabsorbed from the renal tubules and there is a significant increase in urine output.
   b. *Polydipsia*: increased loss of fluids precipitates dehydration, causing thirst.
   c. *Polyphagia*: tissue breakdown and wasting cause hunger.
   d. Weight loss (with type 1 DM): glucose is not available to the cells; body begins to break down fat and protein stores for energy.
B. Classification.
   1. Type 1: lack of insulin secretion (Fig. 9.4).
      a. Absence or minimal insulin production; client is dependent on insulin to prevent ketoacidosis and maintain life.

   b. Generally, affects people under 40 years of age but can occur at any age.
   c. Previously called juvenile diabetes or insulin-dependent DM.
   d. Familial tendencies in transmission.
   e. Client will have type 1 diabetes for the rest of their life.
2. Type 2: combination of insulin resistance and inadequate insulin secretion to compensate (Fig. 9.5).
   a. Insulin deficiency caused by defects in insulin production or by excessive demands for insulin; client is not dependent on insulin.
   b. Ketoacidosis is generally not a problem because of limited insulin production. May have hyperosmolar hyperglycemic syndrome occur as a complication.
   c. May occur at any age in adults. Becoming more common in children due to childhood obesity.
   d. Previously called adult-onset DM (AODM) or noninsulin-dependent DM (NIDDM).
   e. Obesity is a major risk factor; overweight people require more insulin.
   f. There is usually a strong family history.
   g. Blood sugar often controlled by diet and oral hypoglycemics but during episodes of stress may require insulin for control.
3. Prediabetes.
   a. Increased risk for developing type 2 diabetes.
   b. Defined as impaired glucose tolerance test, impaired fasting glucose, or both.
   c. Asymptomatic, although long-term damage may be occurring.
   d. Lifestyle changes can reduce the risk of developing overt type 2 diabetes.
4. Pregestational DM (see Chapter 21).
   a. Woman has either type 1 or type 2 diabetes before becoming pregnant.
   b. Insulin dependent during pregnancy.
   c. Increased risk of intrauterine fetal demise (IUFD), sometimes called *stillbirth*, and congenital

malformations (cardiovascular, CNS, and skeletal system).

5. Gestational DM (GDM) (see Chapter 21).
   a. Develops during pregnancy; usually detected at 24 to 28 weeks' gestation by a screening glucose test; if screen is positive (130–140 mg/dL [7.2–7.8 mmol/L] blood sugar), then an oral glucose tolerance test (OGTT) is ordered.
   b. Higher risk for cesarean delivery, and infants have increased risk for perinatal death, birth injury, and neonatal complications.
   c. Infant may be large for gestational age and may experience hypoglycemia shortly after birth.
   d. Glucose tolerance usually returns to normal soon after delivery.
   e. Commonly occurs again in future pregnancies; client is at increased risk for development of glucose intolerance and type 2 diabetes later in life.

Assessment: Recognize Cues

A. Clinical manifestations.
   1. Types 1 and 2.
      a. Three Ps: polyphagia, polydipsia, polyuria.
      b. Fatigue; increased frequency of infections.
   2. Type 1.
      a. Weight loss; excessive thirst.
      b. Bed-wetting; blurred vision.
      c. Enuresis in children, nocturia in adults.
      d. Complaints of abdominal pain.
      e. Rapid onset, generally over days to weeks.
   3. Type 2 (most clients asymptomatic first 5–10 years).
      a. Weight gain (obese); visual disturbances.
      b. Slow onset; may occur over months.
      c. Fatigue and malaise.
      d. Recurrent vaginal yeast or monilia infections—frequently, this is initial symptom in women.
      e. Older adult assessment considerations (Box 9.1).
B. Diagnostics (the criteria for diagnosis is made using one of the following methods) (see Appendix 9.1).
   1. A1c (glycosylated hemoglobin) of 6.5% or higher.
   2. Fasting blood glucose level: above 126 mg/dL (7 mmol/L) (normal glucose below 100 mg/dL [5.6 mmol/L]) after no caloric intake for at least 8 hours.
   3. Two-hour plasma glucose level greater than or equal to 200 mg/dL (11.1 mmol/L) during an OGTT, using a glucose load of 75 g.
   4. When symptoms of hyperglycemia (polyuria, polydipsia, unexplained weight loss) or hyperglycemic crisis occur, a random plasma glucose greater than or equal to 200 mg/dL (11.1 mmol/L).
   5. Prediabetes: intermediate stage between normal and diabetes.
      a. Impaired glucose tolerance (IGT): 2 hours after a meal, plasma glucose is greater than 140 mg/dL (7.8 mmol/L) to 199 mg/dL (11.0 mmol/L) or higher during an OGTT.
      b. Impaired fasting glucose (IFG): fasting blood glucose is greater than 100 mg/dL (5.6 mmol/L) but less than 126 mg/dL (7 mmol/L).

Box 9.1 OLDER ADULT CARE FOCUS

Diabetic Assessment Considerations and Care

- Determine mental status and manual dexterity to handle injections.
- Determine whether client can access the injection sites.
- Is client alert and mentally capable of making judgments on medications?
- Determine whether the client can pay for supplies.
- What is the client's attitude about needles and injections?
- Assess how many other medications the client is taking. Are there problems with "polypharmacy" (too many medications)?
- Discuss the risk of hypoglycemia unawareness (e.g., does not experience early signs of hypoglycemia related to age and use of beta-adrenergic blockers).
- Determine family's or client's ability to accurately perform serum glucose testing.
- What is the client's support system?

NURSING PRIORITY Glucose stays attached to the red blood cell (RBC) for the life of the cell (about 120 days). The glycosylated hemoglobin A1c level will indicate overall glucose control for approximately the past 120 days. This allows evaluation of control of the blood glucose level, regardless of increases or decreases in the blood glucose level immediately before the sample was obtained.

Analyze Cues and Prioritize Hypotheses

The most important problems are hyperglycemia, acidosis, poor wound healing, diabetic neuropathy, kidney disease, and hypoglycemia.

Generate Solutions

Treatment

A. Factors in diabetes management (Fig. 9.6).
B. ▲ Hypoglycemic agents.
   1. Insulin: may be used in both type 1 and 2 diabetes (Table 9.1).
      a. Insulin may be delivered subcutaneous, IV, inhaled, or via pump.
      b. Only regular insulin can be given intravenously.
      c. Combination premixed insulin therapy eliminates problem of mixing different types (example: NPH/regular 70/30—number refers to percentage of each type of insulin).
      d. Insulin will be used for glucose control during pregnancy.
   2. Oral hypoglycemic agents for type 2 DM (see Appendix 9.2).
   3. Diabetic diet.
      a. Client with type 1 DM should coordinate insulin dosing with eating habits and activity pattern in mind. Food selection is flexible.
      b. Client with type 2 DM should strive for glucose, lipid, and blood pressure goals. Modest weight loss has been associated with improved insulin resistance for those that are overweight or obese.

TRIANGLE OF DIABETIC MANAGEMENT

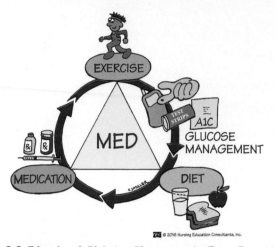

FIG. 9.6 Triangle of Diabetes Management. (From Zerwekh, J., Garneau, A., & Miller, C. J. [2017]. *Digital collection of the memory notebooks of nursing* [4th ed.]. Nursing Education Consultants.)

c. Meal plan.
   (1) Individualized carbohydrate intake (prefer whole grains, fruits, vegetables, low-fat milk). May include carbohydrate counting.
   (2) Fiber intake goal of 25 to 30 g/day.
   (3) Less than 200 mg/day of cholesterol and limited trans fats.
   (4) Protein intake for those with normal kidney function is the same as the general population.
   (5) Alcohol consumption can cause hypoglycemia in clients on insulin or oral hypoglycemic medications.
4. Exercise.
   a. Recommended to exercise 150 min/week (30 min/5 days/week) with moderate-intensity aerobic physical activity.
   b. Those with type 2 diabetes should also perform resistance training three times/week.
   c. Glucose should be monitored before, during, and after exercise.

TEST ALERT Intervene to control symptoms of hypoglycemia or hyperglycemia.

Table 9.1 PROFILE OF INSULINS	
Insulin	*Nursing Implications*
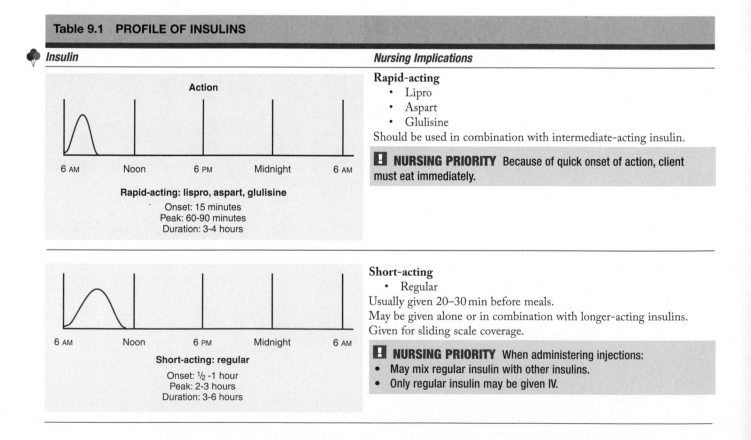 **Rapid-acting: lispro, aspart, glulisine** Onset: 15 minutes Peak: 60-90 minutes Duration: 3-4 hours	**Rapid-acting** • Lipro • Aspart • Glulisine Should be used in combination with intermediate-acting insulin. **❗ NURSING PRIORITY** Because of quick onset of action, client must eat immediately.
Short-acting: regular Onset: ½ -1 hour Peak: 2-3 hours Duration: 3-6 hours	**Short-acting** • Regular Usually given 20–30 min before meals. May be given alone or in combination with longer-acting insulins. Given for sliding scale coverage. **❗ NURSING PRIORITY** When administering injections: • May mix regular insulin with other insulins. • Only regular insulin may be given IV.

Table 9.1   PROFILE OF INSULINS

Insulin	*Nursing Implications*

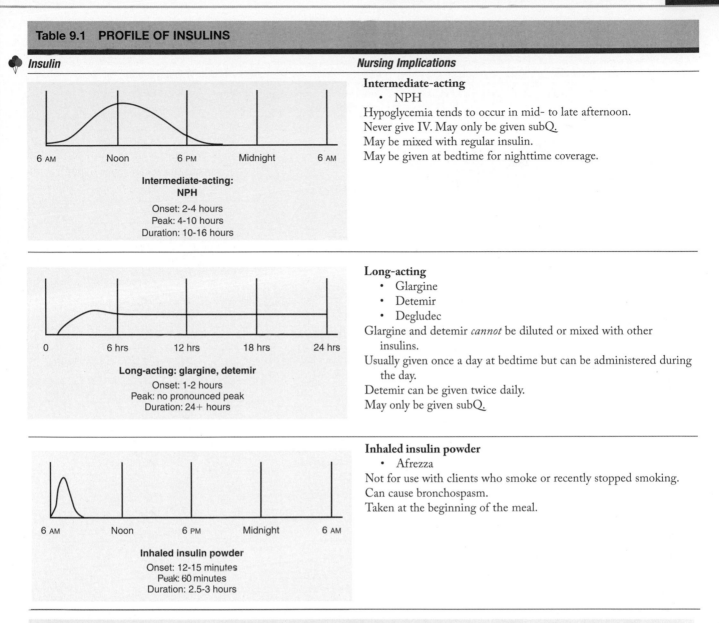

Intermediate-acting: NPH
Onset: 2-4 hours
Peak: 4-10 hours
Duration: 10-16 hours

Long-acting: glargine, detemir
Onset: 1-2 hours
Peak: no pronounced peak
Duration: 24+ hours

Inhaled insulin powder
Onset: 12-15 minutes
Peak: 60 minutes
Duration: 2.5-3 hours

Intermediate-acting
- NPH

Hypoglycemia tends to occur in mid- to late afternoon.
Never give IV. May only be given subQ.
May be mixed with regular insulin.
May be given at bedtime for nighttime coverage.

Long-acting
- Glargine
- Detemir
- Degludec

Glargine and detemir *cannot* be diluted or mixed with other insulins.
Usually given once a day at bedtime but can be administered during the day.
Detemir can be given twice daily.
May only be given subQ.

Inhaled insulin powder
- Afrezza

Not for use with clients who smoke or recently stopped smoking.
Can cause bronchospasm.
Taken at the beginning of the meal.

TEST ALERT Assess client for signs of hypoglycemia/hyperglycemia. Know various insulins and nursing implications for mixing medications from two vials when necessary. Administer insulin according to blood glucose levels.

❗ **NURSING PRIORITY** Remember, every insulin dose must be verified by another nurse as it is drawn up, every time. It is a ▲: high alert medication.

IV, Intravenous; *subQ*, subcutaneous.
(Figures from Harding, M.M., et al. [2023]. *Lewis's Medical-surgical nursing: Assessment and management of clinical problems* [12th ed.]. Elsevier Mosby.)

❗ **NURSING PRIORITY** Metabolic effects of exercise:
1. Reduces insulin needs by decreasing the blood glucose level.
2. Contributes to weight loss or maintenance of normal weight.
3. Helps the body metabolize cholesterol more efficiently.
4. Promotes less extreme fluctuations in blood glucose levels.
5. Decreases blood pressure.

Complications of Insulin Therapy

A. Hypoglycemia (Table 9.2).
B. Allergic reaction.

1. Localized reactions may occur and often resolve in 1 to 3 months.
2. Allergic reactions may also be from the preservatives used or the latex or rubber stoppers of the syringe or vial.
C. Lipoatrophy and lipodystrophy.
1. May result from poor rotation of injection sites.
D. Somogyi effect (Fig. 9.7).
1. Rebound hyperglycemia from an unrecognized hypoglycemic state.
2. Most often occurs at night.
3. May be treated by decreasing the evening insulin dose or by increasing the calories in the bedtime snack.

Table 9.2 COMPARISON OF DIABETIC KETOACIDOSIS, HYPEROSMOLAR HYPERGLYCEMIC SYNDROME, AND HYPOGLYCEMIA

	DKA	HHS	Hypoglycemia
Age	All ages, increased incidence in children.	Adult (usually seen in older adults with underlying chronic disease)	All ages
GI	Abdominal pain, anorexia, nausea, vomiting, diarrhea	Normal	Normal; may be hungry
Mental state	Dull, confusion increasing to coma	More severe neurologic symptoms due to increased osmolarity and high blood glucose level	Difficulty in concentrating, coordinating; eventually coma
Skin temperature	Warm, dry, flushed	Warm, dry, flushed	Cold, clammy
Pulse	Tachycardia, weak	Tachycardia	Tachycardia
Respirations	Initially deep and rapid; lead to Kussmaul respirations	Tachypnea	Shallow
Breath odor	Fruity, acetone	Normal	Normal
Urine output	Increased	Increased	Normal
Laboratory Values			
Glucose	Greater than 250 mg/dL (13.9 mmol/L)	Greater than 600 mg/dL (33.3 mmol/L)	Below 70 mg/dL (3.9 mmol/L)
Ketones	High/large	Normal	Normal
pH	Acidotic (less than 7.3)	Normal	Normal
Hematocrit	High due to dehydration	High due to dehydration	Normal
Laboratory Values: Urine			
Sugar	High	High	Negative
Ketones	High	Negative	Negative
Onset	Rapid (less than 24 hr)	Slow (over many days)	Rapid
Classification of diabetes	Primarily type 1; type 2 in severe distress	Type 2	Type 1 and type 2

DKA, Diabetic ketoacidosis; *GI*, gastrointestinal; *HHS*, hyperosmolar hyperglycemic syndrome.

E. Dawn phenomenon (Fig. 9.8).
  1. Results from nighttime release of growth hormone and cortisol.
  2. Blood glucose elevates from 0500 to 0600 (predawn hours).
  3. May be treated by increasing insulin for overnight period.
  4. Most severe in adolescence and young adulthood with peak growth hormone.
F. Hormones that counteract insulin: glucagon, epinephrine, cortisol, growth hormone.
G. Insulin requirement increases with serious illness, physical trauma, infection, surgery, and growth spurts.

❗ **NURSING PRIORITY** Intensive control of blood glucose levels in clients with type 1 diabetes can prevent or ameliorate many of the complications.

Complications Associated with Poorly Controlled Diabetes

A. Diabetic ketoacidosis.
  1. An extreme increase in the hyperglycemic state.
  2. Occurs predominantly in type 1 diabetes.
B. Clinical manifestations of diabetic ketoacidosis (see Table 9.2).
  1. Onset.
    a. May be acute or occur over several days.
    b. May result from stress, infection, surgery, or lack of effective insulin control.
    c. Results from poorly controlled diabetes.
  2. Severe hyperglycemia (blood glucose levels > 250 mg/dL [13.9 mmol/L]).
  3. Presence of metabolic acidosis (low pH [6.8–7.3] and serum bicarbonate level less than 16 mEq/L [mmol/L]).

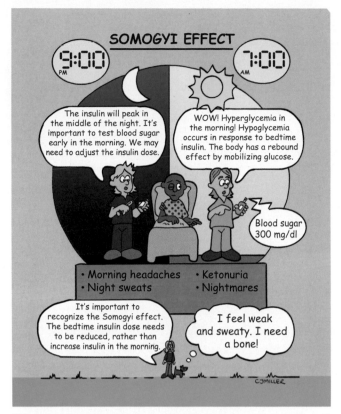

FIG. 9.7 Somogyi Effect. (From Zerwekh, J., Claborn, J., & Gaglione, T. [2011]. *Mosby's pathophysiology memory notecards* [2nd ed.]. Mosby.)

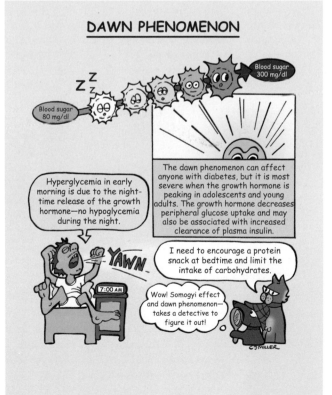

FIG. 9.8 Dawn Phenomenon. (From Zerwekh, J., Claborn, J., & Gaglione, T. [2011]. *Mosby's pathophysiology memory notecards* [2nd ed.]. Mosby.)

4. Hyperkalemia, hypokalemia, or normal potassium level, depending on amount of water loss.
5. Urine ketone and sugar levels are increased.
6. Excessive weakness; increased thirst.
7. Nausea, vomiting.
8. Fruity (acetone) breath.
9. Kussmaul respirations.
10. Decreased level of consciousness.
11. Dehydration.
12. Increased temperature caused by dehydration.

C. Hyperglycemic-hyperosmolar syndrome (HHS).
1. Occurs primarily in older adult clients with type 2 diabetes.
2. Characterized by extreme hyperglycemia (values greater than 600 mg/dL [33.3 mmol/L]).
3. Electrolyte imbalance.
4. Client becomes dehydrated very rapidly.

D. Clinical manifestations of HHS (see Table 9.2).

Complications of Long-Term Diabetes

A. Angiopathy: premature degenerative changes in the vascular system.
1. May affect the large vessels (macroangiopathy, early-onset atherosclerosis, and arteriosclerotic vascular problems).
2. May affect the small vessels (microangiopathy); problems are specific to diabetes.

B. Peripheral vascular disease: combination of both types of angiopathy.

C. Hypertension.

D. Cerebrovascular disease; coronary artery disease.

E. Ocular complications: retinopathy, cataracts, glaucoma.

> **⚠ PEDIATRIC PRIORITY** An ophthalmologic examination should be obtained once the child is 10 years of age and has had diabetes for 3 to 5 years.

F. Nephropathy.
1. Diabetic effects on the kidneys are the single most common cause of end-stage kidney failure.

G. Neuropathy: inadequate blood supply to the nerve tissue and high blood glucose levels cause metabolic changes within the neurons.
1. Peripheral neuropathy: may be general pain and tingling; may progress to painless neuropathy.

> **⚠ NURSING PRIORITY** Painless peripheral neuropathy is a very dangerous situation for the client with diabetes. Severe injury to the lower extremities may occur, and the client will not be aware of it. Clients should be taught to visually inspect their feet and legs daily.

2. Most common chronic complication.

H. Infections: an alteration in immune system response results in impairment of white cells for phagocytosis. Persistent glycosuria potentiates urinary tract infections.

Nursing Interventions: Take Action (All Types)

> ⚠ **NURSING PRIORITY** Evaluating client's control of diabetes:
> 1. Normal fasting blood glucose 70 to 100 mg/dL.
> 2. Two hours after meals or after glucose load, blood glucose is no higher than 140 mg/dL (7.77 mmol/L), less than 150 mg/dL (50–60 years), and less than 160 mg/dL if 60+ years.
> 3. Client is in good general health and is of normal weight.
> 4. Glycosylated hemoglobin A1c is less than 7% (normal range 4–5.9% of total hemoglobin).

Goal: To return serum glucose to normal level.

A. Initially administer regular insulin on a proportional basis according to need (Box 9.2).
B. Administer rapid-acting insulin 15 minutes before and short-acting insulin 30 minutes before a meal or snack; do not administer insulin if there is no carbohydrate intake.
C. Maintain adequate fluid intake.
D. Evaluate serum electrolyte levels.
    1. Do not administer potassium unless client is voiding or if urine output begins to drop.

Box 9.2   IMPLICATIONS IN THE ADMINISTRATION OF INSULIN ▲

1. Do not administer cold insulin; it increases pain and causes irritation at injection site.
2. An open 10-mL vial of unrefrigerated insulin should be discarded after 30 days, regardless of how much was used.
3. Do not allow insulin to freeze and keep it away from heat and sunlight.
4. Insulin pens (NPH and 70/30) should be discarded after 1 week of storage at room temperature. Regular cartridges, which do not contain preservatives, may be left unrefrigerated for up to 1 month.
5. Extreme temperatures (less than 36°F [2.2°C] or greater than 86°F [30°C]) should be avoided.
6. Roll the vial between the palms of the hands to decrease the risk for inconsistent concentration of insulin.
7. The abdomen is the primary site for subcutaneous injections of insulin. Rotate injection sites within one particular anatomic location; injection sites should be 1 inch apart.
8. Abdomen area provides most rapid insulin absorption.
9. Use only insulin syringes to administer insulin.
10. Check expiration date on insulin bottle.
11. When drawing up regular insulin with a long-acting insulin, draw up the regular (clear) insulin before the longer-acting (cloudy) insulin.
12. Regular insulin is used for administration by sliding scale and periods when blood glucose is unstable and difficult to control. *Sliding scale is rarely used today.*
13. Using alcohol to cleanse the skin before injection is not recommended for home care. If used, hold alcohol pad in place for a few seconds but do not massage.
14. Aspirating is not recommended for self-injection.
15. Check dose with another nurse before administering.

E. Evaluate hydration status.
F. *Evaluate and report to the RN clinical manifestations of hypoglycemia and hyperglycemia.*

> **TEST ALERT** Monitor hydration status and electrolyte balance.

Goal: To plan and implement a teaching regimen.

A. Assess current level of knowledge regarding diabetes.
B. Evaluate cultural and socioeconomic parameters.
C. Evaluate client's support system (family, significant others).
D. Instruct regarding sick-day guidelines (Box 9.3).
E. Instruct to wear or carry medic alert information.

> **TEST ALERT** Determine ability of family/support systems to provide care for client. Identify client's and family's strengths.

Box 9.3   DIABETIC "SICK DAY" GUIDELINES

If you do not feel well (not eating regularly or have fever, lethargy, nausea, vomiting, etc.):

1. Check your blood glucose every 3 to 4 hr and urine ketones when voiding.
2. Increase your intake of fluids that are high in carbohydrates; every hour, drink fluids that replace electrolytes: fruit drinks, sports drinks, soups, regular soft drinks (not diet beverages).
3. If you cannot eat and you have replaced four to five meals with liquids, notify your health care provider.
4. Get plenty of rest; if possible, have someone stay with you.
5. Do not omit or skip your insulin injections or oral medications unless specifically directed to do so by your health care provider.
6. Follow your health care provider's instructions regarding blood glucose levels and insulin or oral hypoglycemic agents.
7. Stay warm, stay in bed, and do not overexert yourself.
8. Call your health care provider when:
    a. You have been ill for 1 to 2 days without getting any better.
    b. You have been vomiting or had diarrhea for more than 6 hr.
    c. Your urine self-testing shows moderate to large amounts of ketones.
    d. You are taking insulin and your blood glucose level continues to be greater than 240 mg/dL (13.32 mmol/L) after you have taken two to three supplemental doses of regular insulin (prearranged with your provider).
    e. You are taking insulin and your blood glucose level is less than 60 mg/dL (3.3 mmol/L).
    f. You have type 2 diabetes, you are taking oral diabetic medications, and your premeal blood glucose levels are 240 mg/dL (13.3 mmol/L) or greater for more than 24 hr.
    g. You have signs of severe hyperglycemia (very dry mouth or fruity odor to breath), dehydration, or confusion.
    h. You are sleepier or more tired than normal.
    i. You have stomach or chest pain or any difficulty breathing.
    j. You have any questions or concerns about what you need to do while ill.

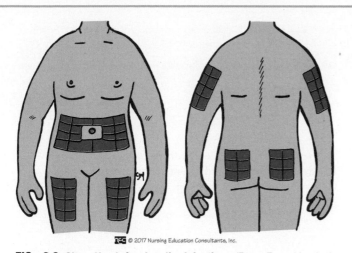

FIG. 9.9 Sites Used for Insulin Injection. (From Zerwekh, J. & Miller, C. J. [2020]. *Review course for the NCLEX.* Nursing Education Consultants.)

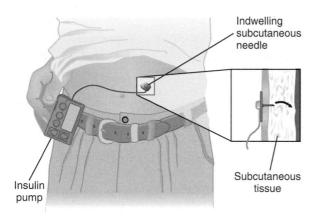

FIG. 9.10 Insulin Pump. (From Black, J. M. & Hawks, J. H. [2009]. *Medical-surgical nursing: Clinical management for positive outcomes* [8th ed.]. Saunders.)

F. Administration of insulin (see Box 9.2).
  1. Correct injection techniques.
  2. Rotate injection site within 1 inch from previous injection site (Fig. 9.9).
  3. Check expiration date on the insulin.
  4. Duration and peak action of prescribed insulin.
  5. Allow for practice time and return demonstration.
  6. Administer at the same time each day.
  7. Clients following an intensive diabetes therapy program may choose to use an insulin pump or to monitor blood glucose levels at least four times a day and take injections at those times (Fig. 9.10).
     a. The insulin pump is battery-operated; insertion site is changed every 2 to 3 days; pump is refilled and reprogrammed when site is changed.
     b. Delivers continuous infusion of short-acting insulin over a 24-hour period, allowing for tight glucose control.
     c. Can deliver bolus of insulin based on excessive carbohydrates ingested.
     d. Monitor insertion site for redness and swelling.

  8. Good handwashing is critical; destroy and dispose of single-use syringe safely.
  9. Insulin pen is a compact portable device that is loaded with insulin and a good option for those that are visually impaired.
G. Oral hypoglycemic agents.
  1. Take medication as scheduled; do not skip or add doses.
  2. Know the signs and symptoms of hypoglycemia.
  3. Anticipate change in medication with pregnancy.
H. Monitoring blood glucose.
  1. Self-monitoring of blood glucose (SMBG)—use soap and water to cleanse site.
  2. Use side of finger pad rather than near the center. If alternative site is used (e.g., forearm), may require different equipment.
  3. Obtain blood drop needed for specific device.
I. Exercise.
  1. Establish an exercise program.
  2. Avoid sporadic exercise.
  3. Review instructions regarding adjustment of insulin and food intake to meet requirements of increased activity.
  4. Extremities involved in activity should not be used for insulin injection (e.g., arms when playing tennis).
J. Diet (Box 9.4).
  1. Regularly scheduled mealtimes.
  2. Understanding of food groups and balanced nutrition.
  3. Incorporate family tendencies and cultural patterns into prescribed dietary regimen.
  4. Provide client and family with written instructions regarding dietary needs.
K. Infection control.
  1. Report infections promptly.
  2. Insulin requirements may increase with severe infections.
  3. Increased problems with vaginitis, urinary tract infections, and skin irritation.
L. Avoid injury.
  1. Decreased healing capabilities, especially in lower extremities.

2. Maintain adequate blood supply to extremities; avoid tight-fitting clothing around the legs.
3. Proper foot care.

Goal: To prepare the client with diabetes for surgery.

A. Oral hypoglycemic agents should not be given the morning of surgery.

B. For clients with NPO (nothing by mouth) status who require insulin, an IV of 5% dextrose in water (D_5W) is frequently started.

C. Obtain a blood glucose reading before sending the client to surgery to make sure there is no developing hypoglycemia.

❗ NURSING PRIORITY Evaluate intake; do not give insulin to a client on NPO status unless an IV is in place.

Goal: To maintain control of diabetic condition in the client who has had surgery.

A. IV fluids and regular insulin until client is able to take fluids orally.

B. Obtain blood glucose level four to six times a day to determine fluctuations.

C. Observe for fluctuation of blood glucose immediately after surgery.

Goal: To identify diabetic ketoacidosis and help client return to homeostasis.

A. Establish IV access.

B. Anticipate rapid infusion of normal saline solution or plasma expanders initially, then at a maintenance rate. Administer with caution to clients with cardiac conditions.

C. Administer insulin: use IV drip (regular insulin only) during the acute phase, then administer subcutaneously as blood glucose level begins to decrease.

D. Frequent monitoring of vital signs.

E. Frequent serum glucose checks.

F. Hourly urine measurements: do not administer potassium if urine output is low or dropping.

G. Monitor blood glucose levels frequently (normally every hour).

H. Cardiac monitor to determine presence of dysrhythmias secondary to potassium levels.

I. Monitor serum electrolyte levels, particularly potassium levels.

Goal: To identify HHS and to help client return to homeostasis.

A. Closely monitor hydration status.

B. Low-dose insulin given intravenously at first to decrease blood glucose level slowly.

C. Evaluate urine output.

D. Monitor serum glucose level.

🔆 Home Care

A. Maintain optimal weight.

B. Continue to receive long-term medical care (Box 9.5).

C. Notify all health care providers of diagnosis of diabetes; wear medical alert identification.

D. Recognize problems of the cardiovascular system.

Box 9.5 "DO NOT" LIST FOR TEACHING CLIENTS WITH DIABETES MELLITUS

When teaching a client and family, the following should be included on the "do not" list.

DO NOT:

- Skip doses of insulin, especially when ill.
- Ignore symptoms of hypoglycemia or hyperglycemia—seek help.
- Forget that exercise will lower blood glucose levels.
- Drink excessive amounts of alcohol, regular soda, or fruit juice.
- Smoke cigarettes or use nicotine products.
- Apply heat or cold directly to your feet.
- Go barefoot.
- Put oil or lotion between your toes.
- Forget to order your insulin, oral hypoglycemic medication, or glucose-monitoring supplies.

---

1. Peripheral vascular disease.
2. Decreased healing.
3. Increased risk for stroke.
4. Increased risk for myocardial infarction.
5. Presence of retinopathy.
6. Increased risk for kidney disease.

E. Recognize problems of peripheral neuropathy.

F. Help client understand problems that diabetes imposes on pregnancy and the subsequent development of a high-risk pregnancy.

G. Help client understand the problem of increased susceptibility to infections.

📋 Hypoglycemia (Insulin Reaction/Shock)

Hypoglycemia **is a condition characterized by a decreased serum glucose level, which results in decreased cerebral function.**

Assessment: Recognize Cues

A. Clinical manifestations.
   1. Lability of mood.
   2. Emotional changes, confusion.
   3. Headache, lightheadedness, seizures, coma.
   4. Impaired vision.
   5. Tachycardia, hypotension.
   6. Nervousness, tremors.
   7. Diaphoresis.

B. Diagnostics: serum glucose below 70 mg/dL (3.89 mmol/L).

Analyze Cues and Prioritize Hypotheses

The most important problems are impaired neurologic function due to low blood glucose and, with clients who have had type 1 diabetes for many years, is *hypoglycemic unawareness*, where the client no longer has early warning signs of hypoglycemia.

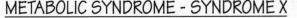

> **Box 9.6 RULE OF 15 (EMERGENCY MANAGEMENT OF HYPOGLYCEMIA)**
>
> **Conscious Client**
> - Have client eat or drink 15 to 20 g of quick-acting carbohydrate (4–6 oz of regular soda, 5–8 LifeSavers, 1 Tbsp syrup or honey, 4 tsp jelly, 4–6 oz orange juice, commercial dextrose products [per label instructions]).
> - Wait 15 min. Check blood glucose again.
> - If blood glucose is still <70 mg/dL, have client repeat treatment of 15 g of carbohydrate.
> - Once the glucose level is stable, give client additional food of carbohydrate plus protein or fat (e.g., crackers with peanut butter or cheese) if the next meal is more than 1 hr away or client is engaged in physical activity.
> - Immediately notify health care provider or emergency service (if client outside hospital) if symptoms do not subside after two or three doses of quick-acting carbohydrate.
>
> **Worsening Symptoms or Unconscious Client**
> - 1 mg glucagon subQ or IM or IV administration of 20 to 50 mL of 50% glucose.
> - Turn the client on the side to prevent aspiration.

METABOLIC SYNDROME - SYNDROME X

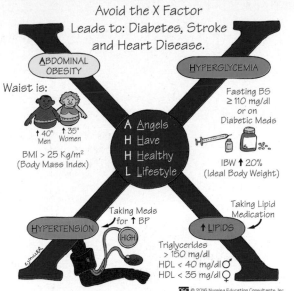

FIG. 9.11 Metabolic Syndrome. (From Zerwekh, J., Garneau, A., & Miller, C. J. [2017]. *Digital collection of the memory notebooks of nursing* [4th ed.]. Nursing Education Consultants.)

Generate Solutions

Treatment

A. Carbohydrates (15–20 g) by mouth if client is alert and can swallow (Box 9.6).
   1. Milk preferred in children with a mild reaction; it provides immediate lactose, as well as protein and fat for prolonged action.
   2. Simple sugars for immediate response: orange juice, honey, candy, glucose tablets.
   3. If simple carbohydrates are taken to increase blood glucose, client should plan on eating protein or complex carbohydrates to prevent rebound hypoglycemia.
B. Glucagon can be given subcutaneously, intramuscularly, or intravenously if client is unconscious. In an acute care setting, hypoglycemia may be treated with 20 to 50 mL of 50% dextrose IV push.

Nursing Interventions: Take Action

Goal: To increase serum glucose level.
A. Glucose/carbohydrate preparations as indicated.

> **⚠ NURSING PRIORITY** When in doubt of diagnosis of hypoglycemia versus hyperglycemia, administer carbohydrates; severe hypoglycemia can rapidly result in permanent brain damage, which is why hypoglycemia is considered an endocrine emergency.

B. Thorough assessment of the client with diabetes for the development of hypoglycemia.
Goal: To help the client identify precipitating causes and activities to prevent the development of hypoglycemia.
A. Instruct the client with diabetes to carry simple carbohydrates.
B. Administer between-meal snacks at the peak action of insulin.

C. Between-meal snacks should limit simple carbohydrates and increase complex carbohydrates and protein.
D. Evaluate the client's understanding of insulin and control of diabetes; reaffirm teaching as appropriate.

📋 Metabolic Syndrome

Metabolic syndrome **(syndrome X or insulin resistance syndrome) is a syndrome that increases a client's chance of developing cardiovascular disease and DM and is characterized by obesity, hypertension, abnormal lipid levels, and high blood glucose.**

Assessment: Recognize Cues

A. Risk factors.
   1. Insulin resistance related to excessive visceral fat.
   2. Obesity, inactivity.
B. Clinical manifestations (Fig. 9.11).
C. Diagnostics.
   1. Elevated fasting blood glucose and triglycerides.
   2. Decreased high-density lipoprotein cholesterol.

Analyze Cues and Prioritize Hypotheses

The most important problems are insulin resistance leading to a high risk for the development of cardiovascular disease.

Generate Solutions

Treatment

A. Medications.
   1. Antihyperlipidemics.
   2. Antihypertensives.
   3. Metformin.

PANCREATITIS
(Inflammatory Condition of the Pancreas)

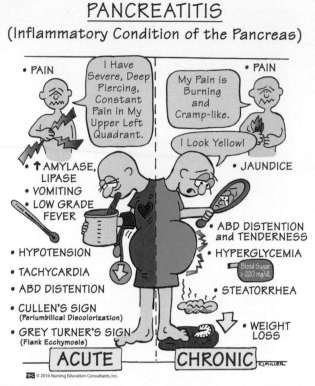

FIG. 9.12 Pancreatitis. (From Zerwekh, J., Garneau, A., & Miller, C. J. [2017]. *Digital collection of the memory notebooks of nursing* [4th ed.]. Nursing Education Consultants.)

Nursing Interventions: Take Action

A. To reduce risk factors—lifestyle modifications.
B. To promote healthy diet—low in saturated fats; promote weight loss.
C. To encourage regular physical activity.

📋 Pancreatitis

Pancreatitis is an inflammatory condition of the pancreas (Fig. 9.12).

Assessment: Recognize Cues

A. Severe constant left upper quadrant or midepigastric pain.
  1. Radiates to the back or flank area.
  2. Exacerbated by eating.
B. Acute.
  1. Persistent vomiting.
  2. Low-grade fever.
  3. Hypotension and tachycardia.
  4. Jaundice, if common bile duct is obstructed.
  5. Abdominal distention.
  6. Cullen sign: bluish periumbilical discoloration.
  7. Gray Turner sign: bluish flank discoloration.
  8. Hypoactive or absent bowel sounds.
C. Chronic.
  1. Decrease in weight.
  2. Mild jaundice.
  3. Steatorrhea.
  4. Abdominal distention and tenderness.
  5. Hyperglycemia.
D. Diagnostics.
  1. Increase in serum amylase (hallmark) and lipase levels.
  2. Increase in urine amylase level.
  3. Hyperglycemia; leukocytosis.
  4. Elevated C-reactive protein.
  5. Hypocalcemia.
  6. Ultrasonography, CT scan.

Analyze Cues and Prioritize Hypotheses

The most important problems relate to acute inflammation of the pancreas, with acute pain and weight loss and the potential for paralytic ileus.

Generate Solutions

Treatment

A. Medications.
  1. Analgesics, antispasmodics.
  2. Antibiotics, carbonic anhydrase inhibitors.
  3. Antacids, proton pump inhibitors.
  4. Chronic pancreatitis may include pancreatic enzyme products and insulin.
B. Decrease pancreatic stimulus.
  1. NPO status; IV fluids.
  2. Nasogastric suction.
  3. Bed rest.
  4. Diet: (if not NPO) low fat, high carbohydrate.
C. Surgical intervention to eliminate precipitating cause (biliary tract obstruction).

Nursing Interventions: Take Action

Nursing interventions are the same for the client with acute pancreatitis and for the client with chronic pancreatitis experiencing an acute episode.
Goal: To relieve pain.
A. Administer analgesics; pain control is essential (restlessness may cause pancreatic stimulation and further secretion of enzymes).
B. Place client in side-lying position with knees drawn up to chest or in semi-Fowler position with knees flexed toward the chest.
C. Evaluate precipitating cause.
Goal: To decrease pancreatic stimulus.
A. Bed rest.
B. Maintain NPO status initially.
C. Maintain nasogastric suctioning.
D. Small, frequent feedings when food is allowed.
E. Pain control.
Goal: To prevent complications.
A. Identify electrolyte imbalances, especially hypocalcemia.
B. Maintain adequate hydration.
C. Maintain respiratory status; problems occur because of pain and ascites.
D. Assess for hypoglycemia and development of diabetes.

Home Care

A. Avoid all alcohol intake.
B. Know signs of hyperglycemia and development of diabetes; understand when to return for evaluation of blood glucose level.
C. Bland diet, low in fat, high in carbohydrates (protein recommendations vary).
D. Replacement of pancreatic enzymes.

Cancer of the Pancreas

The majority of pancreatic tumors occur in the head of the pancreas. As tumors grow, the bile ducts are obstructed, causing jaundice. Tumors in the body of the pancreas frequently do not cause symptoms until growth is advanced. Cancer of the pancreas has a poor prognosis.

Assessment: Recognize Cues

A. Clinical manifestations.
   1. Dull, aching abdominal pain.
   2. Nausea.
   3. Anorexia and progressive weight loss.
   4. Jaundice.
B. Diagnostics—increased cancer-associated antigen 19-9 (CA 19-9) level.

Analyze Cues and Prioritize Hypotheses

The most important problems are preventing tumor spread and decreasing pain, which focus on palliative care.

Generate Solutions

Treatment

A. Surgery: Whipple's procedure (radical pancreatic duodenectomy).
B. Radiation therapy.
C. Chemotherapy.

Nursing Interventions: Take Action

Goal: To maintain homeostasis (see Nursing Interventions for pancreatitis).
Goal: To provide preoperative nursing measures if surgery is indicated.

A. Maintain nasogastric suctioning; assess for adequate hydration.
B. Control hyperglycemia.
C. Assess cardiac and respiratory stability.
D. Assess for development of thrombophlebitis.
Goal: To promote comfort, prevent complications, and maintain homeostasis in client who has undergone Whipple's procedure.
A. General postoperative care (see Chapter 3). Extensive surgical resection of the pancreas and surrounding tissue.
B. Evaluate for hypercoagulable state, as well as bleeding tendencies.
C. Monitor for fluctuation in serum glucose levels.
D. Maintain NPO status and nasogastric suction until peristalsis returns.

E. Encourage adequate nutrition when appropriate.
   1. Decrease fats and increase carbohydrates.
   2. Small, frequent feedings.

Home Care

A. Evaluate for bouts of anxiety and depression caused by severity of illness and prognosis.
B. Assist client in setting realistic goals.
C. Encourage ventilation of feelings.
D. Discuss methods for pain control.

PHYSIOLOGY OF THE ADRENALS

The adrenal glands are located at the apex or top of each kidney.

> **NURSING PRIORITY** Clients experiencing problems of the adrenal medulla have severe fluctuations in blood pressure related to the levels of catecholamines.

System Assessment: Recognize Cues

A. Adrenal medulla.
   1. Evaluate changes in blood pressure.
   2. Assess for changes in metabolic rate.
B. Adrenal cortex.
   1. Evaluate changes in weight.
   2. Evaluate changes in skin color and texture, as well as the presence and distribution of body hair.
   3. Assess cardiovascular system for instability, as evidenced by a labile blood pressure and cardiac output.
   4. Evaluate GI discomfort.
   5. Assess fluid and electrolyte changes from effects of mineralocorticoids and glucocorticoids.
   6. Assess for changes in glucose metabolism.
   7. Assess for changes in reproductive system and in sexual activity.
   8. Evaluate changes in muscle mass.

DISORDERS OF THE ADRENALS

Pheochromocytoma

Pheochromocytoma is a rare disorder of the adrenal medulla characterized by a tumor that secretes an excess of epinephrine and norepinephrine.

Assessment: Recognize Cues

A. Clinical manifestations.
   1. Persistent or paroxysmal hypertension.
   2. Palpitations, tachycardia.
   3. Hyperglycemia, headache.
   4. Diaphoresis.
   5. Nervousness, apprehension.
B. Diagnostics (see Appendix 9.1).
   1. Increase in urinary excretion of total free catecholamine.
   2. Increase in urinary excretion of vanillylmandelic acid and metanephrine.
   3. Magnetic resonance imaging, CT scan.

C. Evaluate client's ability to cope with change in body image.
D. Evaluate for thromboembolic problems.
E. Predisposed to fractures; promote weight bearing; monitor for joint and bone pain; promote home safety.

Home Care

A. Stress the need for continuous health care.
B. Encourage continuation of activities.

C. Have the client demonstrate an understanding of the medication regimen.
D. Help the client identify methods of coping with problems of therapy.
E. Have the client demonstrate an understanding of specific problems for which the client needs to notify the health care provider.

Appendix 9.1	ENDOCRINE DIAGNOSTICS	R
DIAGNOSTIC TEST	**NORMAL**	**CLINICAL/NURSING IMPLICATIONS**
Thyroid		
Thyroxine (T4)	4–12 mcg/dL (51–154 nmol/L) Increased in hyperthyroidism, decreased in hypothyroidism	1. Stimulation of the thyroid gland by TSH will initiate the release of stored thyroid hormone.
Triiodothyronine (T3)	70–205 ng/dL (1.7–5.2 nmol/L) Increased in hyperthyroidism, decreased in hypothyroidism	1. When T_3 and T_4 are low, TSH secretion increases. 2. T_3 and T_4 are used to confirm abnormal TSH.
Thyroid-stimulating hormone (TSH)	0.3–5 mU/L	1. Most common test performed for clients with thyroid problems. 2. With hyperthyroidism, the TSH is low and, with hypothyroidism, the TSH is elevated.
Radioactive iodine uptake	24 hr: 5–35%	1. PO dosing is not harmful. 2. No supplemental iodine for 5 weeks before test. 3. Thyroid medication can interfere with test results. 4. Instruct client to increase fluid intake for 24–48 hr posttest.
Pancreas		
Serum glucose Oral glucose tolerance test	Maintains 70–100 mg/dL (3.9–5.6 mmol/L) (fasting) 1 hr: less than 200 mg/dL (11.1 mmol/L) 2 hr: less than 140 mg/dL (7.8 mmol/L)	1. Test is timed to rule out diabetes by determining rate of glucose absorption from serum. 2. In healthy person, insulin response to large dose of glucose is immediate. 3. Insulin and oral hypoglycemic agents should not be administered before test.
Glucose fasting blood sugar (FBS) Also called *fasting blood glucose (FBG)* and *fasting plasma glucose (FPG)*	Same as serum glucose: 70–100 mg/dL (3.9–5.6 mmol/L)—prediabetes; 101–125 mg/dL (5.6–6.9 mmol/L)—greater than 125 mg/dL (6.9 mmol/L) is diagnostic for diabetes	1. Used as a screening test for problems of metabolism. 2. Maintain client in fasting state for 4–8 hr before blood draw. 3. If client is a known diabetic and experiences dizziness, weakness, or fainting, test glucose level. 4. If client is diabetic, withhold insulin or oral hypoglycemic agents until after blood is obtained.
Glycosylated hemoglobin (Hb A1c)	Nondiabetic range is usually 4–6%; American Diabetes Association treatment goal is less than 6.5%	1. More accurate test of diabetic control because it measures glucose attached to hemoglobin (indicates overall control for past 90–120 days, which is the life span of the RBC).

TEST ALERT Frequently, the level of the FBS is given in a question and it is necessary to evaluate the level and determine the appropriate nursing intervention.

Appendix 9.1   ENDOCRINE DIAGNOSTICS—cont'd

DIAGNOSTIC TEST	NORMAL	CLINICAL/NURSING IMPLICATIONS
Pancreas		
Two-hour postprandial blood sugar	65–139 mg/dL (3.6–7.7 mmol/L)	1. Involves measuring the serum glucose 2 hr after a meal; results are significantly increased with diabetes.
Serum amylase	30–122 U/L (0.53–2.04 ukat/L)	1. Used to evaluate pancreatic cell damage. 2. Other intestinal conditions and inflammatory conditions cause increase.
Serum lipase	31–186 U/L (0.52–3.11 ukat/L) Normal values vary with method; elevated is abnormal	1. Appears in serum after damage to pancreas.
Urine sugar	Negative for glucose	1. Use fresh double-voided specimen. 2. A rough indicator of serum glucose levels. 3. Results may be altered by various medications.
Ketone bodies (acetone)	Negative	1. Ketone bodies occur in the urine before there is significant increase in serum ketones. 2. Use freshly voided urine.
Urinary amylase	2-hr specimen 2–34 U/h 24-hr specimen 24–408 U/24 hr	1. In pancreatic injury, more amylase enters blood and is excreted in urine. 2. May be done on a 2-hr or a 24-hr urine specimen.
Pituitary		
Growth hormone (GH)	Less than 4 ng/mL (ug/L) in men Less than 18 ng/mL (ug/L) in women	1. NPO after midnight. 2. Maintain bed rest until serum sample is drawn.
Osmolarity urine	300–900 mOsm/kg (mmol/kg) of water	1. Used in evaluating ADH.
Osmolarity serum	285–295 mOsm/kg (mmol/kg) of water	1. Do serum and urine tests at same time and compare results. 2. Normally, urine osmolarity should be higher than serum.
Adrenal Medulla		
Urinary vanillylmandelic acid (VMA)	Less than 6.8 mg (34.31 umol/d) in 24 hr Increased with pheochromocytoma	1. Client will need to be on VMA-restricted diet (no coffee, tea, chocolate, aspirin, vanilla, citrus fruits) 2–3 days before the test and during testing. 2. 24-hr urine collection.
Urine Catecholamines		
Epinephrine, norepinephrine Dopamine Metanephrine Normetanephrine ACTH stimulation test	Increased in conditions that precipitate increase in catecholamine secretion Increase in plasma cortisol levels by more than 7 mcg/dL (193.12 nmol/L) above baseline	1. Same as for VMA. 2. ACTH is given as IM or IV bolus and samples are drawn at 30 and 60 min to evaluate ability of adrenal glands to secrete steroids.
Adrenal Cortex		
ACTH suppression (dexamethasone suppression test)	Normal suppression; 50% decrease in cortisone production (cortisol level less than 3 mcg/dL [82.76 nmol/L])	1. An overnight test: a small amount of dexamethasone is administered in the evening and serum and urine are evaluated in the morning; extensive test may cover 6 days. 2. Cushing syndrome is ruled out if suppression is normal.

Continued

Appendix 9.1   ENDOCRINE DIAGNOSTICS—cont'd

DIAGNOSTIC TEST	NORMAL	CLINICAL/NURSING IMPLICATIONS
Adrenal Cortex		
Plasma cortisol levels for diurnal variations	Secretion high in early morning, decreased in evening. 0800: 5–23 mcg/dL (137.94–634.52 nmo/L) 1600: 3–16 mcg/dL 83–441 nmol/L)	1. Elevation in plasma cortisol levels occurs in the morning and significant decrease in evening and night—a diurnal variation.
24-hr urine for 17-hydroxycorticosteroids and 17-ketosteroids	Male: 3–10 mg/24 hr (8.28–27.59 nmol/day) Female: 2–8 mg/24 hr (5.51–22.07 nmol/day) Child under 12 years: less than 4.5 mg/24 hr (12.41 nmol/day)	1. Increase in urine levels indicates hyperadrenal function (Cushing).

ACTH, Adrenocorticotropic hormone; *ADH,* antidiuretic hormone; *IM,* intramuscular; *IV,* intravenous; *NPO,* nothing by mouth; *PO,* by mouth; *RBC,* red blood cell.

Appendix 9.2   MEDICATIONS USED IN ENDOCRINE DISORDERS

MEDICATIONS	SIDE EFFECTS	NURSING IMPLICATIONS
ADH Replacement for Diabetes Insipidus: Promotes kidney conservation of water and increased water reabsorption.		
Desmopressin acetate: metered nasal spray, PO, sublingual "melt," IV, IM, subQ	Excessive water retention, headache, nausea, flushing	1. Monitor daily weight, intake and output, and urine specific gravity. 2. Parenteral form is 10 times stronger than oral form.
Vasopressin: IM, IV	Vasoconstriction	1. Vasopressin more likely to cause adverse cardiovascular and thromboembolic problems.
Vasopressin Receptor Antagonists for SIADH: Block the effects of ADH in the renal collecting ducts, thus increasing the excretion of water and used for the treatment of hyponatremia.		
Tolvaptan: PO Conivaptan: IV	*Tolvaptan:* Thirst, dry mouth, polyuria *Conivaptan:* Infusion site reactions, hypokalemia, orthostatic hypotension	1. Can rapidly increase serum sodium, so are typically administered only in a hospital setting. 2. Note common ending of "vaptan."
Somatostatin Analogs: Suppress growth hormone release and used for long-term therapy for acromegaly.		
Octreotide: PO, subQ, IM Lanreotide: subQ	GI upset, possible gallstones, injection site reaction	1. Monitor for asymptomatic cholesterol gall stones. 2. Monitor injection sites.
Growth Hormone Receptor Antagonist: Normalizes serum growth hormone levels.		
Pegvisomant: subQ	Injection site reactions, nausea, diarrhea, chest pain, and flu-like symptoms Can elevate liver enzymes	1. Most effective drug therapy for acromegaly. 2. Action is reduced by opiate analgesics.
Somatotropin (Human Growth Hormone): Used in children to normalize growth and treat short statute.		
Somatropin: subQ, IM	Hyperglycemia, may suppress thyroid (hypothyroidism)	1. Mix powdered preparations gently; do not shake. 2. Do not inject if the preparation is cloudy or contains particulate matter. 3. Rotate the injection site to avoid localized tissue atrophy. 4. Monitor child's height and weight monthly.

Appendix 9.2 MEDICATIONS USED IN ENDOCRINE DISORDERS—cont'd

Rx

MEDICATIONS	SIDE EFFECTS	NURSING IMPLICATIONS
Antithyroid Agents: Inhibit production of thyroid hormone; do not inactivate thyroid hormone in circulating blood. They are not reliable for long-term inhibition of thyroid hormone production.		
Methimazole: PO Propylthiouracil (PTU): PO	Agranulocytosis; abdominal discomfort; nausea, vomiting, diarrhea; crosses placenta Same; crosses placenta more rapidly	1. May increase anticoagulation effect of heparin and oral anticoagulants. 2. May be combined with iodine preparations. 3. Monitor CBC due to agranulocytosis. 4. Store methimazole in light-sensitive container. 5. May be used before surgery or treatment with radioactive iodine.
Lugol's solution: PO	Inhibits synthesis and release of thyroid hormone	1. Administer in fluid to decrease unpleasant taste. 2. May be used to decrease vascularity of thyroid gland before surgery. 3. Risk of iodism due to strong strength of Lugol's solution; limited use to about 2 weeks.
Radioactive Iodine: Accumulates in the thyroid gland; causes partial or total destruction of thyroid gland through radiation.		
Radioactive iodine: PO	Discomfort in thyroid area; bone marrow depression Desired effect: permanent hypothyroidism	1. Increase fluids immediately after treatment because radioactive isotope is excreted in the urine. 2. Therapeutic dose of radioactive iodine is low; no radiation safety precautions are required. 3. Contraindicated in pregnancy.
Thyroid Replacements: Replacement of thyroid hormone.		
Levothyroxine sodium: PO, IV Liothyronine: PO, IV Liotrix: PO Thyroid: PO	Overdose may result in symptoms of hyperthyroidism: tachycardia, heat intolerance, nervousness	1. Be careful in reading exact name on label of medications; micrograms and milligrams are used as units of measure. 2. Generally taken once a day on an empty stomach before breakfast. 3. Within 3–4 days, begin to see improvement; maximum effect in 4–6 weeks.
Pancreatic Enzyme: Replacement enzyme to aid in digestion of starch, protein, and fat.		
Pancrelipase: PO	GI upset and irritation of mucous membranes	1. Client is usually on a high-protein, high-carbohydrate, low-fat diet. 2. Enteric-coated tablets should not be crushed or chewed. 3. Pancrelipase is given just before or with each meal or snack.
Antihypoglycemic Agents: Increase plasma glucose levels and relax smooth muscles.		
Glucagon: IM, IV, subQ Dextrose 50%: IV	None significant	1. IV glucose is the preferred route. 2. Watch for symptoms of hypoglycemia and treat with food first, if conscious. 3. Client usually awakens in 5–20 min after receiving glucagon.

Oral Hypoglycemic Agents: Stimulate beta cells to secrete more insulin; enhance body utilization of available insulin (see Table 9.1 for insulin).

General Nursing Implications
- Dose should be decreased for older adults.
- Use with caution in clients with kidney and hepatic impairment.
- All clients should be carefully observed for symptoms of hypoglycemia and hyperglycemia.
- Medications should be taken in the morning.
- Long-term therapy may result in decreased effectiveness.

Continued

Appendix 9.2   MEDICATIONS USED IN ENDOCRINE DISORDERS—cont'd

MEDICATIONS	SIDE EFFECTS	NURSING IMPLICATIONS
Sulfonylureas: ▲ Stimulate the pancreas to make more insulin.		
Chlorpropamide: PO Glipizide: PO Glyburide: PO Glimepiride: PO Gliclazide: PO Tolbutamide: PO Tolazamide: PO	Hypoglycemia, jaundice, GI disturbance, skin reactions (fewer side effects with second-generation agents)	1. Tolbutamide has shortest duration of action; requires multiple daily doses. 2. Glyburide has a long duration of action. 3. Interact with calcium channel blockers, oral contraceptives, glucocorticoids, phenothiazines, and thiazide diuretics. 4. Instruct client to avoid alcohol; disulfiram-like reaction may occur (nausea, vomiting, flushing).
Biguanide: Decreases sugar production in the liver and helps the muscles use insulin to break down sugar.		
Metformin: PO	Dizziness, nausea, back pain, possible metallic taste	1. Administered with meals. 2. Has a beneficial effect on lowering lipids. 3. Weight gain may occur. 4. Do not use in clients with liver, kidney, or heart failure and clients who drink excessive amounts of alcohol. 5. *May need to be withheld for 48 hr prior and following a procedure requiring contrast dye and is not given until kidney function is verified.*
Alpha-Glucosidase Inhibitors: Slow down body absorption of sugar after eating; also known as *starch blockers*.		
Acarbose: PO Miglitol: PO	Diarrhea, flatulence, abdominal pain	1. Take at beginning of meals; not effective on an empty stomach. 2. Acarbose is contraindicated in clients with inflammatory bowel disease. 3. Frequently given with sulfonylureas to increase effectiveness of both medications.
Thiazolidinediones (Glitazones): Enhance insulin utilization at receptor sites (they do *not* increase insulin production); also referred to as *insulin sensitizers*.		
Pioglitazone: PO Rosiglitazone: PO	Weight gain, edema	1. May affect liver function; monitor LFTs. 2. Postmenopausal women may resume ovulation; pregnancy may occur. 3. Increased risk of heart disease; should not be used in heart failure.
Meglitinides (Nonsulfonylurea Insulin Secretagogues) (Glinides): Stimulate release of insulin from beta cells.		
Nateglinide: PO Repaglinide: PO	Weight gain, hypoglycemia	1. Rapid onset and short duration. 2. Take 30 min before meals (or right at mealtime). 3. Do not take if meal is missed.
Dipeptidyl Peptidase-4 (DDP-4) Inhibitors (Gliptins): Enhance the incretin system, stimulate release of insulin for beta cells, and decrease hepatic glucose production.		
Sitagliptin: PO Linagliptin: PO Saxagliptin: PO Alogliptin: PO	Upper respiratory tract infection, sore throat, headache, diarrhea	1. Should not be used in type 1 diabetes or for the treatment of diabetic ketoacidosis.
Sodium Glucose Cotransporter Inhibitors (Gliflozins): Transport sodium and glucose into cells using sodium/potassium ATPase pumps.		
Canagliflozin: PO Dapagliflozin: PO Empagliflozin: PO	Genital yeast infections, urinary tract infections, polyuria Hypoglycemia when used with other antidiabetic drugs	1. Inhibit glucose reabsorption. 2. More currently under development. 3. Risk of ketoacidosis.

Appendix 9.2   MEDICATIONS USED IN ENDOCRINE DISORDERS—cont'd

MEDICATIONS	SIDE EFFECTS	NURSING IMPLICATIONS
Combination Therapy: Two oral hypoglycemic medications are combined in one tablet. Most often the combination is metformin with a sulfonylurea.		
Metformin/glyburide: PO Metformin/repaglinide: PO Pioglitazone/glimepiride: PO Rosiglitazone/glimepiride: PO Sitagliptin/simvastatin: PO	See individual drugs for side effects	1. Monitor for cardiac changes, congestive heart failure. 2. May cause GI disturbances.

Injectable Drugs for Diabetes

Amylin Mimetic (Agonist): Complements the effects of insulin by delaying gastric emptying and suppressing glucagon secretion.		
Pramlintide: subQ	Hypoglycemia, nausea, injection site reactions	1. Teach client to take other oral medications at least 1 hr before taking or 2 hr after because of delayed gastric emptying. 2. Injected into thigh or abdomen. 3. Cannot be mixed with insulin.

> **! NURSING PRIORITY** Can cause severe hypoglycemia when used with insulin; usually occurs within 3 h after injection.

Incretin Mimetics

Stimulate release of insulin, decrease glucagon secretion, decrease gastric emptying, and suppress appetite.

Exenatide: subQ Dulaglutide: subQ Liraglutide: subQ Albiglutide: subQ	Hypoglycemia, nausea, vomiting, diarrhea, headache, possible weight loss	1. Used in conjunction with metformin. 2. Monitor weight. 3. Not indicated for use with insulin. 4. Monitor for pancreatitis and kidney problems.

▲ High-alert medication
CBC, Complete blood count; *GI*, gastrointestinal; *IM*, intramuscular; *IV*, intravenous; *LFT*, liver function test; *PO*, by mouth (orally); *subQ*, subcutaneous.

Practice & Next-Generation NCLEX (NGN) Questions

Endocrine: Care of Adult Pediatric Clients

More questions on
evolve

1. The nurse is caring for a client who has Addison disease. How will the nurse assess the client for complications associated with this condition?
   1. Monitor for the presence of fluctuating blood pressure readings.
   2. Assess for the development of fever and purulent drainage.
   3. Perform frequent respiratory checks for decreased movement of air.
   4. Check intake and output records to determine compromised kidney function.

2. A client has type 1 diabetes and is receiving NPH insulin. The health care provider has added pramlintide to the client's medication regimen. What is an important nursing implication when administering pramlintide?
   1. Avoid administering to clients with type 1 diabetes.
   2. Administer with a full glass of water.
   3. Monitor for signs of hypoglycemia.
   4. Administer after meals.

3. A client with diabetes comes into the emergency department with a diagnosis of diabetic ketoacidosis. The nurse would anticipate what symptoms with this client?
   1. Shallow respirations, bradycardia, confusion.
   2. Pallor, diaphoresis, tachycardia.
   3. Elevated pressure, deep respirations, nausea, vomiting.
   4. Rapid and deep respirations, tachycardia, confusion.

4. When a client returns to their room following a thyroidectomy, what equipment is important for the nurse to have readily available?
   1. Oral airway.
   2. Tracheostomy tray and suction.
   3. Paper and pencil.
   4. A small cassette tape recorder.

5. A client with type 1 diabetes is being treated for diabetic ketoacidosis. The client's blood glucose is 450 mg/dL. What other laboratory test would be a priority for the nurse to review?
   1. Magnesium.
   2. Creatinine.
   3. Potassium.
   4. A1c.

6. A client admitted with a pheochromocytoma returns from the operating room after adrenalectomy. Which clinical finding is **most** concerning?
   1. Glucose of 70 mg/dL.
   2. Potassium of 3.4 mEq/L.
   3. Blood pressure of 169/98 mm Hg.
   4. Sodium of 146 mEq/L.

7. The nurse is caring for a postoperative client who had a thyroidectomy. The client develops difficulty breathing from laryngospasms, muscular spasms, and twitching. Which medication should the nurse have available for emergency treatment in the client who has had a thyroidectomy?
   1. Calcium chloride.
   2. Potassium chloride.
   3. Magnesium sulfate.
   4. Propylthiouracil.

8. A nurse is urgently called to a homebound neighbor's house. The neighbor is found unconscious and has a history of insulin-dependent diabetes. After determining there is no functioning glucometer available, what should be the nurse's next action?
   1. Administer 10 units of regular insulin subcutaneously.
   2. Arouse the client to drink 4 to 6 ounces of orange juice.
   3. Administer glucagon 1 mg subcutaneously.
   4. Find a phone to call EMS.

9. What is the nurse's **priority** concern for a client admitted to the hospital with a diagnosis of diabetes insipidus?
   1. Sleep disturbance caused by nocturia.
   2. Decreased physical mobility caused by muscular cramping.
   3. Fluid volume excess caused by water retention.
   4. Skin breakdown caused by generalized edema.

10. A client with diabetes receives a dose of NPH insulin at 0700. The nurse reinforces teaching with the client and would tell the client the **most** likely time for signs of hypoglycemia would occur?
    1. Between 1200 and 1300 hours.
    2. Between 0900 and 1700 hours.
    3. Between 1100 and 1600 hours.
    4. Between 0800 and 1100 hours.

11. The following is a nurse's note of a 25-year-old client recently admitted following a motor vehicle accident. Client has type 1 diabetes and sustained a fracture of the left femur. Client is resting quietly in bed. Pain medication of 5 mg morphine sulfate was given in the emergency department. **Highlight the assessment findings that require follow-up by the nurse.**

| Health History | Nurses' Notes | Vital Signs | Provider Orders |

- Blood pressure 154/92
- Pulse 88, regular
- Respirations 12
- SpO2 95% on room air

LABORATORY

TEST	RESULT	REFERENCE RANGE
Glucose	265 mg/dL (mmol/L) nonfasting	70–100 mg/dL (3.9–5.6 mmol/L)
A1c	9.2%	Less than 5.7% (normal) Less than 7% (client with diabetes)
Cholesterol	155 mg/dL	< 200 mg/dL
Triglyceride	75 mg/dL	Females: 35–135 mg/dL Males: 40–160 mg/dL

URINALYSIS DIPSTICK

TEST	RESULTS	REFERENCE
Bilirubin	Negative	Negative
Blood	Negative	Negative
Ketones	Large	Negative
pH	7.2	4.6–8.0
Specific Gravity	1.016	1.005–1.030
Protein	Negative	Negative
Leukocytes	Negative	Negative
Nitrites	Negative	Negative
Bacteria	Negative	Negative

12. A client has been diagnosed with Cushing syndrome and has a history of asthma.

    Complete the following sentences by choosing the most likely options for the missing information from the drop-down lists of options provided.

    The major problems associated with this disorder are related to _____1_____. The client most likely will experience symptoms of _____2_____, _____2_____, _____2_____, and _____2_____. Laboratory reports would show _____3_____, _____3_____, and _____3_____.

OPTIONS FOR 1	OPTIONS FOR 2	OPTIONS FOR 3
Mineralocorticoid deficiency	Postural hypotension	Hypoglycemia
Glucocorticoid deficiency	Weakness	Hyperglycemia
Mineralocorticoid excess	Bruising	Hypokalemia
Glucocorticoid excess	Bronzing pigmentation	Hyperkalemia
Aldosterone excess	Weight gain	Hyponatremia
	Buffalo hump	Hypernatremia
	Moon face	

⚡ Answers to Practice & Next Generation NCLEX (NGN) Questions

1. **1**
Client Needs: Physiological Integrity/Physiological Adaptation
Clinical Judgment/Cognitive Skill: Analyze Cues
Item Type: Multiple Choice
Rationale & Test-Taking Strategy: Recall that clients with Addison disease have a deficiency of the adrenal hormones. It is not an infection, so there would not be fever or purulent drainage. The client with Addison disease has difficulty maintaining a stable blood pressure. The client may have a significant decrease in blood pressure with activity. The other options (respiratory and kidney problems) are not common complications associated with Addison disease.

2. **3**
Client Needs: Physiological Integrity/Pharmacological Therapies
Clinical Judgment/Cognitive Skill: Take Action
Item Type: Multiple Choice
Rationale & Test-Taking Strategy: First, think about what drug class that pramlintide belongs to – amylin mimetics. Is it injected or given orally? Pramlintide is used along with insulin in clients with type 1 or type 2 diabetes and has a black box warning. This medication has the potential to cause severe hypoglycemia within 3 hrs of administration when combined with insulin therapy. It is critically important that the nurse observe the client closely for any

signs or symptoms of hypoglycemia. Pramlintide is subcutaneously injected via a prefilled dosing pen, usually before each meal that includes at least 250 calories or 30 grams of carbohydrates. It is administered along with the client's insulin and cannot be mixed in the same syringe, because the pH values of the two medications are not compatible. Drinking water after the injection is not necessary.

3. 4
Client Needs: Physiological Integrity/Physiological Adaptation
Clinical Judgment/Cognitive Skill: Recognize Cues
Item Type: Multiple Choice
Rationale & Test-Taking Strategy: It is important to recognize the classic symptoms of ketoacidosis and be able to differentiate them from hypoglycemia. Rapid and deep ventilations, tachycardia, hypotension, nausea, vomiting, and confusion occur in diabetic ketoacidosis. Cool, clammy skin, diaphoresis, normal respirations, tachycardia, confusion, tremors, and nervousness occur with low blood glucose or hypoglycemia.

4. 2
Client Needs: Physiological Integrity/Physiological Adaptation
Clinical Judgment/Cognitive Skill: Generate Solutions
Item Type: Multiple Choice
Rationale & Test-Taking Strategy: Think about where the incision is located for a thyroidectomy – the anterior part of the neck. Airway is critical post-thyroidectomy. A tracheostomy set and suction should be readily available in case of respiratory distress. If swelling occurs at the operative site, an oral airway will not be effective. A paper and pencil and cassette tape recorder have nothing to do with care of thyroidectomy clients, as they should be able to communicate verbally after surgery.

5. 3
Client Needs: Physiological Integrity/Reduction of Risk Potential
Clinical Judgment/Cognitive Skill: Prioritize Hypotheses
Item Type: Multiple Choice
Rationale & Test-Taking Strategy: Note the **key** word, "priority." Clients with hyperglycemia have potassium imbalance (hyperkalemia) from low levels of insulin and osmotic diuresis. When insulin therapy is initiated to treat DKA, serum potassium may decrease rapidly as potassium moves into the cells once insulin is available. This movement of potassium into and out of the extracellular fluid can lead to cardiac conduction problems. Hypokalemia is a common cause of death in the treatment of DKA. Creatinine measures kidney function, which is important to monitor in clients with diabetes; however, in this situation, it is not a priority. The magnesium level and the HbA1C level are not significant priorities at this time.

6. 3
Client Needs: Physiological Integrity/Reduction of Risk Potential
Clinical Judgment/Cognitive Skill: Recognize Cues
Item Type: Multiple Choice
Rationale & Test-Taking Strategy: Note the **key** word, "most." Review each clinical finding and ask yourself is this normal or abnormal. The only abnormal finding is the elevated blood pressure. Pheochromocytoma is a tumor in the adrenal medulla that produces excess catecholamines (epinephrine and norepinephrine).

An excess of these catecholamines can cause severe hypertension. Surgery (an adrenalectomy) alleviates the elevated blood pressure most of the time. In 10% to 30% of clients, hypertension remains and must be monitored and treated. Electrolyte imbalances and blood sugar are not typically affected.

7. 1
Client Needs: Physiological Integrity/Reduction of Risk Potential
Clinical Judgment/Cognitive Skill: Generate Solutions
Item Type: Multiple Choice
Rationale & Test-Taking Strategy: Look at the focus of the test item; what medication should be available for emergency treatment? The client has laryngospasms, muscular spasms, and twitching, which are symptoms of hypocalcemia. Calcium chloride or calcium gluconate should be available to treat tetany caused by accidental removal of the parathyroid glands during surgery. The parathyroid glands regulate calcium metabolism. Potassium chloride replaces the electrolyte potassium. Magnesium sulfate is used in the treatment of preeclampsia (pregnancy-induced hypertension). Propylthiouracil is an antithyroid medication used to block production of thyroid hormone.

8. 3
Client Needs: Physiological Integrity/Pharmacological Therapies
Clinical Judgment/Cognitive Skill: Take Action
Item Type: Multiple Choice
Rationale & Test-Taking Strategy: Note the **key** word, "next." This is a priority question. Go back and read through the question and determine what has occurred. When there is doubt as to whether a client is experiencing hyperglycemia or hypoglycemia, treatment is begun for hypoglycemia until a blood glucose determination is obtained to prevent brain damage from extremely low cerebral glucose levels. Caution should be used to not overtreat with glucose. Glucagon would be administered parenterally because the client is unconscious and unable to drink orange juice. It would take too long to find a phone and call EMS. Giving regular insulin would worsen the condition if the unconscious client was experiencing hypoglycemia.

9. 1
Client Needs: Physiological Integrity/Physiological Adaptation
Clinical Judgment/Cognitive Skill: Prioritize Hypotheses
Item Type: Multiple Choice
Rationale & Test-Taking Strategy: Note the **key** word, "priority." DI is associated with a decrease (or deficiency) in the secretion of antidiuretic hormone (ADH). Lack of ADH leads to increased urinary output (as much as 5-20 L/day). Clients with DI become fatigued from nocturia. Fluid volume deficit can occur because of the excess urine output. There is no edema or muscle weakness.

10. 3
Client Needs: Physiological Integrity/Pharmacological Therapies
Clinical Judgment/Cognitive Skill: Prioritize Hypotheses
Item Type: Multiple Choice
Rationale & Test-Taking Strategy: Note the **key** words, "most likely." NPH (an intermediate-acting insulin) peaks in 4 to 10 hrs. Hypoglycemia would most likely occur between 1100 and 1600.

11. The following is a nurse's note of a 25-year-old client recently admitted after a motor vehicle accident. The client has type 1 diabetes and sustained a fracture of the left femur. The client is resting quietly in bed. Pain medication of 5 mg morphine sulfate was given in the emergency room.

    Highlight the assessment findings that require follow-up by the nurse.

    | Health History | Nurses' Notes | Vital Signs | Provider Orders | Laboratory Results |

    - BP 154/92
    - Pulse 88, regular
    - Respirations 12 breaths/min
    - SpO₂ 95% on room air

LABORATORY

TEST	RESULT	REFERENCE RANGE
Glucose	265 mg/dL H (mmol/L) nonfasting	70-100 mg/dL (3.9-5.6 mmol/L)
A1C	9.2 %	Less than 5.7% (normal) Less than 7% (client with diabetes)
Cholesterol	155 mg/dL	<200 mg/dL
Triglyceride	75 mg/dL	Females: 35-135 mg/dL Males: 40-160 mg/dL

URINALYSIS DIPSTICK

TEST	RESULTS	REFERENCE
Bilirubin	Negative	Negative
Blood	Negative	Negative
Ketones	Large	Negative
pH	7.2	4.6-8.0
Specific gravity	1.016	1.005-1.030
Protein	Negative	Negative
Leukocytes	Negative	Negative
Nitrites	Negative	Negative
Bacteria	Negative	Negative

Client Needs: Physiological Integrity/Physiological Adaptation
Clinical Judgment/Cognitive Skill: Recognize Cues
Item Type: Highlight in Text
Rationale & Test-Taking Strategy: Consider the laboratory values; what is normal or abnormal? Are the abnormal findings related to the client's condition? The client's laboratory findings are an elevation of HbA1c, nonfasting blood glucose, and positive ketones in the urine, which are indicative of poor diabetes control. The nondiabetic range for HbA1c is usually 4% to 6% with 2% to 6.4% considered good diabetic control (goal is 6.5% or less). An HbA1c greater than 7% is considered poor diabetic control. Blood sugar levels should be less than 180 mg/dL for adults when drawn after meals (1-2 hrs after eating). The elevated BP may be a result of the leg pain and needs to be monitored. The low respiratory rate may be associated with the pain medication administration because narcotics, such as morphine, can depress respirations. The respiratory rate should be monitored.

---

12. A client has been diagnosed with Cushing syndrome and has a history of asthma.

    Complete the following sentences by choosing the most likely options for the missing information from the drop-down lists of options provided.

    The major problems associated with this disorder are related to *glucocorticoid excess*. The client most likely will experience symptoms of *buffalo hump*, *moon face*, *weight gain*, and *bruising*.
    Laboratory reports would show *hyperglycemia*, *hypokalemia*, and *hypernatremia*.

Client Needs: Physiological Integrity/Physiological Adaptation
Clinical Judgment/Cognitive Skill: Recognize Cues
Item Type: Drop-Down Rationale
Rationale & Test-Taking Strategy: An understanding of Cushing syndrome is required to answer this question. The nurse understands that, when glucocorticoid excess results from drug therapy for another health problem (such as asthma), it is known as Cushing syndrome. The major symptoms of Cushing syndrome include marked change in personality (emotional lability), irritability, moon face, deposit of fat on the back, thin skin, purple striae, truncal obesity with thin extremities, bruises and petechiae, persistent hyperglycemia, osteoporosis, gastrointestinal distress from increased acid production, increased susceptibility to infection, sodium and fluid retention, potassium depletion, hypertension, amenorrhea (females), hirsutism (females), gynecomastia (males), and impotence or decreased libido. Laboratory findings would include hyperglycemia, hypernatremia, and hypokalemia. Postural hypotension, weakness, and bronzing of the skin pigmentation are associated with Addison disease, along with laboratory values indicating hyponatremia and hyperkalemia.

CHAPTER TEN

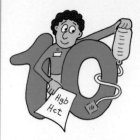

Hematology: Care of Adult Clients

PHYSIOLOGY OF THE BLOOD

A. Components.
1. Plasma (does not contain cellular elements): clear, straw-colored liquid; accounts for about half of the total blood volume.
2. Formed elements (cells): account for about half of the volume.
   a. Erythrocytes (red blood cells [RBCs]).
   b. Leukocytes (white blood cells [WBCs]).
   c. Thrombocytes (platelets).
B. Characteristics of plasma (Fig. 10.1).
1. Plasma is about 90% water.
2. Protein: 6 to 8% of the plasma.
   a. Albumin: most abundant protein; maintains colloid osmotic pressure of the plasma.
   b. Globulins: gamma globulins (immunoglobulins [Ig]) consist primarily of antibodies.
   c. Fibrinogen: necessary for clot formation.
   d. Prothrombin: necessary element for coagulation produced in the liver; production is dependent on vitamin K.
C. Characteristics of erythrocytes (RBCs).
1. Formed in red bone marrow; erythropoiesis is production of RBCs.
2. Vitamin B_{12} and folic acid are necessary for the production of erythrocytes.
3. Erythrocytes: primary function is transportation of oxygen and carbon dioxide.
   a. Hemoglobin is the primary component of the RBC.
      (1) Serves as a buffer in the acid-base balance.
      (2) Hemoglobin combines easily with oxygen to form oxyhemoglobin.
      (3) Iron is a major component of hemoglobin and is necessary for normal oxygen transport.
   b. Hematocrit is a percentage of the blood occupied by the erythrocytes.
   c. Life span of an RBC is 120 days.

> ❗ **NURSING PRIORITY** As a rule of thumb, the hematocrit is usually three times the hemoglobin value.

D. Characteristics of the leukocytes (white blood cells).
1. Function: protect the body against invading microorganisms and remove pathogens.

2. *Leukocytosis* refers to an overall increase in the number of leukocytes; *leukopenia* refers to an overall decrease in leukocytes.
E. Characteristics of thrombocytes (platelets).
1. Function: primarily involved with hemostasis; when vessel wall is damaged, platelets adhere to the area and eventually form a platelet plug to decrease bleeding.
2. *Thrombocytosis* refers to a marked, abnormal increase in the number of thrombocytes; *thrombocytopenia* refers to a marked, abnormal decrease in the number of thrombocytes.
F. Blood classification.
1. Major blood groups: A, B, AB, and O.
2. Although "universal donor" and "universal recipient" types may be used to classify blood in an emergency, blood type tests are always done to prevent transfusion reactions.
   a. O negative is called the *universal donor* because there are no antigens on the RBCs, and Rh (D) is not present.
   b. AB positive is called the *universal recipient* because there are no antibodies in the serum, and Rh (D) is present.
3. Rh System.
   a. Rh system consists of a third antigen, D, which is present on the RBC.
   b. Rh-positive individuals have the D antigen present; this is represented with a (+) sign after the ABO group (e.g., A+).
   c. Rh-negative individuals do not have the D antigen present; this is represented with a (−) sign after the ABO group (e.g., B−).

🔖 System Assessment: Recognize Cues

A. History.
1. Disease of bone marrow and/or RBC-producing organs.
2. Treatment that depresses bone marrow activity (especially chemotherapy or radiation therapy).
3. Familial history and/or genetic predisposition of hematologic disorders (sickle cell anemia, hemophilia, thalassemia, and hemochromatosis).
4. Prior blood transfusions and/or reactions.
B. Bleeding problems occurring during pregnancy, labor and delivery, or immediately after delivery in both mother and infant.

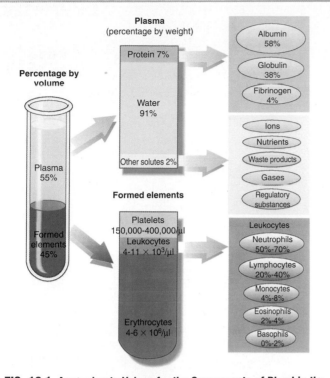

FIG. 10.1 Approximate Values for the Components of Blood in the Adult. Normally, 45% of the blood is composed of blood cells and 55% is composed of plasma. (From Patton, K. T., & Thibodeau, G. A. [2014]. *The human body in health and disease* [6th ed.]. Mosby.)

C. Presence of chronic disorders or disease processes (liver, kidney, or spleen disorders).
D. Effects of aging (Table 10.1).
E. Evaluate effect hematologic disorder has on client's activities of daily living.
   1. How long has client experienced symptoms?
   2. What are the client's current activity levels and metabolic requirements?
   3. Presence or absence of bleeding episodes.
   4. Presence or absence of pain. If pain is present, how well is it controlled?
   5. Presence of appropriate coping/defense mechanisms.
F. Assess client's current nutritional status (especially iron, folic acid, and protein).
G. Evaluate current blood values—complete blood count (CBC).
H. Evaluate status of respiratory and cardiovascular systems in maintaining homeostasis.

DISORDERS OF HEMATOLGY SYSTEM

Anemias

Anemia is characterized by a low RBC count and decreased levels of hemoglobin and hematocrit.
A. Types of anemia (Fig. 10.2).
B. The more rapidly an anemia occurs, the more severe the symptoms will be.
C. Common goal in treatment of all anemias is to identify the origin and correct the problem.

Table 10.1 AGE-RELATED ASSESSMENT FINDINGS FOR THE HEMATOLOGIC SYSTEM

Data Collection Area	Hematologic System Findings	Older Adult Changes and Significance
Nail beds (assess capillary refill)	Pallor, cyanosis, and decreased capillary refill are often noted in hematologic disorders.	Nails are typically thickened and discolored. Use another body area, such as the lips or mucous membrane, to assess for pallor.
Hair distribution	Thin or absent hair on trunk and extremities may indicate poor oxygenation and blood supply to area.	Older adults are losing body hair, but often in an even pattern distribution that has occurred slowly over time. Lack of hair only on lower legs and toes may indicate poor circulation.
Skin moisture and color	Skin dryness, pallor, flushing, and jaundice may occur with anemia, leukemia, rapid hemolysis, or liver disease.	Dry skin is a normal aspect of aging and thus becomes an unreliable indicator of skin moisture. Pigment loss and skin changes along with some yellowing occur with aging.

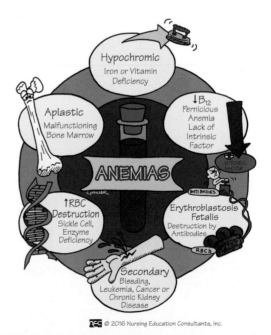

FIG. 10.2 Anemias. (From Zerwekh, J., Garneau, A., & Miller, C. J. [2017]. *Digital collection of the memory notebook of nursing* [4th ed.]. Nursing Education Consultants.)

❗ NURSING PRIORITY Recognize signs of anemia in older adult clients; pallor, confusion, fatigue, peripheral edema, worsening heart failure (HF), and pulmonary congestion.

Assessment: Recognize Cues

A. General symptoms.
1. Pale skin, delayed wound healing, brittle thinning hair, spoon-shaped fingernails, and generalized lymphadenopathy.
2. Shortness of breath, dyspnea on exertion, tachypnea.
3. Tachycardia, palpitations, postural hypotension: cardiac decompensation.
4. Chronic fatigue, weakness, and apathy.
5. Anorexia, nausea, weight loss, constipation, and diarrhea.
6. Headache, dizziness, tingling in extremities.
7. Chronic anemia may result in growth retardation in infants and children.

TEST ALERT Identify client's ability to maintain activities of daily living.

B. Iron-deficiency anemia: characterized by inadequate intake of dietary iron or excessive loss of iron.
1. Common in adolescents due to rapid growth rate.
2. Occurs in infants whose primary diet is milk.
3. May occur in pregnancy.
4. Vegetarians and lacto–ovo vegetarians.
5. Heavy menstrual bleeding.
6. Older adults are more prone to iron-deficiency anemia because of poor dietary iron intake and decreased absorption in the small intestine.
7. Pallor, glossitis, cheilitis (cracking at the corners of the mouth)—most common findings.
8. Diagnostics: decreased iron, hemoglobin, and hematocrit values.

TEST ALERT Evaluate client's nutritional status; adapt a diet to meet special needs of the client; evaluate effect of nutritional status on condition.

C. Pernicious anemia: condition characterized by an inability to absorb vitamin B_{12} (cobalamin). It may be associated with loss of intrinsic factor (e.g., gastrectomy, gastric bypass) or it may be an autoimmune problem.
1. Generally not associated with inadequate dietary intake.
2. More common in older adults; most common age at diagnosis is 60 years.
3. May be precipitated by gastrectomy, gastritis, Crohn disease, or chronic alcoholism.
4. Long-term use of proton pump inhibitors and H_2-histamine receptor blockers prevent the release of the intrinsic factor.
5. General symptoms of anemia, confusion.
6. Paresthesia in the extremities, weakness, reduced vibratory sense.

7. Loss of sense of balance, ataxia.
8. Smooth, beefy, red tongue (glossitis).
9. Diagnostics (see Appendix 10.1).
   a. Homocysteine, cobalamin, and serum folate levels.
   b. Reduced number of RBCs and presence of abnormal RBCs.
   c. Gastric analysis for free hydrochloric acid.

D. Aplastic anemia: characterized by pancytopenia—depression of the bone marrow in production of all blood cell types—RBCs, WBCs, and platelets.
1. Exposure to certain medications and chemicals can precipitate aplastic anemia.
   a. Chemotherapeutic agents, radiation.
   b. Sulfonamides, chloramphenicol, methotrexate.
   c. Anticonvulsant medications (e.g., phenytoin).
   d. Benzene, insecticides, arsenic.
2. Radiation therapy treatment can cause aplastic anemia.
3. General symptoms of anemia.
4. Fever.
5. Infections associated with neutropenia.
6. Bleeding problems associated with thrombocytopenia.
7. Diagnostics: bone marrow biopsy reveals severe decrease in all marrow elements (pancytopenia; see Appendix 10.1).

E. Folic acid deficiency anemia: associated with decreased dietary intake of folic acid.
1. Origin very similar to that of vitamin B_{12} deficiency.
2. Slow, insidious onset.
3. Weight loss, emaciated.
4. May appear ill with malnourishment.
5. Diagnostics.
   a. Differentiate between folic acid deficiency and vitamin B_{12} deficiency.
   b. Serum folate levels less than 3 ng/mL.

Analyze Cues and Prioritize Hypotheses

The most important problems are gas exchange, perfusion and pain (sickle cell anemia), potential for infection and bleeding (leukemia), and bleeding (hemophilia).

Generate Solutions

Treatment

A. Iron-deficiency anemia: supplemental iron intake is necessary for several months to replenish body storage (see Appendix 10-2).
1. Increased dietary iron intake (see Chapter 2).
2. Supplemental folic acid (green, leafy vegetables, fortified cereals, enriched rice and bread, liver, Great Northern beans, black-eyed and green peas, avocado, tomatoes, oranges).

B. Pernicious anemia: injections of vitamin B_{12} or intranasal cyanocobalamin may be required for life.
1. Maintain good nutrition with adequate iron, vitamin C, and folic acid intake.

C. Aplastic anemia: remove causative agent.
1. Hematopoietic stem cell transplant (see Appendix 10.4).
2. Immunosuppressive therapy with antithymocytic globulin (ATG) and cyclosporine.

D. Folic acid anemia.
   1. Oral replacement, 1 mg/day or 5 mg/day for malabsorption syndromes or chronic alcoholism.
   2. Encourage increased dietary intake of folic acid (organ meats, green, leafy vegetables, citrus fruits, whole grains, and beans).

Nursing Interventions: Take Action

For all clients with anemia.
Goal: To assist in establishing a diagnosis.
A. Complete nutritional evaluation.
B. Obtain history of possible causes.
Goal: To decrease body oxygen needs.
A. Assess client's tolerance to activity.
B. Provide diversional activities but also provide for adequate rest.
C. May need supplemental oxygen.
D. Monitor oxygenation with pulse oximetry.
Goal: To prevent infections.
A. Decrease exposure by frequent hand hygiene and limiting visitors.
B. Evaluate for temperature elevations frequently.
C. Observe for elevated WBC count.
D. Maintain adequate hydration.
Goal: To assess for complications of chronic anemic state.
A. Evaluate ability of cardiovascular system to maintain adequate cardiac output.
B. Evaluate for symptoms of hypoxia (see Chapter 17).
Goal: To help client understand implications of disease and measures to maintain health.
A. Explain medical regimen.
B. Discuss importance of continuing medical follow-up.
C. Explain benefits as well as side effects of medications.
D. Identify foods high in vitamin B_{12}, iron, and folic acid (see Chapter 2).

📋 Polycythemia Vera (Primary)

Polycythemia vera **is a chronic disorder characterized by a proliferation of all red marrow cells due to a chromosomal mutation.**

Assessment: Recognize Cues

A. Clinical manifestations.
   1. Usually occurs during middle age; median age is 60 years and is more common in males.
   2. Early: hypertension (that may lead to) headache, vertigo, tinnitus, pruritus, and visual disturbances.
   3. Ruddy complexion (plethora).
   4. Hepatosplenomegaly; peptic ulcer, dyspepsia.
   5. Problems of decreased blood flow.
      a. Angina, hypoxia.
      b. Intermittent claudication (pain in muscles during activity relieved with rest).
      c. Thrombophlebitis, hypertension.
B. Complication: stroke secondary to thrombosis.
C. Diagnostics.

1. Increased RBC, WBC, platelets, and hemoglobin (see Appendix 10.1).
2. Erythropoietin level.
3. Bone marrow biopsy demonstrates an increase in WBCs, RBCs, and platelets.

Analyze Cues and Prioritize Hypotheses

The most important problems are poor gas exchange due to increased number of RBCs and severe hypoxia.

Generate Solutions

Treatment

A. Phlebotomy (2–3 times per week initially, then every 2–3 months).
B. Myelosuppressive agents (busulfan, hydroxycarbamide).
C. Anticoagulants.

Nursing Interventions: Take Action

Goal: To help client's understanding of dietary implications to deal with inadequate food intake due to peptic ulcer pain, dyspepsia, and symptoms of hyperuricemia (gout).
A. Monitor intake and output; avoid fluid overload with rehydration.
B. Avoid foods high in purines—yeast, sweetbreads, some seafood, mutton, veal, liver, bacon, salmon, turkey, trout, and alcohol.
Goal: To help client understand implications of the disease and long-term health care needs (i.e., prevention of deep venous thrombosis [DVT] and stroke, monitoring for signs of leukemia and myelofibrosis as a result of long-term effects of chemotherapy drugs to treat disease).

📋 Leukemia

Leukemia **is an uncontrolled proliferation of abnormal white blood cells; eventual cellular destruction occurs because of the infiltration of the leukemic cells into the body tissue.**

A. Three primary consequences of leukemia.
   1. Anemia from RBC destruction and bleeding.
   2. Infection associated with neutropenia.
   3. Bleeding tendencies caused by decreased platelets.
B. Types of leukemia.
   1. Acute lymphocytic leukemia (ALL) (blast or stem cell).
      a. Peak occurrences: around 4 years of age, then again around 65 years.
      b. Favorable prognosis with chemotherapy.
      c. Leukemic cells will infiltrate the meninges, precipitating increased intracranial pressure; leukemic meningitis.
   2. Acute myelogenous leukemia (AML).
      a. Most common in older adults.
      b. Peak incidence age 60 to 70 years.
   3. Chronic myelogenous leukemia (CML).

a. Uncommon before the age of 20 years; peak incidence age 45 years.

b. Onset is generally slow.

c. Symptoms are less severe than those in acute stages of disease.

d. Presence of Philadelphia chromosome in 90% of cases.

4. Chronic lymphocytic leukemia (CLL).

a. Common malignancy of older adults; rare before age 30 and more common in men.

b. Frequently asymptomatic; often diagnosed in a chronic fatigue workup.

Assessment: Recognize Cues

A. Clinical manifestations (Fig. 10.3).

1. Anemia, fever (infection), and bleeding tendencies occurring together.

2. Anorexia, weight loss, cough.

3. Central nervous system involvement: headache, confusion, increased irritability.

4. Fatigue, lethargy.

5. Petechiae, bruises easily, epistaxis.

6. Complaints of bone and joint pain.

7. Hepatomegaly and splenomegaly.

B. Diagnostics (see Appendix 10.1).

1. Bone marrow aspiration and biopsy: increased numbers of blast (immature) cells (see Appendix 10.1).

2. Lumbar puncture to identify presence of leukemic cells in spinal fluid.

3. CBC.

4. Studies to evaluate liver function (alanine transaminase [ALT], aspartate transaminase [AST]) and kidney function studies (blood urea nitrogen [BUN], serum creatinine); most chemotherapy agents are detoxified in the liver and excreted by way of the kidney system; these systems need to be evaluated before chemotherapy is initiated.

Analyze Cues and Prioritize Hypotheses

The most important problems are potential for infection, poor clotting, and fatigue due to reduced gas exchange.

Generate Solutions

Treatment

A. Medications.

1. Corticosteroids; antineoplastic agents.

2. Allopurinol decreases uric acid levels in clients receiving antineoplastic agents.

3. A combination of chemotherapy agents is used initially to promote remission, which is the absence of leukemic cells and a disappearance of all disease symptoms.

B. Hematopoietic stem cell transplantation [HSCT] (see Appendix 10.4).

C. Radiation therapy (see Chapter 11).

Nursing Interventions: Take Action

Goal: To prevent infection.

A. Systematically assess for evidence of infection: fever, inflammation, pain.

B. Monitor temperature elevation closely; notify health care provider of increase to greater than 100.4°F (38°C).

C. Meticulous skin care, especially oral hygiene and around perianal area.

D. Neutropenic precautions—protect client from exposure to infection; degree of restriction depends on immunosuppression.

E. Initiate protective environment for HSCT clients.

F. Protect client from persons with communicable childhood diseases, especially those with chickenpox.

G. Polio (IPV), varicella, measles-mumps-rubella, and influenza immunizations are not recommended to be given to children or adults during immunosuppression.

H. Avoid urinary catheterization, if possible.

I. Encourage adequate protein and calorie intake, low-bacteria diet (avoid unwashed fruits and vegetables).

J. Maintain adequate hydration.

> **❗ NURSING PRIORITY** Prevention and early treatment of common infections is a priority in the plan of care for this client.

Goal: To prevent or limit bleeding episodes (Box 10.1).

A. Use local measures to control bleeding (pressure to area; cold packs).

B. Restrict strenuous activity.

C. Involve client in evaluating level of activity; decrease activity when platelet counts are low and anemia is present.

Goal: To provide pain relief.

A. Use acetaminophen rather than aspirin or nonsteroidal antiinflammatory drugs (NSAIDs).

B. Maintain environment conducive to rest.

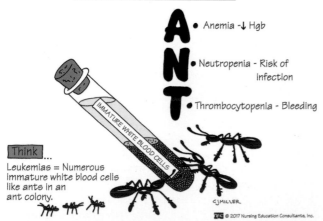

SYMPTOMS OF LEUKEMIA

A • Anemia -↓ Hgb

N • Neutropenia - Risk of infection

T • Thrombocytopenia - Bleeding

IMMATURE WHITE BLOOD CELLS

Think...
Leukemias = Numerous immature white blood cells like ants in an ant colony.

CJMILLER
© 2017 Nursing Education Consultants, Inc.

FIG. 10.3 Symptoms of Leukemia. (From Zerwekh, J., Garneau, A., & Miller, C. J. [2017]. *Digital collection of the memory notebook of nursing* [4th ed.]. Nursing Education Consultants.)

Box 10.1 BLEEDING PRECAUTIONS

Indications: Clients diagnosed with leukemia, hemophilia, DIC, low platelets, or any condition that causes bleeding; clients receiving anticoagulants or thrombolytic medications.

- Limit number of venipunctures and IM injections.
- Use the smallest size needle for all injections or IV infusions.
- Perform guaiac (occult blood) tests on stool as necessary.
- Oral hygiene:
  - Discourage flossing.
  - Use soft-bristle toothbrush; may need to use cotton-tipped swabs while gums are friable.
  - Avoid harsh mouthwashes with alcohol.
  - Rinse mouth frequently with mild nonalcoholic mouthwash.
- Use electric razor for shaving.
- Assess perianal area for fissures and bleeding daily.
- Discourage client from vigorous coughing or nose blowing.
- Prevent constipation.
- Avoid aspirin products; evaluate NSAIDs for bleeding properties.
- Avoid catheters (urinary and suctioning) when possible.
- Avoid enemas and suppositories when possible; use water-soluble lubricant, if indicated.
- Avoid overinflation of blood pressure cuff or leaving cuff inflated for prolonged period of time.
- Provide safe environment and prevent injury according to age (padded side rails, soft toys, nonskid shoes, etc.).
- Monitor for bleeding episode: nosebleed, hematuria, increased bruising, and menstruation.

DIC, Disseminated intravascular coagulation; *IM*, intramuscular; *IV*, intravenous; *NSAIDs*, nonsteroidal antiinflammatory drugs.

C. Position carefully; may coordinate positioning with administration of analgesics.
D. Evaluate effectiveness of pain relief; administer analgesic before pain becomes severe.
E. Do not exercise affected joints.

Goal: To decrease adverse effects of chemotherapy.

Goal: To prevent and recognize complications of transfusions (see Appendix 10.3).

Home Care

A. Do not take aspirin or medications that contain aspirin; caution in use of NSAIDs.
B. Monitor weight gain or loss.
C. Discourage pets (e.g., fish, birds, cats), fresh flowers, and houseplants because of the possibility of bacteria and virus transmission.
D. Teach family methods to stop bleeding.
E. Help parents prepare for their child's return to school.
F. Teach the importance of good handwashing and other infection prevention measures.
G. Teach family members to recognize the early signs of infection and importance of reporting these signs as soon as they are observed.

TEST ALERT Help the family manage care of a client with long-term needs; determine the family's understanding of causes of illness; determine effectiveness of the client's support system.

Lymphomas

Lymphomas **are characterized by malignant neoplasms originating in the bone marrow and lymphocytes.**

Assessment: Recognize Cues

A. Hodgkin lymphoma: characterized by painless enlargement of lymph nodes with progression to involve the liver and spleen. Common metastatic sites are the spleen, liver, bone marrow, and lungs. Disease is spread by extension along the lymphatic system. This is the most curable of the lymphomas.
  1. Increased incidence in immunosuppressed clients (HIV infection).
  2. Initially, painless enlargement of cervical, axillary, inguinal, or mediastinal lymph nodes.
  3. Fever, malaise, night sweats.
  4. Weight loss, fever, and night sweats are associated with a poor prognosis.
  5. Ingestion of small amounts of alcohol causes pain at affected lymph node sites.
  6. Diagnostics: lymph node biopsy specimen showing presence of Reed-Sternberg cells (see Appendix 10.1).
  7. Treatment: chemotherapy and radiation.
B. Non-Hodgkin lymphoma (NHL): a neoplastic growth (derived from B and T cells) that originates in the lymphoid tissue. It spreads malignant cells unpredictably, infiltrating the lymphoid tissue.
  1. Increased incidence in clients with immunodeficiency or autoimmune conditions who have used immunosuppressant medications.
  2. Symptoms are highly variable, depending on where the disease has spread.
  3. Lymphadenopathy that can wax and wane.
  4. Diagnostics: based on classification system of the histopathology of malignant cells.
  5. Magnetic resonance imaging (MRI); lymph node biopsy establishes the cell type and pattern.
  6. Treatment: chemotherapy and radiation.

Analyze Cues and Prioritize Hypotheses

The most important issue is the need for early recognition of large, painless lymph node enlargement so that treatment can be initiated.

Nursing Interventions: Take Action

Goal: To maintain physiologic equilibrium.
A. Maintain hydration and nutrition.
B. Maintain good pulmonary hygiene.
C. Evaluate for shortness of breath; maintain in semi-Fowler position.
D. Decrease body needs for oxygen.
E. Assess ability of cardiovascular system to maintain cardiac output.
F. Manage pain and effects of therapy.

Goal: To prevent infection (see "Goal: To prevent infection" in previous Leukemia section).

Goal: To decrease adverse effects of chemotherapy and radiation therapy.

Goal: To help the client understand the implications of the disease and its prognosis; to have the client demonstrate the ability to cope with the diagnosis and its long-term implications.

Multiple Myeloma (Plasma Cell Myeloma)

Multiple myeloma is a malignancy of plasma cells, specifically the B lymphocytes. Infiltration occurs in the bones and soft tissues.

Assessment: Recognize Cues

A. Clinical manifestations.
  1. Back pain, bone pain (pelvis, spine, and ribs most common).
  2. Pathologic fractures because of diffuse osteoporosis.
  3. Hypercalcemia, high serum protein levels.
  4. Chronic kidney disease.
B. Diagnostics.
  1. Serum and/or protein electrophoresis; increased Bence-Jones protein in urine.
  2. Bone marrow biopsy, showing increased numbers of plasma cells (see Appendix 10.1).
  3. Skeletal bone surveys, MRI, and/or positron emission tomography and computed tomography scans showing areas of bone erosion, thinning, and/or fractures caused by demineralization.

Analyze Cues and Prioritize Hypotheses

The most important problem is the relief of bone pain.

Generate Solutions

Treatment

A. Chemotherapy with corticosteroids and immuno-modulators.
B. Immunotherapy and targeted drug therapy.

Nursing Interventions: Take Action

Goal: To maintain physiologic equilibrium.
A. Careful ambulation to decrease hypercalcemia and improve pulmonary status.
B. Adequate hydration to prevent calcium from precipitating in the kidneys, careful monitoring of hydration status.
C. Comfort measures and analgesics for pain.
D. Safety measures to prevent pathologic fractures.
  1. Do not lift anything weighing more than 10 pounds.
  2. Use proper body mechanics.
E. Braces may be necessary to support the spine.
F. Prevention of infection.
Goal: To help the client understand implications of the disease and measures to maintain health.

DISORDERS OF COAGULATION

Thrombocytopenia

Thrombocytopenia refers to a reduction in platelet levels below 150,000/mL, leading to bleeding episodes that can occur after trauma or injury. Prolonged bleeding is the hallmark feature associated with thrombocytopenia. In some instances, spontaneous bleeding can occur without any precipitating cause or injury sustained to the client.

Types

A. Immune thrombocytopenic purpura (ITP)—most common; considered to be an autoimmune disorder caused by an infection, *H. pylori* or virus.
B. Thrombotic thrombocytopenic purpura (TTP)—closely linked with hemolytic–uremic syndrome; more common in females.
C. Heparin-induced thrombocytopenia (HIT)—Complication associated with heparin therapy where thrombocytopenia develops 5 to 10 days after receiving heparin.

Assessment: Recognize Cues

A. Clinical manifestations.
  1. Petechiae, ecchymosis on skin and mucous membranes.
  2. Epistaxis and gingival bleeding.
  3. Dizziness, hypotension, abdominal pain, tachycardia (internal bleeding).
  4. Internal or external hemorrhage.
B. Diagnostics (see Appendix 10.1).
  1. Low platelet levels.
  2. Specific blood studies to determine type of thrombocytopenia.
  3. Bone marrow biopsy.

Analyze Cues and Prioritize Hypotheses

The most important problem is bleeding.

Generate Solutions

Treatment

A. Corticosteroids (ITP, TTP); immunosuppressant therapy.
B. Platelet transfusions and plasmapheresis based on precipitating cause.
C. Splenectomy (ITP).
D. Warfarin, direct thrombin inhibitors, thrombolytic agents (HIT).
E. Platelet inhibitors (TTP).

Nursing Interventions: Take Action

Goal: To identify the problem early and to decrease potential adverse effects.
A. Assess and monitor for bleeding.
B. Nursing measures to prevent bleeding episodes (see Box 10.1).
C. Assess and support all vital systems.
D. Monitor platelet count and administer platelets when counts are less than 10,000/mm³.

Disseminated Intravascular Coagulation

Disseminated intravascular coagulation (DIC) is a serious secondary coagulation disorder involving widespread clotting in the small vessels, leading to consumption of clotting factors, thereby precipitating a bleeding disorder. It is not a disease, but a result of underlying conditions caused by hemolytic processes, extensive tissue damage, burns, shock, or sepsis.

Assessment: Recognize Cues

A. Clinical manifestations.
1. Thrombocytopenia: petechiae, ecchymosis on skin and mucous membranes.
2. Prolonged bleeding from multiple body areas, such as venipuncture sites.
3. Clots in the lungs, electrocardiogram (ECG) changes, venous distention, abdominal pain, oliguria leading to kidney failure, and tissue necrosis in the skin.
4. Hypotension leading to shock.
5. Multiple organ dysfunction syndrome.
B. Diagnostics (see Appendix 10.1).
1. Low fibrin and platelet levels.
2. Prolonged prothrombin time (PT), partial thromboplastin time (PTT), and activated PTT (aPTT).
3. Elevated fibrin split products (FSPs) and D-dimer assay.

Analyze Cues and Prioritize Hypotheses

The most important problem is the abnormal blood clotting process where clotting and bleeding issues occur.

Generate Solutions

Treatment
A. Correction of the underlying problem.
B. Platelets, fresh frozen plasma transfusions, cryoprecipitate based on precipitating cause.
C. Heparin or low-molecular-weight heparin (enoxaparin).
D. Treatment of shock, as indicated.

Nursing Interventions: Take Action

Goal: To identify the problem early and to decrease potential adverse effects.
A. Thorough assessment of bleeding problems in clients severely compromised by other problems (shock and sepsis).
B. Nursing measures to prevent bleeding episodes (see Box 10.1).
C. Assess and support all vital systems.
Goal: To help the client's family understand the implications of the disease and demonstrate appropriate coping behaviors.
A. Provide emotional support and encourage visiting as intensive care policies and client's condition allow.
B. Encourage ventilation of feelings regarding critical illness of family member.
C. Be available to family members during visiting time.

Disorders of the Spleen

The spleen is a part of the lymphatic system and can be affected by many disorders that result in *splenomegaly* (enlarged spleen). The spleen usually contains approximately 350 mL of blood and about one-third of the platelet volume.

Assessment: Recognize Cues

A. Clinical manifestations.
1. Hypersplenism: splenomegaly with peripheral cytopenias (anemia, leukopenia, thrombocytopenia).
2. Pain due to splenomegaly.
3. Splenic rupture from trauma or inadvertent tearing during other surgical procedures.
B. Diagnostics (see Appendix 10.1).
1. CBC, pitted or pocked RBCs, or Howell-Jolly bodies.
2. Abdominal ultrasound/CT.

Analyze Cues and Prioritize Hypotheses

The most important problem is the relief of pain and monitoring for infection and bleeding.

Generate Solutions

Treatment
A. Splenectomy.
B. Analgesics for pain.
C. Platelets, fresh frozen plasma transfusions.

Nursing Interventions: Take Action

Goal: To identify the problem early (splenomegaly, hypersplenism, or splenic rupture) and to decrease potential adverse effects.
A. Thorough assessment of spleen problem and management to address issues of splenomegaly (pain), hypersplenism, or splenic rupture (emergency surgery).
B. Nursing measures to prevent bleeding episodes in hypersplenism (see Box 10.1).
C. Assess and support all vital systems.
D. Monitor for complications after surgery—hemorrhage, shock, fever, abdominal distention, immunologic deficiencies (IgM), infection.
Goal: To help the client's family to understand the implications of the problem and demonstrate appropriate coping behavior.
A. Provide emotional support and encourage visiting as intensive care policies and client's condition allow.
B. Encourage ventilation of feelings regarding critical illness of family member.
C. Be available to family members during visiting time.
D. Teach about lifelong risk for infection after splenectomy; encourage vaccination for pneumococcus.

Appendix 10.1   HEMATOLOGIC DIAGNOSTICS

R

TEST	NORMAL	CLINICAL AND NURSING IMPLICATIONS
Bone Marrow Aspiration		
Bone marrow aspiration or biopsy	All formed cell elements within normal range Erythrocytes: 4.5–6.0 $10^6/\mu L$ Leukocytes: 4.0–11 $10^3/\mu L$ Platelets: 150–400 $\times 10^3$ units/L 	1. Evaluates presence, absence, or ratio of cells characteristic of a suspected disease (e.g., hematopoiesis pathology, chromosomal abnormalities, staging cancers, anemias). 2. Used to diagnosis leukemia and myeloma. 3. Preferable site is posterior superior iliac spine of pelvis; and proximal tibia (in children). 4. Client preparation: • Position client prone or on the side. • Local anesthetic is used. • Feeling of pressure when bone marrow is entered; pain occurs as marrow is being withdrawn.
		After test: 1. Observe for bleeding at site. 2. Apply pressure to site 5–10 min or longer if client is thrombocytopenic. 3. Bed rest for approximately 30–60 min afterward. 4. Assess for signs of shock (tachycardia, hypotension). 5. Monitor for infection (redness and pain at puncture site).
Lymph node biopsy	No evidence of Reed-Sternberg cells	1. Specimen showing presence of Reed-Sternberg cells indicates lymphoma.
Sickle cell test (SICKLEDEX)	No hemoglobin (Hgb) S present	1. Routine screening test for sickle cell trait or disorder; does not distinguish between them. 2. False-negative result in infants age less than 3 months. 3. False-positive result can occur for up to 3–4 months after a transfusion of RBCs that are positive for the trait.
Hemoglobin electrophoresis	Separates various hemoglobins and allows for identification of specific problem	1. Differentiates between trait or disorder in sickle cell anemia. 2. Diagnosis of thalassemia and hemolytic anemia.
Partial thromboplastin time (PTT) Activated partial thromboplastin time (aPTT)	Normal: 60–70 sec Normal: 30–40 sec	1. Sensitive in monitoring heparin; draw 30 min to 1 h before next heparin dose. 2. May be used to detect circulating anticoagulants. 3. Prolonged in hemophilia because of deficiency of intrinsic clotting.
Prothrombin time (PT) International normalized ratio (INR)	11.0–12.5 sec or 85–100% (each client will have a control value) Normal INR: 0.8–1.0	1. Production of prothrombin depends on adequate intake and utilization of vitamin K. 2. Both tests may be used in management of warfarin therapy. 3. INR should be maintained at 2.0–3.0 for individuals with risk for clots (atrial fibrillation, history of recent DVT) and between 3.0 and 4.0 for individuals with mechanical heart valves or vascular stents. 4. Hemophilia does not alter PT because of no involvement of the extrinsic clotting system.
Homocysteine	Normal: 4–14 $\mu mol/L$	1. An amino acid metabolized through pathways that require vitamin B_{12}. 2. Increased in B_{12} and folic acid deficiency.
D-dimer	Normal: less than 0.4 mcg/mL	1. Used to measure fibrin fragment created by fibrin degradation and clot lysis. 2. Used in management of low-molecular-weight heparin therapy and for diagnosis of DIC and pulmonary embolism. 3. Client must be NPO for 10–12 hr before test, as meat contains increased levels of homocysteine.
Ferritin	Male: 12–300 ng/mL or 12–300 mcg/L (SI units) Female: 10–150 ng/mL or 10–150 mcg/L (SI units) Newborn: 25–200 ng/mL	1. Major iron storage protein reflects iron storage. 2. Diagnoses iron deficiency anemia.

R̲x̲

Appendix 10.1   HEMATOLOGIC DIAGNOSTICS—cont'd

TEST	NORMAL	CLINICAL AND NURSING IMPLICATIONS
Bone Marrow Aspiration		
Bence-Jones protein	Negative	1. Collection of a 24-hr urine specimen. 2. Presence of Bence-Jones protein is diagnostic for multiple myeloma.
Serum folate	5–25 ng/mL or 11–57 mmol/L	1. Needed for erythropoiesis. 2. Decreased in iron deficiency anemia, megaloblastic anemia. 3. Assesses nutritional status; decreased levels in clients with alcoholism.
Spleen scan	A method to evaluate splenic function	1. Injection of a radioactive isotope to evaluate spleen.
Beta2 microglobulin	Can be performed on blood, urine, or cerebrospinal fluid	1. Generally, high beta2 microglobulin and lower levels of albumin are associated with a poorer prognosis in malignancies (multiple myeloma, leukemia, or lymphoma).
Albumin	3.5–5.0 g/dL (35–50 g/L)	1. High albumin levels caused by the disease process in multiple myeloma can result in chronic kidney disease.
Serum and/or protein electrophoresis	Protein spike is abnormal	1. Used to detect hyperglobulinemic states—multiple myeloma, lymphoma.

DIC, Disseminated intravascular coagulation; *DVT*, deep venous thrombosis; *NPO*, nothing by mouth; *RBCs*, red blood cells.

Figure from Pagana, K. & Pagana, T. (2018). *Mosby's manual of diagnostic and laboratory tests* (6th ed., p. 647). Mosby.

Appendix 10.2   HEMATOLOGIC MEDICATIONS

R̲x̲

MEDICATIONS	SIDE EFFECTS	NURSING IMPLICATIONS
Iron Preparations: Replacement.		
Ferrous fumarate: PO Ferrous gluconate: PO Ferrous sulfate: PO Iron dextran injection: IV, IM	GI irritation Nausea Constipation *Toxic reactions:* Fever Urticaria	1. Absorbed better on empty stomach; however, may give with meals if GI upset occurs. 2. Absorption increased if administered with vitamin C. 3. Liquid preparations should be diluted and given through a straw to prevent staining of the teeth. The teeth need to be brushed after administration. 4. Tell client stool may be black and iron may cause constipation. 5. Eggs, milk, cheese, and antacids inhibit oral iron absorption. 6. Iron preparations inhibit oral tetracycline absorption. IM/IV preparations may be used if on oral tetracycline. 7. Anaphylactic reaction can occur; test dose should be given. 8. IM should be avoided because of pain and tissue discoloration. 9. If given IM, use Z-track method to prevent tissue staining. 10. IV route recommended if oral route is not acceptable.
Vitamin K: Necessary for normal prothrombin activity.		
Vitamin K: phytonadione: PO, subQ, IM, IV	GI upset, rash IV not recommended because of hypersensitivity reactions	1. PO and subQ most common routes. 2. Antidote for warfarin. 3. Observe bleeding precautions.
Vitamin B12: Treatment for pernicious anemia.		
Cyanocobalamin: PO, IM, intranasal	Hypokalemia	1. Cyanocobalamin must NOT be given IV. 2. Intranasal doses should not be administered within 1 hour before or 1 hour after consuming hot foods or hot liquids.
Erythropoietic Growth Factor: Stimulates production of RBCs in the bone marrow.		
Epoetin alfa: IV, subQ Darbepoetin: IV, subQ	Hypertension, cardiovascular events (heart failure, thrombotic problems)	1. Monitor BP. 2. Need baseline CBC, BUN, and creatinine.

BP, Blood pressure; *BUN*, blood urea nitrogen; *CBC*, complete blood count; *GI*, gastrointestinal; *IM*, intramuscular; *IV*, intravenous; *PO*, by mouth (orally); *subQ*, subcutaneous.

Appendix 10.3 BLOOD TRANSFUSIONS

BLOOD COMPONENT FOR TRANSFUSION	PURPOSE OF ADMINISTRATION	NURSING IMPLICATIONS
Packed RBCs: 250–350 mL/unit.	To increase oxygen-carrying capacity To decrease risk for incompatible antibodies from the plasma	1. Chart: • Type and amount of blood product infused. • Time started and time completed. • Blood unit identification number. • Rate of infusion—slower rate in older adults. 2. Vital signs are taken immediately before transfusion, at 5 min and 15 min into transfusion, every hour during transfusion, and at completion of transfusion. 3. Closely observe older adult clients for indications of fluid overload.
Platelets: 30–60 mL/unit	To treat thrombocytopenia	1. Chart amount and type of infusion. 2. Infuse rapidly—as fast as client tolerates.
Fresh frozen plasma: 250 mL/unit	Administered for clotting factors, proteins, fluid volume	1. Chart amount and type infused. 2. Infuse immediately after thawing. 3. Infused for 30–60 min or as client tolerates.
Whole blood: 500 mL unit	To provide volume replacement and increase oxygen-carrying capacity. Administered with greater than 25% blood loss	1. Same as with packed RBCs. 2. Observations for fluid volume overload. **TEST ALERT** Monitor transfusion of blood product.

RBC, Red blood cell.

Nursing Guidelines for Monitoring Blood Transfusions

1. The practical nurse should be familiar with the Nurse Practice Act of the individual state and hospital policies regarding the administration of blood and blood products.
2. When blood is brought to the client care unit from the blood bank, it should be started immediately. Blood should never be stored in a unit refrigerator or allowed to sit at room temperature. The maximum amount of time that blood can be out of monitored storage is 30 minutes.
3. *Never add any medication to blood products or to the infusion line of a blood product because they may clot the blood during the transfusion.*
4. The usual rate of infusion in an adult is 1 unit of blood over 3 to 4 hours, depending on the condition of the client. *The registered nurse (RN) should set the initial rate.*
5. Determine whether the client has a history of allergy, specifically a previous reaction to transfused blood.
6. Baseline vital signs must be obtained immediately before starting the infusion. *Notify the RN if the client's temperature is above 101°F or increases more than 2°F, or if any other vital signs have changed significantly from previous readings.* Check vital signs every hour during and 1 hour after transfusion.
7. The client is most likely to experience a reaction during the first 50 mL of blood infused (approximately the first 15 min). Monitor for reaction.
   • Blood deteriorates rapidly after exposure to room temperature. Blood should not hang longer than 4 hours.
8. Transfusion-related acute lung injury (TRALI) reaction—donor blood contains antibodies against the recipient's neutrophil antigens or human leukocyte antigen (HLA) or both.

   • Leading cause of transfusion-related deaths.
   • Arises within 1 to 6 hr of transfusion.
   • Symptoms of dyspnea, hypoxia, and noncardiogenic pulmonary edema.
9. Transfusion-associated *circulatory overload (TACO) reaction occurs when blood is infused too rapidly, especially in the older adult.*
   • *Symptoms include hypertension, bounding pulse, dyspnea, confusion, restlessness.*
   • Place client *in upright position with feet dependent.*

Nursing Guidelines for Platelets and Fresh Frozen Plasma

1. Fresh frozen plasma must be administered immediately.
2. Infuse platelets over 15 to 30 minutes; fresh frozen plasma as rapidly as the client can tolerate, generally over 30 to 60 minutes.
3. Platelets are fragile and are administered with a special transfusion set with a smaller filter and shorter tubing.

Nursing Guidelines for White Blood Cell Transfusions

1. May cause severe reactions because client's immune system recognizes them as nonself.
2. Suspended in plasma, approximately 400 mL and infused slowly over 45 to 60 minutes.
3. Vital signs q15min while WBCs are infusing.
4. Health care provider may need to be in attendance because of the common occurrence of a reaction.

Transfusion Reactions

Types of transfusion reactions (Fig. 10.4).

Appendix 10.3 BLOOD TRANSFUSIONS—cont'd

TYPES OF TRANSFUSION REACTIONS	NURSING MANAGEMENT
Hemolytic transfusion reaction	1. Stop blood transfusion immediately and notify health care provider. 2. Change the IV tubing; do not allow blood in the tubing to infuse into the client; maintain IV access. 3. Obtain first-voided urine specimen to test for blood in the urine. 4. Anticipate blood samples to be drawn by the laboratory. 5. With suspected kidney involvement, treatment with diuretics is initiated to promote diuresis.
Allergic reaction	1. If client has a history of allergic reactions, the antihistamine diphenhydramine may be given before starting the transfusion. 2. Stop transfusion until status of reaction can be determined; if symptoms are mild and transient, the transfusion may be resumed. 3. If anaphylactic/severe allergic reaction, initiate CPR if needed, have epinephrine ready for administration, and do not continue administration of transfusion.
Febrile reaction	1. Keep client covered and warm during transfusion. 2. Give antipyretics as prescribed (acetaminophen). Avoid aspirin and NSAIDs in thrombocytopenic clients. 3. Stop the transfusion until status of reaction can be determined. 4. Transfusion with leukocyte-poor RBCs or frozen washed packed cells may prevent this reaction in clients susceptible to fever. 5. Most common reaction.

CPR, Cardiopulmonary resuscitation; *IV*, intravenous; *NSAIDs*, nonsteroidal antiinflammatory drugs; *RBCs*, red blood cells.

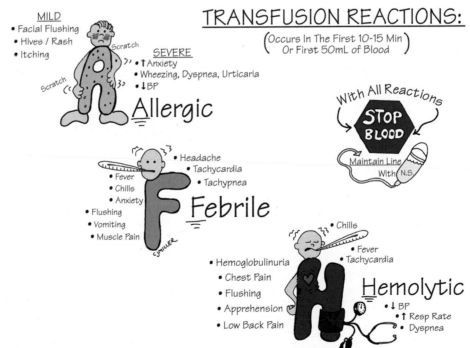

FIG. 10.4 Transfusion Reactions. (From Zerwekh, J., Garneau, A., & Miller, C. J. [2017]. *Digital collection of the memory notebook of nursing* [4th ed.]. Nursing Education Consultants.)

Appendix 10.4   HEMATOPOIETIC STEM CELL TRANSPLANT[a]

Goal: To restore hematologic and immunologic function in clients with immunologic deficiencies, leukemia, congenital or acquired anemias.

Procedure

In the adult client, approximately 400 to 800 mL of bone marrow or harvested stem cells are processed and transfused into the client. (See Appendix 10.1 for care of donor client for bone marrow aspiration.)

Complications

1. Bacterial, viral, or fungal infection from immunosuppressed state.
2. Severe thrombocytopenia resulting in bleeding problems.
3. Graft-versus-host disease (rejection).
   a. Acute rejection generally occurs in 7 to 30 days after transplantation; chronic rejection occurs in 100 days.

[a]Includes bone marrow transplant and stem cell transplant.

b. Erythematous rash on the palms and feet, spreading to the trunk, may be an early symptom.
c. Altered liver enzyme profiles with liver tenderness and jaundice.
d. Gastrointestinal disturbances: anorexia, nausea, vomiting, diarrhea.

Nursing Implications

1. Preparation of the client for immunosuppression with chemotherapy and radiation therapy.
2. Confirmation of rejection is by skin or oral mucosal biopsy.
3. Successful engraftment is indicated by formation of erythrocytes, leukocytes, and platelets, usually 2 to 5 weeks after transplantation.
4. Care of the immunosuppressed client (see Chapter 8).

⚡ Practice & Next Generation NCLEX (NGN) Questions

Hematology: Care of Adult Clients

More questions on
evolve

1. The nurse is assessing a client who has been admitted for treatment of leukemia. What nursing observation should be reported immediately?
   1. Swelling in knees.
   2. Increased bruising.
   3. Nausea and vomiting.
   4. Oral temperature of 101°F (38.3°C).

2. An older client is being discharged after diagnosis and treatment for leukemia. What will be important to reinforce discharge teaching with this client regarding home care?
   1. Maintain a diet that is low in protein and high in carbohydrates.
   2. Check temperature regularly; call health care provider's office if oral temperature is greater than 99°F (37.2°C).
   3. Always thoroughly wash, cook, or peel fresh vegetables and fruits.
   4. Apply warm packs to joints to prevent further bleeding.

3. A client has developed aplastic anemia. What health problem in the client's past would be associated with this condition?
   1. Hemorrhage and shock after surgery.
   2. Poor dietary intake of iron and folic acid.
   3. Treatment for a pulmonary malignancy.
   4. History of stomach resection and loss of intrinsic factor.

4. The nurse is caring for an older client with leukemia. The client is experiencing bleeding into the knees. What is the **best** nursing care regarding joint mobility and activity?
   1. Encourage walking around the unit every 2 hours.
   2. Gently move each leg through active range-of-motion exercises.
   3. Place warm packs on the joints to promote mobility.
   4. Keep the joints immobilized and maintain bed rest.

5. A client has been diagnosed with pernicious anemia. What will the nurse discuss with the client regarding the vitamin B_{12} that will be prescribed at discharge?
   1. The client will need to have monthly injections of vitamin B_{12}.
   2. The client will need to take the medication with milk.
   3. The client should decrease the intake of leafy, green vegetables that are high in vitamin K.
   4. It will be important for the client to have weekly lab studies to evaluate the medication.

6. A client with the diagnosis of multiple myeloma has extreme bone pain. Recently the family reports to the health care provider the client is experiencing increased lethargy and confusion. The nurse would correlate these symptoms with which imbalance?
   1. Hypokalemia
   2. Hypercalcemia
   3. Hyperuricemia
   4. Hypoalbuminemia

7. A client is experiencing a problem with epistaxis. What is the **first** nursing action?
   1. Apply pressure to the nose and have the client lean forward.
   2. Hold the client's head back and put ice on the nose.
   3. Position the client supine and check the blood pressure.
   4. Encourage clear liquids and observe for nausea.

8. What is the **best** method for the nurse to use when assessing for pallor in a client with dark skin?
   1. Assess for changes in the color in the forearm.
   2. Assess the soles of the hands and feet.
   3. Assess the conjunctiva and mucous membranes.
   4. Assess the back of the client's throat.

9. An infusion of packed RBCs is completed at 1000. At 1400 the client is experiencing problems and the nurse suspects a transfusion reaction. What would be the important signs to watch for?
   1. Hypertension.
   2. Pruritus and redness at infusion site.
   3. Flushing and urticaria.
   4. Sudden onset of dyspnea and hypoxia.

10. The nurse is administering platelets to a client who has been diagnosed with disseminated intravascular coagulation. What are the nursing implications in administering platelets?
    1. Use straight intravenous (IV) tubing with 5% dextrose in water as the primary infusion.
    2. Warm the platelets for 15 minutes in warm water prior to infusion.
    3. Initiate a separate IV site with a 22-gauge needle.
    4. Infuse platelets as rapidly as the client will tolerate, usually over 15 to 30 minutes.

11. An older adult client has been diagnosed with anemia. In recent months the client reports having a poor appetite and difficulty driving due to macular degeneration.

    Highlight the laboratory findings that require follow-up by the nurse.

TEST	RESULT	REFERENCE RANGE
White blood cells (WBC)	8800 mm³	WBC count: 5000–10,000/mm³
Red blood cells (RBC)	3.75 μL	RBC count: females: 4.2–5.4 μL; males: 4.7–6.1 μL
Hemoglobin (Hb)	8.2 g/dL	Hemoglobin: females: 12.0–16 g/dL; males: 14.0–18.0 g/dL
Hematocrit (Hct)	27%	Hematocrit: females: 37%–47%; males: 42%–52%
Platelets	175,000 mm³	Thrombocytes (platelets): 150,000–400,000/mm³ of blood
WBC differential	• Band neutrophils: 0% • Segmented neutrophils: 60% • Eosinophils: 1% • Basophils: 0% • Lymphocytes: 35% • Monocytes: 4%	• Band neutrophils: 0%–8% • Segmented neutrophils: 55%–70% • Eosinophils: 1%–4% • Basophils: 0.5%–1% • Lymphocytes: 20%–40% • Monocytes: 2%–8%

12. The nurse is reinforcing the discharge teaching for the client that has just been diagnosed with acute myelogenous leukemia (AML). **For each potential health teaching information about AML listed below, use an X to specify whether the information would be appropriate health teaching for the client at this time.**

POTENTIAL HEALTH TEACHING	APPROPRIATE HEALTH TEACHING
Expect to have repeated phlebotomies.	
Restrict strenuous activities.	
Encourage resting between activities.	
Avoid crowds due to increased risk of infection.	
Low-dose aspirin may be prescribed by your health care provider.	
Add fresh fruits and raw vegetables to the diet.	
Perform hand hygiene frequently.	
Monitor for bleeding episodes.	

Answers to Practice & Next Generation NCLEX (NGN) Questions

1. 4
Client Needs: Physiological Integrity/Physiological Adaptation
Clinical Judgment/Cognitive Skill: Recognize Cues
Item Type: Multiple Choice
Rationale & Test-Taking Strategy: Notice the **key** word, "immediately." This is a priority test item. What is of greatest concern with a client who has leukemia? The abnormal white blood cells from the leukemia affect the ability of the immune system to protect the body from infection. Infections are most often the cause of death because of neutropenia. Any temperature above 100°F (38.3°C) should be reported. Swelling of the knees is not a symptom associated with leukemia. While bruising may occur with decreased platelets, the client is not actively bleeding. Therefore, the priority is to address the elevated temperature. Nausea and vomiting are expected adverse effects of clients with leukemia undergoing treatment such as chemotherapy and do not take priority over the client's infection.

2. 3
Client Needs: Physiological Integrity/Physiological Adaptation
Clinical Judgment/Cognitive Skill: Take Action
Item Type: Multiple Choice
Rationale & Test-Taking Strategy: Prevention of infection is a primary goal – all fruits and vegetables should be thoroughly washed, peeled, or cooked to eliminate bacteria. A temperature above 100.4°F (38°C) should be reported; joints should have cold compresses applied to them, not warm packs. There is no specific diet; it should be well balanced with adequate protein.

3. 3
Client Needs: Physiological Integrity/Physiological Adaptation
Clinical Judgment/Cognitive Skill: Take Action
Item Type: Multiple Choice
Rationale & Test-Taking Strategy: The question is asking about some condition in the client's past medical history that could be related to the current condition. Aplastic anemia is the anemia that results as a serious side effect to some medications. This condition frequently occurs with treatment of chemotherapeutic agents for a malignancy. Poor dietary intake results in iron deficiency anemia. Hemorrhage is loss of blood. Pernicious anemia is caused by lack of the intrinsic factor in the stomach after surgery.

4. 4
Client Needs: Physiological Integrity/Physiological Adaptation
Clinical Judgment/Cognitive Skill: Take Action
Item Type: Multiple Choice
Rationale & Test-Taking Strategy: Note the **key** word, "best." This is a priority nursing care test item. If bleeding is active, it is important to keep the joints immobilized. The client should not be up walking, and the nurse should not perform range-of-motion exercises. Cold packs should be applied to the site, not warm packs. Remember RICE: rest, ice, compression, elevation.

5. 1
Client Needs: Physiological Integrity/Pharmacological Therapies
Clinical Judgment/Cognitive Skill: Take Action
Item Type: Multiple Choice
Rationale & Test-Taking Strategy: Think about how pernicious anemia is treated and how vitamin B12 is administered. Pernicious anemia is treated with injections of vitamin B12 or with an intranasal preparation; it is not effective taken orally. The other options

are not nursing implications for vitamin B12. The client may be taught to do the injections, or they may go to a health care provider. Laboratory results are not done weekly.

6. 2
Client Needs: Physiological Integrity/Physiological Adaptation
Clinical Judgment/Cognitive Skill: Analyze Cues
Item Type: Multiple Choice
Rationale & Test-Taking Strategy: Recall that the continued loss of bone in multiple myeloma causes an increase in calcium, leading to hypercalcemia and symptoms of anorexia, lethargy, confusion, polyuria, seizure, cardiac problems, and death. High protein levels (not hypoalbuminemia) caused by the disease process can result in kidney failure. Uric acid is not elevated. Potassium is usually within normal limits if no indication of kidney failure exists.

7. 1
Client Needs: Physiological Integrity/Physiological Adaptation
Clinical Judgment/Cognitive Skill: Take Action
Item Type: Multiple Choice
Rationale & Test-Taking Strategy: Notice the **key** word, "first" in this priority nursing action test item. The first action to stop the bleeding is to apply pressure. The client should lean forward so they will not swallow the blood and become nauseous. Ice packs to the nose will help, but pressure should be applied while the ice pack is being obtained.

8. 3
Client Needs: Physiological Integrity/Physiological Adaptation
Clinical Judgment/Cognitive Skill: Take Action
Item Type: Multiple Choice
Rationale & Test-Taking Strategy: Notice the **key** word, "best" in this priority nursing assessment test item. Brown or dark skin appears yellow-brown and dull; black skin appears ashen gray and dull. As such, it is best to check the areas with least pigmentation such as the conjunctiva and mucous membranes to detect pallor. Examining the client's throat and roof of the mouth can reveal jaundice. The palms of the hands or soles of the feet may show petechiae. The tongue and back of the client's throat are poor indicators of pallor or cyanosis; however, changes in texture and color may indicate other hematology problems, e.g., a beefy-red tongue (glossitis) with vitamin-B12 deficiency anemia.

9. 4
Client Needs: Physiological Integrity/Physiological Adaptation
Clinical Judgment/Cognitive Skill: Recognize Cues
Item Type: Multiple Choice
Rationale & Test-Taking Strategy: The nurse is suspecting a transfusion reaction. Think about the most likely serious signs to watch for. The client is most likely experiencing a transfusion-related acute lung injury (TRALI), which is the sudden onset (within 6 hrs of a transfusion) of hypoxemic lung disease along with infiltrates on x-ray without cardiac problems. Symptoms include sudden onset of dyspnea, hypoxia, fever, chills, hypotension, frothy sputum, and respiratory failure. TRALI is associated with activation of the inflammatory response caused by a recent transfusion of plasma-containing blood products, such as packed RBCs, platelets, and fresh-frozen plasma. Urticaria and pruritis would be associated with an allergic transfusion reaction. In a hemolytic transfusion reaction, there would be hypotension (not hypertension).

10. 4
Client Needs: Physiological Integrity/Pharmacological Therapies
Clinical Judgment/Cognitive Skill: Take Action
Item Type: Multiple Choice
Rationale & Test-Taking Strategy: Platelets should be administered as rapidly as the client will tolerate, which is generally over 15 to 30 min. It is not necessary to warm the platelets. Because platelets are fragile, a special tubing is required. A straight IV tubing set should not be used, and neither should D5W; it should be normal saline. The IV does not have to be at a separate site, but normal saline should be infusing in the IV when the platelets are started.

11. An older adult client has been diagnosed with anemia. In recent months, the client reports having a poor appetite and difficulty driving due to macular degeneration. **Highlight the laboratory findings that require follow up by the nurse.**

TEST	RESULT	REFERENCE RANGE
White blood cells (WBC)	8800 mm³	WBC count: 5000-10,000/mm³
Red blood cells (RBC)	3.75 µL	RBC count: females: 4.2-5.4 µL; males: 4.7-6.1 µL
Hemoglobin (Hb)	8.2 g/dL	Hemoglobin: females: 12.0-16 g/dL; males: 14.0-18.0 g/dL
Hematocrit (Hct)	27%	Hematocrit: females, 37%-47%; males, 42%-52%
Platelets	175,000 mm³	Thrombocytes (platelets): 150,000-400,000/mm³ of blood
WBC differential	• Band neutrophils: 0% • Segmented neutrophils: 60% • Eosinophils: 1% • Basophils: 0% • Lymphocytes: 35% • Monocytes: 4%	• Band neutrophils: 0%-8% • Segmented neutrophils: 55%-70% • Eosinophils: 1%-4% • Basophils: 0.5%-1% • Lymphocytes: 20%-40% • Monocytes: 2%-8%

Client Needs: Physiological Integrity/Reduction of Risk Potential
Clinical Judgment/Cognitive Skill: Recognize Cues
Item Type: Highlight in Table
Rationale & Test-Taking Strategy: The client has iron deficiency anemia brought on by poor nutrition, which is often observed in the older adult. A poor appetite and difficulty driving (going to a grocery store) are problems for this client. Iron deficiency anemia is characterized by low hemoglobin, low hematocrit, and a low RBC count. In addition, the client would have a low serum iron level. The platelets and WBC count and differential are usually normal unless the anemia is severe, in which case the WBC count would be low and the platelet count

could be either high or low. The following are the normal values for a complete blood count (CBC):

Hemoglobin: females, 12.0-16 g/dL; males, 14.0-18.0 g/dL
RBC count: females, 4.2-5.4 µL; males, 4.7-6.1 µL
Hematocrit: females, 37%-47%; males, 42%-52%
WBC count: 5000-10,000/mm³
Thrombocytes (platelets): 150,000-400,000/mm³ of blood
WBC differential:
  Band neutrophils: 0%-8%
  Segmented neutrophils: 55%-70%
  Eosinophils: 1%-4%
  Basophils: 0.5%-1%
  Lymphocytes: 20%-40%
  Monocytes: 2%-8%

12. The nurse is reinforcing the discharge teaching for the client that has just been diagnosed with acute myelogenous leukemia (AML). **For each potential health teaching about AML listed below, use an X to specify whether the information would be an appropriate health teaching for the client at this time.**

POTENTIAL HEALTH TEACHING	APPROPRIATE HEALTH TEACHING
Expect to have repeated phlebotomies.	
Restrict strenuous activities.	X
Encourage resting between activities.	X
Avoid crowds due to increased risk of infection.	X
Low-dose aspirin may be prescribed by your health care provider.	
Add fresh fruit and raw vegetables to the diet.	
Perform hand hygiene frequently.	X
Monitor for bleeding episodes.	X

Client Needs: Physiological Integrity/Physiological Adaptation
Clinical Judgment/Cognitive Skill: Generate Solutions
Item Type: Matrix Multiple Choice
Rationale & Test-Taking Strategy: Review each potential teaching option and ask yourself if it is accurate regarding the care of a client with leukemia. The client will need to understand the first signs of infection and report them immediately to the health care provider: elevated temperature greater than 100.4°F (38°C). Hand hygiene is important in reducing infection. Restricting strenuous activities and encouraging rest between activities will conserve the client's energy and prevent undue fatigue. Acetaminophen is used rather than aspirin for pain relief and temperature reduction. Caution the client to only eat cooked fruits and vegetables, because raw foods often carry bacteria that could lead to an infection. Anemia, neutropenia, and thrombocytopenia are common problems with clients who have leukemia, so monitoring for bleeding episodes is important. Phlebotomy is the main method of treatment to reduce the hematocrit in clients with polycythemia vera.

CHAPTER ELEVEN

Respiratory: Care of Adult Clients

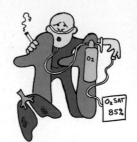

PHYSIOLOGY OF THE RESPIRATORY SYSTEM

Physiology of Respiration

Respiration is a process by which gas is exchanged between the circulating blood and the inhaled air.

A. Organs of the respiratory system (Fig. 11.1).

B. Gases flow from an area of high pressure to an area of low pressure; pressure below atmospheric pressure is designated as negative pressure.

C. Inspiration.
  1. Stimulus to the diaphragm and the intercostal muscles by way of the central nervous system.
  2. Diaphragm moves down and intercostal muscles move outward, thereby increasing the capacity of the thoracic cavity and decreasing intrathoracic pressure to below atmospheric pressure.
  3. Through the airways, the lungs are open to atmospheric pressure; air will flow into the lungs to equalize intrathoracic pressure with atmospheric pressure.

D. Expiration.
  1. Diaphragm and intercostal muscles relax and return to a resting position; therefore, lungs recoil, and capacity is decreased.
  2. Air will flow out until intrathoracic pressure is again equal to atmospheric pressure.

E. Negative pressure is greater during inspiration; therefore, air flows easily into the lungs.

F. Compliance describes how elastic the lungs are or how easily the lungs can be inflated; when compliance is decreased, the lungs are more difficult to inflate.

G. Control of respiration.
  1. Movement of the diaphragm and accessory muscles of respiration is controlled by the respiratory center located in the brainstem (medulla oblongata and pons).
    a. The respiratory center controls respirations by way of the spinal cord and phrenic nerve.
    b. Activity of the respiratory center is regulated by chemoreceptors. These receptors respond to changes in the chemical composition of the cerebrospinal fluid (CSF) and the blood (specifically, the Pao_2, $Paco_2$, and pH).
  2. The medulla contains the central chemoreceptors responsive to changes in CO_2 blood levels.

❗ NURSING PRIORITY The primary respiratory stimulus is CO_2; when the $Paco_2$ is increased, ventilation is initiated.

  3. Carotid and aortic bodies contain the peripheral chemoreceptors for arterial O_2 levels.
    a. Primary function is to monitor arterial O_2 levels and stimulate the respiratory center when a decrease in Pao_2 occurs.
    b. When arterial O_2 decreases to less than 60 mm Hg, stimulation to breathe is initiated by the chemoreceptors.
    c. In a person whose primary stimulus to breathe is hypoxia, this becomes the mechanism of ventilatory control (hypoxic drive).

H. The process of gas exchange.
  1. Ventilation: the process of moving air between the atmosphere and alveoli.
  2. Diffusion: the process of moving O_2 and CO_2 across the alveolar capillary membrane.
  3. Perfusion: the process of linking the venous blood flow to the alveoli.

Oxygen and Carbon Dioxide Transport

A. Internal respiration is the exchange of gases between the blood and interstitial fluid. The gases are measured by an analysis of arterial blood (Table 11.1).

B. O_2 delivered to the tissue is dependent on cardiac output.

C. A decrease in the arterial O_2 tension (Pao_2) and a decrease in the saturation of the hemoglobin with oxygen (Sao_2) results in a state of hypoxemia.

D. At high levels (above 10,000 ft), there is reduced O_2 in the atmosphere, resulting in a lower inspired O_2 pressure and a lower Pao_2. Commercial planes are pressurized to an altitude of 8000 ft.

❗ TEST ALERT Apply knowledge of pathophysiology to monitoring for complications; identify client status based on pathophysiology.

System Assessment: Recognize Cues

A. History.
  1. Determine the frequency of upper respiratory problems and/or surgeries involving respiratory problems.

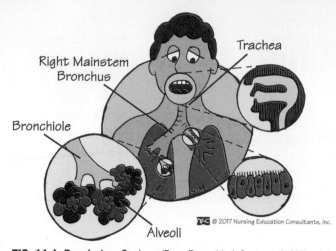

FIG. 11.1 Respiratory System. (From Zerwekh J, Garneau A, Miller CJ. [2017]. *Digital collection of the memory notebooks of nursing* [4th ed.]. Chandler, AZ: Nursing Education Consultants, Inc.)

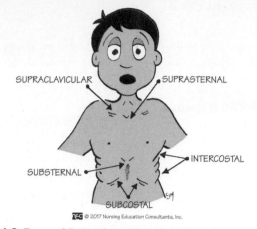

FIG. 11.2 Types of Retractions. (From Zerwekh J, Garneau A, Miller CJ. [2017]. *Digital collection of the memory notebooks of nursing* [4th ed.]. Chandler, AZ: Nursing Education Consultants, Inc.)

Table 11.1 NORMAL ARTERIAL BLOOD GAS VALUES		
Acidity index	pH	7.35-7.45
Partial pressure of dissolved oxygen	Pao2	80-100 mm Hg
Percentage of hemoglobin saturated with oxygen	Sao2	95% or greater
Partial pressure of dissolved carbon dioxide	Paco2	35-45 mm Hg
Bicarbonate	HCO32	22-26 mEq/L (mmol/L)

> **! NURSING PRIORITY** An Sao$_2$ less than 95% indicates respiratory difficulty.

> **! TEST ALERT** Monitor changes in the client's respiratory status. The primary indicators of respiratory disorders are sputum production, cough, dyspnea, hemoptysis, pleuritic chest pain, fatigue, change in voice, and wheezing.

1. Initially observe client's resting position.
   a. Appearance: comfortable or distressed?
   b. Assess client in the sitting position, if possible.
   c. Any dyspnea or respiratory discomfort?
2. Evaluate vital signs.
   a. Appropriate for age level?
   b. Establish database and compare with previous data.
   c. Assess client's pattern of vital signs; normal vital signs vary greatly from one individual to another.
3. Assess upper airway passages and patency of the airway.
4. Inspect the neck for symmetry; check to see whether the trachea is in midline and look for presence of jugular vein distention.
5. Assess the lungs.
   a. Visually evaluate the chest/thorax.
      (1) Do both sides move equally?
      (2) Observe characteristics of respirations and note whether retractions are present (Fig. 11.2).
      (3) Note chest wall configuration (barrel chest, kyphosis, scoliosis).
   b. Palpate chest for tenderness, masses, and symmetry of motion.
   c. Auscultate breath sounds; begin at lung apices and end at the bases, comparing each area side to side. Breath sounds should be present and bilaterally equal.
   d. Determine presence of tactile fremitus: When client says "ninety-nine," there should be equal vibrations palpated bilaterally. Over areas of consolidation (pneumonia), there will be an increase in the vibrations.
   e. Determine presence of adventitious breath sounds (abnormal/extra breath sounds).

2. Status of immunizations.
   a. Tuberculin (TB) skin test (also known as PPD or Mantoux test).
   b. Pertussis, polio, pneumococcal pneumonia vaccine (Pneumovax).
   c. Influenza vaccination.
3. Medications (including over the counter, prescriptions, herbs, and vitamins).
4. Lifestyle and occupational environments.
5. Habits: smoking and alcohol intake.
   a. Pack years are calculated by multiplying the number of packs of cigarettes smoked per day by the number of years the person has smoked.
   b. Example: Smoking one pack a day for the last 20 years or two packs a day for the last 10 years is 20 pack years.
B. Physical Assessment.

(1) Crackles: usually heard during inspiration and do not clear with cough; occur when airway contains fluid (previously also known as *rales*); sounds are not continuous (early cardiac failure, pneumonia, and atelectasis).

(2) Wheezes: may be heard during inspiration and/or expiration; are caused by air moving through narrowed passages; sound is music-like and continuous (asthma, bronchitis, chronic emphysema).

(3) Pleural friction rub: heard primarily on inspiration over an area of pleural inflammation; may be described as a grating sound (pleuritis accompanied by pain with breathing); often uncomfortable with deep breath.

(4) Stridor: high-pitched, inspiratory, crowing sound (croup [laryngotracheobronchitis – LTB], acute epiglottitis).

6. Assess cough reflex and sputum production.
   a. Is cough associated with pain?
   b. What precipitates coughing episodes?
   c. Is cough productive or nonproductive?
   d. Characteristics of sputum.
      (1) Consistency, amount, presence of odor.
      (2) Color (should be clear or white); changes in color indicate infection.

> ❗ **NURSING PRIORITY** When mucus is retained and pools in the lungs, gas diffusion is decreased, providing a medium for bacteria growth.

   e. Presence of hemoptysis – duration and amount.
7. Assess for and evaluate dyspnea.
   a. Onset of dyspnea and precipitating causes.
   b. Presence of orthopnea.
   c. Presence of adventitious breath sounds.
   d. Noisy expiration.
   e. Level of activity tolerance.
   f. Correlate vital signs with dyspnea.
   g. Cyanosis (a very late and unreliable sign of hypoxia).
      (1) For dark-skinned clients, assess less pigmented areas (oral cavity, nail beds, lips, palms).
      (2) Dark-skinned clients may exhibit cyanosis in the skin as a gray hue, rather than blue.
      (3) Assess for prolonged capillary refill time; should be less than 3 secs.
8. Assess for and evaluate chest pain.
   a. Location and character of pain.
   b. Pain associated with cough.
   c. Pain either increased or decreased with breathing.
9. Evaluate fingers for clubbing (characteristic in clients with chronic respiratory disorders) (Fig. 11.3).
10. Evaluate pulmonary diagnostics (Appendix 11.1).
   a. Hemoglobin and hematocrit (presence of polycythemia or anemia).
   b. Electrolyte imbalances.
   c. Arterial blood gases (ABGs), pulse oximetry, end tidal CO^2.

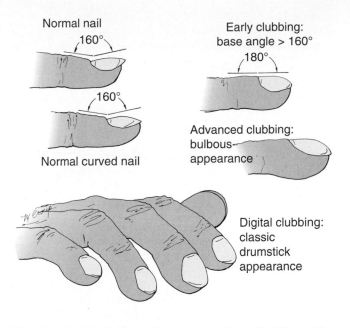

FIG. 11.3 Digital Clubbing (Redrawn from Price SA, Wilson LM. [2003]. *Pathophysiology: Clinical concepts of disease processes* [6th ed.]. St Louis: Mosby.)

RESPIRATORY DISORDERS

📋 Hypoxia

Hypoxia is a condition characterized by an inadequate amount of O_2 available for cellular metabolism.

> ❗ **TEST ALERT** Problems with respiratory status occur in all nursing disciplines. Questions may center around nursing priorities and nursing interventions in maintaining an airway and promoting ventilation in the client with respiratory difficulty. The questions may arise from any client situation (e.g., obstetrics, newborn, surgical, etc.).

A. Hypoxia occurs when signs and symptoms present because of a decrease in Pao_2; hypoxemia occurs when the amount of O_2 in the arterial blood is less than normal.
B. Hypoxia may be caused by inadequate circulation.
   1. Shock.
   2. Cardiac failure.
C. Anemia precipitates hypoxia, caused by a decrease in the O_2-carrying capacity of the blood.
   1. Inadequate red blood cell production.
   2. Deficient or abnormal hemoglobin.

Assessment: Recognize Cues

A. Chronic hypoxia.
   1. Chronic obstructive pulmonary disease (COPD).
   2. Cystic fibrosis, cancer of the respiratory tract.
   3. Heart failure, chronic anemia.

Table 11.2 SYMPTOMS OF RESPIRATORY DISTRESS AND HYPOXIA

Early Symptoms	Late Symptoms
Adults	
Restlessness	Extreme restlessness to
Tachycardia	stupor
Tachypnea, exertional dyspnea	Severe dyspnea
Orthopnea, tripod positioning	Slowing of respiratory rate
Anxiety, difficulty speaking	Bradycardia
Poor judgment, confusion	Cyanosis (peripheral or
Disorientation	central)
	Intercostal retractions
Pediatrics	
Flaring nares (infants)	Mottling, pallor, and
Substernal, suprasternal,	cyanosis
supraclavicular, and intercostal	Sudden increase or sudden
retractions (Fig. 11.2)	decrease in agitation
Stridor – expiratory and inspiratory	Inaudible breath sounds
Increased agitation	Altered level of
	consciousness
	Inability to cry or speak

B. Inflammatory problems affecting alveolar surface area and membrane integrity (e.g., pneumonia, bronchitis).
C. Acute hypoxia.
  1. Acute respiratory failure, sudden airway obstruction.
  2. Conditions affecting pulmonary expansion (e.g., respiratory paralysis).
  3. Conditions causing decreased cardiac output (heart failure, shock, cardiac arrest, etc.).
  4. Hypoventilation (brain attack or stroke, sedation, anesthesia, etc.).
D. Clinical manifestations: underlying respiratory problem, either chronic or acute (Table 11.2).
E. Diagnostics – blood gases, pulmonary function studies (Appendix 11.1).

Analyze Cues and Prioritize Hypotheses

The most important problem is low oxygen saturation.

Generate Solutions

Treatment

Depends on underlying problem.

Nursing Interventions: Take Action

Goal: To maintain good pulmonary hygiene and prevent hypoxic episode
A. Position client to maintain patent airway.
  1. Unconscious client: position on side with the chin extended.
  2. Conscious client: elevate the head of the bed; may position on side as well or in "tripod position" (leaning forward with mouth open).
B. Encourage coughing and deep breathing (Box 11.1).

Box 11.1 EFFECTIVE COUGHING

- Increase activity before coughing: walking or turning from side to side.
- Place client in sitting position, preferably with feet on the floor.
- Client should turn their shoulders inward and bend head slightly forward.
- Take a gentle deep breath in through the nose and breathe out completely.
- Take two deep breaths through the nose and mouth and hold for 5 secs.
- On the third deep breath, cough to clear secretions.
- Sips of warm liquids (coffee, tea, or water) may stimulate coughing.
- Demonstrate to client how to splint chest or incision during cough to decrease pain.
- Premedicate 30-60 min before activity/procedures if very painful (incisions, etc.).

C. Suction client as needed and as indicated by amount of sputum and ability to cough.
D. Maintain adequate fluid intake to keep secretions liquefied.
E. Encourage exercises and ambulation as indicated by condition.
F. Administer expectorants.
G. Administer O_2 if dyspnea is present (Appendix 11.7).

! NURSING PRIORITY Administer fluids very cautiously to a client who is having difficulty breathing. Begin with small sips of water to determine whether the client can swallow effectively – thickened liquids are easier to control. Do not begin with fluids that contain any fat (milk) or caloric value because of the increased risk for aspiration.

Goal: To implement nursing measures to decrease hypoxia (Box 11.2).
A. Assess patency of airway (first/highest priority).
  1. Can client speak? If not, initiate emergency procedures (Appendix 11.3).
  2. If speaking is difficult because of level of hypoxia, place in semi-Fowler position, begin oxygen, obtain assistance, and remain with client.
  3. If client is coherent and able to speak in sentences, continue with assessment of the problem.
  4. Evaluate amount of secretions and ability to cough; suction and administer O_2 as indicated.
B. Assess use of accessory muscles, presence of retractions.
C. Maintain calm approach because increasing anxiety will potentiate hypoxia.
D. Place adult or older child in a semi-Fowler position, if not contraindicated.
E. Place infant in an infant seat or elevate the mattress.

! NURSING PRIORITY Position a client experiencing dyspnea with a pillow placed lengthwise behind the back and head. Do not flex the client's head forward or backward.

OLDER ADULT CARE FOCUS

Respiratory Care Priorities

- The older adult client may not present with respiratory symptoms, but instead with restlessness, confusion, and disorientation.
- Age-related changes that may affect respiratory function include:
  - Decreased cough and laryngeal reflexes
  - Decreased mucociliary function
  - Decreased functioning alveoli
  - Decreased respiratory muscle strength
  - Increased anteroposterior diameter
  - Increased residual volume

Respiratory Care Priorities for the Older Adult

- Provide adequate rest periods between activities, such as bathing, going for treatments, eating.
- Increase compliance with medications by scheduling medication administration with routine activities.
- Encourage annual flu vaccination.
- Evaluate client's response to changes in activity and therapy frequently.
- Position the client upright in a position of comfort to facilitate chest/lung expansion.
- Monitor response of oxygen therapy.
- Maintain adequate hydration but use caution with older adults because of increased tendency for fluid volume overload.

F. Assess color and presence of diaphoresis.
G. Evaluate vital signs: Are there significant changes from previous readings?
H. Evaluate chest movements: Are they symmetric?
I. Evaluate anterior and posterior breath sounds.
J. Assess client for chest pain with dyspnea.
K. Notify health care provider of significant changes in respiratory function.
L. Remain with client experiencing acute dyspnea or hypoxic episodes.
M. Assess response to O_2 therapy.
N. Monitor ABGs and pulse oximetry.

Obstructive Sleep Apnea

Obstructive sleep apnea **(OSA) is a disorder in which an individual frequently stops breathing during sleep (cessation of breathing for 10 secs or longer occurring at least 5 times/hr). The individual may not be aware of snoring or apneic episodes. Apneic episodes cause recurrent arousals from sleep.**

Assessment: Recognize Cues

A. Cardinal symptoms (the three *S*s – snoring, sleepiness, and significant-other report of sleep apnea episodes).
B. Clinical manifestations.
   1. Disruptive snoring, unrefreshing sleep.
   2. Sleeper awakens after 10 secs or longer of apnea.

   3. Short-term memory loss, morning headaches.
   4. Hypersomnia, witness apnea.
   5. Gasping while sleeping, large neck, enlarged tonsils.
   6. Nasal deformity/septal deviation.
   7. Obesity, driving accidents (falling asleep).
   8. Increasing irritability, personality changes, and depression.
C. Diagnostics: overnight polysomnography (PSG) to determine frequency and apneic events.

Analyze Cues and Prioritize Hypotheses

The most important problem is hypoxia due to an abnormal sleep pattern.

Generate Solutions

Treatment

A. Lifestyle changes to include weight loss, smoking cessation, decreased consumption of alcohol, and avoidance of tranquilizer use.
B. Oral appliances designed to keep the throat open during sleep.
C. Change in sleeping position.
D. Continuous positive airway pressure (CPAP) during sleep – pressure helps keep the upper airway open.
E. Uvulopalatopharyngoplasty to remove the tonsils and adenoids and resect the uvula, the posterior part of the soft palate, and any excessive pharyngeal tissue.

Nursing Interventions: Take Action

Goal: To reinforce teaching about proper use of equipment.
A. Have client participate in the selection of mask and equipment.
   1. Teach client how to troubleshoot equipment.
   2. Include spouse or bedpartner in education.
B. If client hospitalized, check hospital policy to see if client can use own equipment.

Pleural Effusion

Pleural effusion **is caused by a collection of fluid in the pleural space. It is generally associated with other disease processes.**

Assessment: Recognize Cues

A. Clinical manifestations.
   1. Symptoms of an underlying problem.
   2. Large quantities of fluid will cause shortness of breath and dyspnea.
   3. Decreased breath sounds.
   4. Pleuritic pain on inspiration.
   5. Asymmetric chest expansion.
B. Diagnostics – chest x-ray, ultrasound, chest computed tomography (CT) scan (Appendix 11.1).

Analyze Cues and Prioritize Hypotheses

The most important problem is the excess fluid, which increases dyspnea, discomfort, and the risk for infection.

Generate Solutions

Treatment

A. Thoracentesis (Appendix 11.1).

B. If empyema develops (purulent fluid in the pleural space), area may have to be opened and allowed to drain. Client will receive antibiotics.

C. Chest tube placement is necessary if fluid buildup is rapid, requiring removal to facilitate respirations.

Nursing Interventions: Take Action

Goal: To recognize problems associated with chest tube placement and prevent an acute episode of hypoxia (see Hypoxia, Nursing Interventions).

Pneumonia

Pneumonia **is an acute inflammatory process caused by a microbial agent; it involves the lung parenchyma, including the small airways and alveoli.**

Assessment: Recognize Cues

A. Predisposing conditions.
   1. Chronic upper respiratory tract infection, prolonged immobility.
   2. Smoking, decreased immunity (disease and/or age).
   3. Aspiration of foreign material or gastric contents.
   4. Chronic health problems: cardiac, pulmonary, diabetes, cancer, stroke.
   5. Nosocomial pneumonia: caused by tracheal intubation, intestinal/gastric tube feedings, ventilator-associated pneumonia (VAP) (Box 11.3).

Box 11.3   STRATEGIES TO PREVENT VENTILATOR-ASSOCIATED PNEUMONIA

Ventilator-associated pneumonia (VAP) is an airway infection that develops at least 48 h after a client is intubated.

- VAP is the leading cause of death related to hospital-acquired infections.
- VAP can develop as a result of aspiration of stomach contents or when bacterial colonies from the oral cavity, sinuses, and trachea develop on the endotracheal tube.

Nursing Implications

1. Practice good hand hygiene/handwashing.
2. Wear gloves when providing oral hygiene.
3. Elevate head of bed between 30 and 45 degrees.
4. Turn client according to agency policy.
5. Minimize sedation with daily spontaneous awakening trials (SATs).
6. Perform daily spontaneous breathing trials (SBTs) as indicated.
7. Suctioning as needed or continuous subglottic secretion drainage.
8. Daily assessment related to readiness to extubate.
9. Use of VAP prevention bundles.

Source: Adapted from Papazian, L., Klompas, M., & Luyt, C.E. (2020). Ventilator-associated pneumonia in adults: A narrative review. *Intensive Care Medicine, 46*(5). 888-986. doi:10.1007/s00134-020-05980-0

B. Clinical manifestations (Fig. 11.4).
   1. Fever, chills, tachycardia, tachypnea, dyspnea.
   2. Productive cough: thick, blood-streaked, yellow, purulent sputum.
   3. Pleuritic chest pain, malaise, altered mental status.
   4. Respiratory distress (hypoxia) (Table 11.2).
   5. Diminished breath sounds, wheezing, crackles, tactile fremitus, dullness to percussion.
   6. Pediatrics.
      a. Feeding difficulty in infants.
      b. Cough initially nonproductive.
      c. Moderate to high fever.
      d. Adventitious breath sounds, tachypnea.
      e. Retractions, nasal flaring.

C. Diagnostics – chest x-ray (Appendix 11.1).

> **! OLDER ADULT PRIORITY** An older adult client may initially present with mental confusion and volume depletion rather than respiratory symptoms and fever (Box 11.2).

Analyze Cues and Prioritize Hypotheses

The most important problems are potential airway obstruction due to inflammation, excessive pulmonary secretions, reduced immunity due to microorganisms, and decreased gas exchange.

Generate Solutions

Treatment

A. Antibiotic according to organism identified.

> **! TEST ALERT** Do not start antibiotics until a good sputum specimen (Appendix 11.9) has been collected. An accurate culture and sensitivity test cannot be done if client has already begun receiving antibiotics.

B. Respiratory precautions: transmitted via airborne droplets.

C. Inhalation therapy.
   1. Cool O_2 mist, incentive spirometer.

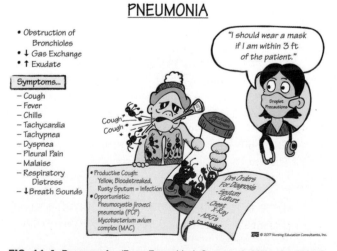

FIG. 11.4 Pneumonia. (From Zerwekh J, Garneau A, Miller CJ. [2017]. *Digital collection of the memory notebooks of nursing* [4th ed.]. Chandler, AZ: Nursing Education Consultants, Inc.)

2. Postural drainage: turn, cough, and deep breathe.

3. Bronchodilators.

D. Chest physiotherapy (CPT) – suctioning, percussion, and postural drainage.

Nursing Interventions: Take Action

Goal: To prevent occurrence.

A. Encourage mobility and ambulation if possible.

B. Good respiratory hygiene: turn, cough, deep breathe, and incentive spirometry.

C. Identify high-risk clients.

D. Encourage pneumococcal vaccine for susceptible clients.

Goal: To decrease infection and remove secretions to facilitate O_2 and CO_2 exchange.

A. Antibiotics.

B. Have client turn, cough, and deep breathe.

C. Liquefy secretions.

1. Adequate hydration (administer PO fluids cautiously to prevent aspiration).

2. Cool mist inhalation.

D. Evaluate breath sounds and changes in sputum.

E. Position for comfort or place in semi-Fowler position.

F. Nursing measures to prevent and evaluate levels of hypoxia (see Hypoxia, Nursing Interventions; also Table 11.2).

G. Provide adequate pain control measures to facilitate coughing and deep breathing.

Goal: To teach client and family how to provide home care when appropriate.

A. Antibiotics.

B. Cool mist humidification.

C. Maintain high oral fluid intake.

D. Antipyretic: acetaminophen.

E. Frequent changes of position.

F. Understand symptoms of increasing respiratory problems and when to notify health care provider.

Tuberculosis

TB is a reportable communicable disease that is characterized by pulmonary manifestations.

A. Characteristics.

1. Organism is primarily transmitted through respiratory droplets; it is inhaled and implants on respiratory bronchioles or alveoli; predominately spread by repeated close contact.

2. Latent TB infection (LTBI): a client in good health is frequently able to resist the primary infection and does not have active disease; these clients will continue to harbor the TB organism.

3. The primary site or tubercle may undergo a process of degeneration or caseation; this area can erode into the bronchial tree, and TB organisms are active and present in the sputum, resulting in further spread of the disease.

4. The area may never erode but may calcify and remain dormant after the primary infection. However, the tubercle may contain living organisms that can be reactivated several years later.

5. The majority of people with a primary infection will harbor the TB bacilli in a tubercle in the lungs and will not exhibit any symptoms of an active infection.

6. May occur as an opportunistic infection in clients who are immunocompromised.

Assessment: Recognize Cues

A. Predisposing conditions.

1. Frequent close or prolonged contact with infected individual.

2. Debilitating conditions and diseases.

3. Poor nutrition and crowded living conditions.

4. Increasing age; prevalent in ethnic minorities and foreign-born people.

B. Cause: *Mycobacterium tuberculosis*, a Gram-positive, acid-fast bacillus.

C. Clinical manifestations (up to 20% of clients may be asymptomatic) (Fig. 11.5).

1. Fatigue, malaise, anorexia, weight loss.

2. May have a chronic cough that progresses to more frequent and productive cough.

3. Low-grade fever and night sweats.

4. Hemoptysis is associated only with advanced condition.

5. May present with acute symptoms.

6. Clients with LTBI will have a positive skin test, but they are asymptomatic.

D. Diagnostics – (Appendix 11.1).

> ❗ **NURSING PRIORITY** A positive reaction to a TB skin test means the person has at some time been infected with the TB bacillus and developed antibodies. It does not mean that the person has an active TB infection.

1. TB skin testing with purified protein derivative (PPD).

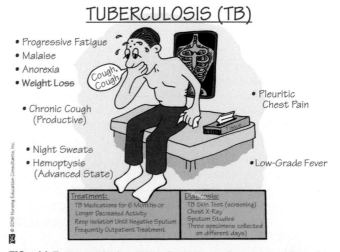

TUBERCULOSIS (TB)

- Progressive Fatigue
- Malaise
- Anorexia
- Weight Loss
- Chronic Cough (Productive)
- Night Sweats
- Hemoptysis (Advanced State)

Cough, Cough

- Pleuritic Chest Pain
- Low-Grade Fever

Treatment:
TB Medications for 6 Months or Longer Decreased Activity
Resp Isolation Until Negative Sputum
Frequently Outpatient Treatment

Diagnosis:
TB Skin Test (screening)
Chest X-Ray
Sputum Studies
Three specimens collected on different days

© 2016 Nursing Education Consultants, Inc.

FIG. 11.5 Tuberculosis. (From Zerwekh J, Garneau A, Miller CJ. [2017]. *Digital collection of the memory notebooks of nursing* [4th ed.]. Chandler, AZ: Nursing Education Consultants, Inc.)

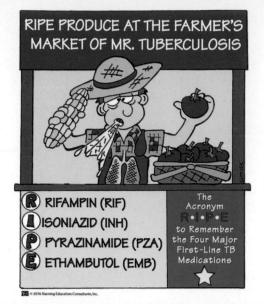

FIG. 11.6 Tuberculosis Medications: RIPE. (From Zerwekh J, Garneau A, Miller CJ. [2017]. *Digital collection of the memory notebooks of nursing* [4th ed.]. Chandler, AZ: Nursing Education Consultants, Inc.)

2. QuantiFERON-TB (QFT) rapid diagnostic: blood test to identify presence of antigens; does not take the place of sputum smears and cultures.
3. New rapid test: nucleic acid amplification test (NAAT); results in 2 hrs.
4. Bacteriologic studies to identify acid-fast bacilli in the sputum; sputum culture is the gold standard (Appendix 11.1).
E. Complications.
   1. Pleural effusion.
   2. Pneumonia.
   3. Other organ involvement.

Analyze Cues and Prioritize Hypotheses

The most important problems are potential for airway obstruction due to thick secretions and weak cough, development of drug-resistant disease leading to a spread of infection, weight loss, fatigue, poor gas exchange.

Generate Solutions

Treatment

A. Medication (Appendix 11.2) (Fig. 11.6).
   1. Medical regimen involves simultaneous administration of two or more medications; this increases the therapeutic effect of medication and decreases development of resistant bacteria.
   2. Sputum cultures are evaluated every 2 to 4 weeks initially, then monthly after sputum is negative. Sputum cultures should be negative within several weeks of beginning therapy; this depends on the medication regimen and the resistance of the bacteria.
   3. Direct observed therapy (DOT): health care personnel provide the medications and observe client swallow the medication; preferred strategy for all clients.

4. Prophylaxis chemotherapy for LTBI.
   a. Close contact with a client with a new TB diagnosis.
   b. Newly infected client with positive skin test reaction.
   c. Client with positive skin test reaction with conditions that decrease immune response (HIV infection, steroid therapy, chemotherapy).
   d. Isoniazid (INH) most often used for prophylaxis.
B. Most often treated on an outpatient basis.

Nursing Interventions: Take Action

Goal: To understand implications of the disease and measures to protect others and maintain own health.
A. Evaluate client's lifestyle and identify needs regarding compliance with treatment and long-term therapy.
B. Identify community resources available to client.
C. Understand medication schedule and importance of maintaining medication regimen.
   1. Nonadherence is a major contributor to the development of multidrug resistance and treatment failure.
   2. DOT recommended to guarantee adherence; may require client to come to public health clinic for nurse to administer medication.
D. Return for sputum checks every 2 to 4 weeks during therapy.
E. Balanced diet and good nutritional status.
F. Avoid alcohol and all medications that may damage the liver.
G. Avoid excessive fatigue; endurance will increase with treatment.
H. Identify family and close contacts who need to report to the public health department for TB screening.
I. Offer client HIV testing.

Goal: To prevent transmission of the disease.
A. When sputum is positive for the organism, implement airborne precautions for hospitalized client.
B. Wear an N95 or high-efficiency particulate air (HEPA) respirator when caring for the client.
C. Home care: teach respiratory precautions.
   1. Cover mouth and nose when sneezing or coughing.
   2. Practice careful handwashing routine.
   3. Wear a surgical mask when in contact with other people.
   4. Discard all secretions (nose and mouth) in plastic bags.
   5. Reevaluate periodically for active disease or secondary infection.

🔲 **NURSING PRIORITY** TB is most likely to be spread by clients who have active, undiagnosed TB.

📋 Chronic Obstructive Pulmonary Disease

COPD **is a group of chronic respiratory disorders characterized by obstruction of airflow, primarily chronic bronchitis and emphysema.**

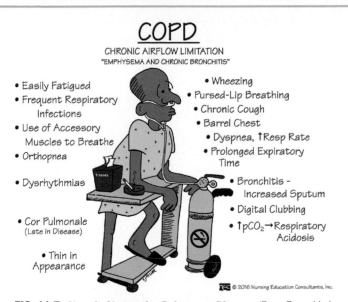

FIG. 11.7 Chronic Obstructive Pulmonary Disease. (From Zerwekh J, Garneau A, Miller CJ. [2017]. *Digital collection of the memory notebooks of nursing* [4th ed.]. Chandler, AZ: Nursing Education Consultants, Inc.)

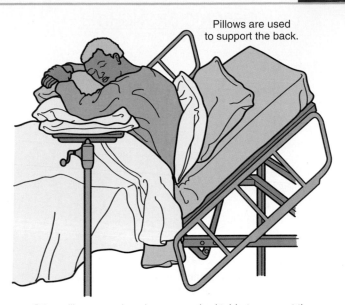

Other pillows are placed on an overbed table to support the weight of the arms, shoulders, and head.

FIG. 11.8 Orthopnea Position. (From Stromberg H. [2023]. *Medical-surgical nursing: Concepts and Practice* [5th ed.]. Elsevier.)

Assessment: Recognize Cues

A. Risk factors/etiology.
  1. Cigarette smoking (including passive smoking) – most common cause.
  2. Chronic infections.
  3. Inhaled irritants (from occupational exposure and air pollution).
  4. Alpha$_1$-antitrypsin deficiency: enzyme deficiency leading to decreased lung elasticity and COPD at an early age.
  5. Aging: changes in thoracic cage and respiratory muscles and loss of elastic recoil.
B. Clinical manifestations common to chronic airflow limitation (Fig. 11.7).
  1. Distended neck veins, ankle edema.
  2. Orthopnea or tripod positioning, barrel chest (Fig. 11.8).
  3. Prolonged expiratory time, pursed-lip breathing.
  4. Diminished breath sounds.
  5. Thorax is hyperresonant to percussion.
  6. Exertional dyspnea progressing to dyspnea at rest.
  7. Increased respiratory rate.
C. As a result of a prolonged increase in Paco$_2$ levels, the normal respiratory center in the medulla is affected; when this occurs, hypoxia will become the primary respiratory stimulus.
D. Emphysema: primarily a problem with the alveoli, characterized by a loss of alveolar elasticity, overdistention, and destruction, with severe impairment of gas exchange across the alveolar membrane (Fig. 11.9).
E. Chronic bronchitis: primarily a problem related to irritation of airway, characterized by excessive mucus production and impaired ciliary function, which decreases mucus clearance. Client may develop polycythemia as a result of the low Pao$_2$. History of productive cough lasting at least 3 months for 2 consecutive years. (Fig. 11.10).

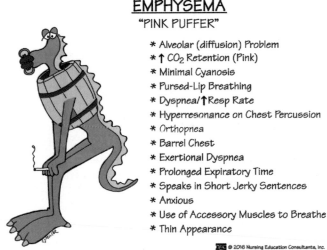

FIG. 11.9 Emphysema. (From Zerwekh J, Garneau A, Miller CJ. [2017]. *Digital collection of the memory notebooks of nursing* [4th ed.]. Chandler, AZ: Nursing Education Consultants, Inc.)

F. Diagnostics (Appendix 11.1).
  1. Pulmonary function studies show increased residual volume (air trapping).
  2. ABGs (Table 11.1).
G. Complications.
  1. Cor pulmonale (right-side heart failure).
  2. Infections (pneumonia).
  3. Peptic ulcer and gastroesophageal reflux disease (GERD).
  4. Acute respiratory failure.

Analyze Cues and Prioritize Hypotheses

The most important problems are associated with alveolar-capillary membrane changes, reduced airway size,

CHRONIC BRONCHITIS
"BLUE BLOATER"

* Airway Flow Problem
* Color Dusky to Cyanotic
* Recurrent Cough & ↑Sputum Production
* Hypoxia
* Hypercapnia (↑pCO_2)
* Respiratory Acidosis
* ↑Hgb
* ↑Resp Rate
* Exertional Dyspnea
* ↑Incidence in Smokers
* Digital Clubbing

* Cardiac Enlargement
* Use of Accessory Muscles to Breathe
* Leads to Right-Sided Heart Failure: Bilateral Pedal Edema, ↑JVD

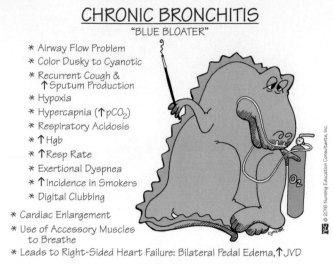

FIG. 11.10 Chronic Bronchitis. (From Zerwekh J, Garneau A, Miller CJ. [2017]. *Digital collection of the memory notebooks of nursing* [4th ed.]. Chandler, AZ: Nursing Education Consultants, Inc.)

ventilatory muscle fatigue, thick and increased mucus production, airway obstruction, diaphragm flattening, fatigue, decreased energy, weight loss, anxiety, decreased endurance due to fatigue and dyspnea, and the potential for pneumonia or other respiratory infections.

Generate Solutions

Treatment
A. Prevention or treatment of respiratory tract infections.
B. Bronchodilators (Appendix 11.2).
C. Mucolytics and expectorants (Appendix 11.2).
D. CPT (suctioning, percussion, and postural drainage).
E. Breathing exercises, humidified low-flow O_2.
F. Exercise to maintain cardiovascular fitness; most common exercise is walking.
G. Corticosteroids.

> **! NURSING PRIORITY** Administer low-flow O_2 for clients with emphysema. High concentrations of O_2 would decrease the client's hypoxic drive and increase respiratory distress. *Always notify the RN or health care provider* if it is necessary to increase the flow of O_2 for clients with COPD.

Nursing Interventions: Take Action

Goal: To improve ventilation.
A. Teach pursed-lip breathing: inhale through the nose and exhale against pursed lips.
B. Avoid activities increasing dyspnea.
C. Humidified O_2 (low flow via nasal cannula at a rate of 1-3 L/min) should be used when clients are experiencing exertional or resting hypoxemia.
   1. Monitor for hypercapnia, hypoxia, and acidosis.
   2. A significant increase in Pao_2 may decrease respiratory drive (O_2 toxicity).
   3. Administer O_2 via nasal cannula or venturi mask (to deliver a more precise fraction of inspired oxygen [Fio_2]).

4. Assess for pressure ulcers on the nares with a nasal cannula and on the top of the client's ears where the elastic holds the mask.

> **! NURSING PRIORITY** Administer O_2 therapy and evaluate results; the risk for inducing hypoventilation should not prevent the administration of O_2 at low levels to the client with COPD who is experiencing respiratory distress. The nurse should be prepared to provide ventilatory assistance if necessary.

D. Assess breath sounds before and after coughing.
E. Avoid cough suppressants.
F. Place client in high-Fowler or sitting position.
G. Maintain adequate hydration to facilitate removal of secretions.

Goal: To improve activity tolerance.
A. Balance activities and dyspnea: gradually increase activities; use portable O_2 tank when walking; avoid respiratory irritants.
B. Encourage pursed-lip and diaphragmatic breathing during exercise and as needed.
C. Schedule activities after respiratory therapy.

Goal: To maintain adequate nutrition.
A. Soft, high-protein, high-calorie, moderate carbohydrate diet – especially for underweight clients with emphysema.
B. Postural drainage completed 30 mins before meals or 3 hrs after meals.
C. Good oral hygiene after postural drainage.
D. Small frequent meals; rest before and after meals.
E. Use a bronchodilator before meals.
F. Encourage at least 2000 to 3000 mL fluid daily unless contraindicated.

Home Care
A. Encourage client and family to verbalize feelings about condition and lifelong restriction of activities.
B. Client teaching.
   1. Include client in active planning for home care.
   2. Instruct client regarding community resources.
   3. Instruct client regarding medication schedule and side effects of prescribed medications.
C. Recognize signs and symptoms of upper respiratory tract infection and know when to call health care provider.
D. Encourage activities such as walking – an increase in respiratory rate and shortness of breath will occur, but if respirations return to normal within 5 mins of stopping activity, it is considered normal.

Cancer of the Upper Airway

Oral/pharyngeal cancer is uncontrollable growth of malignant cells invading and causing damage to areas around the mouth, including the lips, cheeks, gums, tongue, soft and hard palate, floor of the mouth, tonsils, sinuses, and even the pharynx.

Cancer of the larynx may involve the vocal cords or other areas of the larynx. Most lesions are squamous cell

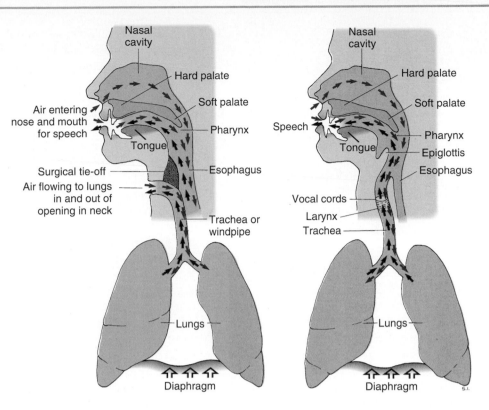

FIG. 11.11 Normal Airflow In and Out of Lungs *(left)* and Airflow In and Out of the Lungs After Total Laryngectomy *(right)*. Clients using esophageal speech trap air in the esophagus and release it to create sound. (From Stromberg H. [2023]. *Medical-surgical nursing: Concepts and Practice* [5ᵗʰ ed.]. Elsevier.)

carcinomas and slow growing. **If detected early, this type of cancer is curable by surgical resection of the lesion.**

Assessment: Recognize Cues

A. Risk factors/etiology.
1. More common in older adult men.
2. History of tobacco and alcohol use.
B. Clinical manifestations of oral cancer.
1. Leukoplakia: whitish elevated patch on oral mucosa or tongue (premalignant lesion).
2. Erythroplasia (erythroplakia): a red velvety patch on the mouth or tongue (premalignant lesion).
3. A sore in the mouth that bleeds and does not heal.
4. A lump or thickening in the cheek.
5. Difficulty chewing or swallowing.
C. Clinical manifestations of laryngeal cancer (may be asymptomatic).
1. Early changes.
a. Voice changes, hoarseness, oral leukoplakia.
b. Persistent unilateral sore throat, difficulty swallowing.
c. Feeling of foreign body in throat.
2. Late changes.
a. Pain.
b. Dysphagia and decreased tongue mobility.
c. Airway compromise.
D. Diagnostics: direct laryngoscopic examination with biopsy.

Analyze Cues and Prioritize Hypotheses

The most important problems are oxygen exchange, eating problems, facial appearance, self-image, speech, and communication before and after surgery.

Generate Solutions

Treatment
Varies with the extent of malignancy.
A. Radiation: brachytherapy – placing a radioactive source into or near the area of the tumor; may also be used with external radiation treatments.
B. Surgical intervention.
1. Partial laryngectomy: preserves the normal airway and normal speech mechanism; if a tracheotomy is performed, it is removed after the risk for swelling and airway obstruction has subsided.
2. Radical neck dissection or total laryngectomy involves resection of the trachea, a permanent tracheotomy for breathing, and an alternative method of speaking (Fig. 11.11).
3. Depending on location of oral lesions, a glossectomy (removal of the tongue) and/or mandibulectomy (removal of mandible) may be performed; cancers of the oral cavity metastasize early to cervical lymph nodes.

Complications

A. Airway obstruction.

B. Hemorrhage.

C. Fistula formation.

Nursing Interventions: Take Action

Goal: To prevent oral and laryngeal cancer.

A. Avoid chemical, physical, or thermal trauma to the mouth.

B. Maintain good oral hygiene: regular brushing and flossing.

C. Prevent constant irritation in the mouth; repair dentures or other dental problems.

D. See a doctor for any oral lesion that does not heal in 2 to 3 weeks.

Goal: To prepare client for surgery.

A. General preoperative preparation.

B. Consult with surgeon as to the anticipated extent of the surgery; determine how airway and nutritional needs will be addressed.

C. Discuss with client the possibility of a temporary tracheotomy or, if anticipated, a permanent tracheotomy.

D. Encourage ventilation of feelings regarding temporary or permanent loss of voice after surgery, as well as alteration in physical appearance.

E. If total laryngectomy is anticipated, schedule a visit from the speech pathologist or member of the laryngectomy club to reassure client of rehabilitation potential.

F. Establish a method of communication for immediate postoperative period.

G. Discuss nutritional considerations after surgery.

Goal: To maintain patent airway after laryngectomy.

A. If tracheotomy is not performed, evaluate for hematoma and increasing edema of the incisional area precipitating respiratory distress.

B. Place in semi-Fowler position.

C. Administer humidified O_2 therapy.

D. Closely monitor for respiratory compromise (hypoxia).

E. Monitor vital signs for hemorrhage.

F. Avoid analgesics that depress respiration.

G. Promote good pulmonary hygiene.

H. If tracheostomy is present, suction as indicated (Appendix 11.6).

Goal: To maintain airway; to prevent complications after tracheotomy (Appendix 11.5).

Goal: To promote nutrition postoperatively.

A. Method of nutritional intake depends on the extent of the surgical procedure (see Appendix 14-5 for tube feedings).

B. IV fluids for first 24 hrs.

C. Gastrostomy, nasogastric, or nasointestinal tubes may be placed during surgery and used until edema has subsided.

D. Provide good oral hygiene; may need to suction oral cavity if client cannot swallow.

E. Evaluate tolerance of tube feedings; treat nausea quickly to prevent vomiting (Appendix 14-5).

F. Closely observe for swallowing difficulty with initial oral feedings.

1. Bland, nonirritating foods.

2. Thicker foods allow more control over swallowing; thin watery fluids should be avoided.

G. For a partial laryngectomy, the possibility of aspiration is a primary concern during the first few days after surgery.

❗ TEST ALERT Identify clients at high risk for aspiration.

Goal: To promote wound healing.

A. Assess pressure dressings and presence of edema formation.

B. Monitor wound suction devices (Hemovac, Jackson-Pratt); drainage should be serosanguineous.

C. Monitor patency of drainage tubes every 3 to 4 hrs; fluid should gradually decrease.

D. If skin flaps are used, the wound is often left uncovered for better visualization of flap and to prevent pressure on area.

E. When drainage tubes are removed, carefully observe area for increased swelling.

F. Type of oral hygiene is indicated by the extent of the procedure.

1. Mouth irrigations.

2. Soothing mouth rinses (cool normal saline or nonirritating antiseptic solutions).

3. If dentures are present, clean mouth well before replacing.

4. Oral hygiene before and after oral intake.

5. Avoid using stiff toothbrushes and metal-tipped suction catheters.

Goal: To identify resources for speech rehabilitation after laryngectomy.

A. If a partial laryngectomy is done, client should have gradual improvement in voice; client is generally allowed to begin whispering 2 to 3 days after surgery.

B. Identify different methods for speech management: esophageal speech, electric/artificial larynx, or tracheoesophageal puncture (closest to normal speech).

Home Care

A. Encourage client to begin own suctioning and caring for the tracheostomy before they leave the hospital.

B. Assist the family in obtaining equipment for home use.

1. System for humidification of air in home environment.

2. Suction and equipment necessary for tracheostomy care.

C. Care of stoma.

1. No swimming.

2. Wear plastic collar over stoma while showering.

3. Maintain high humidification at night to increase moisture in airway.

4. Avoid use of aerosol sprays.

D. Nutritional considerations: client cannot smell; taste will also be affected.

E. Infection.

F. Increased secretions.

G. Client should carry appropriate medical identification.

H. Encourage client to put arm and shoulder on affected side through range-of-motion exercises to prevent functional disabilities of the shoulder and neck.

Cancer of the Lung

Cancer of the lung **is a tumor arising from within the lung. It may represent the primary site or may be a metastatic site from a primary lesion elsewhere.**

Assessment: Recognize Cues

A. Risk factors.
  1. Smoking, including passive smoking.
  2. Occupational exposure to and/or inhalation of carcinogens.
B. Clinical manifestations: nonspecific; appear late in disease.
  1. Persistent chronic cough.
  2. Cough initially nonproductive, then may become productive of purulent and/or blood tinged.
  3. Dyspnea and wheezing with bronchial obstruction.
  4. Recurring fever.
  5. Common sites of metastasis.
    a. Liver, bones, brain, pancreas.
    b. Lymph nodes: mediastinum.
  6. Pain is a late manifestation.
C. Diagnostics: bronchoscopy with biopsy.

Analyze Cues and Prioritize Hypotheses

The most important problems are associated with surgery, which include the gas exchange, the potential for pneumonia or other respiratory infections, and management of pain.

Generate Solutions

Treatment
Varies with the extent of the malignancy.
A. Radiation: may be used preoperatively to reduce tumor mass.
B. Surgery: treatment of choice early in condition.
  1. Lobectomy: removal of one lobe of the lung.
  2. Pneumonectomy: removal of the entire lung.
  3. Lung-conserving resection: removal of a small area (wedge) or a segment of the lung.
C. Chemotherapy.
D. Treatment may involve all three therapies.

Nursing Interventions: Take Action

Goal: To prepare client for surgery.
A. General preoperative preparations.
B. Improve quality of ventilation before surgery.
  1. No smoking.
  2. Bronchodilators.
  3. Good pulmonary hygiene.
C. Discuss anticipated activities in the immediate postoperative period.
D. Encourage ventilation of feelings regarding diagnosis and impending surgery.
E. Establish baseline data for comparison after surgery.
F. Orient client to the intensive care unit, if indicated.

Goal: To maintain patent airway and promote ventilation after thoracotomy.
A. Removal of secretions from tracheobronchial tree, either by coughing or suctioning.
B. Have client cough frequently, deep-breathe, and use incentive spirometer.
C. Assess vital signs; correlate with quality of respirations.
D. Closely observe pulse oximetry – *report levels to RN that are constantly changing or decreasing;* provide supplemental O_2 as indicated.
E. Control pain so that client can take deep breaths and cough.
F. Do not position the client who has undergone a wedge resection or lobe resection on the affected side for extended periods of time; this will hinder the expansion of the lung remaining on that side. If client is in stable condition, place in semi-Fowler position to promote optimal ventilation.

> **! NURSING PRIORITY** Postoperative positioning of a client who has had thoracic surgery is important to remember, especially for a client who has undergone pneumonectomy.

G. If the client who has undergone pneumonectomy experiences increased dyspnea, place them in semi-Fowler position. If tolerated, positioning on the operative side is recommended to facilitate full expansion of lung on unaffected side.
H. Encourage ambulation as soon as possible.
I. Assess level of dyspnea at rest and with activity.
J. Maintain water-sealed drainage system (Appendix 11.4). A client who has undergone pneumonectomy will not have chest tubes for lung reexpansion because there is no lung left in the pleural cavity; however, chest tubes may be used for fluid drainage.

Goal: To assess and support cardiac function after thoracotomy.
A. Monitor for dysrhythmias; assess adequacy of cardiac output.
B. Evaluate urine output.
C. Administer fluids and transfusions with extreme caution; client's condition is very conducive to development of fluid overload.
D. Evaluate hydration and electrolyte status.
E. *Report any significant changes in vital signs, activity tolerance, or respiratory status.*

Goal: To maintain normal range of motion and function of the affected shoulder after thoracotomy.
A. Exercises to increase abduction and mobility of the shoulders.
B. Encourage progressive exercises.

Home Care

A. No smoking; avoid respiratory irritants.
B. Decreased strength is common.
C. Continue activities and exercises.
D. Stop any activity that causes shortness of breath, chest pain, or undue fatigue.

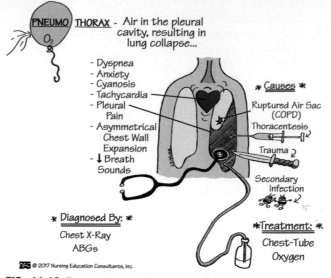

FIG. 11.12 Pneumothorax. (From Zerwekh J, Garneau A, Miller CJ. [2017]. *Digital collection of the memory notebooks of nursing* [4th ed.]. Chandler, AZ: Nursing Education Consultants, Inc.)

E. Avoid lifting heavy objects until complete healing has occurred.

F. Return for follow-up care as indicated.

📋 Pneumothorax

Air in the pleural space results in the collapse or atelectasis of that portion of the lung. This condition is known as *pneumothorax* (Fig. 11.12).

A. Tension pneumothorax: the development of a pneumothorax that allows excessive buildup of pressure (due to air that cannot escape) in the pleural space, causing a shift in the mediastinum toward the unaffected side.

> **❗ NURSING PRIORITY** A tension pneumothorax can rapidly become an emergency situation. It is much easier to treat the client if the pneumothorax is identified *before* it begins to exert tension on the mediastinal area.

Assessment: Recognize Cues

A. Diminished or absent breath sounds on the affected side.

B. Dyspnea, hypoxia, tachycardia, tachypnea.

C. Sudden onset of persistent chest pain, pain on affected side when breathing.

D. Increasing anxiety.

E. Asymmetric chest wall expansion.

F. Hyperresonance on percussion of affected side.

G. Possible development of a tension pneumothorax.
1. Tracheal shift from midline toward unaffected side.
2. Increasing problems of hypoxia.

H. Diagnostics – chest x-ray, CT scan, ultrasound (Appendix 11.1).

> **❗ NURSING PRIORITY** When atmospheric pressure is allowed to disrupt the negative pressure in the pleural space, it will cause the lung to collapse. This requires chest-tube placement to reestablish negative pressure and reinflate the lung.

Analyze Cues and Prioritize Hypotheses

The most important problems are hypoxemia, the potential for a tension pneumothorax, and anxiety due to the life-threatening nature of the condition.

Generate Solutions

Treatment

Placement of chest tubes connected to a water-sealed drainage system (Appendix 11.4).

Nursing Interventions: Take Action

Goal: To recognize the problem and prevent a severe hypoxic episode (see Hypoxia, Nursing Interventions).

A. Begin O_2 therapy.

B. Place in semi-Fowler position.

C. *Notify health care provider or RN and prepare client for insertion of chest tubes.*

Goal: To reinflate lung without complications.

A. Have client cough and deep-breathe every 2 hrs.

B. Encourage exercise and ambulation.

C. Establish and maintain water-sealed chest drainage system (Appendix 11.4).

📋 Open Chest Wound

An *open or "sucking" chest wound* is frequently caused by a penetrating injury to the chest, such as a gunshot or knife wound. If a chest tube is inadvertently pulled out of the chest, a sucking chest wound may be created.

Assessment: Recognize Cues

A. Increase in dyspnea.

B. A chest wound with evidence of air moving in and out via the wound.

Analyze Cues and Prioritize Hypotheses

The most important problems are hypoxemia, hemorrhage, and anxiety due to the life-threatening nature of the condition.

Generate Solutions

Treatment

A. Have the client take a deep breath, hold it, and bear down against a closed glottis. Apply a light occlusive, vented dressing (taped/secured on three sides to allow air to escape) over the wound.

> **❗ NURSING PRIORITY** Immediately occlude the chest wound; do not leave the client to go find a dressing. If necessary, place a towel or whatever is at hand over the wound to stop the flow of air.

B. Prepare for insertion of chest tubes to water-sealed drainage system.

C. After covering the wound with a light occlusive dressing, carefully evaluate the client for development of a tension pneumothorax.

Nursing Interventions: Take Action

Goal: To prevent problems of hypoxia.
Goal: To assess for development of tension pneumothorax.

Flail Chest

Flail chest **is the loss of stability of the chest wall with respiratory impairment because of multiple rib fractures (fractures at two or more points of the ribs involved).**

Assessment: Recognize Cues

A. Paradoxical respirations: the movement of the fractured area (flailed segment) inward during inspiration and outward during expiration, or opposite to the other areas of the chest wall.
B. Symptoms of hypoxia.
C. Diagnostics.
   1. Chest x-ray film showing multiple rib fractures.
   2. Crepitus over the ribs.

Analyze Cues and Prioritize Hypotheses

The most important problems are hypoxemia, hemorrhage, and anxiety due to the life-threatening nature of the condition.

Generate Solutions

Treatment
A. Maintain patent airway.
B. Adequate pain medication to enable client to breathe deeply.
C. O_2.
D. Endotracheal (ET) intubation with mechanical ventilation for severe respiratory distress (Appendixes 11.5 and 11.8).
E. Chest tube placement if pneumothorax occurs as a result of puncture of the lung by the fractured rib.

> **TEST ALERT** Determine changes in client's respiratory status.

Nursing Interventions: Take Action

Goal: To stabilize the chest wall and prevent complications.
A. Prepare client for ET intubation and mechanical ventilation.
B. Assess for symptoms of hypoxia.
C. Assess for symptoms of pneumothorax.

Pulmonary Embolism

A *pulmonary embolism* **(PE) is an obstruction of a pulmonary artery, most often the result of an embolism caused by a blood clot (thrombus), air, fat, amniotic fluid, bone marrow, or sepsis. The severity of the problem depends on the size of the embolus.**

A. Of the clients that die of PE, the majority die because of failure to diagnose.
B. Most pulmonary emboli arise from thrombi in the deep veins of the legs.
C. A PE must originate from the venous circulation, or the right side of the heart.

Assessment: Recognize Cues

A. Common risk factors/etiology.
   1. Conditions or immobility predisposing to venous stasis and/or deep vein thrombosis (DVT): surgery within the past 3 months, stroke, spinal cord injury, or history of DVT, obesity, or advancing age.
   2. Vascular injury: central venous catheters, thrombophlebitis, vascular disease, leg fractures.
   3. DVT: the thrombus spontaneously dislodges secondary to jarring (turbulence) of the area – sudden standing, changes in rate of blood flow (Valsalva maneuver, increased blood pressure).
   4. Hypercoagulability of blood.
B. Clinical manifestations.
   1. Classic triad of symptoms: dyspnea, chest pain, and hemoptysis occur in only 20% of clients.
   2. Other common symptoms.
      a. Increased anxiety, cough.
      b. Sudden, unexplained dyspnea, tachypnea.
      c. Hypotension, tachycardia, syncope.
   3. May result in sudden death if PE is large.
C. Diagnostics (Appendix 11.1).
   1. Pulmonary angiography
   2. Enhanced spiral CT scan (specific for PE).
   3. D-dimer test is elevated (greater than 250 mcg/L [1369 nmol/L]).

Analyze Cues and Prioritize Hypotheses

The most important problems are hypoxemia, hypotension, the potential for excessive bleeding due to anticoagulant therapy or fibrinolytic therapy, and anxiety due to the life-threatening nature of the condition.

Generate Solutions

Treatment
A. Bed rest, high-Fowler position if blood pressure permits.
B. Respiratory support: O_2, intubation (if necessary), ventilator, etc.
C. Anticoagulants (heparin, low-molecular-weight heparin, or warfarin) to prevent further thrombus formation.
D. IV access for fluids and medications to maintain blood pressure.
E. Small doses of morphine sulfate may be used to decrease anxiety, alleviate chest pain, or improve tolerance of ET tube.
F. Thrombolytics if unstable and PE confirmed.
G. Embolectomy or insertion of inferior vena cava filter.

> **TEST ALERT** Assess clients for complications caused by immobility. Immobilized clients have an increased risk for development of a PE. Questions require an understanding of principles for prevention of thrombophlebitis and subsequent embolism formation. It is far easier to prevent the problem than it is to treat the PE.

Nursing Interventions: Take Action

Goal: To identify clients at increased risk and prevent and/or decrease venous stasis.

Goal: To identify problem and implement nursing measures to alleviate hypoxia (see Hypoxia, Nursing Interventions).

Goal: To monitor client's respiratory function and response to treatment and minimize anxiety.

Goal: To minimize bleeding from treatment measures and assess for evidence of bleeding.

Acute Respiratory Distress Syndrome (Adult Respiratory Distress Syndrome)

Acute respiratory distress syndrome (ARDS) or noncardiogenic pulmonary edema, also referred to as shock lung and white lung, is a condition characterized by increased capillary permeability in the alveolar capillary membrane, resulting in fluid leaking into the interstitial spaces and the alveoli and a decrease in pulmonary compliance.

Assessment: Recognize Cues

A. Risk factors/etiology.
  1. Direct lung injury: aspiration, pneumonia, chest trauma, embolism, inhalation injury.
  2. Indirect lung injury: sepsis (most common), severe massive trauma, acute pancreatitis, anaphylaxis, shock.
B. Clinical manifestations.
  1. Restlessness, confusion, tachypnea, dyspnea.
  2. Hypoxemia despite high concentrations of oxygen administered.
  3. Tachycardia, adventitious lung sounds, diaphoresis.
  4. Profound respiratory distress and use of accessory muscles.
  5. Cyanosis or mottling.
C. Diagnostics: chest x-ray, ABGs, and may include CT scan (Appendix 11.1).

Analyze Cues and Prioritize Hypotheses

The most important problems are hypoxemia, hemorrhage, and anxiety due to the life-threatening nature of the condition.

Generate Solutions

Treatment

Care is generally provided in an intensive care setting.

Nursing Interventions: Take Action

Goal: To maintain airway patency and improve ventilation.
A. Frequent assessment for increasing respiratory difficulty; anticipate intubation or tracheotomy (Appendix 11.5).
B. ET tube or tracheotomy suctioning.
C. Evaluate ABG reports, constant monitoring of pulse oximetry.
D. Sedation and paralytic agents are required for clients to tolerate alternative modes of ventilation (Appendix 11.8).
E. Monitor hemoglobin levels and Pao_2 saturation levels.
Goal: To maintain fluid balance and cardiac output.
A. Fluid balance maintained with IV hydration; avoid fluid volume overload.

B. Assess for dysrhythmias.
C. Correlate vital signs with other assessment changes.

Pulmonary Edema

Pulmonary edema or *acute decompensated heart failure* **(ADHF) is caused by an abnormal accumulation of fluid in the lung, in both the interstitial and alveolar spaces.**

A. Origin is most often cardiac: pulmonary congestion occurs when the pulmonary vascular bed receives more blood from the right side of the heart (venous return) than the left side of the heart (cardiac output) can accommodate.
B. Pulmonary edema results from severe impairment in the ability of the left side of the heart to maintain cardiac output, thereby causing an engorgement of the pulmonary vascular bed.

Assessment: Recognize Cues

A. Risk factors/etiology.
  1. Alteration in capillary permeability (inhaled toxins, pneumonia, severe hypoxia).
  2. Cardiac myopathy, heart failure, overhydration.
B. Clinical manifestations: hypoxia (Table 11.2).
  1. Decreasing Pao_2, dyspnea, tachypnea.
  2. Severe anxiety, restlessness, irritability, confusion.
  3. Cool, moist skin.
  4. Tachycardia, S_3, S_4 gallop, dependent edema.
  5. Severe cough producing frothy, blood-tinged sputum.
  6. Noisy, wet breath sounds that do not clear with coughing.

⛑ OLDER ADULT PRIORITY Pulmonary edema can occur rapidly and become a medical emergency.

C. Diagnostics: B-type natriuretic peptide (BNP) level.

Analyze Cues and Prioritize Hypotheses

The most important problems are hypoxemia, frothy, blood-tinged sputum, and anxiety due to the rapid development of this life-threatening condition.

Generate Solutions

Treatment

Condition demands immediate attention; medications are administered intravenously.

A. O_2 in high concentration.
  1. Intubation and mechanical ventilation.
  2. Use of bilevel positive airway pressure (BiPAP).
B. Sedation (morphine) or muscle-paralyzing agents to allow controlled ventilation: decreases preload/vasoconstriction, as well as anxiety and pain.
C. Diuretics to reduce the cardiac preload.
D. Dopamine/dobutamine to facilitate myocardial contractility.

E. Medications to increase cardiac contractility and cardiac output (Appendix 11.2).

F. Vasodilators to decrease afterload.

Nursing Interventions: Take Action

Goal: To assess and decrease hypoxia (see Hypoxia, Nursing Interventions; also Table 11.2).

Goal: To improve ventilation.

A. Place in high-Fowler position with legs dependent.

B. Administer high levels of O_2.

C. Evaluate level of hypoxia and dyspnea; may need ET tube intubation and mechanical ventilation.

D. Problem may occur at night, especially in clients who are on bed rest.

E. IV sedatives/narcotics.
1. To decrease anxiety and dyspnea and to decrease pressure in pulmonary capillary bed.
2. Closely observe for respiratory depression.
3. Administer a sedative to decrease anxiety if client has received a muscle-paralyzing agent.
4. May be used to assist client in tolerating ventilator.

> **⊟ NURSING PRIORITY** Pulmonary edema is one of the few circumstances in which a client with respiratory distress may be given a narcotic. The fear of not being able to breathe is so strong that the client cannot cooperate. When a sedative/narcotic is administered, the nurse must be ready to support ventilation if respirations become severely depressed.

G. Administer bronchodilators and evaluate client's response and common side effects.

H. Closely monitor vital signs, pulse oximetry, hemodynamic changes, and cardiac dysrhythmias.

Goal: To reduce circulating volume (preload) and cardiac workload (afterload).

A. Diuretics (Appendix 12-2).

B. Medications to decrease afterload and increase cardiac output (Appendix 13-2).

C. Carefully monitor all IV fluids and evaluate tolerance of hydration status.

D. Maintain client in semi- to high-Fowler position but allow legs to remain dependent.

Goal: To provide psychological support and decrease anxiety.

A. Approach client in a calm manner.

B. Explain procedures.

C. Administer sedatives cautiously.

D. Remain with client in acute respiratory distress.

Goal: To prevent recurrence of problem.

A. Recognize early stages.

B. Maintain client in semi-Fowler position.

C. Decrease levels of activity.

D. Use extreme caution in administration of fluids and transfusions.

Appendix 11.1 PULMONARY DIAGNOSTICS ℞

X-ray Studies

Chest X-ray Film

An x-ray film of the lungs and chest wall; no specific care is required before or after x-ray study.

Bronchoscopy

Provides for direct visualization of larynx, trachea, and bronchi; client generally receives nothing-by-mouth (NPO) status for 6 hrs before the examination; preoperative medication is given, and the client's upper airway is anesthetized topically.

Nursing Implications
a. After the examination, evaluate the client for return of gag reflex. Maintain client's NPO status until return of gag reflex.
b. Bronchial biopsy may be done to obtain cells for cytologic examination; observe client for development of pneumothorax or frank bleeding.

Pulmonary Angiography

Contrast material (dye) is injected into the pulmonary arteries; the angiography permits visualization of the pulmonary vasculature; definitive diagnosis for pulmonary emboli.

Nursing Implications
1. Client should be well hydrated before procedure.
2. Increase fluid intake postprocedure to flush out the dye.
3. Check puncture site for bleeding, hematoma, or infection.

Contraindications: (1) dye or shellfish allergies, (2) unstable condition, (3) uncooperative client, (4) pregnancy, and (5) bleeding disorders.

Pathology: Laboratory Studies

Sputum Studies (see also Appendix 11.9)

Sputum specimen should come from deep in the lungs and not be contaminated with excessive amounts of saliva. It is best obtained in the morning upon arising; instruct client to rinse mouth out with water before collection to decrease contamination.

Culture and Sensitivity Test: Performed to determine presence of pathogenic bacteria and to which antibiotic the specific organism is sensitive. Should be done before antimicrobial therapy is started.

Acid-Fast Bacilli: Sputum collection and analysis when tuberculosis (TB) is suspected; morning sputum may contain a higher concentration of organisms.

Cytologic Examination: Tumors in pulmonary system may slough cells into the sputum.

Blood Work

D-dimer: Blood test to identify degradation of fibrin; degradation products not commonly found in healthy clients. Elevated in thromboembolism and in disseminated intravascular coagulation (DIC). Normal is less than 0.4 mcg/mL.

Continued

Pulmonary Function Studies

Studies may be done (1) to evaluate pulmonary function before surgery, (2) to evaluate response to bronchodilator therapy, (3) to differentiate diagnosis of pulmonary disease, and (4) to determine the cause of dyspnea.

Client must be alert and cooperative; client should not be sedated. Study is done in the pulmonary function laboratory; client directed to breathe into a cylinder from which a computer interprets and records data in specific values. Client should not smoke or use bronchodilating medications for 6 hrs before the test.

Pulse Oximetry

Measurement is made by placing a sensor on the finger or earlobe; a beam of light passes through the tissue and measures the amount of oxygen-saturated hemoglobin. If probe is placed on the finger, any nail polish should be removed. It provides a method for continuously evaluating the oxygen saturation levels (SpO2). It is noninvasive, and there are no pre- or postoximetry preparations. Readings may be incorrect if severe vasoconstriction has occurred or if Pao_2 is less than 70%. Normal range is 95% or higher.

Nursing Implications

1. Pulse oximetry should be used:
   a. For the client who is on supplemental oxygen and is at increased risk for desaturation.
   b. For the chronically ill client who has a tracheotomy or is on mechanical ventilation for chronic respiratory problems.
   c. For the client who has a critical or unstable airway.
2. Pulse oximetry is not recommended to monitor oxygen saturation:
   a. For clients experiencing problems with hypovolemia or decreased blood flow to extremities.
   b. To evaluate respiratory status when ventilator changes are made.
   c. To monitor progress of client on high levels of oxygen.
   d. During cardiopulmonary resuscitation.

Arterial Blood Gas Studies

ABGs are a measurement of the pH and partial pressures of dissolved gases (oxygen, carbon dioxide) of the arterial blood; it requires at least 0.6 mL of arterial blood, obtained through an arterial puncture. *If client's oxygen concentration or ventilatory settings have been changed, or if a client has been suctioned, blood should not be drawn for at least 30 mins* (Table 11.1). Perform Allen's test to assess collateral circulation before arterial puncture. Pressure should be maintained at the puncture site for a minimum of 5 mins. The arterial blood sample should be tightly sealed, placed on ice, and taken to the laboratory immediately.

Allen's Test: Hold client's hand, palm up. While occluding both the radial and ulnar arteries, have the client clench and unclench their hand several times; the hand will become pale. While continuing to apply pressure to the radial artery, release pressure on ulnar artery. Brisk color return (5-7 secs) to the hand should occur with the radial artery still occluded. If color does not return, the ulnar artery is not providing adequate blood flow, and the cannulation or puncture of radial artery should not be done.

Thoracentesis

Withdrawal of fluid from the pleural cavity/space; used for diagnostic and therapeutic purposes.

Nursing Implications

1. Explain procedure to client.
2. Position client.
   a. Preferably, client should sit upright on the side of the bed with arms and head over the bedside table.
   b. If client is unable to assume sitting position, place on affected side with the head of the bed slightly elevated. Area containing fluid collection should be dependent.
   c. If client has a malignancy, cytotoxic drugs may be infused into the pleural space.
3. Support and reassure the client during the procedure.
4. After the procedure, position the client on their side with puncture side up (or in semi-Fowler position). Monitor respiratory status and breath sounds for possible pneumothorax and assess puncture site.

Mantoux Skin Test (Tuberculin Test)

Mantoux test, or purified protein derivative (PPD) test, is a method of TB skin testing. PPD is injected intradermally in the forearm. Results are read in 48 to 72 hrs. A positive reaction means the individual has been exposed to *M. tuberculosis* recently or in the past and has developed antibodies (sensitized). It does not differentiate between active or latent infection. It may take 2 to 12 weeks after exposure for sensitivity and a positive skin test reaction to develop.

Nursing Implications

1. Intradermal injection: A small (25-gauge) needle is used to inject 0.1 mL of PPD under the skin. The needle is inserted bevel up; a raised area or "wheal" (6-10 mm) will form under the skin. To avoid a false negative, a wheal needs to form.
2. The most common area for injection is the inside surface of the forearm.
3. Do not aspirate; do not massage area.
4. The client should be given specific directions to return, or plans should be made to read the test in 48 to 72 hrs.
5. Interpretation: The area of induration (only the part of the reaction that can be felt; induration may not be visible) is measured, not the area of erythema or inflammation.
   a. An induration of 5 mm or more is a positive reaction in immunosuppressed clients who have been recently exposed to active TB.
   b. An induration of 10 mm is a positive reaction for all nonimmunocompromised persons.
   c. An induration of 15 mm is a positive reaction for individuals who are at low risk.

Nuclear Medicine

Lung Scan (V/Q Scan): A procedure to determine defects in blood perfusion in the lung; particularly useful in the client believed to have a pulmonary embolus or a ventilation/perfusion problem. For the perfusion component, a radioactive dye is injected or is inhaled, and the specific uptake is recorded on x-ray film. For the ventilation component, the client breathes the tracer element through a facemask with a mouthpiece. The ventilation component requires the client's cooperation. Client is not sedated or on dietary restrictions for the examination.

◼ TEST ALERT Monitor laboratory values and notify primary health care provider regarding results; recognize deviations from normal; use critical thinking when evaluating client's diagnostic values.

R̥

Appendix 11.2   RESPIRATORY MEDICATIONS

Bronchodilators: Relax smooth muscle of the bronchi, promoting bronchodilation and reducing airway resistance; also inhibit the release of histamine.

General Nursing Implications

- Metered dose inhalers (MDIs): Handheld pressurized devices that deliver a measured dose of drug with each "puff." When two puffs are needed, 1 min should elapse between them. A spacer may be used to increase the delivery of the medication.
- Dry powder inhalers (DPIs) deliver more medication to lungs and do not require coordination as with an MDI; medication is delivered as a dry powder directly to the lungs; 1 min should elapse between puffs.
- Bronchodilators: β_2 agonists and theophylline are given with caution to the client with cardiac disease, because tachydysrhythmias and chest pain may occur.
- Aerosol delivery systems have fewer side effects and are more effective.

MEDICATIONS	SIDE EFFECTS	NURSING IMPLICATIONS
Beta1 and Alpha agonists ▲Epinephrine: subQ, IV Racemic (nebulized) epinephrine	Headache Dizziness Hypertension Tremors Dysrhythmias	1. Do not administer to clients with hypertension or dysrhythmias. 2. Primarily used to treat acute asthma attacks and anaphylactic reactions. 3. With racemic epinephrine, results should be observed in less than 2 hrs.
Theophylline: PO, IV	Tachycardia Hypotension Nausea/vomiting Seizures	1. Theophylline blood levels should be determined for long-term use; therapeutic levels are between 10 and 20 mcg/mL (56-111 mmol/L); levels greater than 20 mcg/mL (111 mmol/L) are toxic. 2. IV administration may cause rapid changes in vital signs. 3. Considered to be a third-line drug for use with asthma. 4. Avoid caffeine.
		❗ NURSING PRIORITY Monitor blood levels of medications.
Rapid-Acting Control *β2 Agonists* Albuterol: MDI, DPI, PO, aerosol Terbutaline: aerosol, PO Pirbuterol: MDI Levalbuterol: nebulizer Metaproterenol: nebulizer, MDI	Tachycardia, tremors, and angina can occur but are rare with inhaled preparations	1. Used for short-term relief of acute reversible airway problems. 2. Not used on continuous basis in absence of symptoms. 3. Client teaching regarding proper use of MDI and/or DPI.
Anticholinergics Ipratropium bromide: aerosol, MDI	Nasal drying and irritation Minimal systemic effects	1. Nasal spray may be used for clients with allergic rhinitis and asthma. 2. MDI used routinely, not with acute attacks to decrease bronchospasm associated with COPD. 3. Therapeutic effects begin within 30 secs.
Tiotropium: inhalation	Dry mouth	1. For long-term maintenance. 2. Takes effect in 20 min; lasts 24 hrs. 3. Report immediately: blurred vision, eye pain, halos.
Long-Acting Control *β2 Agonists* Salmeterol: DPI	Headache, cough, tremors, dizziness	1. Administered two times daily (every 12 hrs). 2. *Not used for short-term relief:* effects begin slowly and last for up to 12 hrs.
Corticosteroids Beclomethasone: MDI Triamcinolone acetonide: MDI Fluticasone: MDI	Oropharyngeal candidiasis, hoarseness, throat irritation, bad taste, cough, minimal side effects Can slow growth in children and adolescents With prolonged use, can cause adrenal suppression and bone loss	1. Works well with seasonal and exercise-induced asthma. 2. Prophylactic use decreases number and severity of attacks. 3. May be used with β_2 agonist. 4. Gargle after each dose and use a spacer to decrease candidiasis. 5. Do NOT use with acute attacks.

Continued

Appendix 11.2 RESPIRATORY MEDICATIONS—cont'd			℞

MEDICATIONS	SIDE EFFECTS	NURSING IMPLICATIONS
Mast Cell Stabilizers		
Cromolyn sodium: MDI	Inhalation: cough, dry mouth, throat irritation, and bad taste	1. Prophylactic use decreases number and severity of attacks. 2. Prevents bronchoconstriction before exposure to known precipitant (e.g., exercise). 3. Not used for an acute attack.
Nedocromil sodium: MDI	Unpleasant taste	1. Given to children over 6 years of age. 2. Maximal effects develop within 24 hrs. 3. Does not treat an acute asthmatic attack.
Leukotriene Modifiers Montelukast: PO Zafirlukast: PO	Headache, GI disturbance	1. Once daily dose in the evening. 2. Administer within 1 hr before or 2 hrs after eating.

Antitubercular: Broad-spectrum antibiotic specific to TB bacilli.

General Nursing Implications
- Client is not contagious when sputum culture is negative for three consecutive cultures.
- Use airborne respiratory precautions when sputum is positive for bacilli.
- Treatment includes combination of medications for about 6-12 months.
- Monitor liver function studies for clients receiving combination therapy.
- After initial therapy, medications may be administered once daily or on a twice-weekly schedule.
- Teach clients they should not stop taking the medications when they begin to feel better.
- Advise clients to return to the doctor if they notice any yellowing of the skin or eyes or begin to experience pain or swelling in joints, especially the big toe.
- Medication regimens always contain at least two medications to which the infection is sensitive; inadequate treatment is primary cause of increased incidence.

Isoniazid: PO, IM	Peripheral neuritis Hypersensitivity Hepatotoxicity Gastric irritation Weakness	1. Administer with (pyridoxine) vitamin B_6 to prevent peripheral neuritis. 2. Primary medication used in prophylactic and active treatment of TB.
Rifampin: PO Rifapentine: PO (a derivative of rifampin)	Hepatotoxicity – hepatitis Hypersensitivity Gastric upset	1. May negate the effectiveness of birth control pills and warfarin. 2. May turn body secretions orange: urine, perspiration, tears – can stain soft contacts.

Ethambutol: PO	Optic neuritis
	Allergic reactions –
	   dermatitis, pruritus
	Gastric upset
	Hepatotoxicity
	Elevated uric acid –
	   acute gout
		1. Give with food if GI problems occur.
		2. Observe for vision changes.
		3. Do not use in children under 7 years of age.

Pyrazinamide: PO	Hepatotoxicity Increased uric acid levels	1. May take with food to reduce GI upset.

Nasal Decongestants: Produce decongestion by acting on sympathetic nerve endings to produce constriction of dilated arterioles.

Phenylephrine hydrochloride:
   intranasal
Oxymetazoline: nasal spray
Pseudoephedrine: PO, nasal
   aerosol spray
	Large dose will cause
	CNS stimulation,
	anxiety, insomnia,
	increased blood
	pressure, tachycardia
		1. With long-term use of intranasal preparations, rebound congestion may occur.
		2. Not recommended for children under 6 years of age.
		3. Medications are frequently found in OTC combination decongestants.
		4. Caution clients with high blood pressure to check with their health care provider before using.

▪ **TEST ALERT** Evaluate client's use of home remedies and OTC medications.

Antihistamine: Blocks histamine release at H1 receptors (Appendix 6-2).

▪ **NURSING PRIORITY** Monitor for safety concerns related to dizziness and sedation in the older adult.

Appendix 11.2 RESPIRATORY MEDICATIONS—cont'd

MEDICATIONS	SIDE EFFECTS	NURSING IMPLICATIONS
Expectorant: Stimulates removal of respiratory secretions; reduces the viscosity of the mucus.		
Guaifenesin: PO	Nausea GI upset	1. Increase fluid intake for effectiveness. 2. Expect increased cough.
Mucolytic: Breaks down and loosens excessive mucus from the airways.		
Dornase Alfa: aerosol	Dyspnea Chest pain Fever Voice alteration Laryngitis Nasal stuffiness or discharge	1. Do not mix with any other drugs in the nebulizer. 2. Store in the refrigerator and protect from strong light.
Antivirals: Used for treatment of severe respiratory syncytial virus in hospitalized children.		
Ribavirin: aerosol	Anemia, increased respiratory problems	1. Should not be used for infants receiving mechanical ventilation. 2. Carefully monitor respiratory status of infant. 3. Used on hospitalized infants. 4. Pregnant nurses should not have direct contact with medication (Pregnancy Category X).
Prophylaxis: Respiratory syncytial virus (Chapter 22).		
Palivizumab: IM	Hypersensitivity	1. IM injections required once a month (very expensive); pain and erythema at injection site. 2. Dosing for high-risk infants and children should begin in late fall (November) and continue through early spring (April).

▲*CNS*, Central nervous system; *GI*, gastrointestinal; *IM*, intramuscularly; *IV*, intravenously; *OTC*, over the counter; *PO*, by mouth (orally); *subQ*, subcutaneously; *TB*, tuberculosis; *UTI*, urinary tract infection.

Appendix 11.3 SUDDEN AIRWAY OBSTRUCTION

❗ NURSING PRIORITY The procedure to remove airway obstruction is not effective in a child with epiglottitis or sudden airway obstruction caused by inflammation of the upper airways.

Goal: To identify foreign body airway obstruction.

❗ NURSING PRIORITY If the individual is coughing forcefully, do not interfere with attempts to cough and expel the foreign body. Do not administer any forceful blows to the back.

1. If the victim can speak or cry, there is probably adequate air exchange.
2. If the victim cannot speak or cry but is conscious, proceed to implement abdominal thrusts to clear the obstructed airway.
3. If the victim is unconscious:
   a. Call for help: dial 911/announce code blue, etc.
   b. Place client supine.
   c. Start CPR, starting with compressions (do not check for a pulse).
   d. Open the victim's mouth wide each time you prepare to give breaths
   e. Look for the object. If you see the object and can remove it, do so with your fingers.

f. If you do not see the object, continue with CPR using the chest compression-airway-breathing sequence.
g. If efforts to ventilate are unsuccessful, continue with CPR.

❗ TEST ALERT Identify and intervene in life-threatening situations; evaluate and document client's response to emergency procedures.

Goal: To clear obstructed airway – adult and child (conscious and unconscious).

1. Conscious: Perform Heimlich (abdominal thrusts) maneuver (chest thrusts if pregnant or obese) until obstruction is removed or client becomes unconscious.
   a. Stand behind client and wrap arms around waist.
   b. Make a fist and place thumb side against client's abdomen; place fist midline, just above the umbilicus, and below the xiphoid.
   c. Place other hand over fist and press into client's abdomen using quick upward thrusts.
   d. Repeat upward thrusts until foreign body is dislodged or client becomes unconscious.
2. Unconscious – If you see a choking victim collapse or become unresponsive:
   a. Activate the emergency response system.

Continued

b. Lower the victim to the ground and begin CPR, starting with compressions (do not check for a pulse).

c. Open the victim's mouth wide each time you prepare to give breaths. Look for the object.

d. If you see the object and can easily remove it, do so with your fingers.

e. If you do not see the object, continue with CPR using the chest compression-airway-breathing sequence (CAB).

f. If efforts to ventilate are unsuccessful, continue with CPR.

Goal: To clear obstructed airway – infant (conscious and unconscious).

1. Place the infant over the forearm with the head dependent.
2. Deliver up to five forceful back blows between the shoulder blades.

3. Supporting the head, turn the infant back over and administer up to five chest compressions (lower one-third of the sternum, approximately one finger breadth below the nipple line).

4. Attempt to remove foreign body only if it can be visualized.

5. If infant becomes unconscious, check the mouth before giving breaths to see if foreign body can be identified. Start CPR using CAB (compressions, airway, breathing).

> **! PEDIATRIC PRIORITY** Do not do a blind sweep of the infant or child's mouth; the foreign body should be visualized before you attempt to sweep the mouth.

Purposes

1. To remove air and/or fluid from the pleural cavity.
2. To restore negative pressure in the pleural cavity and promote reexpansion of the lung.

Principle of Water-Sealed Chest Drainage

The water seal (or dry seal on some equipment) serves as a one-way valve; it prevents air, under atmospheric pressure, from reentering the pleural cavity. On inspiration, air and fluid leave the pleural cavity via the chest tube; the water or dry seal keeps the air and fluid from reentering (Fig. 11.13).

> **! NURSING PRIORITY** There must be a seal (either water or dry seal) between the client and the atmospheric pressure.

Equipment

Three-chamber disposable chest drainage system: A molded plastic system that provides a collection chamber, a water-sealed chamber, and a suction-control chamber. When suction is applied, there should be a continuous, gentle bubbling in the water in the suction-control chamber (Fig. 11.14). In a dry seal system, a float is visible when the suction is on.

Assessment: Recognize Cues

1. Evaluate for hypoxia.
2. Evaluate character of respirations.
3. Assess for symmetric chest wall expansion.
4. Evaluate breath sounds bilaterally.
5. Palpate around insertion site for subcutaneous emphysema.

Nursing Interventions: Take Action

1. Perform range of motion of the affected arm and shoulder.
2. Encourage coughing and deep breathing every 2 hrs.
3. Encourage ambulation if appropriate.
4. Administer pain medications as indicated.
5. Place in low Fowler or semi-Fowler position.

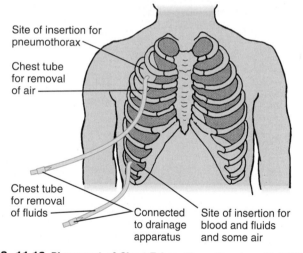

Site of insertion for pneumothorax

Chest tube for removal of air

Chest tube for removal of fluids

Connected to drainage apparatus

Site of insertion for blood and fluids and some air

FIG. 11.13 Placement of Chest Tubes. (From Stromberg H. [2023]. *Medical-surgical nursing: Concepts and practice* [5th ed.]. Elsevier.)

Observe Drainage System for Proper Functioning

1. Water level in the water-seal chamber and in the tubing from the client should fluctuate (tidal): rise on inspiration and fall on expiration. The opposite occurs with positive-pressure mechanical ventilation.

2. Continuous bubbling should not occur in the fluid where water seal is maintained; continuous bubbling indicates an air leak; continuous bubbling should occur only in the system that maintains a third chamber for suction control.

3. Initial bubbling may occur in the water-sealed chamber with coughing or with deep respiration as air is moved out of the pleural cavity, and intermittent bubbling may occur with respirations until the lung is reexpanded.

Maintain Water-Sealed System

1. Keep all drainage equipment below the chest-tube insertion site.

Appendix 11.4 WATER-SEALED CHEST DRAINAGE—cont'd

2. Evaluate for dependent loops in the tubing; this increases resistance to drainage. All extra tubing should be coiled in the bed and flow in a straight line to the system.
3. Tape all connections.
4. Note characteristics and amount of drainage. Mark level on the collection chamber of the drainage system as needed and every 8 hrs.
5. Vigorous "milking" or stripping chest tubes should not be done routinely on clients, because it increases pleural pressures.
6. Change the disposable chest drainage system when the collection chamber is approximately half full. The nurse can change the closed chest drainage system.
7. Do not clamp chest tubes during transport.

> ❗ **TEST ALERT** Monitor effective functioning of therapeutic devices; determine whether chest drainage is functioning properly; adjust tubes to promote drainage; identify abnormal chest tube drainage and *report to RN*.

Chest Tube Removal

1. Criteria for removal of the tube:
   a. Minimum or less than 50 mL drainage per day.
   b. Fluctuations/tidaling/bubbling stop in the water-seal chamber.
   c. Chest x-ray film reveals expanded lung.
   d. Client has good breath sounds and is breathing comfortably.
2. Procedure.
   a. Provide appropriate analgesia about 30 mins before procedure.
   b. Generally, the health care provider will want the client in a low Fowler or semi-Fowler position, unless contraindicated.
   c. The health care provider will ask the client to exhale and hold it or to exhale and bear down (a Valsalva maneuver). Either of these procedures will increase the intrathoracic pressure and prevent air from entering the pleural space.
   d. With the client holding their breath, the health care provider will quickly remove the tube and place an occlusive bandage over the area; the client can then breathe normally.

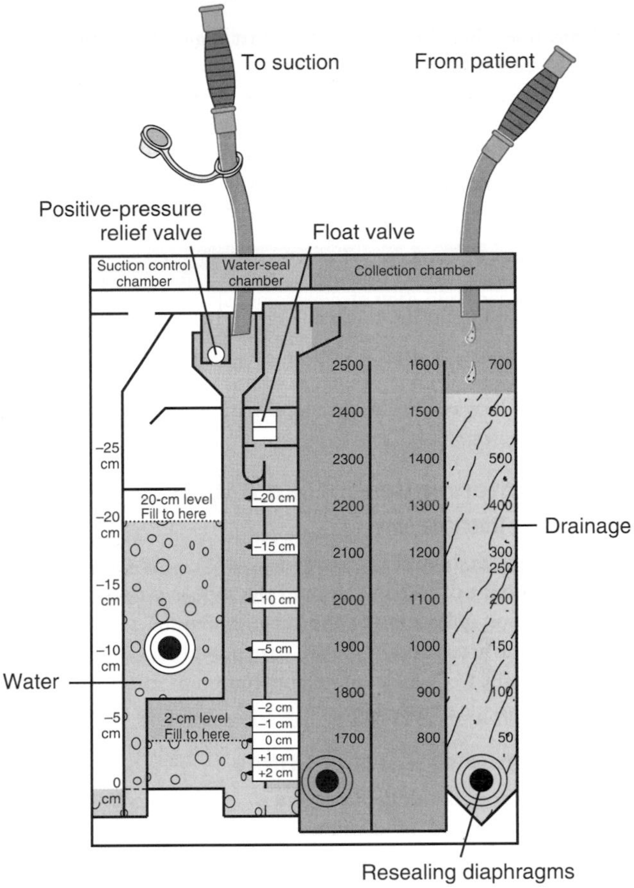

FIG. 11.14 Water-Sealed Chest Drainage. (From Harkreader H, Hogan MA. [2004]. *Fundamentals of nursing: Caring and clinical judgment* [2nd ed.]. Saunders.)

   e. Assess the client's tolerance of the procedure; check breath sounds, and a chest x-ray film may be obtained to determine the lungs remain fully expanded.

Appendix 11.5 ARTIFICIAL AIRWAYS

Endotracheal Intubation

Placement of an ET tube through the mouth or nose into the trachea (Fig. 11.15).

Purpose

To provide an immediate airway; to maintain a patent airway; to facilitate removal of secretions and provide method for artificial ventilation.

Nursing Interventions: Take Action

1. Provide warm, humidified oxygen.
2. Establish method of communication, because the client cannot speak; child is unable to cry.
3. Maintain safety measures.
   a. Prevent client from accidentally removing tube: soft hand/wrist restraints or mittens.
   b. Secure ET tube to the face.
   c. Child with an ET tube requires constant attendance.
4. As soon as tube is inserted, assess symmetry of chest expansion and bilateral breath sounds. Assess for presence of bilateral breath sounds every 2 hrs. If tube slips farther into the trachea, it may pass into the right mainstem bronchus, obliterating the left mainstem bronchus. Determine placement by checking breath sounds.
5. Cuff must remain inflated if client is on a volume ventilator. If the client has adequate spontaneous respiration and is not on a ventilator, the cuff may be left deflated.
6. Minimal occluding volume (MOV) should be used when inflating the cuff to prevent aspiration or to maintain mechanical ventilation. This is accomplished by placing a stethoscope over the trachea or by listening to the client's breath sounds to

Continued

Appendix 11.7   OXYGEN—cont'd

4. Use oxygen with caution in clients with chronic airway disease; most often administered via mask or nasal cannula at 2 to 4 LPM unless client is in severe distress.
5. Oxygen supports combustion but is not explosive.

Oxygen Toxicity

A medically induced condition produced by inhalation of high concentrations of oxygen over a prolonged period. Toxicity is directly related to concentration of oxygen, duration of therapy, and degree of lung disease present.
1. Tracheal irritation and cough.
2. Dyspnea and increasing cough.
3. Decrease in vital capacity.
4. The Pao_2 continues to decrease, even with an increasing Fio_2.
5. Atelectasis.

Appendix 11.8   VENTILATORS

TEST ALERT Monitor and maintain clients on a ventilator.

Ventilators

Ventilators deliver air and/or oxygen at a predetermined tidal volume. The ventilator delivers the volume of air and/or oxygen within safe ranges of pressure. A pressure limit is set, and an alarm will sound if the tidal volume cannot be delivered within the set pressure limits. The intrathoracic pressure is increased with the ventilator; this decreases the venous blood return (preload) to the right side of the heart and subsequently decreases cardiac output.

Patterns of Ventilation

1. **Control ventilation:** Delivers a predetermined rate and volume of gas (air/oxygen) independent of client's effort. This mode of ventilation is rarely used.
2. **Assist-control ventilation (AC):** The client may initiate the cycle with inspiration. All initiated breaths are supported with the preset tidal volume or pressure.
3. **Synchronized intermittent mandatory ventilation (SIMV):** Delivers preset tidal volume or pressure and rate allowing for spontaneous breaths between; synchronizes with the client's efforts. Used as a weaning mode.
4. **Positive end-expiratory pressure (PEEP):** Maintains positive pressure at alveolar level at end of expiration to facilitate the diffusion of oxygen. PEEP will increase the intrathoracic pressure, thus further decreasing the venous return and causing a decrease in preload.
5. **Indications for use:** ARDS; clients unable to maintain patent airway; neuromuscular diseases causing respiratory failure.
6. **Continuous positive airway pressure (CPAP):** Used to augment the functional residual capacity (FRC) during spontaneous breathing. Used to wean clients from ventilators and may be administered by face mask. Clients must have spontaneous respirations.
7. **High-frequency ventilation:** Small amounts of gas (air/oxygen) are delivered at a rapid rate. Requires sedation and pharmacologic paralysis.

TEST ALERT Identify changes in respiratory status and intervene to improve it; assess client for unexpected response to therapy.

Nursing Interventions: Take Action

1. All alarms should be set and checked each shift, especially low pressure and low exhaled volume.

2. A bag and valve mask resuscitator is placed in the client's room in case of mechanical failure of equipment.
3. Central venous pressure (CVP) and pulmonary artery pressure readings will be affected by the ventilator; readings should be determined in a consistent manner.
4. Ventilator setting for Fio_2, tidal volume, respiratory rate, pattern of control (AC/SIMV, etc.), and PEEP should be checked and charted in the nurses' notes.
5. Assess client's tolerance of the ventilator; IV medications such as propofol, a short-acting hypnotic that produces amnesia, or fentanyl, a central nervous system depressant, may be used. If weaning or removal of the ventilator is anticipated, do not medicate the client.
6. Clients frequently experience a high level of anxiety and fear. Explain equipment and alarms to the client and to the family. Maintain a calm, reassuring approach to the client.
7. When ventilator changes are made, carefully assess the client's response (pulse oximetry, ABGs, vital signs).
8. Never allow the condensation in the tubing to flow back into fluid reservoir.
9. Adequate nutrition is mandatory and will facilitate weaning. The GI tract is preferred, if functioning.
   a. Nutritional support provided via the GI tract preserves mucosal integrity, improves intestinal blood, and decreases the incidences of sepsis.
   b. The use of a small-bore transpyloric tube emptying in the duodenum is the recommended route to administer either bolus or continuous feedings. (Elevate the head of the bed 30 degrees during feeding.)

Common Ventilator Alarms

1. High pressure alarm: Sounds when tidal volume cannot be delivered at set pressure limit.
   Nursing Care: Increased secretions – suction; client biting tube – place oral airway; coughing and increased anxiety – administer sedative.
2. Low pressure alarm: Sounds when the machine cannot deliver the tidal volume because of a leak or break in the system.
   Nursing Care: Disconnection – check all connections for break in system; client stops breathing on the SIMV mode – evaluate client's tolerance; tracheostomy or ET tube cuff is leaking – check for air escaping around cuff, may need to replace tracheostomy tube if cuff is ruptured.

Weaning From Ventilators

Weaning may be done via a spontaneous breathing trial using a T-piece with heated mist and oxygen or by SIMV mode or CPAP

Appendix 11.8   VENTILATORS—cont'd

Ⓡ

on the ventilator. During weaning, it is imperative for the nurse to maintain close observation for increasing fatigue, dyspnea, and hypoxia. If client experiences dyspnea, they should be returned to the ventilator at whatever parameters were being used, and the doctor should be notified; anticipate drawing blood to determine of ABG values.

> **❗ NURSING PRIORITY** Focus on the client, not on the ventilator. In case of problems with the ventilator, assess the client; if adequate ventilation is not being achieved, take client off the ventilator, maintain respirations via a bag and valve mask resuscitator, and call for assistance.

Appendix 11.9   NURSING PROCEDURE: SPUTUM SPECIMEN COLLECTION

Ⓡ

Sputum Specimen Collection

This test analyzes sputum samples (material expectorated from client's lungs and bronchi during deep coughing) to diagnose respiratory disease, identify the cause of pulmonary infections, identify abnormal lung cells, and assist in managing pulmonary disease.

Nursing Interventions: Take Action

1. Sputum for culture and sensitivity should be collected as soon as possible (before administration of antibiotics, if possible) to facilitate identification of bacteria and treatment.
2. Specimens for cytology and for acid-fast bacilli for TB diagnostics should be collected in the morning when bacteria and cells are most concentrated.
3. No mouthwash should be used before collection of specimen; have client rinse their mouth with water or brush their teeth with water, but do not use toothpaste.
4. Aerosol mist will assist in decreasing thickness of sputum and increasing effectiveness of coughing.
5. Maintain strict asepsis and standard precautions in collecting and transporting specimen; use sterile specimen collection container.

6. Acid-fast bacillus: Sputum collection should be done on 3 consecutive days.
7. Culture and sensitivity: Initial specimen should be obtained before antibiotics are administered.

Clinical Tips for Problem Solving

If client experiences pain while coughing:
- Support painful area with roll pillows to minimize pain and discomfort.
- Encourage client to take several deep breaths before beginning. This assists in triggering the cough reflex and aerates the lungs (Box 11.1).
- If client is unable to produce sputum specimen:
  - Attempt procedure early in the morning when mucus production is greatest.
  - Notify health care provider to obtain orders for a bronchodilator or nebulization therapy.

Practice & Next Generation NCLEX (NGN) Questions
Respiratory: Care of Adult Clients

More questions on
evolve

1. The nurse reviews the written orders for a client admitted with a respiratory problem. The nurse is to obtain a sputum specimen for culture and sensitivity. How should the specimen be obtained?
   1. Ask the respiratory therapist to suction the client.
   2. Instruct the client to spit in a clean specimen container.
   3. Restrict fluids for 4 hrs before the specimen is to be collected.
   4. Obtain the specimen in the morning after the client rinses the mouth with water.

2. Clients with COPD are usually on low levels of oxygen via nasal cannula. What problem would occur if these clients received too high an oxygen concentration?
   1. Increased sputum production with decreased oxygen exchange.
   2. Respiratory rate greater than 30 breaths per minute.
   3. Decrease in rate and depth of respirations.
   4. Increased wheezing and irritability.

3. A thoracentesis procedure is to be done in the client's room. The nurse would place the client in which position for this procedure?
   1. Prone position with feet elevated.
   2. Sitting with upper torso over bedside table.
   3. Lying on left side with right knee bent.
   4. Semi-Fowler with lower torso flat.

4. What findings would the nurse expect to find in a client who is developing pneumonia as a complication of immobility?
   1. Diminished breath sounds.
   2. Use of accessory respiratory muscles.
   3. Dry hacking cough at night.
   4. Bradypnea and lethargy.

5. An expectorant has been ordered for a client. How will the nurse evaluate the client to determine the effectiveness of the medication?
   1. Decrease in the viscosity of the sputum, making it easier to cough up sputum.
   2. Decrease in the amount of mucus by drying the mucous membrane.
   3. Decrease in respiratory rate with a decrease in dyspnea.
   4. Increased depth and quality of respirations.

6. Which client would be at an increased risk for development of a deep vein thrombosis (DVT) and potential for pulmonary emboli?
   1. Client in chronic kidney failure on hemodialysis.
   2. Client with history of hypertension and current BP 180/110 mm Hg.
   3. Older adult client with kyphosis from osteoporosis and respiratory difficulty.
   4. Client who is immobile after repair of a fractured femur.

7. A client is experiencing progression of a chronic obstructive pulmonary condition. What characteristic finding would be discovered on assessment of this client?
   1. Increased temperature and headache.
   2. Hyperventilation and bradycardia.
   3. Increasing dyspnea with cough and fatigue.
   4. Production of sputum and frequent cough.

8. What is important for the nurse to anticipate in providing care for a client who is 2 days postoperative for a total laryngectomy?
   1. The client will have a hoarse voice and difficulty speaking.
   2. The tracheostomy stoma will require cleansing and protection.
   3. The client will experience respiratory fatigue with activity.
   4. Hourly suctioning will be required to reduce secretions.

9. A client is 3 days postoperative from a thoracotomy. What would be a normal finding when assessing the chest tube?
   1. Dark drainage with no fluctuation of the fluid in the tubing.
   2. Bubbling in the collection chamber on expiration.
   3. 300 mL daily of serosanguineous drainage.
   4. Moderate amount of bright red drainage in tubing.

10. When transporting a client to the radiology department, how should the nurse provide for the water-sealed chest drainage system?
    1. Hang the drainage apparatus on the head of the bed.
    2. Clamp the chest tube until the client reaches the radiology department.
    3. Keep the collection system below the level of the client's chest.
    4. Disconnect chest tube from drainage collection chamber.

11. A client is admitted to the emergency room with difficulty breathing. The client's history reveals they are a 40 pack-year cigarette smoker. The following are the admitting nurses' notes.

Health History	Nurses' Notes	Vital Signs	Laboratory Results

1500: A 66-year-old client is admitted with difficulty breathing and reports a 40 pack-year history of cigarette smoking. Client states they cough all the time; however, it has become worse. Expectorating blood-tinged sputum and reporting slight tightness and pain in the chest. Color is pale and client appears weak and thin. Wheezing and diminished breath sounds bilaterally on auscultation.

- Temperature: 99 °F (37.2 °C)
- BP: 148/78 mm Hg
- Heart rate: 104 beats/min and regular
- Respirations: 24 breaths/min
- SpO2: 89% on room air

For each client finding, use an X to specify whether the finding is consistent with the disease process of lung cancer, bacterial pneumonia, or tuberculosis. Each finding may support more than one disease process.

CLIENT FINDING	LUNG CANCER	BACTERIAL PNEUMONIA	TUBERCULOSIS
Productive cough			
Wheezing			
Persistent cough			
Dyspnea			
Unintended weight loss			
Fever			
Purulent sputum			
Night sweats			
Blood-tinged sputum			

12. The following are the nurses' notes for a client who is admitted to the emergency department.

Health History	Nurses' Notes	Vital Signs	Laboratory Results

1500: An adult client was in a motor vehicle collision and reports the airbag deployed in the car when the left side of the car was hit. Admission vital signs are pulse oximetry (SPO2) 93%, pulse 88, respirations 28, BP 112/77. The client has lacerations on the left arm and bruising across the left side of the chest.
1530: After returning from radiology, the client suddenly develops shortness of breath, reports chest tightness, feels as though they can't get a deep breath, and appears anxious. Vital signs are: SpO2 89%, pulse 100, respirations 34, BP 115/80. Lung sounds diminished and absent over the left upper lobe.
1545: Chest x-ray confirms a pneumothorax on the right side with no shifting of the mediastinum or trachea. Client is prepared for placement of a chest tube on the left side.
1600: Chest tube inserted and placed to water seal without suction.

For each assessment finding listed below, use an X to specify whether the finding indicates the chest-tube insertion intervention was effective (helped to meet expected outcomes), ineffective (did not help meet expected outcomes), or unrelated (not related to the expected outcome).

ASSESSMENT FINDING	EFFECTIVE	INEFFECTIVE	UNRELATED
Persistent bubbling in water-seal bottle			
Chest dressing dry and intact			
Drainage system placed above chest tube entry site.			
SpO_2 88%, respirations 32			
Reports nausea			
Chest tubing is pinned to the client's bed clothes			
Tidaling noted in the water-seal bottle			

⚡ Answers to Practice & Next Generation NCLEX (NGN) Questions

1. 4

Client Needs: Physiological Integrity/Reduction of Risk Potential

Clinical Judgment/Cognitive Skill: Take Action

Item Type: Multiple Choice

Rationale & Test-Taking Strategy: Think about when pulmonary secretions are the most abundant. Obtain the specimen early in the morning after the client rinses the mouth with water, because secretions collect during the night. Suctioning would be indicated if the client could not cough effectively to produce a sputum specimen. The client needs to expectorate sputum into a container after coughing deeply. Spitting usually involves the removal of saliva from the mouth. Hydration is necessary to produce a sputum specimen, so restricting fluids would not be indicated. A sterile collection container should be used to collect a sputum specimen.

2. 3

Client Needs: Physiological Integrity/Physiological Adaptation

Clinical Judgment/Cognitive Skill: Analyze Cues

Item Type: Multiple Choice

Rationale & Test-Taking Strategy: Ask yourself, "Are there specific problems with receiving too high a concentration of oxygen by nasal cannula?" The client with COPD is dependent on their lower level of oxygen saturation for the stimulus to breathe, because they have adjusted to the high levels of CO_2 circulating in their body. Increasing the client's oxygen level too much will decrease their stimulus to breathe, and they will begin to hypoventilate with a decreased respiratory rate and depth of respirations. Apnea can develop. Sputum production, wheezing, and irritability are not necessarily indicative of problems with increased inspired levels of oxygen.

3. 2

Client Needs: Physiological Integrity/Reduction of Risk Potential

Clinical Judgment/Cognitive Skill: Take Action

Item Type: Multiple Choice

Rationale & Test-Taking Strategy: Consider the thoracentesis procedure. Where would the needle most likely be inserted: the front or back of the body? The client needs to be in an upright position, leaning over a bedside table for easier access to the thoracic cavity. An alternative position for the client who is unable to sit upright may be with the client in a side-lying position with the head of the bed elevated. Lying on the side is okay, but the client needs the head of the bed elevated, not the right knee bent. Prone position would restrict respirations and would be contraindicated in a client who needs fluid removed from the pleural space.

4. 1

Client Needs: Physiological Integrity/Physiological Adaptation

Clinical Judgment/Cognitive Skill: Analyze Cues

Item Type: Multiple Choice

Rationale & Test-Taking Strategy: Recall what you know about the complications of immobility and how they affect different body systems, specifically the lungs. Regardless of the precipitating cause of pneumonia, there is a decrease in breath sounds over the area of consolidation. The use of accessory muscles indicates difficulty breathing, not necessarily pneumonia. The cough is usually productive, and the client has an increased respiratory rate (tachypnea).

5. 1

Client Needs: Physiological Integrity/Pharmacological Therapies

Clinical Judgment/Cognitive Skill: Evaluate Outcomes

Item Type: Multiple Choice

Rationale & Test-Taking Strategy: Recall how expectorants work; they liquefy respiratory secretions to stimulate coughing and to make the mucus easier to cough up. Antihistamines and decongestants dry up the mucus and make it difficult to remove by coughing. A bronchodilator will decrease difficulty breathing by opening the airways. Expectorants do not increase the depth or quality of respirations.

6. 4

Client Needs: Physiological Integrity/Physiological Adaptation

Clinical Judgment/Cognitive Skill: Analyze Cues

Item Type: Multiple Choice

Rationale & Test-Taking Strategy: Pulmonary embolus is a common complication of immobility (venous pooling of blood) and DVT (increased incidence of venous pooling and clot formation). Pulmonary emboli are secondary to venous pooling, which most often occurs from immobility. The only client listed that is immobilized is the client with the fractured femur. The other clients can be up and about.

7. 3

Client Needs: Physiological Integrity/Physiological Adaptation

Clinical Judgment/Cognitive Skill: Recognize Cues

Item Type: Multiple Choice

Rationale & Test-Taking Strategy: Dyspnea and fatigue are characteristic in the progression of COPD. Cor pulmonale (right-sided heart failure) commonly occurs as the condition progresses. Production of sputum and cough are common and not indicative of progression of the disease. Temperature and headache may be indicative of an infection. An infection would be a complication, not progression of the condition.

8. 2

Client Needs: Physiological Integrity/Physiological Adaptation

Clinical Judgment/Cognitive Skill: Analyze Cues

Item Type: Multiple Choice

Rationale & Test-Taking Strategy: Note the **key** word, "total." In a total laryngectomy, the client will have a permanent tracheostomy and will have lost normal voice. The tracheostomy should be suctioned as necessary; however, not every hour. The client may or may not experience respiratory fatigue with activity. The client's lungs were not the site of the malignancy; it was in the throat or larynx.

9. 1

Client Needs: Physiological Integrity/Reduction of Risk Potential

Clinical Judgment/Cognitive Skill: Recognize Cues

Item Type: Multiple Choice

Rationale & Test-Taking Strategy: Recall the purpose of inserting a chest tube after a thoracotomy. Three days after surgery, the lung should be expanded, which means there will be a minimum amount of dark drainage and no fluctuation of the fluid level in the tubing; 300 mL of serosanguineous drainage would be expected on the operative day, as well as the first postoperative day. There should be no bubbling in the collection chamber. There should not be any bright red blood at this time.

10. **3**
Client Needs: Physiological Integrity/Reduction of Risk Potential
Clinical Judgment/Cognitive Skill: Take Action
Item Type: Multiple Choice
Rationale & Test-Taking Strategy: Remember the principles of chest tube function. The chest collection bottle should always be kept below the level of the chest to prevent drainage from going back into the pleural cavity. The chest tube should not be clamped, and the chest tubes are not disconnected from the drainage collection chambers. The drainage collection should never be placed on the head of the bed.

11. A client is admitted to the emergency room with difficulty breathing. The client's history reveals a 40 pack-year cigarette smoker. The following is the admitting nurses' notes.

| Health History | Nurses' Notes | Vital Signs | Laboratory Results |

1500 A 66-year-old client is admitted with difficulty breathing and reports a 40 pack-year history of cigarette smoking. Client states they cough all the time; however, it has become worse, expectorating blood-tinged sputum and reporting slight tightness and pain in the chest. Color is pale, and client appears weak and thin. Wheezing and diminished breath sounds bilaterally on auscultation.

- Temperature: 99°F (37.2°C)
- BP: 148/78 mmHg
- Heart rate: 104 bpm and regular
- Respirations: 24 breaths/min
- SpO$_2$: 89% on room air

For each client finding, use an X to specify whether the finding is consistent with the disease process of lung cancer, bacterial pneumonia, or tuberculosis. Each finding may support more than one disease process.

CLIENT FINDING	LUNG CANCER	BACTERIAL PNEUMONIA	TUBERCULOSIS
Productive cough		X	X
Wheezing	X		
Persistent cough	X		
Dyspnea	X	X	X
Unintended weight loss	X		X
Fever	X	X	X
Purulent sputum		X	X
Night sweats			X
Blood-tinged sputum	X	X	X

Client Needs: Physiological Integrity/Physiological Adaptation
Clinical Judgment/Cognitive Skill: Analyze Cues
Item Type: Matrix Multiple Response
Rationale & Test-Taking Strategy: Remember that each client finding may be consistent with other disease processes. Cigarette smoking is the cause of the majority of cases of lung cancer. The most common symptom, and often the one that is reported first, is a persistent cough. Dyspnea, wheezing, and blood-tinged sputum may be present because of bleeding caused by the cancer. Chest pain may be present. Later manifestations include nonspecific systemic symptoms, such as anorexia, nausea and vomiting, fatigue, and weight loss. Hoarseness may be present due to laryngeal nerve involvement. The most common signs and symptoms of bacterial pneumonia are cough, fever, chills, dyspnea, tachypnea, and pleuritic chest pain. The cough often is productive, and the sputum may be green, yellow, or even rust colored (blood-flecked), depending on the microorganism responsible for the infection. The primary manifestation of tuberculosis (TB) is an initial dry cough that often becomes productive with mucoid or mucopurulent sputum; however, sometimes there is blood in the sputum (hemoptysis). Clients with active TB may initially present with fatigue, malaise, anorexia, unexplained weight loss, low-grade fevers, and night sweats. Dyspnea is a late symptom that may signify considerable pulmonary disease or a pleural effusion.

12. The following are the nurses' notes for a client who is admitted to the emergency department.

| Health History | Nurses' Notes | Vital Signs | Laboratory Results |

1500 An adult client was in a motor vehicle collision and reports the airbag deployed in the car when the left side of the car was hit. Admission vital signs are pulse oximetry (SPO$_2$) 93%, pulse 88 bpm, respirations 28 breaths/min, BP 112/77. The client has lacerations on the left arm and bruising across the left side of the chest.

1530 After returning from radiology, the client suddenly develops shortness of breath, reports chest tightness, feels as though they cannot get a deep breath, and appears anxious. Vital signs are: SpO$_2$ 89%, pulse 100, respirations 34, BP 115/80. Lung sounds are diminished and absent over the left upper lobe.

1545 Chest x-ray confirms a pneumothorax on the right side with no shifting of the mediastinum or trachea. Client is prepared for placement of a chest tube on the left side.

1600 Chest tube inserted and placed to water seal without suction.

For each assessment finding listed below, use an **X** to specify whether the finding indicates the chest tube insertion intervention was effective (helped to meet expected outcomes), ineffective (did not help to meet expected outcomes) or unrelated (not related to the expected outcome).

ASSESSMENT FINDING	EFFECTIVE	INEFFECTIVE	UNRELATED
Persistent bubbling in water seal bottle		X	
Chest dressing dry and intact	X		
Drainage system placed above chest tube entry site		X	
SpO$_2$ 88%, respirations 32 bpm		X	
Reports nausea			X
Chest tubing is pinned to the client's bed clothes		X	
Tidaling noted in the water-seal bottle	X		

Client Needs: Physiological Integrity/Reduction of Risk Potential
Clinical Judgment/Cognitive Skill: Evaluate Outcomes
Item Type: Matrix Multiple Choice
Rationale & Test-Taking Strategy: Review each assessment finding and determine if it indicates the chest tube insertion was effective. Because the client has a pneumothorax, probably due to the deployment of the air bag causing direct blunt trauma to the chest wall, there should not be any drainage or blood noted in the chest tube. The chest tube is functioning to remove the air that is in the pleural space. There should be no dependent loops of the chest tubing. The drainage system must always remain below the client's chest level, as it works by gravity. The nurse can loop the tubing on the bed to prevent dependent loops from forming. Never pin the chest tubing to the client's clothes. Never clamp the chest tubing unless searching for an air leak or specifically instructed to do so by a provider. The nurse can expect tidaling, which is the movement of fluid in the water-seal bottle, when the client breathes. Persistent bubbling in the water-seal bottle indicates an air leak. Occasional bubbles may appear with breathing, sneezing, and coughing. The SpO$_2$ 88% and respirations of 32 bpm indicate the client's condition is not improving, and the interventions are ineffective. Nausea is unrelated to the functioning of the chest tube system and resolving the pneumothorax. Other nursing actions include making sure the tubing is covered with an occlusive dressing and taped securely to the client's chest and ensuring all connections are tightly secured to prevent leaks.

Vascular: Care of Adult Clients

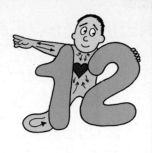

CHAPTER 12
VASCULAR

PHYSIOLOGY OF THE VASCULAR SYSTEM

Vessels

A. Arteries: primary function is to transport nutrients and oxygen to the cellular level.

B. Capillaries: allow the exchange of fluid and nutrients between the blood and the interstitial fluid.

C. Veins: primary function is to return blood to the heart.

D. Lymphatic system: primary function is to return fluid and protein to the blood from the interstitial fluid.

Blood Pressure

A. Peripheral resistance is resistance of arterioles to flow of blood.
   1. *Dilation* decreases peripheral resistance, thereby *decreasing* blood pressure (BP).
   2. *Vasoconstriction* increases peripheral resistance, thereby *increasing* BP.

B. Systolic pressure represents the ejection of blood from the heart.

C. Diastolic pressure represents the pressure remaining in the arteries at the end of systole.

D. Pulse pressure is the difference between the systolic and diastolic pressures.

E. Mean arterial pressure (MAP) is the average pressure within the arterial system.

F. Autonomic nervous system influence on BP:
   1. Parasympathetic system stimulates the vagus nerve.
   2. Sympathetic nervous system controls BP by:
      a. Maintaining peripheral resistance through constriction and dilation of the vessels.
      b. Increasing heart rate and force of contraction.
      c. Causing constriction of the large veins, which promotes an increase in venous return to the heart, thereby increasing cardiac output.

G. Kidney influence on BP:
   1. Renin, a strong vasoconstrictor, increases BP.
   2. Activation of the renin-angiotensin system increases secretion of aldosterone, thus precipitating sodium and water retention and increasing vascular volume.

H. Vasopressin (antidiuretic hormone) is released when BP falls below normal; this increases the blood volume, which increases BP.

System Assessment: Recognize Cues

A. Health history.

1. Identify risk factors for peripheral vascular disease (PVD) and shock.

B. Physical assessment.
   1. Inspection.
      a. Inspect extremities for edema, color changes, varicosities, ulcers, hair distribution.
      b. Monitor for jugular venous distention (JVD).
   2. Palpation.
      a. Monitor temperature, moisture, pulses, and edema in extremities.
      b. Neurovascular assessment (Fig. 12.1).
   3. Auscultation.
      a. Evaluate BP (Box 12.1).
      b. Monitor for bruit (buzzing or humming heard over blood vessel).

DISORDERS OF THE VASCULAR SYSTEM

Atherosclerosis

A *gradual thickening and narrowing of the arterial lumen*; sometimes referred to as "hardening of the arteries" (Fig. 12.2).

A. Process is slow and can gradually lead to a significant decrease in blood supply to tissue.

B. Arteries commonly affected by atherosclerosis and the ensuing problems:
   1. Coronary arteries – myocardial infarction (MI).
   2. Cerebrovascular arteries – stroke, brain attack.
   3. Aorta – aortic aneurysm, PVD.
   4. Renal arteries – hypertension, chronic kidney disease.
   5. Peripheral arteries – PVD.

Assessment: Recognize Cues

A. Modifiable risk factors:
   1. Elevated serum cholesterol and triglyceride levels.
   2. Sedentary lifestyle, obesity.
   3. Stress, smoking.

B. Nonmodifiable risk factors:
   1. Familial tendencies, age.
   2. Race, gender (men at greater risk than women until age 60).

C. Conditions accelerating atherosclerotic development:
   1. Diabetes mellitus (DM).
   2. Hypertension.
   3. High cholesterol/triglyceride levels.

NEUROVASCULAR ASSESSMENT

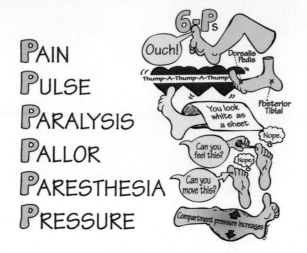

FIG. 12.1 Neurovascular Assessment. (From Zerwekh J, Garneau A, Miller CJ. [2017]. *Digital collection of the memory notebooks of nursing* [4th ed.]. Chandler, AZ: Nursing Education Consultants, Inc.)

Box 12.1	OLDER ADULT CARE FOCUS

Evaluation of Blood Pressure

- If a client has had hypertension for a long time, the client's "normal" blood pressure (BP) may need to be higher to maintain adequate blood flow and allow the client to perform activities of daily living (ADLs).
- Teach the client how to avoid problems with orthostatic hypotension.
- Obtain BP reading while client is standing, lying, and sitting. Make sure client has not had any nicotine or caffeine for about 1 hr before BP is measured.
- Palpate for disappearance of the brachial or radial pulse when assessing BP to avoid the auscultatory gap.
- Compliance problems occur when client must take several medications for BP and cope with other chronic health problems.

D. Clinical manifestations: depends on artery involved.
E. Diagnostics – serum lipids (Appendix 12.1).

Analyze Cues and Prioritize Hypotheses

The most important problems are need for health teaching to minimize risk factors, especially hyperlipidemia, and making necessary lifestyle changes.

Generate Solutions

Treatment

A. Decrease risk factors (exercise, stop smoking, decrease weight, decrease stress, and decrease fat in diet).
B. Antihyperlipidemic and peripheral vasodilating medications (Appendix 12.2).
C. Vascular surgery.

PROGRESSION OF ATHEROSCLEROSIS

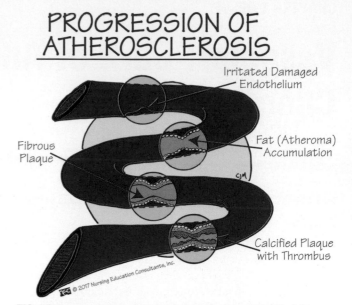

FIG. 12.2 Progression of Atherosclerosis. (From Zerwekh J, Garneau A, Miller CJ. [2017]. *Digital collection of the memory notebooks of nursing* [4th ed.]. Chandler, AZ: Nursing Education Consultants, Inc.)

Table 12.1	CHOLESTEROL AND LIPOPROTEIN LEVELS
Cholesterol (total)	<200 mg/dL (5.18 mmol/L)
Low-density lipoprotein (LDL)	<130 mg/dL (3.37 mmol/L)
High-density lipoprotein (HDL)	>40 mg/dL (1.04 mmol/L) in males; >50 mg/dL (1.30 mmol/L) in females
Triglycerides	<150 mg/dL (1.69 mmol/L)

Nursing Interventions: Take Action

Goal: To identify individuals at high risk.

A. Screen for and recognize modifiable and nonmodifiable risk factors.
B. Recognize significant deviations of laboratory values (Table 12.1).
C. Identify and control conditions that accelerate atherosclerotic development.
D. Recognize common signs and symptoms of atherosclerosis.

Hypertension

Hypertension or high BP is an elevation above the normal limit.

A. Definitions.
   1. Normal BP is defined as less than 120/80 mm Hg.
   2. Elevated BP (high-normal) is a systolic BP (SBP) of 120 to 129 mm Hg and diastolic BP (DBP) less than 80 mm Hg.

HYPERTENSION

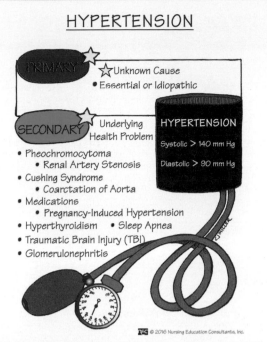

FIG. 12.3 Hypertension. (From Zerwekh J, Garneau A, Miller CJ. [2017]. *Digital collection of the memory notebooks of nursing* [4th ed.]. Chandler, AZ: Nursing Education Consultants, Inc.)

Table 12.2 RISK FACTORS FOR ESSENTIAL HYPERTENSION

Nonmodifiable Factors	
Age	Develops between 30 and 50 years of age. Poorer prognosis when it develops at younger age.
Gender	More prevalent in men under 55 years of age; after age 55, more prevalent in women.
Ethnic group	The incidence of hypertension is twice as high among African Americans as among whites.
Family history	Clients with parents or siblings who have hypertension are at greater risk for high blood pressure at a younger age.
Modifiable Factors	
Obesity	Weight gain is associated with increased frequency of hypertension. Central abdominal obesity poses greatest risk.
Stress	Sustained or repeated stressors.
Substance abuse	Drug abuse, drinking more than 1 oz (30 mL) of alcohol per day, use of tobacco products.
Excess sodium intake	Can cause water retention and hypertension, especially in those who are already overweight.
Elevated serum lipids	Elevated levels of cholesterol and triglycerides are primary risk factors in atherosclerosis, which is a contributing factor to hypertension.
Sedentary lifestyle	Regular physical activity helps decrease risk.
Diabetes mellitus	Blood vessel disease associated with diabetes mellitus leads to a high risk for hypertension.
Diet	Diet high in saturated fats and salt leads to atherosclerotic plaque buildup.

Data from the American Heart Association: *Hypertension Guideline Toolkit*. (2019). http://aha-clinical-review.ascendeventmedia.com/books/aha-high-blood-pressure-toolkit/

3. Stage 1 hypertension is defined as SBP 130 to 139 mm Hg and/or DBP 80 to 89 mm Hg.
4. Stage 2 hypertension is defined as SBP ≥140 mm Hg and/or DBP ≥ 90 mm Hg.
5. Recommends a target BP of <130/80 mm Hg for older clients (aged ≥65).

B. Classification (Fig. 12.3).
   1. Primary hypertension (essential or idiopathic): exact cause unknown.
   2. Secondary hypertension: elevated BP with a specific cause that can be identified and corrected.
   3. Hypertensive crisis (malignant hypertension): a sudden and severely elevated BP, often above 180/120 mm Hg with clinical evidence of target organ disease, which may be life threatening.

Assessment: Recognize Cues

A. Risk factors (Table 12.2).
B. Clinical manifestations of primary hypertension:
   1. Most often asymptomatic ("the silent killer").
   2. Increase in BP.
   3. Cardiac effects:
      a. Angina, fatigue, activity intolerance.
      b. Acute coronary syndrome (ACS), heart failure.
      c. Left ventricular hypertrophy, palpitations.
   4. Cerebrovascular effects:
      a. Transient ischemic attack (TIA).
      b. Stroke (cerebrovascular accident [CVA], brain attack).
      c. Dizziness, visual disturbances.
   5. Peripheral vascular effects:
      a. Intermittent claudication.
      b. Arterial insufficiency, venous stasis.
C. Diagnostics:
   1. Increase in BP (using correct BP cuff size) on two separate occasions, even repeated readings at the same visit (Table 12.3).
   2. Diagnostic tests to rule out problem of secondary hypertension.

Analyze Cues and Prioritize Hypotheses

The most important issue is the need for health teaching to minimize risk factors, such as the potential lack of adherence to medication therapy because of side effects and making necessary lifestyle changes.

Table 12.3 COMPARISON OF ARTERIAL AND VENOUS PERIPHERAL DISEASE

Characteristic	Arterial	Venous
Peripheral pulses	Decreased or absent	Present; may be difficult to palpate with edema
Capillary refill	>3 secs	<3 secs
Ankle-brachial index	≤0.90	>0.90
Edema	Absent unless leg constantly in dependent position	Lower leg edema
Hair growth	Loss of hair on legs, feet, toes	Hair may be present or absent
Ulcer location	Tips of toes, foot, or lateral malleolus	Near medial malleolus
Ulcer margin	Rounded, smooth, looks "punched out"	Irregularly shaped
Ulcer drainage	Minimal	Moderate to large amount
Ulcer tissue	Black eschar or pale pink granulation	Yellow slough or dark red, "ruddy" granulation
Pain	Intermittent claudication or rest pain in foot; ulcer may or may not be painful	Dull ache or heaviness in calf or thigh; ulcer often painful
Nails	Thickened; brittle	Normal or thickened
Skin color	Dependent rubor; elevation pallor	Bronze-brown pigmentation; varicose veins may be visible
Skin texture	Thin, shiny, taut	Skin thick, hardened, and indurated
Skin temperature	Cool, temperature gradient down the leg	Warm, no temperature gradient
Dermatitis	Rarely occurs	Frequently occurs
Pruritus	Rarely occurs	Frequently occurs

Adapted from Harding M, Kwong J, Roberts D, Hagler D, Reinisch C. (2023). *Lewis's medical-surgical nursing: Assessment and management of clinical problems* (12th ed.). Mosby.

Generate Solutions

Treatment

A. Dietary and stress management.
B. Antihypertensive and diuretic medications (Appendix 12.2).

Nursing Interventions: Take Action

Goal: To identify and educate high-risk individuals.

A. Encourage participation in community BP screening programs.
B. Educate the public regarding risk factors (Table 12.2).
C. Identify health-promoting behavior for high-risk individuals (Box 12.2).

❗ TEST ALERT Identify side effects and adverse effects or contraindications of medications.

Goal: To reduce BP and help client maintain control.

A. BP should be monitored frequently during initial medication dosage adjustments and at least twice a week thereafter, if not daily.

❗ NURSING PRIORITY BP should be evaluated with the client lying, sitting, and standing; readings should be obtained from both arms. Legs should not be crossed.

Box 12.2 LIFESTYLE MODIFICATIONS FOR THE PREVENTION AND CONTROL OF HYPERTENSION

- Lose weight if indicated.
- Limit alcohol and caffeine intake.
- Follow a regular program of aerobic exercise (30-45 mins; 3-4 days a week).
- Limit sodium intake.
- Maintain adequate potassium intake.
- Maintain adequate intake of dietary calcium, magnesium, and fiber.
- Stop smoking.
- Reduce intake of dietary saturated fat and cholesterol.
- Control diabetes.

B. Instruct client regarding possible side effects (Fig. 12.4):
   1. Do not suddenly stop taking medications; report side effects to health care provider.
   2. Assure client that side effects are often temporary.
   3. Sexual problems such as impotence should be reported.
C. When BP is initially decreased, evaluate client for:
   1. Postural (orthostatic) hypotension.
   2. Decreased urinary output.
   3. Decrease in energy level and mental alertness.

ANTIHYPERTENSIVES

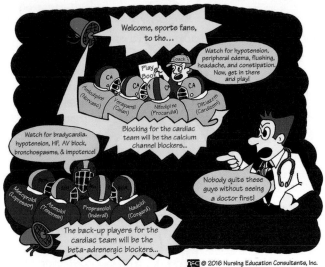

FIG. 12.4 Antihypertensives. (From Zerwekh J, Garneau A, Miller CJ. [2017]. *Digital collection of the memory notebooks of nursing* [4th ed.]. Chandler, AZ: Nursing Education Consultants, Inc.)

⚠ TEST ALERT Compare client's current vital signs and baseline vital signs; intervene when abnormal.

🌅 Home Care

A. DASH (**D**ietary **A**pproaches to **S**top **H**ypertension) diet; low-sodium/low-cholesterol diet.
B. Educate client and family members on how to take BP:
   1. Client should be seated with arm at heart level.
   2. No tobacco products or caffeine 30 mins before measurement of BP.
   3. Use appropriate cuff size.
   4. Can use either upper arm or forearm for accurate reading.
   5. Do not cross legs.
C. Adhere to medication regimen:
   1. Take medication at regular times.
   2. Do not suddenly stop taking medications; call health care provider if experiencing problems with medication regimen; continue taking despite BP within normal ranges and check with physician for further recommendations.
   3. Plan with client a method to keep track of medications (e.g., using daily pill box or marking on calendar).
   4. Notify health care provider if unable to afford medications.
   5. Learn to recognize and report the most common side effects of medications.
   6. Limit alcohol intake: one drink a day for women and two drinks a day for men (one drink = 12 oz. [360 mL] beer, 5 oz. [150 mL] wine, or 1.5 oz. [45 mL] liquor [such as vodka or gin]).

HYPERTENSIVE CRISIS

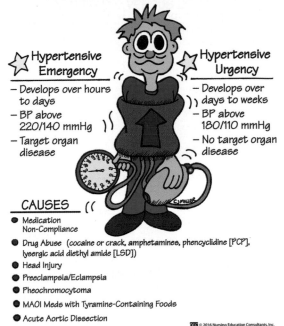

FIG. 12.5 Hypertensive Crisis. (From Zerwekh J, Garneau A, Miller CJ. [2017]. *Digital collection of the memory notebooks of nursing* [4th ed.]. Chandler, AZ: Nursing Education Consultants, Inc.)

⚠ TEST ALERT Instruct client about self-administration of prescribed medications; evaluate client's compliance with prescribed therapy; evaluate and document client's response to therapy.

D. Avoid hot baths, steam rooms, and spas (these increase vasodilation).
E. Decrease and/or prevent problems of orthostatic hypotension:
   1. Get up slowly, sit at the bedside to regain equilibrium, then slowly stand.
   2. Wear elastic support hose.
   3. Lie or sit down when dizziness occurs.
   4. Do not stand or sit for prolonged periods of time.
F. Monitor and record BP regularly; take records to physician visits.

📋 Hypertensive Crisis

Hypertensive crisis **is a term used to indicate either a hypertensive urgency (develops over days to weeks; no target organ damage) or a hypertensive emergency (develops over hrs to days). BP is severely elevated, over 180/120 (often >220/140 mm Hg) (Fig. 12.5).**

Assessment: Recognize Cues

A. Hypertensive emergency – sudden rise in BP with severe headache, nausea, vomiting, seizures, confusion, coma.
B. Renal insufficiency to chronic kidney disease.
C. Rapid cardiac decompensation – unstable angina, MI, pulmonary edema possible.
D. Neurologic symptoms similar to a stroke (typical no focal or lateralizing signs).

C. Nonsurgical:
1. Percutaneous transluminal angioplasty (PTA): use of a balloon catheter to compress the plaque against the arterial wall.
2. Laser-assisted angioplasty: a probe is advanced through a cannula to the area of occlusion; a laser is then used to vaporize the atherosclerotic plaque.
3. Intravascular stent: placement of a stent within a narrowed vessel to maintain patency.

Nursing Interventions: Take Action

> ❗ **TEST ALERT** Identify client with a condition that increases the risk for insufficient vascular perfusion; assess client for abnormal peripheral pulses.

Goal: To assess for characteristics of arterial versus venous disease (Table 12.3).
A. Assess and compare quality of peripheral pulses (Fig. 12.6).
B. Evaluate skin of the affected extremity:
1. Color, warmth, capillary refill.
2. Condition of the skin and nail beds.
3. Presence of ulcers or lesions and stages of healing.
C. Assess tolerance to activity; determine at what point claudication occurs and whether pain at rest is present.

> ❗ **TEST ALERT** Interpret client data that needs to be reported immediately.

Goal: To prevent injury and infection:
A. Avoid vigorous rubbing of the extremity.
B. Prevent skin breakdown at pressure sites. Use heel covers and bed cradle to prevent pressure on the toes and heels.
C. Visually inspect extremities for discolored areas, breaks in skin, and signs of infection.
D. Maintain good skin hygiene and proper care of toenails.
1. Encourage clients to see a podiatrist to trim toenails rather than doing this themselves.
2. Do not trim calluses or corns.
3. *Advise RN or health care provider if client has an ingrown toenail or ulceration formation.*
4. Keep feet clean and dry, do not soak feet, use lubricating lotion without alcohol to prevent skin cracks.
5. Teach client to always wear well-fitting shoes, wear cotton socks, and avoid shoes or socks that are too tight.

Goal: To increase arterial blood supply.
A. Encourage moderate exercise (e.g., walking).
1. Level of pain should be a guide to exercise; activity should be stopped when pain occurs.
2. Goal is 30 to 60 mins per day, 3 to 5 days a week.
B. Promote blood flow to legs:
1. Avoid standing in one position for prolonged periods.
2. Avoid crossing legs at the knees or ankles while in bed. Do not raise the knee area or lower section of the bed without raising the foot of the bed to eliminate pressure behind the knee.
3. Swelling may develop. Teach to avoid raising legs above the heart level, as this decreases arterial blood

flow to the feet. Hanging affected leg from the bed or sitting in an upright chair may decrease discomfort.
4. Provide warmth (room temperature, extra clothing, blankets). Never apply external heat or cold to the extremities.
5. Avoid pressure in the posterior popliteal area; avoid positions, clothing, or bandages that restrict circulation to the lower extremities (hose, girdles, elastic bandages, etc.).
6. When client is sitting in a chair, make sure the feet are flat on the floor to decrease pressure from the edge of the chair behind the knee.
7. Inspect feet daily for color changes or development of skin irritation/sores.
C. Prevent vasoconstriction:
1. Decrease caffeine intake.
2. Stop all tobacco use.
3. Avoid becoming chilled; keep lower extremities warm.

Goal: To evaluate and promote circulation in affected extremity after vascular surgery.
A. Frequent assessment to determine adequacy of circulation and patency of graft.
1. Circulation checks distal to the graft every 15 mins four times and then hourly for 24 hrs; notify health care provider immediately of any changes in the neurocirculatory status of the extremities.
2. Monitor for compartment syndrome (Chapter 17) and graft thrombosis.
3. Monitor for bleeding at arterial puncture site, which is sealed with a special collagen plug.
B. Encourage movement of the extremity as soon as client is awake; avoid flexion in the area of the graft (femoral or popliteal area).
C. Help client to ambulate as soon as possible; perform pulse checks when client returns to bed.
D. Do not raise the knee area of the bed.
E. Monitor anticoagulation medications; maintain bleeding precautions.
F. Assess for development of dependent edema; may require compression dressings or diuretic.
G. Notify surgeon or health care provider immediately of any symptoms suggestive of a further decrease in circulation or occlusion of graft.

Home Care

A. Take steps to lose weight if appropriate.
B. Avoid:
1. Standing or sitting for prolonged periods of time.
2. Tight socks, stockings, or clothing.
3. Tobacco products and caffeine.
4. Trauma to the extremities – always wear shoes.
C. Care of extremities:
1. Wash and visually inspect feet daily; dry well between toes. Use a mirror to observe bottoms of feet.
2. Do not apply any type of direct heat or cold to the legs.
3. Lubricate dry skin; do not use lotions that contain alcohol on open lesions or between the toes.

4. Seek professional care for calluses, corns, blisters, ulcers, etc.
5. File toenails straight across or see podiatrist for nail care and assessment of fcct.
6. Wear cotton socks and shoes that fit well; avoid shoes/nylon socks that cause feet to perspire.
D. Teach client methods to increase circulation during normal workday (do not cross legs; use a good chair; get up and walk every hour if working at a desk).
E. Notify health care provider of:
1. Presence of lesions or blisters that do not heal or infections on an extremity.
2. Any increase in pain or decrease in exercise tolerance.

Raynaud Phenomenon

Raynaud phenomenon **consists of intermittent episodic spasms of the arterioles, most frequently in the fingers, toes, ears, and tip of the nose. Spasms are not necessarily correlated with other peripheral vascular problems.**

Assessment: Recognize Cues

A. Clinical manifestations.
1. Raynaud phenomenon is more often seen in women 20 to 40 years of age (Fig. 12.8).
2. Symptoms are precipitated by:
   a. Exposure to cold.
   b. Emotional upset.
   c. Nicotine and caffeine intake.
3. Decreased perfusion leads to:
   a. Pallor and waxy appearance of tissue in the vasoconstrictive phase.
   b. Numbness and tingling.
   c. Throbbing, aching, tingling, and burning in the hyperemic phase.
4. Pulses are usually unaffected.
5. Involvement is bilateral.
6. Attacks are intermittent and last only a few mins.
B. Diagnostics.
1. Based on history.
2. Presence of clinical manifestations.
C. Complications: may progress to ulceration/gangrene in severe cases.

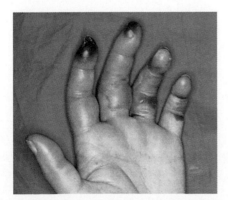

FIG. 12.8 Raynaud Disease. (From Kamal A, Brockelhurst JC. [1991]. *Color atlas of geriatric medicine* [2nd ed.]. Mosby.)

Analyze Cues and Prioritize Hypotheses

The most important problems are a decreased peripheral perfusion and pain cause by spasm of the arterioles.

Generate Solutions

Treatment
A. Medical.
1. No cure; treatment is based on symptoms.
2. Medications: vasodilators, calcium channel blockers.
B. Surgical: sympathectomy.

Nursing Interventions: Take Action

Goal: Help client to understand implications of the disease and measures to decrease episodic attacks.
A. Prevent vasospasms.
1. Wear gloves when handling cold objects (items from the refrigerator or freezer).
2. Protect feet, hands, nose, and ears when exposed to cold weather.
3. Maintain warm environment.
4. Avoid caffeine and tobacco products.
5. Manage stress.
6. Avoid vasoconstrictive drugs.

Thromboangiitis Obliterans (Buerger Disease)

Thromboangiitis obliterans **is a condition that causes vasculitis of the small- and medium-size arteries and veins of the extremities.**

Assessment: Recognize Cues

A. Clinical manifestations.
1. Intermittent claudication; pain at rest in advanced stages; pain is the predominant symptom.
2. Ischemic ulcerations and gangrene may develop in fingers and toes and then progress upward.
3. Temperature changes occur in the affected limb.
4. The extremity becomes more sensitive to cold.
5. The peripheral pulses may be diminished or absent.
6. The extremity develops cyanosis and redness.
B. Diagnostics.
1. Based on clinical manifestations.
2. Sometimes difficult to distinguish from peripheral arterial disease (PAD).
C. Complications: ulcerations and gangrene.

Analyze Cues and Prioritize Hypotheses

The most important problems are the relief of pain and the prevention of ulcerations and gangrene of the feet and lower extremities.

Generate Solutions

Treatment
A. No cure; treatment is based on symptoms. Cessation of all tobacco use early in the disease can stop symptoms and progression of the disease. Exercise is also recommended to promote circulation in the lower extremities.

B. Medications: vasodilators, antiplatelets, calcium channel blockers.
C. Surgical therapy.
1. Sympathectomy, revascularization.
2. Amputation in extreme cases.

Nursing Interventions: Take Action

Goal: To evaluate level of involvement and increase circulation to the extremity.
A. Decrease or stop all tobacco use (also exposure to secondhand smoke).
B. Evaluate tolerance to activity.
C. Inspect feet for vascular changes.
D. Avoid extreme cold.
E. Perform circulatory checks of the affected extremity.

> **!** **NURSING PRIORITY** The vascular problem has a direct relationship to cigarette smoking. For the condition to be controlled, the client must quit smoking.

Peripheral Venous Disease (Chronic Venous Insufficiency; Venous Stasis Ulcers)

Peripheral venous disease **(PVD), or** *chronic venous insufficiency* **(CVI), is an alteration of the natural flow of blood through the veins of the peripheral circulation. Caused by thrombus formation and/or defective valves, it leads to the regurgitation of blood, venous pooling, and edema in the lower extremities, eventually resulting in the development of venous leg ulcers.**

Assessment: Recognize Cues

A. Risk factors:
1. Advancing age, increased venous pressure.
2. Diabetes, obesity.
3. Varicosities, prolonged immobility.
4. Virchow triad (Box 12.3).
5. Previous episode of deep vein thrombosis (DVT).
6. Incompetence of the valves in the lower extremities.
B. Clinical manifestations (Table 12.3; Fig. 12.9).
1. Stasis eczema leading to chronic itching. Trauma to the skin from scratching leads to breakdown and ulceration.
2. "Brawny," leathery appearance to skin of lower leg.
3. Sclerosis occurs as a result of long-standing edema; leg becomes larger at the calf.
4. Ulcerations more commonly seen near the outer ankle.
5. Ulcer appearance: irregular margins, copious exudate.

Box 12.3 VIRCHOW TRIAD

Three Factors Contributing to Venous Thrombosis

- Venous stasis
- Damage to the endothelium of the vein
- Hypercoagulability of the blood

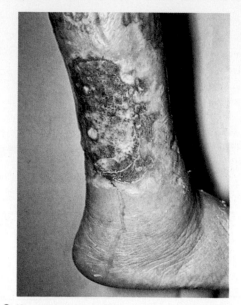

FIG. 12.9 Venous Leg Ulcer. (From Kamal A, Brockelhurst JC. [1991]. *Color atlas of geriatric medicine* [2nd ed.]. Mosby.)

6. Very painful.
C. Diagnostics: history and clinical manifestations.

> **!** **NURSING PRIORITY** It is essential to distinguish between arterial and venous ulcers, as treatment methods differ.

D. Complications.
1. Infection, cellulitis.
2. Delayed or poor healing caused by stasis of blood in the lower extremities.

Analyze Cues and Prioritize Hypotheses

The most important problems are decreased tissue perfusion leading to stasis ulcers, the potential for infection, poor wound healing, and pain.

Generate Solutions

Treatment
A. Medical therapy:
1. Compression therapy.
   a. Elastic compression stockings.
   b. Sequential compression devices.
   c. Unna boot (a paste bandage).
2. Moist dressings.
3. Good nutritional status.
4. Treatment of varicose veins.
5. Use of a wound vacuum in difficult cases.
B. Surgical therapy: excision of ulcer with skin grafting.

Nursing Interventions: Take Action

Goal: To prevent and treat venous stasis (Box 12.4).
A. Compression devices: prevention of venous stasis is key to healing.
1. Compression boots/stockings: extremity may be continuously covered with compression bandage, boot, or stocking.

Box 12.4 NURSING MEASURES TO DECREASE VENOUS STASIS

- Encourage mobility; even standing at the bedside promotes venous tone.
- Elastic support stockings:
  - Hospitalized clients should wear them all the time.
  - Home clients generally wear them during the day. They should be put on before getting out of bed and removed when going to bed.
  - Toe hole should be under the toes and heel patch over the heel.
  - Make sure stockings are not causing increased pressure behind the knee; do not allow stocking to bunch up and cause constriction behind the knee.
  - Do not hang feet dependently when putting stockings on; elevate the legs or put them parallel on the bed.
  - Make sure stockings are the correct fit by measuring the legs and ordering the appropriate size and length.
- Teach client to elevate legs for about 20 mins every 4 or 5 hrs.
- Avoid prolonged sitting; walk around every 1-2 hrs.
- Do not cross legs when sitting or lying in bed.
- Do not wear restrictive clothing.
- Maintain adequate fluid intake; avoid dehydration.
- Pneumatic sequential compression devices (SCDs) may be used in the hospital on clients at increased risk for complications secondary to venous stasis.
  - Remove compression device every 8 hrs to inspect skin.
  - If client is at high risk for development of thrombophlebitis, measure area to determine whether there is an increase in size of calf or thigh.
  - Assess legs for areas of warmth, tenderness, or inflammation.

2. Intermittent or sequential pneumatic compression devices: always check arterial circulation with any type of compression device.
3. Always assess adequacy of arterial circulation before compression therapy.

> **! TEST ALERT** Implement measures to promote venous return, to manage potential circulatory complications, and to monitor wounds for signs and symptoms of infection.

Goal: To prevent infection and promote healing:

A. Keep feet clean and dry; assess for development of venous ulcers and signs of infection.
B. Apply moist oxygen permeable dressings (e.g., hydrocolloids, foams).
C. Change dressings as needed for excessive wound drainage.
D. Prevent itching and breaks in skin from scratching.
E. Encourage increase in protein and vitamins to promote healing.
F. Maintain adequate blood perfusion and oxygen levels to tissue.

> **! TEST ALERT** Perform or assist with dressing changes; provide wound care (e.g., central line dressing or wound dressings).

📋 Venous Thromboembolism

Venous thromboembolism (VTE) is the presence of a clot in a vein; it may be a *superficial vein thrombosis* (SVT) or a *deep vein thrombosis* (DVT). Phlebitis is inflammation of a superficial vein without the presence of a clot (thrombus).

Assessment: Recognize Cues

A. Risk factors (Virchow triad – Box 12.3).
  1. Venous stasis.
     a. Surgery (especially hip, pelvic, and orthopedic surgery).
     b. Pregnancy, obesity, prolonged immobility.
     c. Heart disease (atrial fibrillation, heart failure).
  2. Hypercoagulability.
     a. Malignancies, dehydration.
     b. Blood dyscrasias.
     c. Oral contraceptives, hormone replacement therapy (HRT).
     d. Pregnancy and postpartum.
  3. Endothelial damage.
     a. Intravenous fluids and drugs (intravenous catheterization, drug abuse, caustic solutions or drugs).
     b. Fractures and dislocations (especially of the pelvis, hip, or leg).
     c. History of VTE/diabetes.

> **! TEST ALERT** Provide measures to prevent complications of immobility.

B. Clinical manifestations.
  1. Firm, palpable, cordlike vein.
  2. Area around vein is tender to touch, reddened, and warm.
  3. Temperature elevation (>100.4°F [38.0°C]).
  4. Extremity pain and edema.
  5. Elevated white blood cell count and positive blood culture.
C. Diagnostics.
  1. D-dimer testing.
  2. Ultrasound, magnetic resonance venography.
D. Complications.
  1. Pulmonary emboli.
  2. CVI, venous stasis ulcers.

Analyze Cues and Prioritize Hypotheses

The most important problems are the potential for injury and death caused by complications of the VTE and anticoagulation therapy.

Generate Solutions

Treatment

A. Medical:
  1. Elevation of the affected extremity.
  2. Anticoagulant, anti-inflammatory, and fibrinolytic medications.

Appendix 12.1 VASCULAR DIAGNOSTICS

TEST	NORMAL VALUE	THERAPEUTIC VALUE	NURSING IMPLICATIONS
Serum Studies			
Fragment D dimer (D-dimer test)	Less than 250 ng/mL	Less than 250 ng/mL	1. Produced by the action of plasma on fibrin, verifies fibrinolysis has occurred. 2. Used in diagnosis of DIC and to screen for venous thromboembolism, acute MI, and PE.
Prothrombin time (PT)	10- to 13-sec range	1.5-2.5 times normal	1. Sensitive to alterations in vitamin K. 2. Limit intake of foods with vitamin K. 3. Used to evaluate liver function and response to warfarin medications. 4. Watch for blood dyscrasias.
Activated partial thromboplastin time (aPTT)	Activated: 24-36 secs	1.5-2.5 times normal	1. Indicator of adequacy of anticoagulation with heparin. 2. Do not draw sample from extremity with a heparin lock or infusion. 3. Watch for blood dyscrasias.
International normalized ratio (INR)		2-3 (anticoagulation)	1. Calculated level based on PT; method of standardizing values. 2. Used to evaluate warfarin.
Activated coagulation time (ACT)	80-135 secs	180-240 secs or twice normal	1. Used to evaluate anticoagulation with heparin.

DIC, disseminated intravascular coagulation; *MI*, myocardial infarction; *PE*, pulmonary embolism.

Invasive Studies

Magnetic Resonance Angiography

Involves contrast medium injected to help visualize blood flow through peripheral arteries. Most common test used.

Venography (Phlebography)

Involves injection of a radiopaque dye into either the artery or the vein; x-ray films are obtained to identify atherosclerotic plaque, occlusion, injury, or presence of an aneurysm. *Once the gold standard, but now rarely done.*

Nursing care should include:
1. Explain procedure to client. Mild sedative may be indicated.
2. Requires an informed consent be signed.
3. Postprocedure:
   a. Frequent circulatory checks distal to the puncture site.
   b. Monitor for allergic reactions to the dye.
   c. Apply pressure dressing to arterial puncture site and monitor for bleeding.

Noninvasive Studies

Doppler Ultrasonography

Handheld Doppler device used to detect flow of blood in PAD; is not sensitive to early disease changes.

Ankle-Brachial Index

Calculated index using a handheld Doppler; divide the ankle systolic blood pressure (SBP) by the highest brachial SBP; normal = 1.00 to 1.30; moderate PAD = 0.41 to 0.70.

Venous/Arterial Duplex Scan

Uses a color Doppler to trace blood flow through an artery or vein. Has become the primary diagnostic tool for VTE, because it allows for visualization of the vein.

Computed Tomography

Allows for visualization of the arterial wall and adjacent structures; used for diagnosis of AAA, graft occlusions.

Trendelenburg Test

To test for venous incompetence. Client lies supine with leg elevated to promote venous drainage; a tourniquet is applied at midthigh, and client is asked to stand. Veins normally fill from below or distally; a varicose vein will fill from above or proximally because of the incompetent valves. Do not leave tourniquet in place longer than 1 min.

Antihyperlipidemic Medications: These decrease low-density lipoprotein (LDL) cholesterol but preferably not high-density lipoprotein (HDL) cholesterol. Antihypertensive medications should be used in combination with dietary restrictions, exercise, and smoking cessation to reduce blood lipid levels.

General Nursing Implications
- Serum liver enzymes should be monitored throughout therapy.
- Medications should be taken before the evening meal or at bedtime.
- Medications should be used in conjunction with other lipid-lowering therapies (exercise, low-cholesterol diet, smoking cessation).
- Serum cholesterol and triglyceride levels should be monitored before and periodically throughout therapy.
- When statins are being taken, one should avoid grapefruit and grapefruit juice in the diet.

Primary Prevention Guidelines
- Clients with LDL-C levels equal to or greater than 190 mg/dL should be evaluated for secondary causes.
- Diabetic clients aged 40 to 75 years should be treated with high-intensity statin therapy.
- Adults 40 to 75 years of age with an LDL-C between 70 and 189 mg/dL without clinical signs of acute sclerotic cardiovascular disease (ASCVD) or DM should be treated with moderate- to high-intensity statins.

MEDICATION	SIDE EFFECTS	NURSING IMPLICATIONS
Colesevelam: PO Colestipol: PO Cholestyramine: PO	Constipation Bloating Indigestion	1. Increase fiber and fluid intake to prevent constipation. 2. Administer other medications 1 hr before or 6 hrs after these meds.
Nicotinic acid: PO	Flushing GI disturbances Hyperglycemia Gouty arthritis	1. Immediately report signs of hepatotoxicity (darkening of urine, light colored stools, anorexia). 2. Flushing can be decreased by premedicating with a nonsteroidal antiinflammatory drug (NSAID) 30 mins before administration.
Gemfibrozil: PO Fenofibrate: PO	Diarrhea GI disturbances Hematuria Gallstones	1. Assess for increase in muscle pain. 2. Will potentiate warfarin-derivative anticoagulants.
Lovastatin: PO Simvastatin: PO Fluvastatin: PO Atorvastatin: PO Pravastatin: PO Rosuvastatin: PO Pitavastatin: PO	Rhabdomyolysis Elevated liver enzymes GI disturbances	1. Give with evening meal. 2. Should not be given to clients with preexisting liver disease. 3. Assess for increase in muscle pain. 4. Monitor liver enzymes closely. 5. Do not confuse pravastatin with lansoprazole. 6. Simvastatin has multiple drug interactions.
Ezetimibe: PO	Hepatotoxic Cholecystitis	1. Assess for increase in muscle pain. 2. Monitor liver enzymes closely.
Combination drugs- Ezetimibe and simvastatin: PO Amlodipine and atorvastatin: PO Niacin and lovastatin: PO	Hepatotoxic May interact with other drugs such as warfarin, cyclosporine, and some antibiotics Watch for drug combinations and potential effects not related to lipids (e.g., BP)	1. Combination drugs may assist with compliance to drug regime. 2. Monitor liver enzymes, BP, and muscle discomfort depending on drug combination.
Icosapent ethyl: PO	Arthralgias	1. Used for clients with hypertriglyceridemia levels greater than 500.
Evolocumab: SQ Alirocumab: SQ Taken every 2-4 weeks	Injection site discomfort, muscle/limb pain, fatigue	1. Used with familial hypercholesterolemia to lower LDL in those who cannot take statins.

Ŗ

▲**Anticoagulants:** Reduce formation of fibrin, warfarin inhibits the synthesis of clotting factors, including factor X and thrombin. All other anticoagulants (e.g., heparin inhibit the activity of clotting factors: either factor Xa or thrombin, or both.

General Nursing Implications
- Increased risk for bleeding when used concurrently with other drugs, herbal remedies, or foods affecting coagulation.
- Maintain bleeding precautions.
- Review laboratory results – complete blood count (CBC) with attention to hemoglobin and hematocrit (H & H) and platelets.
- A second health care provider should always check order, calculation of dosage, and/or infusion pump settings when medications are being administered intravenously.
- Do not automatically discontinue according to "automatic stop" policies (procedures, surgery) without verifying the order; reevaluate all clients whose anticoagulants are being held for procedures; and assess the need to reorder the anticoagulant therapy.
- Client should wear a medical alert bracelet.

❗ NURSING PRIORITY Clarify all anticoagulant dosing for clients. Caution should be taken when reading labels for heparin concentrations, especially for intravenous bolus doses.

MEDICATION	SIDE EFFECTS	NURSING IMPLICATIONS
▲ Heparin: IV, SQ May not be given PO Short-term anticoagulation	Visible or occult blood in emesis, urine, stool, or sputum Bleeding from trauma site, surgical site, or intracranially Heparin-induced thrombocytopenia: associated with increase in thrombosis	1. Check the activated partial thromboplastin time (APTT) for normal levels versus therapeutic levels. 2. Protamine sulfate is the antidote. 3. Intravenous administration should occur via infusion pump to ensure accurate dosage. 4. Will not dissolve established clots. 5. Evaluate client for decreased platelet count. 6. Effective immediately after administration; anticoagulation effect has short half-life. 7. Before starting infusion and with each change of the container or rate of infusion, have second practitioner check drug, dosage, route, and rate. 8. Do not store in same area as insulin; both are given by units.
Low-Molecular-Weight Heparin (LMWH)		
▲ Enoxaparin: SQ ▲ Dalteparin: SQ ▲ Tinzaparin: SQ	Similar to those with heparin	1. **Use:** prophylaxis for thromboembolic problems in high-risk clients (immobility, hip, or knee replacement). 2. Dosage *is not* interchangeable with heparin. 3. Leave the air lock in the prefilled syringe to prevent leakage. 4. Should be injected into the "love handles" of the abdomen.
▲ Warfarin sodium: PO Long-term anticoagulation	Bleeding ranging from bruising to major hemorrhage	1. Check the prothrombin time (PT) and international normalized ratio (INR) to evaluate level of anticoagulation; INR greater than 3 may indicate adverse drug reaction. 2. Vitamin K is the antidote. 3. Client teaching: a. Bleeding precautions. b. Advise all health care providers of medication. c. Not recommended if client is pregnant or lactating. d. Maintain routine checks on coagulation studies. e. Client must not stop taking medication unless told to do so by health care provider. 4. Check drug literature when administering with other medications; drug interactions are common. 5. Oral contraceptives may decrease effectiveness. 6. Half-life is 3-5 days; discontinue 3 days before an invasive procedure.
Direct Thrombin Inhibitors		
▲ Argatroban: IV ▲ Dabigatran: PO	Bleeding, dizziness, shortness of breath, fever, urticaria, dyspepsia	1. Due to potential breakdown and loss of potency from moisture, should not be stored in pillboxes or organizers. 2. Does not require INR/PT monitoring. 3. Idarucizumab is an antidote to reverse bleeding caused by dabigatran. 4. Do not double up on doses at the same time if a dose is missed.

Appendix 12.2   MEDICATIONS—cont'd

℞

MEDICATION	SIDE EFFECTS	NURSING IMPLICATIONS
Factor Xa Inhibitors		
▲ Apixaban: PO ▲ Rivaroxaban: PO	Has same potential for bleeding, as with warfarin Does not have the dietary and drug interactions that warfarin has	1. Inform health care provider if client is having surgery or dental surgery. 2. Does not require INR/PT monitoring. 3. Andexanet Alfa is an antidote to reverse bleeding for apixaban or rivaroxaban.

> ⚠ **TEST ALERT** Questions about anticoagulant medications are consistently found on the examination.

Antiplatelet Medications: Inhibit platelet aggregation and prolong bleeding time. Used to prevent and treat thromboembolism events such as stroke, MI, and peripheral artery disease.

General Nursing Implications
- Use with caution in clients at risk for bleeding.
- Concurrent use with NSAIDs, heparin, thrombolytics, or warfarin may increase risk of bleeding.
- Teach bleeding precautions to client and family.
- Monitor bleeding times throughout therapy.

MEDICATION	SIDE EFFECTS	NURSING IMPLICATIONS
Aspirin: PO	GI bleeding, hemorrhagic stroke, ecchymosis Tinnitus	1. Given in small doses (e.g., 81 mg qd). 2. Prophylactic therapy for prevention of myocardial infarction (MI) and thrombotic stroke in clients with transient ischemic attacks (TIAs). 3. Take with food.
Clopidogrel: PO Prasugrel: PO Ticagrelor: PO Vorapaxar: PO	Abdominal pain, dyspepsia, diarrhea Blood dyscrasias	1. Prophylactic treatment for prevention of MI, strokes in clients with established peripheral artery disease, or after stent placement. 2. Effect is decreased significantly when combined with omeprazole. 3. Should be taken with food.
Cilostazol: PO	Headache, dizziness, GI bleeding, flatus, diarrhea	1. Monitor for relief of intermittent claudication. 2. Grapefruit juice inhibits metabolism. 3. Administer on an empty stomach.
Ticlopidine: PO	Diarrhea, bleeding, aplastic anemia	1. Monitor coagulation studies throughout therapy. 2. Monitor cholesterol/triglyceride levels. 3. Older adults may have increased sensitivity.
Blood Viscosity Reducing Agent		
Pentoxifylline: PO	GI disturbances, dizziness	1. Monitor for relief of intermittent claudication in lower extremities. 2. Therapeutic effect may not be noted for 2-4 weeks. 3. Do not chew, crush, or break tablets.

Antihypertensive Medications: Lower blood pressure.

General Nursing Implications
- Advise client that postural hypotension may occur and explain how to decrease effects.
  - Advise client to sit on side of bed before standing.
  - Client should not stand for prolonged periods.
  - Older clients are at increased risk.
  - Symptoms may occur with first dose ("first dose effect") or subsequent doses.
  - Problem is most often temporary.
- Hypotension may be increased by hot weather, hot showers, hot tubs, and alcohol ingestion.
- Client should not abruptly discontinue medication or change dosage without consulting health care provider. Abrupt withdrawal can cause rebound hypertension.
- Encourage a low-sodium diet, weight maintenance or reduction, and limitations of caffeine.
- Discourage use of all tobacco products.
- Have client report unpleasant side effects related to sexual dysfunction.
- Advise client to not take over-the-counter cough medications or decongestants that contain pseudoephedrine; these medications cause an increase in BP.
- Administer with meals to enhance absorption.
- Client should monitor BP and pulse frequently during initial dosage adjustments and daily/weekly during therapy; record results and take along when visiting health care provider.

Continued

Appendix 12.2   MEDICATIONS—cont'd

®

MEDICATION	SIDE EFFECTS	NURSING IMPLICATIONS

Vasodilators: Act directly on vascular smooth muscle to produce vasodilation.

MEDICATION	SIDE EFFECTS	NURSING IMPLICATIONS
Hydralazine HCl: PO, IM, IV	Tachycardia, headache, sodium retention, drug-induced lupus syndrome	1. Advise client that postural hypotension may occur. 2. Vitamin B₆ may be used to prevent peripheral neuritis with long-term therapy. 3. May be used in combination with other antihypertensive medications.
▲Nitroprusside: IV	Nausea/vomiting, headache, abdominal pain, dizziness, excessive hypotension	1. Used to treat hypertensive crisis; very rapid response. 2. Solution must be prepared immediately before use and protected from light during administration; use within 24 hrs. 3. Administer via infusion pump to ensure accurate flow rate. 4. Maintain continuous electrocardiographic (ECG) and BP monitoring, preferably in a critical-care setting.
Minoxidil: PO	Tachycardia, fluid retention, nausea, headache, fatigue	1. Used to treat severe hypertension in clients unresponsive to other antihypertensives.
Nitroglycerin: PO, SL, topical, IV, spray	Hypotension, headache, flushing, skin irritation	1. Evaluate BP prior to administration. 2. If given intravenously, use infusion pump and dosage to titrate for BP or chest pain per health care provider's guidelines. 3. Sublingual dose/spray given for episodes of angina. Administer one dose every 5 mins for a total of three doses. If no relief, transport to health care facility for further treatment and evaluation.

Centrally Acting Inhibitors (Antiadrenergics): Decrease sympathetic effect (norepinephrine), resulting in decreased BP and peripheral resistance, decrease in heart rate, and no change in cardiac output.

Methyldopa: PO Methyldopate: IV Clonidine: PO or topical Guanabenz: PO Guanfacine: PO	Hepatotoxicity, hemolytic anemia, sexual dysfunction, orthostatic hypotension, dry mouth, sedation	1. If withdrawn abruptly, may precipitate a hypertensive crisis. 2. Do not confuse methyldopa with levodopa or L-dopa. 3. Older adult clients may have increased sensitivity to methyldopa. Monitor for depression or altered mental status.

ACE Inhibitors: Reduce peripheral resistance without increasing cardiac output, rate, or contractility; angiotensin antagonists.

Captopril: PO Enalapril: PO, IV Lisinopril: PO Ramipril: PO Moexipril: PO Trandolapril: PO	Postural hypotension, hyperkalemia, insomnia, nonproductive cough, loss of taste	1. Monitor closely on first dose; hypotension and first-dose syncope may occur. 2. Can cause hyperkalemia; *may not require* a potassium supplement when given with a diuretic. 3. Skipping doses or stopping drug may result in rebound hypertension. 4. Aspirin and NSAIDs may reduce effectiveness. 5. Not to be used with potassium-sparing diuretics.

Beta-Adrenergic Blockers: See Appendix 13.2.

Calcium Channel Blockers: See Appendix 13.2.

Diuretics (Fig. 12.10)

General Nursing Implications

- In hospitalized clients, evaluate daily weights for fluid loss or gain.
- Maintain intake and output ratios.
- Monitor for hypokalemia, anorexia, muscle weakness, numbness, tingling, paresthesia, confusion, and excessive thirst.
- Advise client of foods that are rich in potassium.
- Administer medications in the morning to allow diuresis to occur during the day.
- Teach client how to decrease effects of postural hypotension.
- Monitor BP response to medication.
- Interactions:
  - Digitalis action is increased in the presence of hypokalemia.
  - Lithium levels may be increased in the presence of hyponatremia.

Loop Diuretics: Block sodium and chloride reabsorption, which causes water and solutes to be retained in the nephrons. Prevention of reabsorption of water back into the circulation causes an increase in excretion of the water and thus diuresis.

Appendix 12.2   MEDICATIONS—cont'd

MEDICATION	SIDE EFFECTS	NURSING IMPLICATIONS
Furosemide: PO, IM, IV Bumetanide: PO, IM, IV Torsemide: PO, IV	Dehydration, hypotension; excessive loss of potassium, sodium, chloride; hyperglycemia, hyperuricemia; muscle weakness	1. Furosemide is a strong diuretic that provides rapid diuresis. 2. Use with caution in older adults; can cause central nervous system (CNS) problems of confusion, headache. 3. Monitor closely for tinnitus/hearing loss. 4. Do not confuse **Bumex** (trade name for bumetanide) with buprenorphine (**Buprenex**). 5. Do not confuse furosemide with torsemide. 6. Intravenous push should occur over 1-2 min, depending on dose to be administered.

Thiazide Diuretics: Increase the kidney excretion of NaCl, K, and water. Require adequate urine output to be effective.

Chlorothiazide: IV, PO Chlorthalidone: PO Hydrochlorothiazide: PO Metolazone: PO (a thiazide-like diuretic: may give 2–4 times per week depending on client need and tolerance)	Dehydration, hypotension; excessive loss of potassium, hyperglycemia, hyperuricemia; muscle weakness, dry mouth, lethargy	1. Frequently used as first-line drug to control essential hypertension. 2. Increased risk for digitalis toxicity if digoxin products are also being taken. 3. If client is allergic to thiazides or sulfonamides, metolazone may be contraindicated. 4. Potassium supplements may be needed.

Aldosterone Antagonist (Potassium-Sparing Diuretics): Blocks the effect of aldosterone; inhibits the renal-angiotensin-aldosterone system (RAAS); blocks receptors in the renal tubules, heart, and blood vessels. Used in treatment of heart failure and hypertension.

Spironolactone: PO Triamterene: PO	Hyperkalemia, hyponatremia, impotence, hypotension	1. May be used in combination with other diuretics to reduce potassium loss. 2. Potassium-sparing effects may result in hyperkalemia. 3. Not used for clients experiencing chronic kidney disease. 4. Avoid salt substitutes and foods containing large amounts of sodium or potassium.

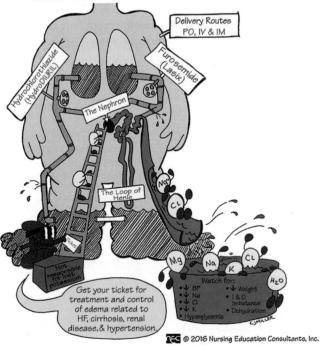

FIG. 12.10 Diuretic Water Slide. (From Zerwekh J, Garneau A, Miller CJ. [2017]. *Digital collection of the memory notebooks of nursing* [4th ed.]. Chandler, AZ: Nursing Education Consultants, Inc.)

Continued

12. A client with a history of arteriosclerotic heart disease (ASHD) is seen in the clinic. The client has a history of peripheral arterial disease (PAD) and hypertension. The health care provider prescribed bumetanide and benazepril, which have maintained the client's BP within normal limits over the past 6 months. The client has hypercholesterolemia and hypertriglyceridemia and has been prescribed lovastatin. The client follows a DASH diet plan and exercises 3 times a week for 1 hr.

For each potential complication listed below, drop down to select the potential nursing intervention that would be appropriate for the client at this time. Each complication may support more than one potential nursing intervention, but a least one option in each category needs to be selected.

POTENTIAL COMPLICATION	APPROPRIATE NURSING ACTION
Chest pain	
Edema	
Dyspnea	

NURSING ACTIONS FORPOTENTIAL CHEST PAIN	NURSING ACTIONS FOR POTENTIAL EDEMA	NURSING ACTIONS FOR POTENTIAL DYSPNEA
Check BP daily. Administer nitroglycerin sublingually. Change position q2h.	Encourage fluid intake. Daily electrolyte lab test. Monitor daily weight.	Maintain a supine position. Assess vital signs. Auscultate lungs.

⚡Answers to Practice & Next Generation NCLEX (NGN) Questions

1. 4
Client Needs: Physiological Integrity/Physiological Adaptation
Clinical Judgment/Cognitive Skill: Take Action
Item Type: Multiple Choice
Rationale & Test Taking Strategy: Note the key word, "priority." Although all of these options are important, consider what is the priority after an aortic femoral bypass graft. Peripheral pulse checks are priority. After ambulation, it is important to determine the quality of the peripheral pulses to assess the integrity of the graft. The pulse rate and blood pressure are important to evaluate if there is any indication of difficulty with the activity or ambulation. The temperature of the affected extremity is another method to determine adequacy of circulation.

2. 3
Client Needs: Physiological Integrity/Reduction of Risk Potential
Clinical Judgment/Cognitive Skill: Analyze Cues
Item Type: Multiple Choice
Rationale & Test Taking Strategy: When looking at the four options, laboratory studies measuring clotting are a priority rather than total cholesterol. The INR is used to monitor warfarin therapy, and the desired outcome is usually to maintain the client's INR between 2.0 and 3.0 regardless of the actual PT in seconds. A client with an INR of 5.2 is at risk for bleeding. Although the total cholesterol is slightly elevated (normal value should be less than 200 mg/dL), it is not a priority concern. The other coagulation studies are within normal limits. Normal range of PT is 11 to 12.5 seconds; normal range of aPTT is 30 to 40 seconds; normal range of INR is 0.8 to 1.1.

3. 1
Client Needs: Physiological Integrity/Physiological Adaptation
Clinical Judgment/Cognitive Skill: Recognize Cues
Item Type: Multiple Choice
Rationale & Test Taking Strategy: Think about what you know regarding peripheral artery disease and peripheral venous disease. This client has compromised circulation. With peripheral arterial occlusion, there is a decrease in the quality of the pulse, and the feet are frequently pale and cool to touch with dependent rubor, not a dusky gray color. The pedal pulses are significantly diminished or absent prior to the changes in the color of the feet. Muscle spasms are not associated with arterial disease. Rather, intermittent claudication is present with walking and the pain is relieved with rest. Healing ability is significantly diminished. Edema is associated with peripheral venous disease.

4. 1
Client Needs: Physiological Integrity/Physiological Adaptation
Clinical Judgment/Cognitive Skill: Analyze Cues
Item Type: Multiple Choice
Rationale & Test Taking Strategy: Note the **key** word, "immediately." The surgery puts the client at an increased risk for kidney complications because an aortic aneurysm is commonly in the area of the renal arteries. A normal urinary output should be around 30 mL/hr. A urinary output of 80 mL over 4 hours is too low, and the health care provider should be contacted immediately. If the feet are cool, a blanket should be placed over them, and they can be checked again later. The nurse would not expect to hear bowel sounds in this early postoperative period. Development of a paralytic ileus is common following surgery; a nasogastric tube is placed, and the nurse assesses for the return of bowel sounds. There is presence of the pulses, and they are equal in both extremities. Because the pulses are weak, they will need to be monitored but are not a priority at this time.

5. 3
Client Needs: Physiological Integrity/Physiological Adaptation
Clinical Judgment/Cognitive Skill: Take Action
Item Type: Multiple Choice
Rationale & Test Taking Strategy: The client would be on bed rest to prevent dislodgement of a thrombus. The client will also be on an anticoagulant. Active range of motion would not be done on the affected extremity. Any contraction and flexion of muscles in the leg should be avoided to prevent pressure on the area of the deep vein thrombosis.

6. 4
Client Needs: Physiological Integrity/Physiological Adaptation
Clinical Judgment/Cognitive Skill: Recognize Cues
Item Type: Multiple Choice
Rationale & Test Taking Strategy: Think about what intermittent means—something that is not continuous. Intermittent claudication is the term used to describe pain in the legs that is relieved by resting the muscle, which is characteristic of peripheral artery disease (PAD). The other options are not characteristic of intermittent claudication. Pain in the leg at rest is indicative of advanced arterial disease. When sitting down there is stasis of blood leading to congestion and pain in the lower extremities, which is a venous problem, not arterial as in PAD. Analgesics are usually not necessary as pain decreases significantly or goes away when the client is at rest. Pain in the hands is often noted in Raynaud disease.

7. 2, 4
Client Needs: Physiological Integrity/Pharmacological Therapies
Clinical Judgment/Cognitive Skill: Analyze Cues
Item Type: Select All That Apply
Rationale & Test Taking Strategy: Recall what "first-dose effect" means. The first-dose effect is the result of severe postural hypotension. Drugs that typically have this effect are selective (alpha$_1$) adrenergic antagonists (alpha blocker), such as prazosin, and angiotensin-converting enzyme (ACE) inhibitors, such as lisinopril. To minimize the first-dose effect, the initial dose should be small (1 mg or less). Subsequent doses can be gradually increased with little risk of fainting. Clients who are starting treatment should be forewarned about the first-dose effect and advised to avoid driving and other hazardous activities for 12 to 24 hours. Administering the initial dose immediately before going to bed eliminates the risk of a first-dose effect. Lovastatin is an antihyperlipidemic medication that does not have this effect, nor does ticlopidine, which is an antiplatelet medication. Thiazides are diuretics that can cause hypotension but do not have a first-dose effect.

8. 4
Client Needs: Physiological Integrity/Physiological Adaptation
Clinical Judgment/Cognitive Skill: Recognize Cues
Item Type: Multiple Choice
Rationale & Test Taking Strategy: The typical symptoms of deep vein thrombosis are venous pooling, pain on dorsiflexion of the foot, and swelling, warmth, and tenderness over the affected area. The condition is most often unilateral; redness and swelling occur only on the affected extremity.

9. 1
Client Needs: Physiological Integrity/Physiological Adaptation
Clinical Judgment/Cognitive Skill: Analyze Cues
Item Type: Multiple Choice
Rationale & Test Taking Strategy: Look at the options and determine if they are normal or abnormal. The only option that indicates a decrease in tissue perfusion that occurs with hypovolemic shock is the decrease in urine output. Jugular vein distention is present with an increase in venous pressure and blood volume overload. The chest tube output is expected, and the vital signs can be a result of anxiety or stress. The urine output should be at least 30 mL/hr. Urine output is a critical indicator of the adequacy of kidney perfusion.

10. 3
Client Needs: Physiological Integrity/Pharmacological Therapies
Clinical Judgment/Cognitive Skill: Generate Solutions
Item Type: Multiple Choice
Rationale & Test Taking Strategy: Think about what you can modify to change habits. Hyperlipidemia is a major modifiable risk factor of CAD and can be treated with an HMG-CoA reductase inhibitor, often referred to as a "statin." Atorvastatin is a statin medication used to treat hyperlipidemia. Statins reduce low-density lipoprotein cholesterol levels, reduce triglycerides, and increase high-density lipoprotein cholesterol levels. Fluticasone/salmeterol and budesonide are used in the treatment of asthma. Amlodipine is a calcium channel blocker and does not treat a modifiable risk factor.

11. A client tells the nurse that they have a diagnosis of peripheral vascular disease (PVD). The nurse is preparing to assess the client and assist in understanding the disease process.

For each client finding, use an X to specify whether the assessment finding is consistent with the disease process of peripheral arterial disease (PAD) or chronic venous insufficiency. Each assessment finding is consistent with only one condition.

CLIENT FINDING	PAD	CHRONIC VENOUS INSUFFICIENCY
Diminished, weak popliteal pulse	X	
Intermittent claudication	X	
Dull, achy pain		X
Mottling with brown pigmentation at ankles		X
Severe ankle and foot edema		X
Pallor, dependent rubor	X	
Necrosis and gangrene of foot	X	
Ulcers at ends of toes	X	

Client Needs: Physiological Integrity/Physiological Adaptation
Clinical Judgment/Cognitive Skill: Analyze Cues
Item type: Matrix Multiple Choice
Rationale & Test Taking Strategy: Peripheral vascular disease (PVD) includes disorders that involve both arteries and veins of the peripheral circulation, which leads to decreased perfusion to body tissues. More often, PVD affects the legs more frequently than the arms. In general, a diagnosis of PVD implies arterial disease (peripheral arterial disease [PAD]) rather than venous involvement or chronic venous insufficiency. Some clients may have both arterial and venous disease. The following are associated with peripheral arterial occlusive disease (PAD): gangrenous wounds, diminished peripheral

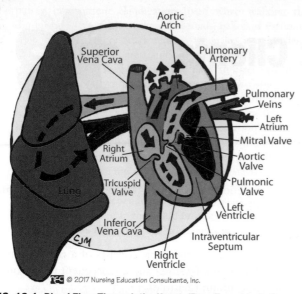

FIG. 13.1 Blood Flow Through the Heart. (From Zerwekh, J., Garneau, A., & Miller, C. J. [2017]. Digital collection of the memory notebooks of nursing [4th ed.]. Nursing Education Consultants.)

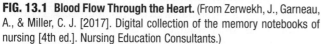
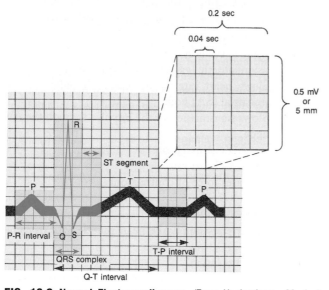

FIG. 13.2 Normal Electrocardiogram. (From Hockenberry, M. J. & Duffy, E.A., & Gibbs, K. [2024]. Wong's nursing care of infants and children [12th ed.]. Mosby.)

C. Relationship of conducting pathways to the ECG (Fig. 13.2; Appendix 13.4).
1. P wave: indicative of the impulse generated from the SA node; initiates atrial depolarization.
2. PR interval: delay of the impulse at the AV node and bundle of His to promote ventricular filling.
3. QRS complex: passage of the impulse through the bundle of His, down the bundle branches, through the Purkinje fibers; depolarization of the ventricle occurs.
4. T wave: ventricular repolarization and return to the resting state.
5. ST segment: above the baseline in cardiac injury (ST elevation) and below the baseline with ischemia (ST depression).

System Assessment: Recognize Cues

A. Health history.
1. Identify presence of risk factors for the development of arteriosclerotic disease.
2. Coping strategies.
3. Respiratory history.
   a. History of difficulty breathing.
   b. Medications taken for respiratory problems.
   c. Determine normal activity level.
4. Circulation.
   a. History of chest discomfort (Table 13.1).
   b. History of edema, weight gain, syncope.
   c. Skin temperature and pulses.
5. Medications taken for the heart or for high blood pressure.
B. Physical assessment.
1. What is the general appearance of the client; is there any evidence of distress? What is the client's level of orientation and ability to think clearly?
2. Evaluate blood pressure.
   a. Pulse pressure: the difference between systolic and diastolic pressure.
   b. Assess for postural (orthostatic) hypotension (decrease in blood pressure when client stands).
   c. Take blood pressure sitting, standing, and lying if client is having problems with pressure changes (see Chapter 3 for accurate blood pressure measurement).
   d. Paradoxical blood pressure (paradoxical pulse): a decrease in systolic blood pressure of at least 10 mm Hg that occurs during inspiration.
3. Evaluate quality and rate of pulse; assess for dysrhythmias (see Appendix 13.3 for determining dysrhythmias).
   a. Pulse deficit: the radial pulse rate is less than the apical pulse rate; occurs in atrial fibrillation and atrial flutter.
   b. Pulsus alternans: regular rhythm but quality of pulse alternates with strong beats and weak beats.
   c. Thready pulse: weak and rapid; difficult to count.
4. Assess quality and pattern of respirations and evidence of respiratory difficulty.
5. Auscultation of the heart (Fig. 13.3).
   a. Heart sounds heard during the cardiac cycle:
      (1) S_1: closure of the AV valves—mitral and tricuspid.
      (2) S_2: closure of the semilunar valves—aortic and pulmonic.
      (3) S_3: represents rapid ventricular filling; normal in children and young adults; in adults older than 30 years, it may be an indication of volume overload, ventricular dysfunction secondary to hypertension.
      (4) S_4: caused by the atria contracting forcefully in an effort to overcome an abnormally stiff or hypertrophic ventricle.

Table 13.1 ASSESSING CHEST PAIN (PQRST)

P: Precipitating Factors	Q: Quality of Pain	R: Region and Radiation of Pain	S: Severity Symptoms/Signs (Associated with Chest Pain)	T: Timing and Response to Treatment
May occur without precipitators Physical exertion Emotional stress Eating a large meal	Pressure Squeezing Heaviness Smothering Burning Severe pain Increases with movement	Substernal or retrosternal Spreads across the chest Radiates to the inside of either or both arms, the neck, jaw, back, upper abdomen	Severity—scale from 1–10 Diaphoresis, cold clammy skin Nausea, vomiting Dyspnea Orthopnea Syncope Apprehension Dysrhythmias Palpitations Auscultation of extra heart sounds Auscultation of crackles Weakness	Sudden onset Constant Duration more than 30 min Not relieved with nitrates or rest Relief with narcotics

5 AREAS FOR LISTENING TO THE HEART

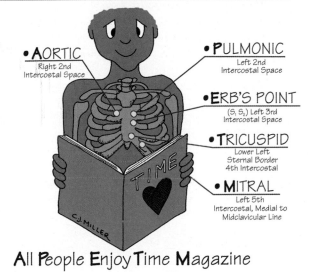

- **AORTIC** Right 2nd Intercostal Space
- **PULMONIC** Left 2nd Intercostal Space
- **ERB'S POINT** (S₁ S₂) Left 3rd Intercostal Space
- **TRICUSPID** Lower Left Sternal Border 4th Intercostal
- **MITRAL** Left 5th Intercostal, Medial to Midclavicular Line

All People Enjoy Time Magazine

© 2017 Nursing Education Consultants, Inc.

FIG. 13.3 Five Areas for Listening to the Heart. (From Zerwekh, J., Garneau, A., & Miller, C. J. [2017]. Digital collection of the memory notebooks of nursing [4th ed.]. Nursing Education Consultants.)

b. Presence of murmurs created by turbulent blood flow: graded on a scale of loudness from 1 to 6.
   (1) Abnormal flow through diseased valves: stenosis and insufficiency.
   (2) Abnormal flow of blood between cardiac chambers (congenital heart disease).
c. Presence of a pericardial friction rub: a scratchy, high-pitched sound usually heard over the left lower sternal border during S₁ and S₂; can be heard best with client sitting and leaning forward.

TEST ALERT Identify common abnormal heart sounds (e.g., S₃, S₄).

6. Evaluate adequacy of peripheral vascular circulation and check for presence of peripheral edema.

7. Evaluate for presence of chest pain or discomfort (see Table 13.1).
   a. Location.
   b. Intensity of pain.
   c. Precipitating causes.

TEST ALERT Perform focused assessment or reassessment; interpret data that need to be reported immediately.

DISORDERS OF THE CARDIAC SYSTEM

Coronary Artery Disease

Coronary artery disease (CAD), also called *arteriosclerotic heart disease* (ASHD), occurs as a result of the atherosclerotic process in the coronary arteries. The buildup of plaque or fatty material in the coronary artery causes a narrowing of the lumen of the artery and precipitates myocardial ischemia, causing chest pain.

A. Pain (angina) occurs when the oxygen demands of the heart muscle exceed the ability of the coronary arteries to deliver it.
B. Temporary ischemia does not cause permanent damage to the myocardium. Pain frequently subsides when the precipitating factor is removed.
C. Risk factors for CAD (Box 13.1).
D. CAD treatment: health promotion, physical activity, nutritional therapy, lipid-lowering drug therapy, antiplatelet therapy.

Chronic Stable Angina

Chest pain that occurs intermittently over a long period of time with a similar pattern of onset, duration, and intensity of symptoms.

Box 13.1   RISK FACTORS FOR CORONARY ARTERY DISEASE

Major Modifiable Risk Factors
Elevated Lipids
- Total cholesterol greater than 200 mg/dL (5.18 mmol/L)
- Triglycerides greater than or equal to 150 mg/dL (1.7 mmol/L)
- Low-density lipoprotein (LDL) cholesterol greater than 130 mg/dL (4.14 mmol/L)
- High-density lipoprotein (HDL) cholesterol less than 40 mg/dL (1.0 mmol/L) in men or 50 mg/dL (1.3 mmol/L) in women
- Blood pressure greater than or equal to 120/80 mm Hg
- Tobacco use
- Physical inactivity
- Diabetes
- Obesity: waist circumference greater than or equal to 102 cm (40 inches) in men and 88 cm (35 inches) in women
- Metabolic syndrome

Contributing Modifiable Risk Factors: Elevated homocysteine, C-reactive protein, and lipoprotein levels; psychosocial factors (stress, hostility, depression); substance use

Nonmodifiable Risk Factors
- Genetic predisposition
- Positive family history of heart disease
- Increasing age
- Gender: after age 55, the incidence of myocardial infarction in men and women equalizes
- Ethnicity: more common in White men than in African Americans

TEST ALERT Teach health promotion information. Know the coronary artery disease risk factors and be able to teach the client how to effectively reduce their risk factors.

Assessment: Recognize Cues

A. Episodic pain lasting a few minutes that is relieved by rest or nitroglycerin.
B. Provoked by a stressor.
  1. Physical exertion; temperature extremes.
  2. Strong emotions; consumption of heavy meal.
  3. Tobacco use; sexual activity.
  4. Stimulants (cocaine, amphetamines).
  5. Circadian rhythm patterns.

Generate Solutions

Treatment
A. Short- and long-acting nitrates.
B. Angiotensin-converting enzyme inhibitors (ACEIs) and angiotensin receptor blockers (ARBs).
C. Beta-adrenergic blockers, calcium channel blockers.
D. Lipid-lowering drugs.
E. Sodium current inhibitor.
F. Cardiac catheterization.

Acute Coronary Syndrome

Prolonged ischemia that is not immediately reversible. *Acute coronary syndrome* (ACS) includes unstable angina, non-ST-segment-elevation myocardial infarction (NSTEMI), and ST-segment-elevation myocardial infarction (STEMI).

A. Unstable angina is chest pain that is new in onset, occurs at rest, or occurs with increasing frequency, duration, or with less effort than chronic stable angina.
B. Myocardial infarction (MI) is a dynamic process, occurring over several hours and most often in the area of the LV.
C. The severity of the situation depends on the area of the heart involved and the size of the infarction.

Assessment: Recognize Cues

A. Risk factors/etiology: CAD.
B. Clinical manifestations of MI (Fig. 13.4).
  1. Pain at varying levels of severity (PQRST) (see Table 13.1).
  2. Pain not relieved by rest, position changes, or nitrate administration.
  3. Pain most often located behind or just to the left of the sternum or epigastric area.
  4. Pain may radiate to neck, jaw, and shoulders.
  5. Client may describe pain as squeezing, choking, constricting, or as a vague feeling of pressure and indigestion.
  6. Client will frequently deny the seriousness of the pain.
  7. Accompanying symptoms may include diaphoresis, weakness, dyspnea, pallor, anxiety, nausea and/or vomiting.
  8. Women's typical clinical manifestations.
    a. Indigestion, interscapular pain, aching jaw, choking sensation with exertion.
    b. Fatigue, sleep disturbance, dyspnea.

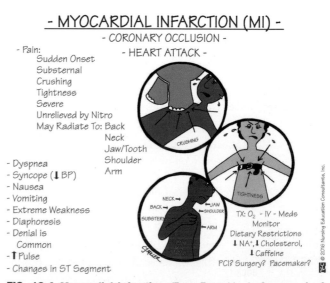

FIG. 13.4 Myocardial Infarction. (From Zerwekh, J., Garneau, A., & Miller, C. J. [2017]. Digital collection of the memory notebooks of nursing [4th ed.]. Nursing Education Consultants.)

! OLDER ADULT PRIORITY The only symptom of MI in older adults may be shortness of breath or indigestion. Those older than 80 years of age may present with acute confusion or disorientation, which can indicate inadequate cardiac output and tissue perfusion.

C. Diagnostics (see Appendix 13.1)
   1. 12-lead ECG.
   2. Elevated cardiac troponin T and I, which begin to rise with bedside "point of care" testing results available within 15 to 20 minutes.
   3. Elevated creatinine kinase isoenzyme MB (CK-MB).
D. Complications of myocardial infarction.
   1. Dysrhythmias (see Appendix 13.3).

! NURSING PRIORITY Dysrhythmia, especially ventricular fibrillation, is the most frequent cause of death in the client with an MI. The greatest risk for death from MI is during the first 4 hours.

   2. Heart failure, cardiogenic shock.

Analyze Cues and Prioritize Hypotheses

The most important problems are acute pain, decreased perfusion, and potential for dysrhythmias and heart failure.

Generate Solutions

Treatment
A. Immediate treatment of an MI.
B. Restricted activity, supplemental oxygen.
C. Fibrinolytic (reperfusion) therapy (Appendix 13.2).
D. Procedures/surgical interventions.
   1. Percutaneous coronary intervention (PCI).
      a. Balloon angioplasty: a balloon-tipped catheter is inserted into an artery in the groin leading to the affected coronary artery. The balloon is then inflated in an effort to compress the plaque and dilate the narrowed artery, reestablishing blood flow to the myocardium.
      b. Stent: expandable wire mesh that can be inserted during a PCI. A stent serves as a scaffold to maintain patency of the coronary artery. Stents may be bare metal or drug-clotting types and will require extended treatment with aspirin and clopidogrel after they are placed.
   2. Cardiac revascularization: coronary artery bypass graft (CABG) surgery, open heart surgery.
      a. Transmyocardial laser revascularization (TMR): laser probe is inserted into the wall of the LV; channels are created to promote the development of revascularization. Used for clients with advanced CAD who are not candidates for CABG surgery.

! NURSING PRIORITY Immediate reperfusion with an invasive intervention (stent or CABG) is used to save the life of the client in cardiogenic shock.

E. Control of modifiable risk factors (see Box 13.1).

Nursing Interventions: Take Action

Goal: To decrease pain and increase perfusion and myocardial oxygenation.

A. Begin supplemental oxygen.
B. Position client in reclining position with head elevated.
C. Assess characteristics of pain: administer morphine for pain control.
D. *Immediately report presence of chest pain and/or any changes in characteristics of chest pain to the registered nurse (RN).*
E. Administer medications—nitroglycerin, analgesics, antiplatelets.
F. Maintain a calm, reassuring atmosphere.
G. Establish venous access for fluids and intravenous (IV) medications.
H. Notify health care provider if pain does not respond to medication or if vital signs deteriorate.

! NURSING PRIORITY To relieve chest pain and decrease cardiac damage resulting from an inadequate blood and oxygen supply to the myocardium, there must be an immediate reduction in the workload of the heart that results in a decrease in oxygen consumption: rest, nitroglycerin, oxygen therapy.

Goal: To evaluate characteristics of anginal pain and client's overall response.
A. Does pain increase with breathing? (Anginal pain is generally not affected by breathing or changes in position.)
B. Assess activity tolerance or precipitating factor.
C. Assess changes in characteristics of pain (see Table 13.1).
D. Evaluate response of pain to treatment or progression to more severe level.
E. Assess vital signs.
F. Continuous ECG monitoring: assess for presence of dysrhythmia and effect on cardiac output.
G. Monitor troponin levels (see Appendix 13.1).
H. Assess client's psychosocial response: denial is common; anger, fear, and depression occur in both client and family.

Goal: To provide care after PCI (with or without stent).
A. Monitor for chest pain and hypotension; reocclusion is a primary complication.
B. Assess for bleeding or hematoma formation at vascular site.
C. Frequently assess status of circulation distal to area of cannulation.
D. A sheath may be left in place; monitor area for bleeding; *if bleeding occurs, put manual pressure on the area and notify the RN or health care provider.*
E. Prevent flexion of affected extremity and maintain bed rest for 6 to 8 hours.
F. Client is to avoid heavy lifting; may return to work in 1 to 2 weeks.
G. Notify the health care provider of any chest pain, syncope, or bleeding at the site.
H. Assess ECG for evidence of ST-segment changes.

❗ **NURSING PRIORITY** As long as chest pain persists, cardiac ischemia continues. If client experiences tachycardia, decrease activity whether client has chest pain or not.

Goal: To evaluate characteristics of cardiac pain and client's overall response.

A. Continuous cardiac monitoring to identify and treat dysrhythmias affecting cardiac output.
B. Frequent assessment for dysrhythmias, murmurs, and presence of S_3 and S_4.
C. Maintain IV access.
D. Maintain bed rest for the first 24 hours.

TEST ALERT Meet client's pain management needs; provide medication for pain relief; use clinical decision making when administering medications; monitor for effects of pain medication.

E. Frequent assessment of chest pain.
F. Evaluate urinary output and kidney response.
G. Assess respiratory system for pulmonary congestion.
H. Evaluate peripheral circulation; assess for dependent edema.
I. Maintain NPO (nothing by mouth) status initially, then allow clear liquids; progress to light meals that are low in sodium and cholesterol.
J. Promote normal bowel pattern.
  1. Stool softeners, bedside commode.
  2. Caution against stimulation of the vagus nerve (Valsalva maneuver).
  3. Increase fiber in diet.

TEST ALERT Identify potential/actual stressors for the client; implement measures to reduce environmental stress; promote methods to reduce stress.

K. Decrease anxiety.
L. Monitor for changes in neurologic status: confusion, disorientation, etc.
M. Monitor progressive activity: walking in hallway three to four times a day with gradual increasing increments.

TEST ALERT Determine changes in client's cardiovascular system.

Home Care

A. Participate in organized cardiac rehabilitation program.
  1. Progressive monitored exercise.
  2. Dietary modifications.
  3. Stress management.
  4. Continued education regarding ACS and decreasing personal risk factors.
B. Understand medication regimen.

C. Teach client how to take the pulse and check for rate and regularity.
D. Teach client how to evaluate response to exercise (dyspnea, tachycardia, chest pain, etc.).
  1. Remain close to home to begin walking program.
  2. Client should always carry nitroglycerin when walking or exercising.
  3. Client should check pulse rate before, halfway through, and at the end of activity.
  4. Stop activity for pulse increase of more than 20 beats/min, shortness of breath, chest pain, nausea, or dizziness.
E. Call the health care provider for pain not controlled by nitroglycerin, significant changes in pulse rate, decreased tolerance to activity, syncope, or an increase in dyspnea.
F. Sexual intercourse can generally be resumed in 4 to 6 weeks after MI or when the client can walk one block or climb two flights of stairs without difficulty.
  1. Do not drink any alcohol before sexual activity.
  2. Take nitroglycerin before sexual activity.
  3. Do not have sex after a heavy meal.
  4. Position for intercourse does not influence cardiac workload but depends only on client comfort.
  5. Do not take erectile dysfunction medications (see Appendix 22.2) if taking nitrates.

TEST ALERT Assess client's ability to perform self-care. Determine whether the client with cardiac disease understands the illness and whether knowledge of care can be demonstrated.

📋 Heart Failure

Heart failure **(HF) includes cardiac decompensation, cardiac insufficiency, and ventricular failure; it ultimately results in the heart's inability to pump adequate amounts of blood into the systemic circulation, resulting in impaired tissue perfusion.**

Physiology of Ventricular Failure

A. Systolic (left-sided) failure.
  1. LV unable to maintain adequate cardiac output and generate needed pressure to eject blood through the aorta effectively.
  2. Left-ventricular hypertrophy (LVH) develops; increasing pressure in the pulmonary capillary bed causes lungs to become congested, resulting in impaired gas exchange.
B. Diastolic (right-sided) failure.
  1. Ventricles unable to relax during diastole (filling).
  2. Cardiac output is decreased.
  3. Venous engorgement in both systemic and pulmonary systems.
C. Cardiac compensatory mechanisms will attempt to maintain the body's requirements for cardiac output; when these mechanisms become ineffective, cardiac decompensation or failure ensues.

LEFT SIDED ♥ FAILURE

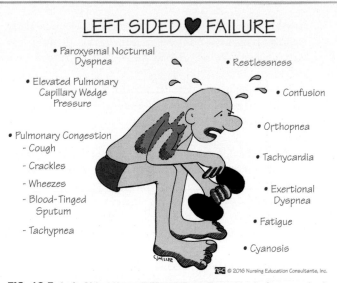

- Paroxysmal Nocturnal Dyspnea
- Elevated Pulmonary Capillary Wedge Pressure
- Pulmonary Congestion
  - Cough
  - Crackles
  - Wheezes
  - Blood-Tinged Sputum
  - Tachypnea
- Restlessness
- Confusion
- Orthopnea
- Tachycardia
- Exertional Dyspnea
- Fatigue
- Cyanosis

FIG. 13.5 Left-Sided Heart Failure. (From Zerwekh, J., Garneau, A., & Miller, C. J. [2017]. Digital collection of the memory notebooks of nursing [4th ed.]. Nursing Education Consultants.)

RIGHT SIDED ♥ FAILURE
(Cor Pulmonale)

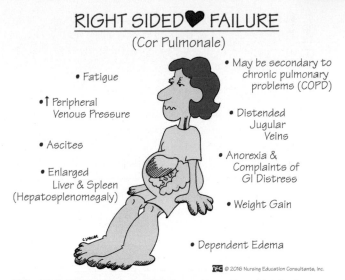

- Fatigue
- ↑ Peripheral Venous Pressure
- Ascites
- Enlarged Liver & Spleen (Hepatosplenomegaly)
- May be secondary to chronic pulmonary problems (COPD)
- Distended Jugular Veins
- Anorexia & Complaints of GI Distress
- Weight Gain
- Dependent Edema

FIG. 13.6 Right-Sided Heart Failure. (From Zerwekh, J., Garneau, A., & Miller, C. J. [2017]. Digital collection of the memory notebooks of nursing [4th ed.]. Nursing Education Consultants.)

D. Edema development in HF.
  1. Decreased cardiac output leads to decreased kidney perfusion; the kidneys respond by stimulating the adrenal cortex to increase the secretion of aldosterone, thus increasing the retention of sodium and water.
  2. With an increase in venous pressure from the increased circulating volume, there is an increase in the capillary pressure and dependent pitting edema occurs.
E. In children, HF occurs most often as the result of a structural or congenital problem of the heart.
F. Particularly in older adults, decreased cardiac output and reduction in cerebral perfusion can cause confusion, memory loss, and slow verbal responses.

Assessment: Recognize Cues

A. Risk factors/etiology.
  1. MI, CAD, valvular disease.
  2. Hypertension, congenital heart disease.
B. Clinical manifestations.
  1. Types of HF (Figs. 13.5 and 13.6).
    a. Left-sided failure—pulmonary symptoms.
    b. Right-sided failure—systemic symptoms.
  2. Acute decompensated heart failure (ADHF)—pulmonary edema due to left-ventricular failure secondary to CAD.
  3. Chronic HF.
    a. FACES acronym (Fig. 13.7).
    b. Tachycardia, nocturia, chest pain, weight changes.
    c. Skin changes: cool, damp, diaphoretic, absent hair growth, and a brown or brawny skin discoloration on lower extremities.
    d. In infants, difficulty with feeding causes failure to thrive and to gain adequate weight.
C. Diagnostics—B-type natriuretic peptide, chest x-ray, echocardiogram, ECG, magnetic resonance imaging (MRI) (see Appendix 13.1).

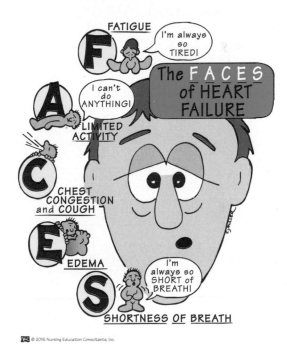

FIG. 13.7 FACES of Chronic Heart Failure. (From Zerwekh, J., Garneau, A., & Miller, C. J. [2017]. Digital collection of the memory notebooks of nursing [4th ed.]. Nursing Education Consultants.)

D. Complications.
  1. Pleural effusion, cardiogenic shock, chronic kidney disease.
  2. Left-ventricular thrombus, hepatomegaly.

Generate Solutions
Treatment

A. Treatment of the underlying problem.
B. Prevention.
  1. Administration of prophylactic antibiotics to clients with rheumatic heart disease before medical procedures to prevent mitral valve damage.

2. Effective early treatment of hypertension.

3. Early treatment of dysrhythmia.

C. Position client in high Fowler with feet horizontal in bed or dangling at beside.

D. Oxygen.

E. Activity limitations.

F. Medications: treatment for HF includes reduction of the preload and afterload as well as improvement of the myocardium's contractility.

   1. Cardiac glycosides, beta-adrenergic agonists (see Appendix 13.2).

   2. Diuretics, aldosterone antagonists.

   3. Vasodilators, morphine.

   4. ACEIs.

   5. Classified as high-alert drugs, beta-blockers are contraindicated in acute HF; when used for chronic HF, they are started slowly at a very low dose.

   6. Electrolyte replacement; carefully monitor serum potassium levels.

   7. Antidysrhythmic drugs, calcium channel blockers.

   8. Anticoagulants (see Appendix 12.2).

G. Dietary restriction of sodium; fluid restriction for moderate to severe HF and renal insufficiency. Sodium and fluids may not be restricted for infants and children; infants seldom need fluid restriction because of difficulty feeding and their need to be adequately hydrated.

❗ NURSING PRIORITY The goals for therapeutic intervention in clients with HF are to:

- Decrease symptoms: dyspnea and fatigue.
- Improve cardiac output: digitalis and oxygen.
- Decrease activity; administer vasodilator.
- Administer diuretics; decrease sodium and fluid intake.

Nursing Interventions: Take Action

Goal: To decrease cardiac demands and improve cardiac output.

A. Assess vital signs and compare with other physical assessment data.

B. Conserve energy.

   1. Encourage rest alternated with activity.

   2. Monitor pulse, respiratory rate, and dysrhythmias during periods of activity.

C. Avoid chilling; it increases oxygen consumption, especially in infants.

D. Provide supplemental oxygen, especially when needed with increased activity.

E. Provide uninterrupted sleep when possible.

F. Take steps to minimize crying in children and infants.

G. Decrease stress and anxiety; encourage parents to remain with child.

Goal: To decrease circulating volume.

A. Assess breath sounds; check for distended neck veins and peripheral edema.

B. Low-sodium diet and fluid restriction in adults and older children.

C. Evaluate fluid retention by determining accurate daily weight (1-kg or 2.2-lb weight gain = 1 L of fluid loss or retention). *Notify RN if client gains 2 to 4 lb over 24 hours.*

D. Accurate intake and output; monitor electrolyte balance and therapeutic effect of fluid loss.

Goal: To reduce respiratory distress.

A. Position.

   1. Adult may be placed in Fowler or semi-Fowler position or may sit in an armchair.

   2. When client is in semi-Fowler position, do not elevate client's legs; this increases venous return (preload).

   3. An infant or small child may breathe better in a side-lying position with the knees drawn up to the chest.

   4. An infant may be placed in an infant seat, especially after feeding.

   5. Make sure diapers are loosely pinned and that safety restraints do not hinder maximal expansion of the chest.

   6. Hold infant upright over your shoulder with the infant's knees flexed (knee-chest position).

B. Administer oxygen: use oxygen hood for infants and nasal cannula for adults and older children; provide supplemental oxygen to *keep saturation levels at or greater than 90%.*

C. Evaluate breath sounds; evaluate adventitious breath sounds and presence of congestion.

D. Do not allow infants to cry for extended periods.

E. For clients who smoke, encourage them to stop and/or provide smoking cessation advice.

Goal: To monitor for development of hypoxia. (See Chapter 11.)

Goal: To maintain nutrition.

A. Provide small, frequent meals of easily digestible foods; give client enough time to eat.

B. Help client with cultural implications in dietary management.

C. An infant will require more calories because of increased metabolic rate.

   1. May require tube feedings.

   2. An infant does not generally require fluid restriction because of decreased fluid intake secondary to the dyspnea.

   3. Do not prop the bottle; burp the infant frequently.

   4. Decreased calorie intake will result in decreased strength, decreased weight gain, and failure to meet developmental motor skills.

🔆 Home Care

A. Client should begin walking short distances, 250 to 300 feet (72–91 m), at least three to four times per week; distance can be increased as tolerated (no shortness of breath, dizziness, chest pain, or tachycardia).

B. Teach client how to take pulse.

C. Teach client to do daily weights every morning, before breakfast and with similar clothes on (nightgown, pajamas, etc.).

D. Discuss use of and safety factors for home oxygen.
E. Contact health care provider for:
1. Weight gain of 3 to 5 lb (1.4–2.3 kg) over a week or 1 to 2 lb overnight (0.5–0.9 kg).
2. Increase in dyspnea or angina, especially with decreased activity or at rest.
3. Waking up breathless at night.
4. Nausea with abdominal swelling, pain, and tenderness.
5. Increased urination at night; presence or increase in peripheral edema.
6. Cough (especially when lying down) or respiratory congestion.
7. Fatigue or weakness.
F. Provide written instructions for medications, especially in the case of digitalis.
G. Assess client's home situation and ability of home caregivers.

Rheumatic Fever and Heart Disease

(See Chapter 22.)

Infective Endocarditis

Infective endocarditis (IE) is an infection of the valves and inner lining or endocardium of the heart.
A. Bacteria may enter from any site of localized infection; most common are *Staphylococcus aureus* and *Streptococcus viridans*.
B. Organisms grow on the endocardium and produce a characteristic vegetation consisting of fibrin deposits, leukocytes, and microbes; the vegetation may then invade adjacent valves.
C. Vegetation is fragile and may break off, resulting in emboli.

Assessment: Recognize Cues

A. Risk factors/etiology.
1. History of endocarditis, prosthetic valves, or acquired valvular disease.
2. Aging, kidney dialysis, IV drug abuse.
3. History of recent invasive procedures.
4. Hospital-acquired bacteremia.
B. Clinical manifestations.
1. Symptoms of systemic infection: low-grade intermittent fever, chills, weakness, malaise.
2. Murmur develops or there are changes in previous murmurs.
3. Symptoms associated with HF.
4. Vascular symptoms.
a. Splinter hemorrhages causing black longitudinal streaks in the nailbeds.
b. Petechiae in conjunctiva, lips, buccal mucosa; on the ankle; and in the antecubital and popliteal areas.
c. Small, flat, painless red spots on the palm and soles.

d. Infants may have feeding difficulties, respiratory distress, tachypnea, tachycardia, HF, or septicemia.
5. Symptoms associated with emboli.
a. Spleen: splenomegaly, upper left quadrant pain.
b. Kidney: flank pain, hematuria.
c. Brain: hemiplegia, decreased level of consciousness, visual changes.
C. Diagnostics.
1. Echocardiography, ECG.
2. Blood cultures, drawn 30 minutes apart from two sites.
D. Complications.
1. HF secondary to valve damage.
2. General systemic emboli.

Analyze Cues and Prioritize Hypotheses

The most important problems are heart valve damage and systemic emboli.

Generate Solutions

Treatment
A. IV antibiotic therapy for 4 to 6 weeks.
B. Bed rest if high fever or evidence of HF is present.
C. IV antibiotic therapy for 2 to 8 weeks and only prophylactic antibiotics for high-risk children having congenital heart disease, prosthetic heart valve, cardiac transplant, or previous IE infection.
D. Surgical intervention for severe valvular damage.

Nursing Interventions: Take Action

Goal: To help parents understand the need for long-term prophylaxis.
Goal: To maintain homeostasis and prevent complications.
A. Intravenous antibiotic medications.
B. Assess activity tolerance.
C. Evaluate for occurrence of emboli and HF.

Home Care

A. Good oral hygiene: daily care and regular dental visits.
B. Avoid excessive fatigue; plan rest periods and activity.
C. Client and family must understand the need for continued antibiotics.
D. Report temperature elevations, fever, chills, anorexia, weight loss, and increased fatigue.
E. Advise all health care providers of history of endocarditis.
F. Teach parents of high-risk children to receive prophylactic antibiotic treatment 1 hour before dental procedures, invasive procedures, or when there is an infection of the skin.

Pericarditis

Pericarditis is an inflammation of the pericardium. The pericardial space is a cavity between the inner and outer layers of the pericardium.

Assessment: Recognize Cues

A. Risk factors/etiology.

1. Acute pericarditis may occur within 48 to 72 hours after an MI.
2. Dressler syndrome occurs about 4 to 6 weeks after an MI.
3. Chronic constrictive pericarditis usually begins with acute episode; fluid is gradually absorbed, with scarring and thickening.

B. Clinical manifestations.
  1. Acute.
     a. Pericardial friction rub caused by myocardium rubbing against inflamed pericardium.
     b. Pain increases with deep inspiration and lying supine; sitting may relieve pain; pain may radiate, making it difficult to differentiate from angina.
  2. Chronic: symptoms are characteristic of gradually occurring HF and decreased cardiac output; chest pain is not a prominent symptom.

C. Diagnostics: acute and chronic (see Appendix 13.1).
  1. Increased leukocytes.
  2. Inflammation: increased C-reactive protein (CRP), increased erythrocyte sedimentation rate (ESR).

D. Complications.
  1. Pericardial effusion (fluid in pericardial space) can result in cardiac tamponade.

Analyze Cues and Prioritize Hypotheses

The most important problems are pain, pericardial effusion, and possible cardiac tamponade.

Generate Solutions

Treatment

A. Acute episode.
  1. Treat underlying problem.
  2. Bed rest.
  3. Nonsteroidal antiinflammatory drugs (NSAIDs) and corticosteroids.

B. If pleural effusion and tamponade occur, pericardiocentesis (aspiration of fluid from the pericardial sac) is performed.

Nursing Interventions: Take Action

Goal: To maintain homeostasis and promote comfort.

A. Assess characteristics of pain; administer appropriate analgesics.

B. Upright position, with client leaning forward, may relieve the pain.

C. Client often associates problem with an MI; decrease anxiety by teaching the difference.

D. In a client with chronic pericarditis, evaluate for symptoms of HF and initiate appropriate nursing interventions.

Heart Valve Disorders

A. Causes of valve disease.
  1. Congenital heart disease.
  2. Rheumatic heart disease.
  3. Infective endocarditis.
  4. Ischemia caused by ACS.

B. Mitral valve is the most common area of involvement because of high pressures in left side of heart, followed by the aortic valve.

C. *Valvular stenosis:* a narrowing of the valve opening and progressive obstruction to blood flow; increase in workload of the cardiac chamber pumping through the stenosed valve.

D. *Valvular insufficiency* (incompetency, regurgitation): impaired closure of the valve allows blood to flow back into the cardiac chamber, thereby increasing the workload of the heart.

Assessment: Recognize Cues

A. Risk factors: associated with history of rheumatic fever, endocarditis, cardiovascular disease.

B. Clinical manifestations—mitral valve disorders.
  1. Exertional dyspnea progressing to orthopnea.
  2. Progressive fatigue caused by decrease in cardiac output.
  3. Cardiac murmur (diastolic); palpitations.
  4. Systemic embolization.
  5. Atrial fibrillation (concern is maintaining cardiac output).

C. Clinical manifestations—aortic valve disorders.
  1. Syncope and vertigo.
  2. Nocturnal angina with diaphoresis (condition interferes with coronary artery filling).
  3. Dysrhythmia; systolic murmur in stenosis.
  4. Dyspnea and increasing fatigue; HF (exertional dyspnea, orthopnea, and paroxysmal nocturnal dyspnea).
  5. With severe disease, the nurse notes a "bounding" arterial pulse and widened pulse pressure; client feels palpitations and may have nocturnal angina with diaphoresis.
  6. Upon auscultation, a high-pitched, blowing, decrescendo diastolic murmur with aortic regurgitation.

D. Diagnostics—transesophageal echocardiogram (TEE), transthoracic echocardiogram (TTE), exercise stress test, chest x-ray, ECG (see Appendix 13–1).

Analyze Cues and Prioritize Hypotheses

The most important problems are decreased perfusion, potential for emboli, dysrhythmias, and HF.

Generate Solutions

Treatment

A. Prevention of HF, pulmonary edema, thromboembolism, and endocarditis.
  1. Oxygen as needed to maintain O2 sat at 95%.
  2. Digitalis; diuretics.
  3. Beta blockers to decrease cardiac rate.

B. Prophylactic anticoagulation to prevent thrombus formation.

C. Prophylactic antibiotics before invasive procedures.

D. Open heart surgery for valve replacement when there is evidence of progressive cardiac failure; two types: mechanical or biologic (tissue).

E. Percutaneous transluminal balloon valvuloplasty (PTBV): performed in cardiac catheterization laboratory; balloon is threaded through the affected valve in an attempt to separate the valve leaflets.

! NURSING PRIORITY Monitor respiratory status closely with clients with mitral stenosis who often have pulmonary hypertension and stiff lungs. Postop clients with aortic valve replacements are at high risk for hemorrhage. Carefully monitor heart rate and blood pressure.

Nursing Interventions: Take Action

Goal: To prevent development of rheumatic heart disease and provide prophylactic treatment to individuals with history of rheumatic heart disease.

Goal: To teach importance of recommended long-term anticoagulant therapy for clients with mechanical valve replacement or clients with biologic valve replacement who have atrial fibrillation.

Goal: To prevent and/or to identify early development of HF (see Heart Failure, Nursing Interventions).

! NURSING PRIORITY Primary care for the client with cardiac valve disease consists of maintaining homeostasis and preventing the development of HF. The client should be advised to avoid excessive fatigue and should be assessed according to the level of activity tolerance.

TEST ALERT Client education for valvular disease includes the importance of taking prophylactic antibiotic therapy before invasive dental or respiratory procedures but is *not* recommended before gastrointestinal procedures.

Cardiac Surgery

A. CABG, aortic and mitral valve replacements: open heart surgery is performed with the use of the cardiopulmonary bypass machine; this machine allows for full visualization of the heart while maintaining perfusion and oxygenation.
B. Closed heart surgery is performed without the use of the bypass machine.
  1. Minimally invasive direct CABG (MIDCABG): one of the most common procedures; involve grafts to the left anterior descending artery.
  2. Aortic and mitral balloon valvuloplasty.
C. Intensive care unit (ICU) for 24 to 36 hours after surgery for intensive monitoring of client's hemodynamic status.

Analyze Cues and Prioritize Hypotheses

The most important problems are hemorrhage, pain, and perfusion alterations.

Nursing Interventions: Take Action

Goal: To prepare the client psychologically and physiologically for surgery.

A. Evaluate client's history for other chronic health problems.
B. Establish baseline data for postoperative comparison.
C. Provide appropriate preoperative teaching according to age level; frequently includes a visit to the ICU (parents should accompany the child on the visit).
D. Discuss immediate postoperative nursing care and anticipated nursing procedures.
E. Correct metabolic and electrolyte imbalances.
F. Establish and maintain adequate hydration.
G. Anticipate adjustments in medication schedule before surgery.
  1. Digitalis dosage is usually decreased.
  2. Diuretics may be discontinued 48 hours before surgery.
  3. Long-acting insulin will be changed to regular insulin.
  4. Antihypertensive medication dosage may be modified.
H. Eliminate possible sources of infection.

Goal: To evaluate and promote cardiovascular function after surgery.

A. Maintain adequate blood pressure.
B. Evaluate for dysrhythmia.
C. Maintain client in semi-Fowler position.
D. Evaluate fluid and electrolyte balances.
  1. Record daily weight and compare with previous weight.
  2. Evaluate electrolyte balance, especially potassium levels.
  3. Measure urine output hourly to evaluate adequacy of kidney perfusion.
  4. Administer IV fluids, as indicated.
E. Observe for hemorrhage: most often identified by increase in mediastinal chest tube drainage.
F. Evaluate adequacy of peripheral circulation.
  1. Mark location of pedal pulses preoperatively; assess postoperatively.
  2. If saphenous vein harvested, monitor incision for wound edge approximation, drainage, and signs of infection. Keep incision clean; apply antibacterial ointment to site.
G. Mediastinal chest tubes are frequently placed in the pericardial sac to prevent tamponade.

Goal: To evaluate and promote respiratory function.

A. Mechanical ventilation via an endotracheal tube may be used for approximately 12 to 24 hours after surgery. Children are generally extubated sooner than adults.
B. Maintain water-sealed drainage for mediastinal/chest tubes.
C. Pulmonary hygiene via endotracheal tube; carefully assess pulse oximetry during suctioning.
D. Promote good respiratory hygiene after extubation (fluids, incentive spirometry, activity).

E. Evaluate ABGs for adequate oxygenation; also check acid-base balance.

F. Encourage activity as soon as possible; client should be out of bed on the first postoperative day.

G. Monitor pulse oximetry levels.

Goal: To evaluate neurologic status for complications after surgery.

A. Recovery from anesthesia within appropriate time frame.

B. Assess for changes in neurologic status.

Goal: To prevent complications of immobility after surgery. (See Chapter 3.)

Goal: To decrease anxiety and promote comfort after surgery.

A. Frequent orientation to surroundings.

B. Prevent sensory overload.

C. Promote uninterrupted sleep.

D. Administer pain medications as appropriate.

Common Complications after Cardiac Surgery

A. Dysrhythmia.

B. Hypovolemia.

1. Observe client closely for response to fluid replacement because fluid overload occurs very rapidly, especially in children and older adults.

C. Emboli.

D. Cardiac tamponade.

1. Pressure on the heart caused by a collection of fluid in pericardial sac.

2. May be caused by fluid collecting postoperatively or from pericarditis; be sure pericardial chest-drainage system is functioning. Report output that is greater than 150 mL/hr.

E. ICU delirium (most common in adults); incorrectly called ICU psychosis because client is *not* psychotic.

1. Alterations in mentation (delusions, short attention span, loss of memory).

2. Psychomotor behavior (restlessness, lethargy).

3. Disrupted sleep-wake cycle (daytime sleepiness, nighttime agitation).

Appendix 13.1 CARDIAC DIAGNOSTICS

Serum Laboratory Studies

Cardiac Markers

The contents of the injured cells are released into the bloodstream.

Cardiac Troponin T and Cardiac Troponin I

A myocardial muscle protein released into the bloodstream with myocardial muscle damage; normal level is less than 0.2 ng/mL (mg/L) (for T) and less than 0.03 ng/dL (mg/L) (for I). Levels are elevated early—within 4 to 6 hours after an MI—and peak within 10 to 24 hours. Any rise in values indicates cardiac necrosis or acute MI.

Creatinine Kinase Isoenzyme MB

CK-MB is specific to heart muscle. Increases greater than 5% of total CK are highly indicative of MI. Increases occur within 4 to 6 hours after an MI, peak in 12 to 24 hours, and return to normal in 24 to 36 hours.

Nursing Implications

1. Enzymes must be drawn on admission and obtained in a serial manner thereafter. There is a characteristic pattern to the increases and decreases of enzyme levels in a client with an MI.

2. The larger the infarction, the larger the enzyme response.

3. Evaluate serial levels of the enzymes; increased levels of troponin are the most significant and diagnostic of myocardial damage.

4. Cardiac-specific troponin helps discriminate from other tissue injury.

⚠ **NURSING PRIORITY** For a client with an increase in CK-MB (CK_2) and an increase in cardiac troponin levels, it is important to monitor closely for symptoms of ACS. In a client with ACS, serum levels may be checked every 6 to 8 hr during the acute phase.

C-Reactive Protein, Highly Sensitive C-Reactive Protein

CRP is synthesized by the liver and is not normally present in the blood except when there is inflammation from tissue trauma. The response to the test helps to determine the severity and course of inflammatory conditions. Highly sensitive CRP (hs-CRP) is an independent risk factor for the development of CAD and ACS.

Normal: Less than 1 mg/L (9.52 nmol/L); a level greater than 3 mg/L (28.57 nmol/L) is significant and may indicate some degree of inflammatory response caused by plaque formation. It is used to determine treatment options for those at risk for CAD and to manage statin therapy after an acute MI.

B-Type Natriuretic Peptide

Natriuretic peptides promote vasodilation and diuresis through sodium loss. Fluid overload caused by HF stretches the ventricles, leading to a release of the **B-type natriuretic peptide (BNP)**. Serial BNP values may be determined to evaluate left-ventricular function and help to identify HF versus respiratory failure as the cause of dyspnea. Normal is less than 100 pg/mL (ng/L). Values increase with age and in women and are lower in people who are obese.

Noninvasive Diagnostics

Electrocardiogram

A graphic representation of the electrical activity of the heart, generally conducted by using a 12-lead format. Test to identify conduction in rhythm disorders and the occurrence of ischemia, injury, or death of myocardial tissue.

Holter Monitor

Client is connected to a small portable ECG unit with recorder that records the client's heart activity for approximately 24 to 48 hours.

The client keeps a log of activity, pain, and palpitations. Client should not remove leads but is encouraged to maintain normal activity; client should not shower or bathe while the monitor is in place. The recording is analyzed and compared with the client's activity log.

Event Monitor (Transtelephonic Event Recorder)

Client is connected to portable ECG unit with a recorder. The client can activate the recorder whenever any type of dizziness or palpitations occurs. Monitor may be worn for extended periods of time. Monitor leads and battery are removed for showering but should be reconnected immediately. Recordings are transmitted over the phone.

Exercise Stress Test

This test involves the client exercising, usually on a treadmill, which increases speed and incline to increase the heart rate. ECG leads are attached to the client, and the response of the heart to exercise is evaluated. If the client is unable to walk on the treadmill, medications may be administered to simulate exercise.

Nursing Implications

1. Provide appropriate pretest preparation; establish baseline vital signs and cardiac rhythm.
2. Client should
   a. Avoid smoking, eating, or drinking any caffeinated beverages for 3 hours before the test.
   b. Avoid stimulants, eating, and extreme temperature changes immediately after the test.
3. Cardiac monitoring is done constantly during test.
4. Reasons for terminating an exercise stress test: chest pain, significant increase or decrease in blood pressure, or significant ECG changes.
5. If any of these changes occurs, the test is terminated and the stress test result is said to be positive.

Echocardiogram

An ultrasound procedure to evaluate valvular function, cardiac chamber size, ventricular muscle, and septal motion. The ultrasound waves are displayed on a graph and interpreted.

Transesophageal Echocardiography

Provides a higher-quality picture than a regular echocardiogram. The throat is anesthetized, and a flexible endoscope is passed into the esophagus to the level of the heart. Sedation is used during the procedure.

Nursing Implications

1. Maintain NPO for 4 to 8 hours before test.
2. Check for gag-and-swallow reflex before client resumes oral intake of fluids.

Invasive Diagnostics

Cardiac Catheterization

An invasive procedure in which a catheter is passed through the brachial or femoral artery for left-side cardiac catheterization; the brachial or femoral vein for right-side cardiac catheterization. Cardiac catheterization will provide data regarding status of the coronary arteries, as well as cardiac muscle function, valvular functions, and left-ventricular function (ejection fraction).

Nursing Implications

1. Pretest preparation.
   a. Maintain NPO status for 6 hours before test.
   b. Check for dye allergy, especially allergy to iodine and contrast media.
   c. Record quality of distal pulses for comparison after test.
   d. Determine whether any medications need to be withheld.
   e. Appropriate client education (feeling of warmth when dye is injected; will be awake during procedure; report any chest pain; need to lie still).
2. After the test.
   a. Evaluate catheterization entry site (most often femoral) for hematoma formation. Notify health care provider immediately for excessive bleeding at the site, dramatic changes in blood pressure.
   b. Evaluate neurovascular status (pulses distal to catheterization site, color, sensation of the extremity). *Notify health care provider immediately for a decrease in peripheral circulation or neurovascular changes in affected extremity.*
   c. Assess for dysrhythmias.
   d. Maintain bed rest; avoid flexion; keep extremity straight for 3 to 6 hours.
   e. Keep head of bed elevated at 30 degrees or less.
   f. Encourage oral intake of fluids; IV access may be maintained.

Positron Emission Tomography

Very sensitive in identifying viable and nonviable cardiac tissue. The procedure takes about 2 to 3 hours. A radioactive dye is injected intravenously, followed by glucose. A client's glucose must be between 60 and 140 mg/dL (3.3–7.8 mmol/L) before the test.

Appendix 13.2 CARDIAC MEDICATIONS

Nitrates: Increase blood supply to the heart by dilating the large coronary arteries; cardiac workload is reduced due to decrease in venous return because of peripheral vasodilation (decreases preload).

MEDICATIONS	SIDE EFFECTS	NURSING IMPLICATIONS
Nitroglycerin: sublingual Nitroglycerin extended release: buccal tablets Nitroglycerin: topical (patch) Nitroglycerin IV Nitroglycerin ointment: topical, by the inch Nitroglycerin translingual spray Isosorbide dinitrate: PO, extended release	Headaches (diminish with therapy), postural hypotension, syncope, blurred vision, dry mouth, reflex tachycardia	1. Advise client that alcohol will potentiate postural hypotension. 2. Educate client regarding self-medication (Box 13.2). 3. Do not take with erectile dysfunction drugs. 4. Topical or transdermal application is used for sustained protection against anginal attacks. 5. Avoid skin contact with topical form; remove all previous applications when applying topical form. 6. Sublingual tablets and translingual spray given for an immediate response.

Continued

Box 13.2   CLIENT EDUCATION FOR NITROGLYCERIN ADMINISTRATION

1. Keep in a tightly closed dark glass container.
2. Carry a supply at all times—either sublingual (SL) tablets or translingual spray; do not swallow SL tablets or inhale the translingual spray.
3. Fresh tablets should cause a slight tingling under the tongue.
4. Date all opened containers and discard all medication that is 6 months old.
5. Take nitroglycerin prophylactically to avoid pain—before sexual intercourse, exercise, walking, etc.
6. Take nitroglycerin when pain begins; stop all activity.
7. If pain is not relieved in 5 minutes, call 911 and activate EMS.
8. While waiting for EMS response, if chest pain remains unrelieved, take another SL pill and then a third 5 minutes later.
9. Remain lying down; orthostatic hypotension can be a problem.
10. Long-acting preparations should not be abruptly discontinued; this may precipitate vasospasm.
11. To decrease development of tolerance in long-acting preparations, schedule an 8-hour nitro-free period each day, preferably at night.
12. Do not take erectile dysfunction drugs with nitroglycerin.

TEST ALERT Instruct clients about the self-administration of medications.

Appendix 13.2   CARDIAC MEDICATIONS—cont'd   ℞

MEDICATIONS	SIDE EFFECTS	NURSING IMPLICATIONS

Calcium Channel Blockers: Blockade of calcium channel receptors in the heart causes decreased cardiac contractility and a decreased rate of sinus and AV nodal conduction. Used to treat chronic stable angina, hypertension, atrial fibrillation, and atrial flutter.

MEDICATIONS	SIDE EFFECTS	NURSING IMPLICATIONS
Diltiazem: PO, IV Nifedipine: PO Clevidipine: IV for severe hypertension Verapamil: IV, PO	Constipation (verapamil—especially in older adults), exacerbation of HF, hypotension, bradycardia, peripheral dilation, edema, and headaches	1. Monitor heart rate and blood pressure. 2. Nifedipine is less likely to exacerbate preexisting cardiac conditions; is not effective in treating dysrhythmias. 3. Intensifies cardio-suppressant effects of beta-blocker medications. 4. Client education includes reporting dyspnea, orthopnea, JVD, or swelling of the legs; changing positions slowly.

Beta-Adrenergic Blocking Agents (Adrenergic Antagonists): Blockade of beta$_1$ receptors in the heart causes decreased heart rate and decreased rate of AV conduction. Used to treat hypertension as well as angina. Beta blockers should be administered to all clients experiencing unstable angina or having an MI unless contraindicated.

MEDICATIONS	SIDE EFFECTS	NURSING IMPLICATIONS
▲ Labetalol: PO, IV ▲ Metoprolol: PO, IV ▲ Propranolol: PO, IV ▲ Atenolol: PO, IV Carvedilol: PO *Note: Carvedilol, bisoprolol, and metoprolol sustained release are used to treat HF* Cardioselective—atenolol, carteolol, metoprolol, betaxolol, bisoprolol, nebivolol at low dose	Bradycardia, hypotension, depression, lethargy, and fatigue	1. High-alert medications. 2. Closely monitor cardiac client—may precipitate HF but is also used to treat HF. 3. Teach client how to decrease effects of postural hypotension. 4. Teach client not to stop taking medication when not feeling better. 5. Bradycardia is common adverse effect. 6. If client has diabetes, blood glucose control may be impaired.

Antidysrhythmics: Decrease cardiac excitability; delay cardiac conduction in either the atrium or ventricle. Atropine is a cardiac stimulant for bradycardia.

General Nursing Implications
- Assess client for changes in cardiac rhythm and effect on cardiac output.
- Evaluate effect of medication on dysrhythmia and resulting effects on cardiac output.
- Client should be on bed rest and have a cardiac monitor attached during IV administration.
- Have atropine available for cardiac depression resulting in symptomatic bradycardia.
- All cardiac depressant medications are contraindicated in clients with sinus node or AV node blocks.
- Digitalis will enhance cardiac depressant effects.
- *RN or health care provider will administer intravenous medications*; licensed practical nurse (LPN) may assist in monitoring the client.
- See Appendix 13.3: Cardiac Dysrhythmias.

Appendix 13.2   CARDIAC MEDICATIONS—cont'd

Rx

MEDICATIONS	SIDE EFFECTS	NURSING IMPLICATIONS
Quinidine sulfate: PO	Hypotension Diarrhea, nausea, vomiting	1. *Use:* Supraventricular tachycardia and ventricular dysrhythmias. 2. Monitor for ECG changes for toxicity—widened QRS and prolonged QT. 3. Administer with food.
Atropine: SQ, IV	Tachycardia Dry mouth, blurred vision, dilated pupils, urinary retention	1. *Use:* Symptomatic bradycardia 2. Monitor heart rate and rhythm after administration. 3. Can cause chest pain in clients with ischemic CAD. 4. Contraindicated in clients with acute angle-closure glaucoma.
Adenosine: IV	Common—facial flushing, shortness of breath, dyspnea, and chest pain Significant hypotension, AV heart block	1. *Not* used for irregular wide complex tachycardias because it can degenerate to VF and has a rapid half-life. 2. Causes a brief period of asystole after administration; monitor for bradycardia and hypotension. 3. Monitor heart rate and rhythm closely after administration.
▲ Amiodarone hydrochloride: PO, IV	Bradycardia, AV heart block, hypotension, worsening dysrhythmias Toxicity—lung, visual, liver, and thyroid Muscle-related side effects usually develop early in treatment	1. *Use:* Life-threatening ventricular arrhythmias (pulseless VT/Vfib), atrial fibrillation. 2. Can cause cardiac and respiratory arrest.
▲ Lidocaine hydrochloride: IV	Drowsiness, confusion, paresthesias, slurred speech, seizures, severe depression of cardiac conduction	1. *Use:* Ventricular dysrhythmias (PVCs, VT, VF). 2. Must use IV preparation for IV infusion. 3. Given as a bolus loading dose then continual drip 1–4 mg/min drip.
Mexiletine hydrochloride: PO	Hypotension and bradycardia CNS (common): blurred vision, dizziness, ataxia, confusion GI disturbances—nausea/vomiting, diarrhea; CNS disturbances—tremor, dizziness	1. *Use:* Prevent/control ventricular dysrhythmias (PVCs, VT, VF). 2. Monitor blood pressure and heart rate.
Procainamide: PO, IV	Abdominal pain, cramping, hypotension, prolonged QT interval Long-term use: systemic lupus erythematosus–like syndrome (pain and inflammation of joints) Blood dyscrasias	1. *Use:* Short- and long-term control of ventricular and supraventricular dysrhythmias. 2. Client should report any joint pain and inflammation. 3. Closely monitor for bradycardia and hypotension. 4. Do not take OTC cold preparations.
▲ Propranolol hydrochloride: PO, IV	See previous discussion of beta-adrenergic blockers	1. *Use:* Short- and long-term treatment and prevention of tachycardia (arterial fibrillation, atrial flutter, PVCs).

▲ **Fibrinolytics:** Work by different actions to initiate fibrinolysis of a clot. Medications are not clot specific; they will break up a clot on a surgical incision as well as a clot from an MI.

General Nursing Implications
- Therapy should begin as soon as the MI is diagnosed or when there is a history of prolonged angina. For best results, from admission in the emergency department until medication is administered is 30 minutes (door to needle) or within 60 minutes of onset of symptoms.
- Fibrinolytics can be given within 6 hours from onset of symptoms for a client with an MI and within a 3-hour time frame for a client with a nonhemorrhagic cerebrovascular accident (CVA).
- "Door-to-needle goal" of 30 minutes for most optimum results.
- If a client has any of the following, fibrinolytic therapy may be contraindicated:
  - Systolic blood pressure (BP) greater than 180 mm Hg or diastolic BP greater than 110 mm Hg.
  - Significant closed head or facial trauma within the past 3 months.
  - History of intracranial hemorrhage, currently on anticoagulants, cardiopulmonary resuscitation (CPR) longer than 10 minutes.
  - Pregnancy, serious systemic disease (liver, kidney).
- Bleeding precautions (see Box 10.1).

Continued

Appendix 13.2   CARDIAC MEDICATIONS—cont'd

MEDICATIONS	SIDE EFFECTS	NURSING IMPLICATIONS
▲ Alteplase: IV ▲ Reteplase: IV ▲ Tenecteplase (TNKase): IV	Bleeding and hypotension	1. First-line therapy for clots caused by an MI, limited arterial thrombosis, and thrombotic strokes. 2. Given within the first 2–4 hr after the onset of an MI and within 3 hr following a stroke. 3. Obtain base vital signs and coagulation studies. 4. Avoid venipunctures during and after infusion. 5. *Use:* MI, PE, DVT; contraindicated in clients with active bleeding.

▲ **Cardiac Glycosides:** Increase myocardial contractility, thereby increasing cardiac output. Decrease heart rate by slowing conduction of impulses through the AV node. Enhance diuresis by increasing kidney perfusion.

General Nursing Implications

- Take the apical pulse for a full minute; if the rate is less than 60 beats/min in an adult, less than 90 to 110 beats/min in an infant or young child, or less than 70 beats/min in an older child, hold the medication and notify the health care provider.
- Evaluate for tachycardia, bradycardia, and irregular pulse. If there is significant change in rate and rhythm, hold the medication and notify the health care provider.
- Evaluate serum potassium levels and response to diuretics; hypokalemia potentiates the action of digitalis.
- GI symptoms are frequently the first indication of digitalis toxicity.
- Teach client not to increase or double a dose in the case of a missed dose; if client vomits, do not give an additional dose.
- To achieve maximum results rapidly, an initial loading dose is administered, then the medication is reduced to a maintenance dose.
- *Digibind* is a digitalis antagonist and may be used for digitalis toxicity; watch for decreased potassium levels and client's response to decreased digitalis levels.

MEDICATION	SIDE EFFECTS	NURSING IMPLICATIONS
▲ Digoxin: PO, IV	Most common: anorexia, nausea, vomiting Most serious: drug-induced dysrhythmias Visual disturbances, fatigue 🍦 Children/infants: frequent vomiting, poor feeding, or slow heart rate may indicate toxicity	1. Therapeutic plasma levels of digoxin are 0.5–2.0 ng/mL (0.64–2.56 nmol/L). 2. First sign of toxicity is usually GI symptoms. 3. Slowed heart rate or rhythm changes may indicate toxicity. 4. Withhold digoxin for up to 48 hr before elective cardioversion as it increases the risk for VF. 5. Increased risk of digitalis toxicity when client has hypokalemia. 6. *Use:* Supraventricular tachycardia, HF.

▲ High-alert medications

AV, Atrioventricular; *CAD*, coronary artery disease; *CNS*, central nervous system; *DVT*, deep venous thrombosis; *ECG*, electrocardiogram; *GI*, gastrointestinal; *HF*, heart failure; *IV*, intravenous; *JVD*, jugular venous distention; *MI*, myocardial infarction; *OTC*, over the counter; *PE*, pulmonary embolism; *PO*, by mouth (orally); *PVCs*, premature ventricular contractions; *SQ*, subcutaneous; *VF*, ventricular fibrillation; *VT*, ventricular tachycardia.

Appendix 13.3   CARDIAC DYSRHYTHMIAS

A dysrhythmia is defined as an interruption in the normal conduction of the heart, either in the rate or the rhythm.

> **TEST ALERT** Recognize and report basic abnormalities on a client's cardiac monitor strip.

Characteristics of Normal Sinus Rhythm (Fig. 13.8)

Rate: 60 to 100 beats/min
Rhythm: regular
P waves: present, precede each QRS complex
P-R interval: 0.12 to 0.20 second

QRS complex: present and under 0.10 second
Dysrhythmias may be classified according to rate—either bradycardia or tachycardia. They are also classified according to their origin—atrial or ventricular. Ventricular dysrhythmias are more life-threatening than atrial dysrhythmias. (See Common Dysrhythmias further on.)

Nursing Implications

1. Identify dysrhythmia and evaluate client's tolerance.
2. Monitor adequacy of cardiac output; keep on bed rest and oxygen.
3. Convert abnormal rhythm to normal sinus rhythm—via medications or cardioversion.
4. Prevent complications.

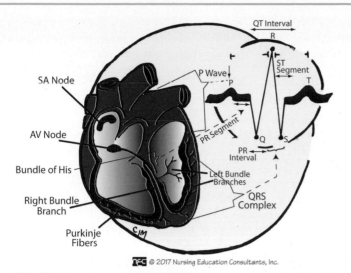

FIG. 13.8 Cardiac Conduction System. (From Zerwekh, J. & Miller, C. J. [2017]. Review course for the NCLEX. Nursing Education Consultants.)

Interpretation of Electrocardiogram

1. Determine heart rate. Count the P waves in a 6-second strip to determine the atrial rate and count the R or Q waves to determine the ventricular rate.
2. Are the QRS complexes occurring at regular intervals?
3. Are P waves present for each QRS complex?
4. Measure the P-R interval.
5. Measure the QRS interval.
6. Identify the T wave and ST segment.
7. Analyze any abnormalities.
8. Correlate findings with the characteristics of normal sinus rhythm.

Common Dysrhythmias

RHYTHM	CHARACTERISTICS	INTERVENTIONS/IMPLICATIONS
Sinus bradycardia	Sinus rhythm less than a rate of 60 beats/min	Assess client for tolerance of the rate. If hypotension or decreasing LOC occurs, the rhythm is treated. *Treatment:* Atropine (can be given via endotracheal tube). If atropine is effective, chronotropic drug infusions are recommended as alternative to external transcutaneous pacing.
Sinus tachycardia	Regular rhythm; P waves present. Rate: 100–150 beats/min	Assess client for tolerance of the rate. Most often caused by caffeine, alcohol, or physiologic response to stimuli. Treatment based on underlying cause. *Treatment:* Vagal maneuvers, adenosine, beta blockers, calcium channel blockers, or synchronized cardioversion.
Atrial fibrillation	Grossly irregular rate; cannot identify P waves or P-R interval on ECG. Controlled rate: 60–100 beats/min. Uncontrolled rate: greater than 100 beats/min	Assess client for tolerance to rapid cardiac rate. Most common dysrhythmia. Evaluate client for systemic emboli (pulmonary emboli or an embolic stroke) from clots that tend to form in fibrillating atrium; a decrease in cardiac output will occur with tachycardia; maintain bed rest until rate is controlled. Pulse deficit will occur with rapid rate. Anticoagulation should precede cardioversion if client is in AF for longer than 48 hours. *Treatment:* Digitalis, calcium channel blockers, beta blockers, cardioversion, or dronedarone; anticoagulants such as warfarin, dabigatran, rivaroxaban, or apixaban.

Continued

Appendix 13.3 CARDIAC DYSRHYTHMIAS—cont'd

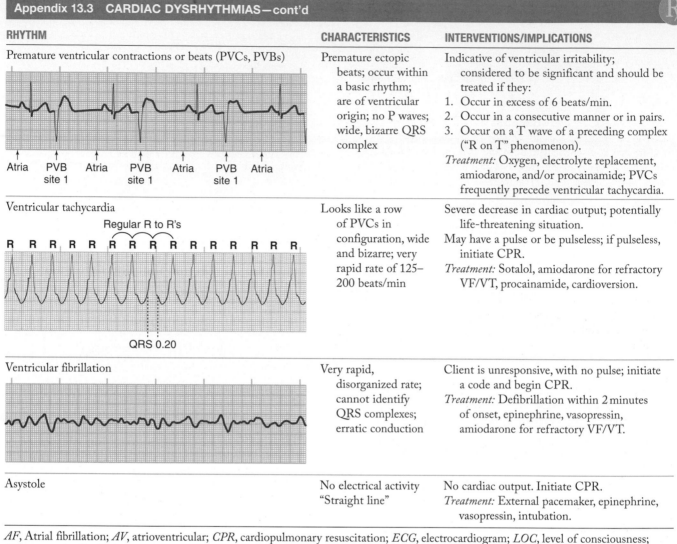

RHYTHM	CHARACTERISTICS	INTERVENTIONS/IMPLICATIONS
Premature ventricular contractions or beats (PVCs, PVBs) Atria PVB site 1 Atria PVB site 1 Atria PVB site 1 Atria	Premature ectopic beats; occur within a basic rhythm; are of ventricular origin; no P waves; wide, bizarre QRS complex	Indicative of ventricular irritability; considered to be significant and should be treated if they: 1. Occur in excess of 6 beats/min. 2. Occur in a consecutive manner or in pairs. 3. Occur on a T wave of a preceding complex ("R on T" phenomenon). *Treatment:* Oxygen, electrolyte replacement, amiodarone, and/or procainamide; PVCs frequently precede ventricular tachycardia.
Ventricular tachycardia Regular R to R's R R R R R R R R R R R R R R R QRS 0.20	Looks like a row of PVCs in configuration, wide and bizarre; very rapid rate of 125–200 beats/min	Severe decrease in cardiac output; potentially life-threatening situation. May have a pulse or be pulseless; if pulseless, initiate CPR. *Treatment:* Sotalol, amiodarone for refractory VF/VT, procainamide, cardioversion.
Ventricular fibrillation	Very rapid, disorganized rate; cannot identify QRS complexes; erratic conduction	Client is unresponsive, with no pulse; initiate a code and begin CPR. *Treatment:* Defibrillation within 2 minutes of onset, epinephrine, vasopressin, amiodarone for refractory VF/VT.
Asystole	No electrical activity "Straight line"	No cardiac output. Initiate CPR. *Treatment:* External pacemaker, epinephrine, vasopressin, intubation.

AF, Atrial fibrillation; *AV*, atrioventricular; *CPR*, cardiopulmonary resuscitation; *ECG*, electrocardiogram; *LOC*, level of consciousness; *VF*, ventricular fibrillation, *VT*, ventricular tachycardia.

Illustrations from Monahan, F. D., Sands J., Neighbors M., Marek J., & Green-Nigro C. (2007). *Phipps' medical-surgical nursing: Health and illness perspectives* (8th ed.). Mosby.

Appendix 13.4 PACEMAKERS

Temporary Pacing

Noninvasive: Application of two large external electrodes attached to an external pulse generator.

Invasive: Wire electrodes are placed in contact with the heart and attached to a battery-operated pulse generator. Wires may be placed on the epicardium during heart surgery; leads are passed through the chest wall. Wires may also be placed via a catheter inserted in the antecubital vein and lodged in the RA and/or ventricle. Used in emergency situations and in severe cases of bradycardia. Anticipate placement of permanent pacemaker (PM).

Permanent: An internal generator is inserted into soft tissue of the upper chest or abdomen and electrodes are positioned in the atrium and ventricles. PM may synchronize pacing between atrium and ventricle (Fig. 13.9). Procedure is planned and conducted under optimal conditions; used in persistent chronic heart block, dysrhythmias, and/or severe bradycardia.

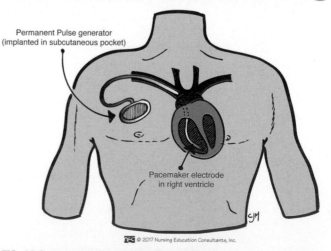

Permanent Pulse generator (implanted in subcutaneous pocket)

Pacemaker electrode in right ventricle

© 2017 Nursing Education Consultants, Inc.

FIG. 13.9 Permanent Pacemaker Placement. (From Zerwekh, J. & Miller, C. J. [2017]. Review course for the NCLEX. Nursing Education Consultants.)

Pacing Modes

Synchronous demand: The heart is stimulated to beat when the client's pulse rate falls below a set value or rate (majority of PMs have a set rate between 60 and 72 beats/min; if client's pulse rate falls below the set value, the PM initiates a heartbeat). The PM "senses" the normal heartbeat and the following conduction. If a normal cardiac beat is initiated and conducted, the PM does not initiate an impulse.

Atrioventricular: The ventricle is sensed and the atrium is paced. If the ventricle does not depolarize, it is also paced.

Universal atrioventricular: Both the atrial and ventricular circuits sense and pace in the respective chambers. This most closely resembles the normal conduction system.

Pacemaker Failure

A cardiac monitor or an ECG must be available to verify PM failure.

Failure to sense: The PM fails to recognize spontaneous heartbeats and will fire inappropriately. This is dangerous because the pacer impulse may be discharged during a critical time in the cardiac cycle and cause a lethal arrhythmia.

Failure to pace: A malfunction in the PM generator; it may also be due to dislodgment of the leads.

Failure to capture: May occur with a low battery or poor connection. The PM is discharging the impulse; however, there is no responding cardiac contraction.

Nursing Implications
1. Assess for dysrhythmias; rate should not fall below preset level.
2. Maintain bed rest if pulse rate drops below preset level.
3. Hypotension, syncope, and bradycardia should not occur.

Client Education
1. Client must notify all health care providers of PM placement and parameters; should also wear a medical alert identification.
2. Avoid constrictive clothing that puts pressure on or irritates the site; report any signs of infection.
3. Safe environment: Avoid areas of high voltage, magnetic force fields (MRI units), or arc welding equipment.
4. Avoid activity that requires vigorous movement of arms and shoulders or any direct blows to PM site.
5. Teach client to check pulse and report if pulse rate is less than 60 beats/min and client is experiencing symptoms; if this occurs, the PM is not functioning properly; this must be reported immediately.
6. Advise client to immediately report episodes of dizziness or syncope, difficulty breathing, chest pain, weight gain, or prolonged hiccupping.
7. Follow-up care and monitoring of PM are important.
8. Client may travel without restrictions.

TEST ALERT Perform check of client's pacemaker.

Appendix 13.5 CARDIOPULMONARY RESUSCITATION FOR HEALTH CARE PROVIDERS

The American Heart Association (AHA) has established standards for cardiopulmonary resuscitation (CPR) for the health care provider. For further delineation of the procedure, consult the 2020 AHA CPR Guidelines. For health care providers, the AHA uses the term *infant* to refer to individuals between birth and 1 year of age; *child* is used to refer to those who are between 1 year of age and the onset of puberty.
1. Verify scene safety.
   - Check for responsiveness.
   - Shout for nearby help.
   - Activate emergency response system via mobile device.
   - Get automated external defibrillator (AED) and emergency equipment.
2. Assessment
   - Check the person for no breathing, abnormal breathing (adult), or only gasping.
   - Simultaneously check the pulse for no more than 10 seconds. If no pulse, start CPR.
   - Adult and child: check the carotid pulse.
   - Infant: check the brachial or femoral pulse.
3. Start CPR
   - Place the victim on a firm surface. If the client is in a bed, put a cardiac board behind the client. *Do not* attempt to remove the victim from the bed.
   - Locate the lower half of the sternum in the adult. For the adult, place one hand over the lower sternum; place the other hand on top of the previous hand. For a child (age 1 year to puberty), use the heel of one hand, or two hands based on the size of the child, and press on the center of the chest at the nipple line. For an infant, locate the nipple line; the area for compression is one finger's width below the line.
   - Depress the sternum at least 2 inches (5 cm) in the adult; in children, at least ½ anterior-posterior (AP) diameter, about 2 inches (5 cm); in infants, at least ¼ diameter, about ½ inch (1.3 cm).

- Push hard and fast—allow complete chest recoil.
- If the pulse is absent, begin chest compressions—cycles of 30 compressions and 2 breaths.
- If the pulse is present, continue rescue breathing and recheck pulse every 2 min. If, despite adequate ventilation, the heart rate of an infant or child remains under 60 beats per min, chest compressions should be started.
- Use AED as soon as it arrives.
- Minimize interruptions to less than 10 seconds.
- Rotate health care provider compressors every 2 minutes.

Adult: One rescuer and two rescuers: 30 compressions (rate of 100 per min) to 2 ventilations.

Pediatric: One rescuer and two rescuers: 30 compressions (rate of 100–120 per min) to 2 ventilations.

Infant: One rescuer: 30 compressions (rate of 100–120 per min) to 2 ventilations. Two rescuers: 15 compressions to 2 ventilations.

4. Rescue breathing.
   - Open the airway: head-tilt/chin-lift maneuver. Use jaw thrust if trauma is suspected.
   - Maintain the open airway.
   - Pinch nostrils closed.
   - Adult: 1 breath every 5 to 6 secs, 10 to 12 breaths per min.
   - Child and infant: 1 breath every 2 to 3 secs, 20 to 30 breaths per min.
   - Advanced airway present (laryngeal mask airway, endotracheal tube): 1 breath every 6 to 8 secs without trying to synchronize breaths with compressions, 8 to 10 breaths per min.

PEDIATRIC NURSING PRIORITY Be careful not to hyperextend the infant's head; this may block the airway. Don't pinch the infant's nose shut; cover the nose with your mouth instead. Breathe slowly, just enough to make the chest rise.

Continued

11. The nurse is reviewing the nurses' notes for a client who presents at the local emergency department. **Highlight the assessment findings that require immediate follow-up by the nurse.**

| Health History | Nurses' Notes | Provider Orders | Laboratory Results |

1700 : A 50-year-old female presents to a local emergency department following a 15-minute episode of diaphoresis, extreme fatigue, and moderate substernal chest pressure. The chest pain was central and did not radiate. The client reports a history of occasional brief episodes of angina lasting 15–20 seconds that are precipitated by emotional upsets with her ex-husband. The client has a history of 20 cigarettes (1 pack) daily (35 pack-years) and is not aware of any other cardiovascular risk factors. On examination the client appears anxious and worries about having a heart attack. There were no heart murmurs present on cardiac auscultation. Breath sounds clear on auscultation.

- Temperature: 98°F (37°C)
- BP: 168/98 mm Hg
- Heart rate: 104 bpm and regular
- Respirations: 24 breaths/min
- SpO2: 97% on room air

12. Stat laboratory tests are ordered. The ECG confirms an ST-segment-elevation myocardial infarction MI (STEMI). The client's troponin, CPK, and CK-MB levels are elevated, which support the diagnosis of an acute MI.

Complete the following sentences by choosing from the list of options.

As a result of the ECG diagnosis of MI, the nurse is aware that ____**1**____ is the most common complication after an MI, especially ____**2**____. The greatest risk of death from an MI is during the first ____**3**____.

OPTIONS FOR 1	OPTIONS FOR 2	OPTIONS FOR 3
Respiratory failure	Heart block	1 hour
Dysrhythmia	Asystole	24 hours
Hypovolemic shock	Ventricular fibrillation	48 hours

⚡Answers to Practice & Next Generation NCLEX (NGN) Questions

1. 1
Client Needs: Physiological Integrity/Reduction of Risk Potential
Clinical Judgment/Cognitive Skill: Take Action
Item Type: Multiple Choice
Rationale & Rationale & Test Taking Strategy: Think about where the insertion site is for the procedure—either the brachial or the femoral artery or vein area. Bleeding from the area is a concern. After a cardiac catheterization, the client will be required to lie flat. The client is usually awake and alert, and pain should not be a problem. The client will not be allowed out of bed for several hours; however, a urinary catheter is not used unless he cannot void from a supine position.

2. 4
Client Needs: Physiological Integrity/Reduction of Risk Potential
Clinical Judgment/Cognitive Skill: Prioritize Hypotheses
Item Type: Multiple Choice
Rationale & Rationale & Test Taking Strategy: Note the **key** words, "highest priority" to reduce cardiac risk factors. One of the highest priority interventions to reduce risk factors is for the client to stop smoking because of its effect on has arterial vasoconstriction and atherosclerosis. Although the other interventions are important considerations, the immediate effects of smoking cessation are generally felt to be the initial most important step in reducing risk factors followed by weight reduction and increasing exercise and physical activity.

3. 4
Client Needs: Physiological Integrity/Pharmacological Therapies
Clinical Judgment/Cognitive Skill: Recognize Cues
Item Type: Multiple Choice
Rationale & Test Taking Strategy: The question is asking about a common side effect of a vasodilator medication. The primary action of nitroglycerin is vasodilation of the arteries. This may precipitate a headache because the cerebral arteries are dilated as well as the coronary arteries, which is often a sign that this medication is working. The other options are not characteristic of nitroglycerin because it causes hypotension and tachycardia. Nausea and vomiting are not common side effects.

4. 1
Client Needs: Physiological Integrity/Physiological Adaptation
Clinical Judgment/Cognitive Skill: Analyze Cues
Item Type: Multiple Choice
Rationale & Test Taking Strategy: The test item asks for "atypical" symptoms. Atypical symptoms in women having a myocardial infarction include shortness of breath, pressure or pain in the lower

chest or upper abdomen, dizziness, light-headedness or fainting, upper back pressure, or extreme fatigue. Pain on inspiration may be related to pleurisy symptoms and manifested with pulmonary problems. Substernal pressure and a feeling of heaviness on the chest and diaphoresis with exertion are typical signs.

5. 4
Client Needs: Physiological Integrity/Physiological Adaptation
Clinical Judgment/Cognitive Skill: Take Action
Item Type: Multiple Choice
Rationale & Test Taking Strategy: Note the **key** word, "immediate." The client is having difficulty breathing and respiratory rate is elevated. High-Fowler, if tolerated, or Fowler (45 degrees) position with the legs dependent will help to decrease venous return. This position will decrease the workload of the heart and increase cardiac efficiency. Increasing cardiac efficiency will help to improve the quality of ventilation. Oxygen should be started immediately as well. Dyspnea and tachycardia are indications that the heart failure is progressing. When the client last had prescribed medications is not a priority at this time. A supine position with the feet elevated will increase the cardiac workload, venous return, and dyspnea. The nursing supervisor or health care provider should also be notified.

6. 2
Client Needs: Physiological Integrity/Pharmacological Therapies
Clinical Judgment/Cognitive Skill: Generate Solutions
Item Type: Multiple Choice
Rationale & Test Taking Strategy: Review the vital signs and ask yourself if any of these are abnormal. The client has a significantly low pulse of 48 beats/min and so the metoprolol should be held and the health care provider notified. Metoprolol is used to treat angina and hypertension. Side effects include bradycardia, drowsiness, dizziness, tiredness, diarrhea, reduced cardiac output, AV block, and precipitation of heart block, even though some beta blockers are used to treat heart failure. The client would need to receive the clopidogrel to prevent platelet aggregation and clotting and acetaminophen for the slight temperature elevation. The blood pressure is in normal range, along with the respiratory rate.

7. 4
Client Needs: Physiological Integrity/Pharmacological Therapies
Clinical Judgment/Cognitive Skill: Take Action
Item Type: Multiple Choice
Rationale & Test Taking Strategy: Think about how nitroglycerin is administered. Nitroglycerin should be taken at the first sign of any chest pain; if the pain is not relieved within 5 minutes, another tablet should be taken, and emergency medical services should be called. If the client continues to experience chest pain prior to the arrival of assistance, another sublingual nitroglycerin should be taken. The medication should be stored in a dark container and, after dosing, should be allowed to dissolve under the tongue. It does have a rapid onset, but it is most important to tell the client to take it at the first indication of chest pain. If possible, the client should lie down when taking the nitroglycerin.

8. 1, 3
Client Needs: Physiological Integrity/Pharmacological Therapies
Clinical Judgment/Cognitive Skill: Take Action
Item Type: Select All That Apply
Rationale & Test Taking Strategy: The nurse should reinforce the teaching to avoid drinking grapefruit juice or eating grapefruit because it can inhibit intestinal and hepatic metabolism of the drug, thereby raising the drug level. Because constipation is a common side effect of verapamil, the nurse should encourage the client to increase fluids and dietary fiber to prevent this common side effect. When a sustained-release formulation is prescribed, the client should not crush or chew the medication, but instead the client should swallow the pill intact because chewing or crushing could result in a bolus effect. Monitoring liver enzymes and electrolytes is not indicated.

9. 2
Client Needs: Physiological Integrity/Physiological Adaptation
Clinical Judgment/Cognitive Skill: Take Action
Item Type: Multiple choice
Rationale & Test Taking Strategy: Note the **key** word, "first." When a client reports having chest pain, the client should immediately be returned to bed and oxygen started. After this is done, assessment of the chest pain and possibly administration of nitroglycerin can be accomplished. *The charge nurse should be notified immediately.* The health care provider can be notified after further assessment of the client. What the client last ate is not immediately relevant to the situation.

10. 3
Client Needs: Physiological Integrity/Physiological Adaptation
Clinical Judgment/Cognitive Skill: Generate Solutions
Item Type: Multiple Choice
Rationale & Test Taking Strategy: The right arm must remain abducted to prevent inadvertent movement of the pacemaker wires that were inserted via the right subclavian vein. Checking the radial pulse does not determine if the pacemaker is functioning or if the client is maintaining his own rhythm. There are no external wires on a permanent pacemaker. The status of the incision is not of high importance in preventing immediate complications.

11. The nurse is reviewing the nurses' notes for a client who presents at the local emergency department. **Highlight the assessment findings that require immediate follow-up by the nurse.**

Health History	Nurses' Notes	Provider Orders	Laboratory Results

1700 A 50-year-old female presents to a local emergency department following a 15-minute episode of diaphoresis, extreme fatigue, and moderate substernal chest pressure. The chest pain was central and did not radiate. The client reports a history of occasional brief episodes of angina lasting 15–20 seconds that are precipitated by emotional upsets with her ex-husband. The client has a history of 20 cigarettes (1 pack) daily (35-pack-years) and is not aware of any other cardiovascular risk factors. On examination the client appears anxious and states she is worried she is having a heart attack. There were no heart murmurs present on cardiac auscultation. Breath sounds clear on auscultation.

- Temperature: 98°F (37°C)
- BP: 168/98 mmHg
- Heart rate: 104 bpm and regular
- Respirations: 24 breaths/min
- SpO2: 97% on room air

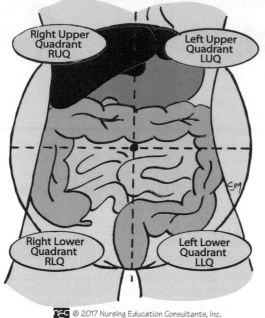

FIG. 14.1 Abdominal Quadrants. (From Zerwekh, J. & Miller, C. J. [2017]. *NCLEX review course.* Nursing Education Consultants.)

Box 14.1 OLDER ADULT CARE FOCUS

Changes in Gastrointestinal System Related to Aging

- Decreased hydrochloric acid and decreased absorption of vitamins; encourage frequent, small feedings that are high in vitamins.
- Decreased peristalsis and decreased sensation to defecate; encourage diet high in fiber and minimum of 2000 mL of fluid daily; encourage physical activity.
- Decreased lipase from pancreas to aid in fat digestion; encourage smaller meals because diarrhea may be caused by increased fat intake.
- Decreased liver activity with decreased production of enzymes for drug metabolism; tendency toward accumulation of medications; instruct clients not to double up on their medications, especially cardiac medications.
- Increased disorders causing acute and/or chronic pain such as osteoarthritis may lead to increased use of aspirin, NSAIDs, and/or opioid medications as analgesics; monitor for side effects such as GI bleeding or constipation/fecal impaction.

GI, Gastrointestinal; *NSAID,* nonsteroidal anti-inflammatory drug.

Analyze Cues and Prioritize Hypotheses

The most important problems are electrolyte, fluid, and acid-base balance problems.

Generate Solutions

Treatment

A. Eliminate the precipitating cause.
B. Antiemetics (see Appendix 14.2).
C. Parenteral replacement of fluid if loss is excessive.

Nursing Interventions: Take Action

Goal: To prevent recurrence of nausea and vomiting and ensuing complications.

A. Prophylactic antiemetics for the client with a tendency to vomit.
B. Prompt removal of unpleasant odors, used emesis container, and soiled linens.
C. Good oral hygiene.
D. Place conscious client on side or in semi-Fowler position; place unconscious client on side with head of bed slightly elevated to promote drainage of oral cavity.
E. Withhold food and beverages initially after vomiting; begin oral intake slowly; for adults, begin with tea, water, or oral rehydrating solutions (ORSs) at room temperature; for infants and children, begin with ORSs.
F. Gastric decompression with a nasogastric (NG) tube may be used for prolonged vomiting.
G. Assess surgical client for presence of bowel sounds and distention; do not begin oral administration of fluids if abdomen is tender or distended or no bowel sounds are present.
H. Support abdominal and thoracic incisions during vomiting.

Assessment: Recognize Cues

A. Precipitating causes.
  1. GI obstruction, toxic substances, infection, etc.
  2. Chemotherapy/radiation, medications.
  3. Surgery (postoperative complication).
  4. Pregnancy: vomiting most often occurs in the morning.
B. Clinical manifestations.
  1. Identify precipitating cause.
  2. Assess frequency and amount of vomiting and contents of vomitus.
  3. Vomiting in children is common.
  4. Further investigation and intervention are needed for progressively severe vomiting, persistent vomiting over 24 hours, and/or symptoms of dehydration.
  5. Hematemesis: presence of blood in vomitus.
    a. Bright red blood is indicative of active bleeding.
    b. Coffee-ground material is indicative of blood retained in the stomach; the digestive process has broken down the hemoglobin.
  6. Projectile vomiting: vomiting, which may not be preceded by nausea in which vomitus is expelled with excessive force; often seen with increased intracranial pressure.
  7. Presence of fecal odor and bile in vomitus indicates a backflow of intestinal contents into stomach.
  8. Vomiting in children is usually self-limiting; assess for fever, diarrhea, and abdominal pain accompanying nausea and vomiting.
C. Diagnostics: clinical manifestations.

TEST ALERT Identify client potential for aspiration; intervene to prevent aspiration.

Goal: To assess client's response to prolonged vomiting.

A. Monitor fluid and electrolyte status.
B. Assess for continued presence of gastric distention.
C. Assess for adequate hydration.

TEST ALERT Monitor client's hydration status.

Constipation

Constipation **exists when there is a decrease in frequency of bowel movements; stool is hard and difficult to pass, and there is less than one bowel movement every 3 days.**

Assessment: Recognize Cues

A. Precipitating causes.
   1. Decreased fiber and fluid intake.
   2. Immobility, inadequate exercise.
   3. Medications: opioids, antidepressants, iron supplements, anticonvulsants.
   4. Older adult client.
   5. Overuse of laxatives or enemas.
   6. Ignoring the urge to defecate.
   7. Diverticulosis, tumors, intestinal obstructions, irritable bowel syndrome.

TEST ALERT Evaluate client's use of home remedies and OTC drugs. Assess what the client is using to treat constipation; frequently, the older adult client is using harsh laxatives.

B. Clinical manifestations.
   1. Abdominal distention.
   2. Decreased amount and/or frequency of stool.
   3. Dry, hard stool; straining to pass stool.
   4. Impaction.
      a. Constipation; rectal discomfort.
      b. Anorexia, nausea, vomiting.
      c. Diarrhea around impacted stool.
C. Diagnostics: clinical manifestations, colonoscopy.

Analyze Cues and Prioritize Hypotheses

The most important problems are difficulty with passing stool (abdominal or gas pains), inability to pass stool (impaction).

Generate Solutions

Treatment

A. Change dietary intake: increase intake of high-fiber foods and fluids.
B. Bulk laxatives, stool softeners, or enemas (see Appendix 14.2).
C. Instruct client to maintain normal bowel schedule and not to ignore urge to defecate.
D. Discourage overuse or misuse of laxatives and enemas.
E. Encourage regular exercise.

Nursing Interventions: Take Action

TEST ALERT Assess and intervene when a client has a problem with elimination.

Goal: To identify client at risk for developing constipation and institute preventive measures (Box 14.2).
Goal: To implement treatment measures for fecal impaction removal.

A. An impaction may be present if client has had no bowel movement for 3 days or has passed only small amounts of semisoft or liquid stool.
B. Steps in removing impaction:
   1. Follow facility policy and procedure.
   2. Manually check for presence of impaction with nonsterile, lubricated gloved finger.
   3. Gently attempt to break up impaction using a scissor motion with the fingers.
   4. Emphasis is on *prevention* of impaction (see Box 14.2).
   5. Suppositories inserted into rectum may be given between attempts to clear the stool.

! NURSING PRIORITY Monitor client's heart rate during and after digital removal of feces; vagal stimulation can precipitate bradycardia.

Diarrhea

Diarrhea is the rapid movement of intestinal contents through the small bowel.

A. Infants and older adults are most susceptible to complications of dehydration and hypovolemia.
B. Acute diarrhea is most often caused by an infection and is self-limiting when all causative agents or irritants have been evacuated.

Box 14.2   OLDER ADULT CARE FOCUS

Preventing Fecal Impaction

- Increase intake of high-fiber foods: raw vegetables, whole-grain breads and cereals, fresh fruits.
- Increase fluid intake.
- Maintain regular activity: daily walking, swimming, or biking. If confined to wheelchair, change position frequently, perform leg raises and abdominal muscle contractions.
- Avoid overuse and misuse of laxatives and enemas.
- Encourage use of bulk-forming products to provide increased fiber (methylcellulose, psyllium).
- Encourage bowel movement at same time each day.
- Try to position client on bedside commode rather than on a bedpan to facilitate defecation.
- If client is experiencing diarrhea, check to see if stool is oozing around an impaction.

4. Pain may radiate to back and neck.
5. Regurgitation not associated with belching or nausea.

C. Diagnostics: 24-hour pH monitoring, esophageal manometry, esophagogastroduodenoscopy (EGD) (see Appendix 14.1).

Analyze Cues and Prioritize Hypotheses

The most important problems are acute pain due to gastrointestinal reflux and potential compromised nutrition due to dietary selection.

Generate Solutions

Treatment

A. Medications: histamine$_2$-receptor antagonists (H$_2$R blockers), proton pump inhibitors (PPIs), and GI stimulants or promotility drugs (see Appendix 14.2).
B. Surgical: fundoplication or antireflux surgery.

Nursing Interventions: Take Action

Goal: To decrease esophageal reflux.

A. Dietary.
   1. Eat four to six small meals per day (at 3-hour intervals) and avoid foods that precipitate discomfort (fats, caffeine, chocolate, spicy food, tomato products).
   2. Consume a high-protein, low-fat diet and avoid temperature extremes in foods.
   3. Avoid drinking beverages during meals, including alcohol and carbonated drinks.
   4. Avoid drinking fluids 3 hours before bedtime.
B. Lifestyle.
   1. If overweight, lose weight to decrease abdominal pressure gradient.
   2. Do not lie down for 2 to 3 hours after eating.
   3. Elevate the head of the bed on 4- to 6-inch (10–15 cm) blocks.
   4. Avoid tobacco, nonsteroidal anti-inflammatory drugs (NSAIDs), and salicylates.

> **! OLDER ADULT PRIORITY** GERD is often underreported in the older client; clients who awaken from coughing should be evaluated for GERD; clients are also at increased risk for aspiration.

Gastritis

Gastritis is an inflammation and breakdown of the normal gastric mucosa barrier. Acute gastritis is generally self-limiting with no residual damage.

Assessment: Recognize Cues

A. Risk factors/etiology.
   1. Primary cause of chronic gastritis is *Helicobacter pylori*.
   2. Often caused by dietary indiscretion (gastric irritants: coffee, alcohol) and medications (corticosteroids, aspirin, NSAIDs).

3. Acute gastritis is a common problem in ICUs because of stress.

B. Clinical manifestations (may be asymptomatic).
   1. Epigastric tenderness.
   2. Anorexia, nausea, vomiting, bloating, dyspepsia.
C. Diagnostics (see Appendix 14.1).
   1. Endoscopy with biopsy to rule out gastric carcinoma.
   2. Stool examination for occult blood.
   3. Gastric analysis for decreased acid production (achlorhydria).
   4. Serum, stool, and gastric biopsy for *H. pylori*.

Analyze Cues and Prioritize Hypotheses

The most important problems are indigestion and potential fluid and electrolyte imbalance due to vomiting.

Generate Solutions

Treatment

A. Eliminate cause.
B. Medical management.
   1. Antiemetics, antacids, PPIs, and H$_2$R blockers (see Appendix 14.2).
   2. Treatment for *H. pylori* with antibiotics and PPIs.
C. Surgical intervention, if medical treatment fails or hemorrhage occurs.

Nursing Interventions: Take Action

Goal: To decrease gastric irritation.

A. Nothing-by-mouth (NPO) status initially, with intravenous (IV) fluid and electrolyte replacement.
B. Begin ORSs as client tolerates them.

Goal: To monitor fluid status and prevent dehydration. (See Chapter 6.)

Goal: To assist client to identify and avoid precipitating causes.

Gastroenteritis

Gastroenteritis is the irritation and inflammation of the mucosa of the stomach and small bowel.

Assessment: Recognize Cues

A. Risk factors/etiology.
   1. Salmonella: fecal oral transmission by direct contact or via contaminated food.
   2. Staphylococcal: transmission via foods that were handled by contaminated carrier.
   3. Dysentery: *E. coli* and *Shigella*.
B. Clinical manifestations.
   1. Abdominal cramping, distention, and pain.
   2. Nausea, vomiting, and diarrhea.
   3. Anorexia, fever, and chills.
C. Diagnostics: stool culture.

Analyze Cues and Prioritize Hypotheses

The most important problems are indigestion and potential fluid and electrolyte imbalance due to vomiting and diarrhea.

Generate Solutions

Treatment
A. Nothing by mouth until nausea subsides.
B. Rehydrate with water and ORSs.
C. Client resumes eating with bland, easily digestible foods.
D. Appropriate medication for causative agents.

Nursing Interventions: Take Action

See Nursing Interventions section under Nausea and Vomiting.

Obesity

Obesity **is an imbalance between energy expenditure and caloric intake that results in an abnormal increase in fat cells.**

A. According to the Centers for Disease Control and Prevention, approximately 40% of people in the United States over age 20 are overweight or obese.
B. Children are considered overweight if their weight is in the 95th percentile or higher for their age, gender, and height on the growth chart.
C. Classified according to the body mass index (BMI).

Assessment: Recognize Cues

A. Risk factors.
   1. Genetic predisposition.
   2. Sedentary lifestyle: energy intake (food) exceeds energy expenditure.
   3. Obesity puts client at increased risk for cardiovascular, respiratory, and musculoskeletal problems, as well as increased risk for development of diabetes.
B. Clinical manifestations.
   1. A BMI of 25 to 29.9 kg/m^2 is considered overweight; a BMI of more than 30 kg/m^2 is considered obese; and a BMI greater than 40 kg/m^2 is considered severe/morbid obesity.
   2. Android obesity *(apple-shaped)* is considered to be a higher risk for obesity-related problems than those whose fat is primarily located in the upper legs and hips (gynecoid obesity or *pear-shaped*), especially elevated triglycerides, hypertension, and type 2 diabetes.

Analyze Cues and Prioritize Hypotheses

The most important problems are weight gain due to increased intake of calories and potential for problems associated with being overweight (e.g., diabetes, coronary artery disease, hypertension).

Generate Solutions

Treatment
A. Lifestyle changes and modification of dietary intake.
B. Bariatric surgery.
   1. Restrictive surgery.
      a. Vertical banded gastroplasty (VBG): adjustable gastric banding (AGB) involves placing a band around the fundus of the stomach; band may or may not be inflatable.
      b. Vertical sleeve gastrectomy (VSG): removes up to 85% of the stomach.
   2. Malabsorptive: biliopancreatic diversion (BPD): 70% of stomach removed; stomach and small intestine connected.
   3. Combination of restrictive and malabsorptive surgery: Roux-en-Y gastric bypass (RYGB) connects a small stomach pouch with the jejunum; first part of small intestine is bypassed.

Nursing Interventions: Take Action

Goal: To prepare client for surgery. (See Chapter 3.)
Goal: To maintain homeostasis postoperatively.
A. Immediately postoperative airway may be a problem; maintain good pulmonary hygiene; ventilator support may be necessary.
   1. If continuous positive airway pressure (CPAP) was used at home, client will need it in hospital.
   2. Elevate the client's upper body at a 35- to 45-degree angle to reduce abdominal pressure and increase lung expansion.
B. Increased risks for thromboembolic problems: encourage use of sequential compression stockings and early ambulation and administer thromboprophylaxis with low-molecular-weight heparin.
C. Do not adjust an NG tube and do not insert NG tube even if there is protocol to do so for nausea and vomiting; *notify registered nurse (RN) or surgeon.*
D. Observe client for development of anastomotic leaks: increasing back, shoulder, or abdominal pain; unexplained tachycardia or decreased urine output; *notify RN or surgeon of these findings.*
E. Extra attention is needed to skin care because of large folds of skin and extra weight.
F. In client with diabetes, assess for fluctuations in serum blood glucose; may require less hypoglycemics.
G. Client with malabsorption surgery may experience dumping syndrome (Box 14.4; Fig. 14.3).

Home Care

A. Diet.
   1. Eat at least four to six small meals a day; chew food completely.
   2. Drink fluids throughout the day, but do not drink fluids with meals.
   3. Avoid high-calorie, high-sugar, high-carbohydrate, and high-fat foods.
   4. Stop eating when a full feeling occurs.
   5. Try to get 50 to 60 g of protein daily; may need to take a protein supplement.
   6. Learn how to avoid dumping syndrome.
B. Take a chewable or liquid multivitamin with iron.
C. For women, do not try to get pregnant for about 18 months after surgery.
D. Develop a daily routine for exercise.

Peptic Ulcer Disease

Peptic ulcer disease (PUD) **is an erosion of the GI mucosa by hydrochloric acid and pepsin. Any location in the GI tract that comes in contact with gastric secretions is susceptible to ulcer development.**

PERITONITIS

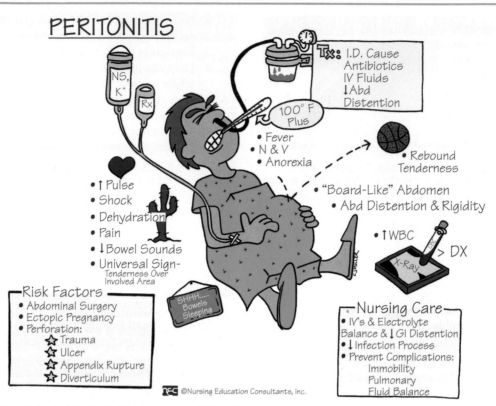

FIG. 14.5 Peritonitis. *GI*, Gastrointestinal; *IV*, intravenous; *WBC*, white blood cell. (From Zerwekh, J., Garneau, A., & Miller, C. J. [2017]. *Digital collection of the memory notebooks of nursing* [4th ed.]. Nursing Education Consultants.)

1. Presence of precipitating cause (ulcer perforation, ruptured appendix or diverticulum, trauma).
2. Sharp or knifelike pain and/or dull and deep-seated pain over involved area; rebound tenderness; pain may radiate to back, shoulder, or scapula.
3. Sudden, excruciating pain suggests the possibility of rupture.
4. Abdominal mass or distention.
5. Abdominal muscle rigidity ("boardlike" abdomen), guarding.
6. Unexplained persistent or labile fever.
7. Anorexia, nausea, vomiting, hiccups.
8. Tachycardia, hypotension, shallow respirations.
9. Decreased or absent bowel sounds.
10. Hypovolemia, dehydration.
11. Shallow respirations in an attempt to avoid pain.

C. Diagnostics.
   1. CBC for elevated WBC count.
   2. Abdominal x-ray, CT, and ultrasonography.
   3. Peritoneal lavage (aspiration) to evaluate abdominal fluid.

Analyze Cues and Prioritize Hypotheses

The most important problems are infection, abdominal pain, and risk for sepsis.

Generate Solutions

Treatment

A. Identify and treat precipitating cause; frequently requires surgical intervention.
B. Antibiotics.
C. IV fluids and electrolyte replacement.

D. Decrease abdominal distention: NPO, NG tube.

Nursing Interventions: Take Action

Goal: To provide pain control, wound care, prevent complications of immobility, and monitor postoperative progress (see Chapter 3).

Goal: To maintain fluid and electrolyte balances and reduce gastric distention.

A. Maintain NG suction (see Appendix 14.4).
B. Maintain IV fluid replacement and hydration status.
C. Assess level of distention and return of peristalsis and bowel function.
D. Maintain intake and output records.
E. Assess for problems of dehydration and hypovolemia.
F. Encourage activities to facilitate return of bowel function (i.e., ambulation).

Goal: To reduce infectious process.

A. Assess client's tolerance of antibiotics and status of infusion site.
B. Evaluate vital signs and correlate with progress of infectious process.
C. Assess wound for signs of infection, purulent/foul-smelling drainage.
D. Maintain in semi-Fowler position to enhance respirations, as well as to localize drainage and prevent formation of subdiaphragmatic abscess.

Diverticular Disease

When a diverticulum (a pouchlike herniation of superficial layers of the colon through weakened muscle of the bowel wall) becomes inflamed, it is known as *diverticulitis*. Multiple diverticula are known as *diverticulosis*.

Meckel diverticulum is a congenital diverticulum present in about 2% of the population, usually presenting with symptoms before age 2 years.

Assessment: Recognize Cues

A. Risk factors/etiology.
  1. Increased risk in clients over 45 years old.
  2. Low-fiber diet and chronic constipation.
  3. Most frequently occurs in sigmoid colon.
  4. Indigestible fibers (corn, seeds, etc.) may precipitate diverticulitis, but they do not contribute to the development of diverticula.
B. Clinical manifestations.
  1. Diverticular disease is frequently asymptomatic; symptoms vary with degree of inflammation.
  2. Diverticulitis occurs when undigested food and bacteria are trapped in the diverticula.
      a. Symptoms of infection (fever, leukocytosis).
      b. Acute left lower quadrant pain; may be accompanied by nausea and vomiting.
      c. Abdominal distention and increased pain on palpation.
      d. May progress to abscess, intestinal obstruction, and/or perforation.
C. Diagnostics (see Appendix 14.1).
  1. Computed tomography (CT) scan and/or ultrasound.
  2. Barium enema or colonoscopy is contraindicated in acute diverticulitis.

Analyze Cues and Prioritize Hypotheses

The most important problems are abdominal pain, risk of intestinal obstruction or perforation, and dietary changes.

Generate Solutions

Treatment

A. Management of uncomplicated diverticulum.
  1. High-fiber diet, mainly fruits and vegetables.
  2. Decreased intake of fat and red meat.
  3. Stool softeners, bulk laxatives.
  4. Increased activity: walking, exercise.
B. Treatment for acute diverticulitis.
  1. Antibiotics, antispasmodics.
  2. May be NPO or on a low-residue diet.
  3. IV fluids for hydration, if needed.
  4. Possible surgery and colon resection if abscess, obstruction, bleeding, or perforation.

Nursing Interventions: Take Action

Goal: To assist client to understand dietary implications and maintain prescribed therapy to prevent exacerbations.

A. Teach client to gradually reintroduce fiber after an acute episode of diverticulitis.
B. Maintain high fluid intake.

TEST ALERT Monitor and provide for nutritional needs of client.

C. Weight reduction, if overweight or obese.
D. During acute diverticulitis, avoid activities that increase intraabdominal pressure (e.g., straining at stool, bending, lifting); avoid wearing tight restrictive clothing; maintain NPO status or clear liquids only.
E. Use bulk laxatives to prevent acute episodes of diverticulitis but not during an episode; avoid enemas and harsh laxatives.

Inflammatory Bowel Disease

Inflammatory bowel disease (IBD) **is an autoimmune disease characterized by chronic inflammation of the GI tract with periods of remission and exacerbation. It is considered an autoimmune disease; tissue damage is due to overactive sustained inflammatory response.**

A. *Crohn disease* (ileitis or enteritis) is inflammation occurring anywhere along the GI tract, from the mouth to the anus; patches of inflammation occur next to healthy bowel tissue; most frequently affecting the terminal ileum and colon.
B. *Ulcerative colitis* is an inflammation and ulceration that most commonly occurs in the sigmoid colon and rectum; inflammation frequently begins in the rectum and spreads in a continuous manner up the colon; seldom is the small intestine involved.
C. Clients frequently experience periods of complete remission that alternate with exacerbations.

Assessment: Recognize Cues

A. Risk factors/etiology.
  1. Familial tendency.
  2. Commonly occurs in the teenage years, with a second peak in occurrence in clients age 60 and older.
  3. Altered inflammatory response.
B. Clinical manifestations—Crohn disease.
  1. Diarrhea; bloody stools.
  2. Weight loss; nutritional deficiencies; impaired absorption of vitamin B_{12} (cobalamin).
  3. Intermittent fever.
  4. Entire thickness of bowel wall is involved; fistulas are not uncommon.
  5. Nausea, abdominal pain, flatulence.
C. Clinical manifestations—ulcerative colitis.
  1. Abdominal pain.
  2. Bloody diarrhea.
  3. Number of stools increases with exacerbation of condition; 10 to 20 stools per day in acute exacerbation.
  4. Increase in systemic symptoms (fever, malaise, anorexia) with exacerbation.
  5. Anemia.
  6. Minimal small-bowel involvement.
D. Diagnostics (see Appendix 14.1).
  1. Stool analysis to rule out bacterial or parasitic infection.

A. Monitor all stools; passage of normal stool may indicate reduction of the obstruction, especially an intussusception.

B. Classic signs and symptoms of intussusception may not be present; observe child for diarrhea, anorexia, vomiting, and episodic abdominal pain.

Goal: To decrease gastric distention and to maintain hydration and electrolyte balance.

A. Maintain NPO status.

B. Maintain NG suction.

C. Monitor IV fluid replacement: most often normal saline or lactated Ringer solution.

D. Evaluate peristalsis, presence of any bowel function.

E. Maintain accurate intake and output records.

F. Assess for dehydration, hypovolemia, and electrolyte imbalance.

G. Measure abdominal girth to determine whether distention is increasing.

H. Encourage activities to facilitate return of bowel function.
1. Encourage physical activity, as tolerated.
2. Attempt to decrease amount of medication (especially opioids) required for effective pain control.
3. Maintain hydration.

I. Frequently, the position of comfort is side-lying with knees flexed.

Goal: To provide appropriate preoperative preparation when surgery is indicated (see Chapter 3).

Goal: To maintain homeostasis and promote healing after abdominal laparotomy (see Chapter 3).

Goal: To decrease infection and promote healing after surgery.

A. Monitor client's response to antibiotics.

B. Monitor vital signs frequently and evaluate for presence or escalation of infectious process.

C. Provide wound care. Evaluate drainage and healing from abdominal drains, as well as from abdominal incisional area.

TEST ALERT Empty and reestablish negative pressure of portable wound suction devices (Hemovac and Jackson-Pratt drains).

Goal: To reestablish normal nutrition and promote comfort after abdominal laparotomy.

A. Evaluate tolerance of liquids when NG tube is removed.

B. Begin administration of clear liquids initially and continue to evaluate for peristalsis and/or distention, nausea, and vomiting.

C. Progress diet as tolerated.

D. Administer analgesics as needed.

E. Promote psychological comfort.
1. Keep client and family informed and involved in plan of care and procedures.
2. Encourage parents of child to room-in with child and ask questions.

Hernia

A *hernia* is a protrusion of the intestine through an abnormal opening or weakened area of the abdominal wall.

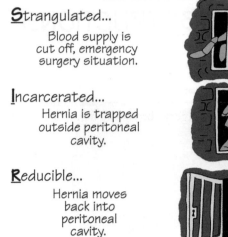

"SIR" HERNIA

Strangulated...
Blood supply is cut off, emergency surgery situation.

Incarcerated...
Hernia is trapped outside peritoneal cavity.

Reducible...
Hernia moves back into peritoneal cavity.

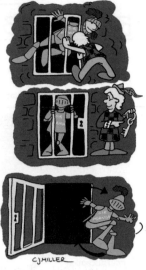

CJMILLER

© 2017 Nursing Education Consultants, Inc.

FIG. 14.7 Hernia. (From Zerwekh, J., Garneau, A., & Miller, C. J. [2017]. *Digital collection of the memory notebooks of nursing* [4th ed.]. Nursing Education Consultants.)

A. Types.
1. Inguinal: a weakness in which the spermatic cord in men and the round ligament in women passes through the abdominal wall in the groin area; more common in men; most common type of hernia in children.
2. Femoral: protrusion of the intestine through the femoral ring; more common in women.
3. Incisional or ventral: weakness in the abdominal wall caused by a previous incision.
4. Umbilical: occurs most often in children when the umbilical opening fails to close adequately; most common hernia in infants; may occur in adults when the rectus muscle is weak from surgical incision.
5. Classification (Fig. 14.7).
   a. Reducible: hernia may be replaced into the abdominal cavity by manual manipulation.
   b. Incarcerated or irreducible: hernia cannot be pushed back into place.
   c. Strangulated: blood supply and intestinal flow in the herniated area are obstructed; this leads to intestinal obstruction and possible perforation or necrosis.

Assessment: Recognize Cues

A. Risk factors.
1. Obesity or weakened abdominal musculature.
2. Straining during bowel movement or lifting heavy objects.
3. Pregnancy.

B. Clinical manifestations.
1. Hernia protrudes over the involved area when the client stands or strains or when the infant cries.
2. Severe pain occurs if hernia becomes strangulated.

3. Strangulated hernia produces symptoms of intestinal obstruction.

C. Diagnostics—ultrasound, CT scan (see Appendix 14.1).

Analyze Cues and Prioritize Hypotheses

The most important problem is the risk of strangulation.

Generate Solutions

Treatment

A. Preferably elective surgery through abdominal incision (herniorrhaphy).

B. Laparoscopic hernia repair.

C. Emergency surgery for strangulated hernias.

Nursing Interventions: Take Action

Goal: To prepare client for surgery, if indicated (see Chapter 3).

Goal: To maintain homeostasis and promote healing after herniorrhaphy.

A. General postoperative nursing care (see Chapter 3).

B. Assess male clients for development of scrotal edema; may require the use of a scrotal support with application of an ice bag.

C. Encourage deep breathing and activity.

D. If coughing occurs, teach client how to splint the incision.

E. Refrain from heavy lifting for approximately 6 to 8 weeks after surgery.

F. Wound care.

   1. Keep wound clean and dry: use occlusive dressing or leave open to air.

   2. Change diapers frequently and/or prevent irritation and contamination in incisional area.

Cancer of the Stomach

Stomach or *gastric cancer* is usually an adenocarcinoma of the stomach wall.

Assessment: Recognize Cues

A. Risk factors/etiology.

   1. Peak incidence in seventh decade.

   2. Presence of *H. pylori* is considered an increased risk factor.

   3. Diet including smoked foods, salted fish and meat, and pickled vegetables.

B. Clinical manifestations.

   1. Early symptoms (may be asymptomatic until disease has far advanced).

      a. Loss of appetite; persistent indigestion.

      b. Early satiety; dyspepsia.

      c. Nausea, vomiting; fatigue, weakness.

      d. Blood in stool.

   2. Later symptoms.

      a. Pain often exacerbated by eating.

      b. Weight loss; anemia.

      c. Nausea and vomiting due to impending GI obstruction.

      d. Presence of a palpable mass in the stomach; ascites from involvement of peritoneal cavity.

C. Diagnostics (see Appendix 14.1).

   1. Gastroscopy and biopsy.

   2. CT and full-body imaging for metastasis.

Analyze Cues and Prioritize Hypotheses

The most important problems are the risk of metastasis to other organs, need for surgery, and managing chemotherapy and/or radiation therapy side effects.

Generate Solutions

Treatment

A. Partial or complete gastrectomy is the preferred method of treatment.

B. Chemotherapy and radiation usually follow surgery.

Nursing Interventions: Take Action

See Nursing Interventions for gastric resection under Peptic Ulcer Disease.

Colorectal Cancer

***Colorectal cancer* (cancer of the colon and/or the rectum) is the third most common cancer in the United States and the second leading cause of cancer-related deaths.**

Assessment: Recognize Cues

A. Risk factors/etiology.

   1. Family history (first-degree relative) of colorectal cancer.

   2. Incidence increases significantly after age 50.

   3. History of IBD.

   4. High-fat, high-calorie, low-residue diet with high intake of red meat increases anaerobic bacteria in bowel, which convert bile acids into carcinogens.

   5. Alcohol, tobacco use, and obesity are also associated with increased risk.

B. Clinical manifestations.

   1. Symptoms are vague early in disease state and may take years to present.

   2. Bloody stools, melena (dark tarry) stools.

   3. Change in bowel habits: constipation and diarrhea.

   4. Change in shape of stool (pencil- or ribbon-shaped in sigmoid or rectal cancer).

   5. Weakness and fatigue from iron deficiency anemia and chronic blood loss.

   6. Pain, anorexia, and unexpected weight loss are late symptoms.

   7. Bowel obstruction may lead to perforation and peritonitis.

C. Diagnostics (see Appendix 14.1).

   1. Sigmoidoscopy and colonoscopy with biopsies.

   2. Carcinoembryonic antigen (CEA) tumor marker detected in blood.

Analyze Cues and Prioritize Hypotheses

The most important problems are the risk of metastasis to other organs, need for surgery, and managing chemotherapy and/or radiation therapy side effects.

Generate Solutions

Treatment

A. Colon resection: may have resection with or without a colostomy or may have an abdominal-perineal resection that includes the sigmoid colon, rectum, and anus.

B. Laser photocoagulation: destroys small tumors; palliative for large tumors obstructing bowel.

C. Endoscopic excision or electrocoagulation for small, localized tumors or for clients who are poor surgical candidates.

D. Radiation therapy, chemotherapy.

Nursing Interventions: Take Action

Goal: To provide information to high-risk clients.

A. Diet: high-fiber, low-fat diet with a decreased intake of red meat.

B. Digital rectal examinations yearly after age 40.

C. Annual fecal occult blood testing after age 50.

D. Colonoscopy every 3 or 5 years after age 40 for high risk; otherwise, every 10 years for average risk.

Goal: To provide preoperative care.

A. Determine extent of surgery anticipated; colostomy is not always done.

B. Bowel preparation: low-residue diet, cathartics 24 hours before surgery.

C. Oral neomycin to decrease bacteria in the bowel.

D. If colostomy is to be done, discuss implications and identify appropriate area for stoma on abdomen (see Appendix 14.7).

Goal: To provide appropriate wound care after abdominal-perineal resection.

A. Client will have three incisional areas:
   1. Abdominal incision.
   2. Incisional area for colostomy.
   3. Perineal incision.

B. Perineal wound.
   1. Wound may be left open to heal by secondary intention: provide warm sitz baths for 10 to 20 minutes.
   2. Wound may be partially closed with drains (Jackson-Pratt and/or Hemovac) in place: assess the wound for integrity of suture line and presence of infection; drainage should be serosanguineous; drains remain in place until drainage is less than 50 mL/24 hours.
   3. Wound may be open and packed: drainage is profuse first several hours after surgery; may require frequent reinforcement and dressing change; drainage is serosanguineous.

C. Position client with a perineal wound on side; do not allow client to sit for prolonged period until wound is healed.

D. Assess status of stoma and healing of abdominal incision (see Appendix 14.8).

Goal: To maintain homeostasis and promote healing after abdominal-perineal resection or colon resection.

A. Infection, hemorrhage, wound disruption, thrombophlebitis, and stoma problems are the most common complications.

Home Care

A. Recovery period is long, especially for the older adult.

B. Help client and family identify resources and obtain equipment for colostomy care.

C. Assess client's ability to care for stoma; help client begin self-care before discharge.

Hemorrhoids

Dilated hemorrhoidal veins of the anus and rectum; may be internal (above the internal sphincter) or external (outside of the external sphincter).

Assessment: Recognize Cues

A. Risk factors/etiology: conditions that increase anorectal pressure.
   1. Pregnancy, obesity, prolonged constipation.
   2. Prolonged standing or sitting.
   3. Portal hypertension.
   4. Straining at bowel movement.

B. Clinical manifestations.
   1. External hemorrhoids appear as protrusions at the anus.
   2. Thrombosed hemorrhoid: a blood clot in a hemorrhoid that causes inflammation and pain.
   3. Rectal bleeding during defecation.

C. Diagnostics: rectal examination.

Analyze Cues and Prioritize Hypotheses

The most important problems are pain and discomfort with defecation and possible rectal bleeding.

Generate Solutions

Treatment

A. Conservative treatment.
   1. Sitz baths, stool softeners, ointments, topical anesthetics.
   2. Prevent constipation: diet high in fiber (bran) and roughage with increased water intake.
   3. Avoid straining with bowel movement; keep anal area clean.

B. Surgical treatment.
   1. Ligation of prolapsed, thrombosed hemorrhoids with small rubber band.
   2. Infrared coagulation for bleeding hemorrhoids.
   3. Surgery for painful, large, bleeding hemorrhoids.

Nursing Interventions

Goal: To provide appropriate information to help client manage problem at home.

A. Avoid prolonged standing or sitting.

B. Take sitz baths to decrease discomfort.

C. Use OTC ointments to decrease discomfort.

D. Apply ice pack, followed by a warm sitz bath, if severe discomfort occurs.

E. Avoid constipation and straining at stool.

F. Encourage bulk laxatives and increased fluid intake to promote soft stool for first bowel movement.

Celiac Disease

Celiac disease is a type of malabsorption syndrome also known as sprue or gluten-sensitive enteropathy. This disease is an immune reaction to rye, wheat, barley, and oat grains that leads to an inflammatory response, causing damage to the villi of the small intestines and resulting in the inability to absorb nutrients (malabsorption).

A. Previously considered a disease of childhood with symptoms beginning between the ages of 1 year and 5 years; celiac disease is now commonly seen at all ages, with mean age of diagnosis being 40 years.

B. Symptoms frequently begin in early childhood but condition may not be diagnosed until adulthood.

C. Development of celiac disease is dependent on genetic predisposition, ingestion of gluten, and immune-mediated response.

Assessment: Recognize Cues

A. Cause: congenital defect or an autoimmune response in gluten metabolism.

B. Clinical manifestations.
1. Symptoms may begin when child has increased intake of foods containing gluten: cereals, crackers, breads, cookies, pastas, etc.
2. Foul-smelling diarrhea with abdominal distention and anorexia in infants and toddlers.
3. Poor weight gain in children; failure to thrive.
4. Constipation, vomiting, and abdominal pain may be the initial presenting symptoms in adults.

5. Vitamin deficiency leads to central nervous system impairment and bone malformation or decreased bone density and osteoporosis.

C. Diagnostics: endoscopy with biopsy, upper and lower GI series.

Analyze Cues and Prioritize Hypotheses

The most important problem is the need for dietary change.

Generate Solutions

Treatment: Primarily dietary management: gluten-free diet.

Nursing Interventions: Take Action

Goal: To help client and family understand diet therapy and promote optimal nutrition intake.

A. Written information regarding a gluten-free diet; corn, rice, potato, flax, and soy products may be substituted for wheat in diet.

B. Diet should be well balanced and high in protein.

C. Teach client and/or family how to read food and medication labels for gluten content; thickenings, soups, instant foods, and some medications may contain hidden sources of gluten.

D. Important to discuss the necessity of maintaining a lifelong gluten-restricted diet; problems may occur in clients who relax their diet and experience an exacerbation of the disease state.

E. Lack of adherence to dietary restrictions may precipitate growth retardation, anemia, bone deformities, and lymphomas.

> **TEST ALERT** Adapt the diet to meet client's specific needs.

Appendix 14.1 GASTROINTESTINAL SYSTEM DIAGNOSTICS

X-ray

Upper Gastrointestinal Series or Barium Swallow

X-ray examination in which barium or Gastrografin is used as a contrast material; used to diagnose structural abnormalities and problems of the esophagus, stomach, and small intestine.

Nursing Implications

1. Explain procedure to client (usually not done on client with acute abdomen until possibility of perforation has been ruled out).
2. Maintain client's NPO status 8 hours before procedure.
3. Client will swallow barium to coat the GI tract for visualization of various landmarks and structures and assume various positions on the x-ray table.
4. After examination, promote normal excretion of barium to prevent impaction. Barium can cause constipation, so encourage extra fluids. It may be necessary to use a stool softener or laxative to promote evacuation of the barium.
5. Stool should return to normal color within 72 hours.

Lower Gastrointestinal Series or Barium Enema

X-ray examination of the colon in which barium is used as a contrast medium; barium is administered rectally.

Nursing Implications

1. Maintain client's NPO status for 8 hours before test. Client may have clear liquids the evening before the test.
2. Colon must be free of stool; laxatives and enemas are administered the evening before the test.
3. Explain to client that cramping and the urge to defecate may be experienced during the procedure.
4. After the procedure, increase fluids and administer a laxative to assist in expelling the barium.

Endoscopy

Gastroscopy, Esophagogastroduodenoscopy, Colonoscopy, Sigmoidoscopy, Capsule Endoscopy

Endoscopy is the direct visualization of the GI tract via a flexible fiber-optic lighted scope. The endoscope is capable of obtaining biopsy specimens and clipping benign polyps.

Nursing Implications Before Procedure

1. Upper GI: NPO for up to 12 hours before procedure.
2. Lower GI: bowel prep—cathartics and/or enemas, clear liquid diet for 24 hours before test.
3. Client should avoid aspirin, NSAIDs, iron supplements, and gelatin containing red coloring for a week before procedure.

Continued

4. May give preoperative medication for relaxation and to decrease secretions.
5. Upper GI studies: a topical anesthesia will be used to anesthetize the throat before insertion of the scope.
6. Upper GI studies: assess client's mouth for dentures and removable bridges.
7. Lower GI studies: help client into the left side-lying, knee-chest position; explain the need to take a deep breath during the insertion of the scope; client may feel urge to defecate as scope is passed.
8. Conscious sedation frequently used for upper and lower GI studies or colonoscopy.

Nursing Implications During Procedure
1. Verify informed consent and client identification.
2. For upper GI studies, confirm NPO status for past 8 hours; for lower GI studies, confirm bowel preparation.
3. Assess for presence of GI bleeding; *notify RN or health care provider if any bleeding is present.*
4. Maintain safety: airway precautions during sedation; positioning, monitor level of sedation (see Chapter 3).

Nursing Implications After Procedure
1. Upper GI: *maintain client's NPO status until the gag reflex returns*; position client on side to prevent aspiration until gag or cough reflex returns; use throat lozenges or warm saline solution gargles for relief of sore throat.
2. Monitor vital signs and O_2 saturation during recovery.
3. Observe for signs of perforation: upper GI bleeding—dysphagia, substernal or epigastric pain; lower GI bleeding—rectal bleeding, increasing abdominal distention.
4. Assist client to upright position: observe for orthostatic hypotension.
5. Warm sitz bath for any anal discomfort.

Analysis of Specimens

Capsule endoscopy requires client to swallow a capsule with a camera that transmits photos of the GI tract.

Nursing Implications Before Procedure
1. Bowel prep according to health care provider.
2. Explain client will swallow capsule and wear an external monitor to capture pictures.

Nursing Implications During Procedure
1. Keep client NPO for 4 to 10 hours.
2. Remove monitoring device after 6 to 10 hours.

Paracentesis, Diagnostic Peritoneal Lavage

Procedure: A catheter is inserted into the peritoneal cavity, most often just below the umbilicus.

Purposes
1. To determine effect of blunt abdominal trauma.
2. To assess for presence of ascites.
3. To identify cause of acute abdominal problems (e.g., perforation, hemorrhage).

Nursing Implications
1. An NG tube may be used to maintain gastric decompression during procedure.
2. Have the client void before the procedure; if client has a full bladder at the time of insertion of the catheter, risk for bladder perforation and peritonitis is increased.
3. In clients with chronic liver problems, assess coagulation laboratory values before procedure.
4. Place client in semi-Fowler position.
5. Maintain sterile field for puncture.
6. Weigh the client before and after the paracentesis and document the weights.
7. Measure the drainage and record accurately.

Complications
1. Perforation of bowel: peritonitis.
2. Introduction of air into abdominal cavity; client may complain of right referred shoulder pain (caused by air under the diaphragm).
3. Contraindicated in pregnancy and in clients with coagulation defects or possible bowel obstruction.
4. Hypotension/hypovolemia if too much fluid is removed.

Stool Examination

Stool is examined for form and consistency and to determine whether it contains mucus, blood, pus, parasites, or fat. Stool will be examined for presence of occult blood.

Nursing Implications
1. Collect stool in sterile container if examining for pathologic organisms.
2. A fresh, warm stool is required for evaluation of parasites or pathogenic organisms.
3. Collect the sample from various areas of the stool.
4. The result of the guaiac test for occult blood is positive when the paper turns blue.
5. Document medications and OTC drugs client is taking when sample is obtained.
6. Sample should be approximately the size of a walnut or 30 mL, if soft.
7. Take the specimen immediately to the laboratory. Do not allow specimen to remain on the unit.

Appendix 14.2 MEDICATIONS

℞

Antiemetics

MEDICATIONS	SIDE EFFECTS	NURSING IMPLICATIONS
Dopamine Antagonists: Depress or block dopamine receptors and chemoreceptor trigger zone of the brain.		
Phenothiazines—suppress emesis Chlorpromazine hydrochloride: PO, suppository, IM Promethazine: PO, IM, IV, suppository ▲ High-Alert Medication for injection routes Prochlorperazine: PO, suppository, IM Thiethylperazine maleate: PO, suppository, IM	Central nervous system depression, drowsiness, dizziness, blurred vision, hypotension, photosensitivity	1. SubQ injection or IV administration may cause tissue irritation and necrosis. 2. Use with caution in children. 3. Thorazine should be used only in situations of severe nausea or vomiting. Can also be used for intractable hiccups. 4. Thiethylperazine: Cautious use in clients with liver and kidney diseases. 5. Promethazine can cause fatal respiratory depression, especially in the young. Do not give promethazine to children under 2 years of age and use it with caution in children older than 2 years.
Prokinetics—stimulate motility Metoclopramide: PO, IM, IV	Restlessness, drowsiness, fatigue, anxiety, headache	1. Used to decrease problems with esophageal reflux, gastroparesis, and nausea and vomiting associated with chemotherapy. 2. Contraindicated in GI obstruction, perforation, or hemorrhage.
Antihistamines: Depress the chemoreceptor trigger zone, block histamine receptors.		
Hydroxyzine: PO, IM Dimenhydrinate: PO, suppository, IM	Sedation; anticholinergic effects—blurred vision, dry mouth, difficulty in urination, and constipation; paradoxical excitation may occur in children	1. Caution client regarding sedation: should avoid activities that require mental alertness. 2. Administer early to prevent vomiting. 3. Use with caution in clients with glaucoma and asthma. 4. SubQ injection may cause tissue irritation and necrosis; use Z-track injection technique.
Serotonin Receptor Antagonists: Act on specific serotonin (5-HT) receptors to decrease nausea and vomiting.		
Ondansetron: IV, PO Granisetron: IV Dolasetron: PO	Headache, diarrhea, rash, bronchospasm	1. Assess baseline vitals. 2. Use caution in clients with liver dysfunction. 3. Ondansetron prolongs the QT interval and poses a risk of torsades de pointes, a potentially life-threatening dysrhythmia. 4. Use cautiously in clients with electrolyte abnormalities, heart failure, or bradydysrhythmias.
Neurokinin–1 Receptor Inhibitor Antagonists: Neurokinin–1 (NK1) binds to the NK1 receptor and stops the signal for vomiting from being transmitted.		
Aprepitant: PO, IV Fosaprepitant: IV Rolapitant: PO Fixed-dose combination: netupitant and palonosetron: PO, IV	Fatigue, hiccups, constipation, diarrhea, neutropenia	1. Assess type, amount, and frequency of emesis. 2. Identify underlying causes. 3. Assess bowel patterns prior to administration due to potential for diarrhea and constipation.

General Nursing Implications
- Laxatives should be avoided in clients who have nausea, vomiting, undiagnosed abdominal pain and cramping, and/or any indications of appendicitis or peritonitis.
- Dietary fiber should be taken for prevention of, and as first-line treatment for, constipation.
- Daily intake of fluids should be increased.
- Constipation is determined by stool firmness and frequency.
- Increasing activity will increase peristalsis and decrease constipation.
- Opioid analgesics and anticholinergics will cause constipation.
- A laxative should be used only briefly and in the smallest amount necessary.
- Use laxatives with caution during pregnancy.

Laxatives

MEDICATIONS	SIDE EFFECTS	NURSING IMPLICATIONS
Bulk-forming—stimulate peristalsis and passage of soft stool Methylcellulose Psyllium Fibercon Bran	Esophageal irritation, impaction, abdominal fullness, flatulence	1. Not immediately effective; 12–24 hr before effects are apparent. 2. Use with caution in clients with difficulty swallowing. 3. Administer with full glass of fluid to prevent problems with irritation and impaction.
Surfactants—decrease surface tension, allowing water to penetrate feces Docusate sodium	Occasional mild abdominal cramping	1. Do not use concurrently with mineral oil. 2. Not recommended for children less than 6 years old.
Stimulants—stimulate and irritate the large intestine to promote peristalsis and defecation Bisacodyl: PO, suppository Senna concentrate: PO, suppository	Diarrhea, abdominal cramping	1. Use for short period of time. 2. Do not use in presence of undiagnosed abdominal pain or GI bleeding.
Osmotics—osmotic agents that pull fluid into the bowel Polyethylene glycol: PO, NG Magnesium hydroxide: PO	Nausea, bloating, abdominal fullness	1. Primary use is in preparing the bowel for examination. 2. Clear liquids only (no gelatin with red coloring) after administration. 3. Polyethylene glycol requires the client to drink a large amount of fluid (4 L); provide 8–10 oz (240–300 mL) chilled at a time to increase client consumption and enhance taste. 4. Best if consumed over 3–4 hr. 5. Hyperosmotics and saline cause frequent bowel movements; advise client to plan accordingly. 6. Most osmotic laxatives cause problems with loss of water, whereas sodium phosphate can lead to fluid retention.

Antidiarrheal Agents: Slow intestinal transit time to relieve diarrhea.

MEDICATIONS	SIDE EFFECTS	NURSING IMPLICATIONS
Anhydrous morphine: PO	Light-headedness, dizziness, sedation, nausea, vomiting, paralytic ileus, abdominal cramping	1. Opioid derivative; suppresses peristalsis. 2. Not recommended during pregnancy or breastfeeding. 3. Can produce drug dependence and mild withdrawal symptoms. 4. Encourage increased fluids. 5. Avoid activities that require mental alertness.
Diphenoxylate/Atropine: PO Loperamide HCl: PO Bismuth subsalicylate: PO	May precipitate constipation and an impaction	1. Absorbent, has soothing effect, and absorbs toxic substances. 2. May interfere with absorption of oral medications. 3. Should not be given to clients with fever greater than 101°F (38.3°C). 4. Do not give in presence of bloody diarrhea. 5. Bismuth may cause black stools and a blackish colored tongue that is harmless.

Antiulcer Agents

MEDICATIONS	SIDE EFFECTS	NURSING IMPLICATIONS

Antacid: An alkaline substance that will neutralize gastric acid secretions; nonsystemic. Some combination antacids also relieve gas, and some work as laxatives. Several antacids form a protective coating on the stomach and upper GI tract.

Appendix 14.2   MEDICATIONS—cont'd   ℞

Antiulcer Agents

MEDICATIONS	SIDE EFFECTS	NURSING IMPLICATIONS
Aluminum hydroxide: PO Aluminum hydroxide and magnesium salt combinations: PO	Constipation, phosphorus depletion with long-term use Constipation or diarrhea, hypercalcemia, renal calculi	1. Avoid administration within 1–2 hr of other oral medications; should be taken frequently—before and after meals and at bedtime. 2. Instruct clients to take medication even if they do not experience discomfort. 3. Clients on low-sodium diets should evaluate sodium content of various antacids. 4. Administer with caution to the client with cardiac disease because GI symptoms may be indicative of cardiac problems.
Sodium preparations Sodium bicarbonate: PO	Rebound acid production, alkalosis	1. Discourage use of sodium bicarbonate because of occurrence of metabolic alkalosis and rebound acid production.

Histamine H2 Receptor Antagonists: Reduce volume and concentration of gastric acid secretion.

Cimetidine: PO, IV, IM	Rash, confusion, lethargy, diarrhea, dysrhythmias, gynecomastia, reduced libido and impotence (binds to androgen receptors), and pneumonia (decreased gastric pH leads to bacterial colonization of respiratory tract)	1. Take 30 min before or after meals. 2. May be used prophylactically or for treatment of PUD. 3. Do not take with oral antacids.
Famotidine: PO, IV	Anemia, dizziness Headache, dizziness, constipation, diarrhea	1. Use with caution in clients with kidney or hepatic problems. 2. Dosing may be done without regard to food or to mealtime. 3. Caution clients to avoid aspirin and other NSAIDs.

Proton Pump Inhibitors (PPIs): Inhibit the enzyme that produces gastric acid.

Omeprazole: PO Lansoprazole: PO Pantoprazole: PO, IV Esomeprazole: PO Rabeprazole: PO Dexlansoprazole: PO	Headache, diarrhea, dizziness, increased risk of fractures, hypomagnesemia	1. Administer before meals. 2. Do not crush or chew; do not open capsules. 3. Sprinkle granules of lansoprazole over food; do not chew granules. 4. The combination of omeprazole with clarithromycin effectively treats clients with *H. pylori* infection in duodenal ulcer.

Cytoprotective Agent: Binds to diseased tissue to provide a protective barrier to acid.

Sucralfate: PO	Constipation, GI discomfort	1. Avoid antacids. 2. Inhibits absorption of PPIs. 3. Used for prevention and treatment of stress ulcers, gastric ulceration, and PUD. 4. May impede the absorption of medications that require an acid medium (phenytoin, digoxin, warfarin, and fluoroquinolone antibiotics).

Prostaglandin Analog: Suppresses gastric acid secretion; increases protective mucus and mucosal blood flow.

Misoprostol: PO	GI problems, headache, diarrhea	1. Contraindicated in pregnancy but may be used to start labor. 2. Indicated for prevention of NSAID-induced ulcers.

Continued

this method may not be accurate if the client is on medications that alter the pH of gastric secretions.

   c. It is *not recommended to* determine placement by injecting air and listening with a stethoscope for sound of air in the stomach.

   d. Always validate placement of an NG tube before instilling anything into tube.

- Once tube placement is validated, mark the tube to indicate where the tube exits the nose.
- Label the tube for use only for enteral feedings and/or oral medication administration.
- Characteristics of nasogastric drainage.
  a. Normally greenish yellow, with strands of mucus.
  b. Coffee-ground drainage: old blood that has been broken down in the stomach.
  c. Bright red blood: indicates bleeding in the esophagus, the stomach, or the lungs.
  d. Foul-smelling (fecal odor): occurs with reverse peristalsis in bowel obstruction; increase in amount of drainage with obstruction.
- If duodenal placement is required, have client lay in right lateral position for several hours. Provide enough excess in the tube to allow the tube to migrate down into duodenum.

Clinical Tips for Problem Solving

- *Abdominal distention:* Check for patency and adequacy of drainage, determine position of tube, assess presence of bowel sounds, and assess for respiratory compromise from distention.
- *Nausea and vomiting:* Place client in semi-Fowler position or turn to side to prevent aspiration; suction oral pharyngeal area. Attempt to aspirate gastric contents and validate placement of tube. Tube may not be far enough into stomach for adequate decompression and suction; try repositioning. If tube patency cannot be established, tube may need to be replaced.
- *Inadequate or minimal drainage:* Validate placement and patency; tube may be in too far and be past pyloric valve or not in far enough and in the upper portion of the stomach. Reassess length of tube insertion and characteristics of drainage; request x-ray for validation.

❗ NURSING PRIORITY *ALWAYS check the placement of an NG tube before irrigating it or administering medications; placement should be checked each shift; do not adjust or irrigate the NG tube on a client after a gastric resection or bariatric surgery because of the risk of disruption of the anastomosis or staple line.*

Short Term

1. *Nasogastric:* Provides alternative means of ingesting nutrients for clients.
2. *Nasointestinal:* A weighted tube of soft material is placed in the small intestine to decrease chance of regurgitation. A stylet or guide wire is used to progress the tube into the intestine. Do not remove stylet until tube placement has been verified via x-ray. Do not attempt to reinsert stylet while tube is in place; this could result in perforation of the tube.

Long Term

1. *Percutaneous endoscopic gastrostomy (PEG):* A tube is inserted percutaneously into the stomach; local anesthesia and sedation are used for tube placement.
2. *Percutaneous endoscopic jejunostomy (PEJ):* A tube is inserted percutaneously into the jejunum.
3. *Gastrostomy:* A surgical opening is made into the stomach and a gastrostomy tube is positioned with sutures.

Methods of Administering Enteral Feedings

- *Continuous:* Controlled with a feeding pump. Decreases nausea and diarrhea and decreases the risk of aspiration.
- *Intermittent/bolus:* Prescribed amount of fluid infuses via a gravity drip or feeding pump over specific time. For example, 350 mL is given over 30 minutes.
- *Cyclic:* Involves feeding solution infused via a pump for a part of the day, usually 12 to 16 hours. This method may be used for weaning from feedings.

Nursing Implications

- Determine the correct tubing by tracing from the client to point of origin.
- Do not use IV tubing or IV pumps for enteral feedings.
- Make sure enteral tube line is labeled prior to starting a feeding.
- The client should be sitting or lying with the head elevated 30 to 45 degrees. Head of bed should remain elevated for 30 to 60 minutes after feeding if intermittent or cyclic feeding is used; for continuous feeding, maintain semi-Fowler position at all times.
- If feedings are intermittent, tube should be irrigated with water before and after feedings.
- Aspirate gastric contents to determine residual. If residual is more than 200 mL and there are signs of intolerance (nausea, vomiting, distention), hold next feeding for 1 hour and recheck residual or, if residual is greater than half of last feeding, delay next feeding for 1 to 2 hours and recheck the residual volume. If gastric residual volume continues high after the second residual check, consider a promotility agent.
- Return aspirated contents to stomach to prevent electrolyte imbalance.
- Flush the tube with 30 to 50 mL of water:
  a. After each intermittent feeding.
  b. Every 4 to 6 hours for continuous feeding.
  c. Before and after each medication administration.
- When a PEG or PEJ tube is placed, immediately after insertion measure the length of the tube from the insertion site to the distal end and mark the tube at the skin insertion site. This tube should be routinely checked to determine whether the tube is migrating from the original insertion point.
- For continuous or cyclic feeding, add only 4 hours of product to the bag at a time to prevent bacterial growth. A closed system is preferred, with each set being used no longer than 24 hours.
- Prevent diarrhea:
  a. Slow, constant rate of infusion.
  b. Keep equipment clean to prevent bacterial contamination.

c. Check for fecal impaction; diarrhea may be flowing around impaction.
d. Identify medical conditions that would precipitate diarrhea.
- For continuous feeding, change feeding reservoir every 24 hours.

> **! NURSING PRIORITY** If in doubt of a tube's placement or position, stop or hold the feeding and obtain x-ray confirmation of location.

> **TEST ALERT** Change rate and amount of tube feeding based on client's response.

Appendix 14.6 NURSING PROCEDURE: ENEMAS

Types of Enemas

Soap suds enema: Castile soap is added to tap water or normal saline. Dilute 5 mL of castile soap in 1 L of water.

Tap water enema: Request order for specific quantity when administered to infants or children; should not be repeated because of risk for water toxicity. Use caution when administering to adults with altered cardiac and renal reserve.

Saline enema: Safest enema to administer; safe for infants and children.

Retention enema: Oil-based solution that will soften the stool. Should be retained by client 30 to 60 minutes. Typically 150 to 200 mL. May be mineral oil or similar oil or may include antibiotics or nutritive solution.

Hypertonic enema: Used when only a small amount of fluid is tolerated (120–180 mL). Commercially prepared Fleet enema.

Carminative enema: Agent used to expel gas from the GI tract. Example is magnesium sulfate/glycerin/water (MGW).

✓Key Points: Administering an Enema

- Fill enema container with warmed solution.
- Allow solution to run through the tubing before inserting into rectum so that air is removed.
- Place client in modified left lateral recumbent position.

- Generously lubricate the tip of the tubing with water-soluble lubricant.
- Gently insert tubing into client's rectum (3–4 inches [8–10 cm] for adults, 2–3 inches [5–8 cm] for children, 1 inch [2.5 cm] for infants), past the external and internal sphincters.
- Raise the solution container no more than 12 to 18 inches (30–46 cm) above the client.
- Allow solution to flow slowly. If the flow is slow, the client will experience fewer cramps. The client will also be able to tolerate and retain a greater volume of solution.

Clinical Tips for Problem Solving

If client expels solution prematurely:
- Place client in supine position with knees flexed.
- Slow the water flow and continue with the enema.

If the enema returns contain fecal material before surgery or diagnostic testing, repeat enema. If, after three enemas, returns still contain fecal material, *notify health care provider.*

If client complains of abdominal cramping during instillation of fluid, slow the infusion rate by lowering the fluid bag.

> **TEST ALERT** Assist and intervene with client who has an alteration in elimination.

Appendix 14.7 NURSING PROCEDURE: CARE OF THE CLIENT WITH AN OSTOMY

Types of Ostomies (Fig. 14.8)

Colostomy: Opening of the colon through the abdominal wall; stool is generally semisoft and bowel control may be achieved.

Ileostomy: Opening of the ileum through the abdominal wall; stool drainage is liquid and excoriating; drainage is frequently continuous; it is therefore difficult to establish bowel control. Fluid and electrolyte imbalances are common complications.

Kock ileostomy: May be referred to as a "continent" ileostomy; an internal reservoir for stool is surgically formed. Decreases problem of skin care caused by frequent irritation of stoma by drainage. Primary complications are leakage at the stoma site and peritonitis; rarely used today.

Goals

1. Maintain physiologic and psychological equilibrium.
2. Assist client to maintain total care of colostomy or ileostomy before discharge.

Preoperative Care

1. Preoperative education: Actively involve family and client; encourage questions concerning the procedure.

2. Placement of stoma is evaluated and site is selected with client standing.

✓Key Points: Postoperative Nursing Implications—Initial Care

- Evaluate stoma every 8 hours after surgery. It should remain pink and moist; dark blue stoma indicates ischemia and *should be reported immediately to the RN.*
- Measure the stoma and select an appropriately sized appliance. Mild to moderate swelling is common for the first 2 to 3 weeks after surgery, which necessitates changes in size of the appliance.
- Appliance should fit easily around the stoma and cover all healthy, abdominal skin.
- Keep the skin around the stoma clean, dry, and free of stool and intestinal secretions. Prevent contamination of the abdominal incision.
- Ostomy bags should be changed when about one-third full to avoid weight of bag dislodging skin barrier.

✓Key Points: Pouching an Ostomy

- A pouching system consists of a pouch and skin barrier.

Continued

Appendix 14.7 NURSING PROCEDURE: CARE OF THE CLIENT WITH AN OSTOMY—cont'd

R̃x

- Pouches come in one- and two-piece systems and are flat or convex.
- Pouches may have the opening precut by the manufacturer; others require the stoma opening to be cut by the nurse or client to fit stoma.
- Pouch may have an integrated closure or may need a clip (older types).
- Change the pouching system approximately every 3 to 7 days.
- Carefully remove used pouch and skin barrier gently by pushing skin away from barrier; may need to use an adhesive remover to facilitate removal of skin barrier.
- Measure stoma by using measurement tool provided with pouch.

! NURSING PRIORITY Stoma measurement may change, especially 2 to 4 weeks after surgery, so remeasurement will be required.

- Trace measured stoma pattern from tool onto pouch/skin barrier and cut the opening.
- Remove protective backing and apply pouch over stoma.

✓Key Points: Irrigation

- Do not irrigate an ileostomy or maintain regular irrigations in child with colostomy.
- Irrigate colostomy at same time each day to assist in establishing a normal pattern of elimination.
- Involve client in care as early as possible.
- In adults, irrigate with 500 to 1000 mL of warm tap water.

! NURSING PRIORITY
- Use a cone-tipped ostomy irrigator; do not use an enema tube/catheter.
- Do not irrigate more than once a day.
- Do not irrigate in the presence of diarrhea or severe abdominal pain.

- Place the client in a sitting position for irrigation, preferably in the bathroom with the irrigation sleeve in the toilet.
- Elevate the solution container approximately 12 to 20 inches (30–51 cm) and allow solution to flow in gently. If cramping occurs, lower fluid or clamp the tubing.
- Allow 25 to 45 minutes for return flow. Client may want to walk around before the return starts.
- Encourage client to participate in care of colostomy. Have client perform return demonstration of colostomy irrigation before leaving the hospital.
- Assist the client to control odors: diet and odor-control tablets.
- Kock ileostomy is drained when client experiences fullness. A nipple valve is created in surgery and drained by insertion of a catheter.

Clinical Tips for Problem Solving

If water does not flow easily into colostomy stoma:
- Check for kinks in tubing from container.

- Check height of irrigating container.
- Encourage client to change positions, relax, and take a few deep breaths.

If client experiences cramping, nausea, or dizziness during irrigation:
- Stop flow of water, leaving irrigation cone in place.
- Do not resume until cramping has passed.
- Check water temperature and height of water bag; if water is too hot or flows too rapidly, it can cause dizziness.

If client has no return of stool or water from irrigation:
- Be sure to apply drainable pouch; solution may drain as client moves around.
- Have client increase fluid intake; may be dehydrated.
- Repeat irrigation the next day.

If diarrhea occurs:
- Do not irrigate colostomy.
- Check client's medications; sometimes they may cause diarrhea.
- If diarrhea is excessive and/or prolonged, notify health care provider.

TEST ALERT Provide ostomy care.

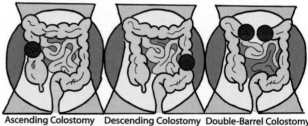

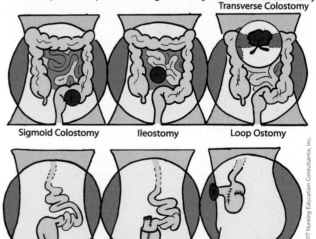

FIG. 14.8 Types of Colostomies. (From Zerwekh, J., Garneau, A., & Miller, C. J. [2017]. *Digital collection of the memory notebooks of nursing* [4th ed.]. Nursing Education Consultants.)

⚡ Practice & Next Generation NCLEX (NGN) Questions

Gastrointestinal: Care of Adult Clients

More questions on
evolve

1. On the second day after gastric resection, the client's nasogastric (NG) tube is draining bile-colored liquid containing coffee-ground material. What is the **best** nursing action?
   1. Continue to monitor the amount of drainage and correlate it with any change in vital signs.
   2. Reposition the NG tube and irrigate the tube with normal saline solution.
   3. Call the health care provider and discuss the possibility that the client is bleeding.
   4. Irrigate the NG tube with iced saline solution and attach the tube to gravity drainage.

2. A nurse is changing the ileostomy bag on a client the day after surgery. What is a normal characteristic of the stoma?
   1. Pitting edema around base.
   2. Dusky gray color.
   3. Red with some edema.
   4. Tissue sloughing in the area.

3. The nurse is caring for a client who has been diagnosed with a bleeding duodenal ulcer. What clinical findings identified on a nursing assessment would indicate an intestinal perforation and require immediate nursing action?
   1. Increasing abdominal distention with increased pain and vomiting.
   2. Decreasing hemoglobin and hematocrit with bloody stools.
   3. Diarrhea with increased bowel sounds and hypovolemia.
   4. Decreasing blood pressure with tachycardia and disorientation.

4. The nurse is admitting a client with a diagnosis of "rule out intestinal obstruction." Nursing assessment reveals a distended abdomen, minimal bowel sounds in the right upper quadrant, and nausea and vomiting. The client is NPO and an IV of normal saline is infusing at 100 mL/hr. Which medication would the nurse question administering to this client?
   1. Hydroxyzine IM q 6 hours.
   2. Cimetidine IVPB q 6 hours.
   3. Cephalexin IVPB q 6 hours.
   4. Metoclopramide IVPB q 4 hours.

5. A client has just returned to the nursing unit following a gastrectomy. A nasogastric (NG) tube is in place and the client begins to report nausea. What is the **priority** nursing action?
   1. Gently irrigate the NG tube with normal saline.
   2. Clamp the tube for 30 minutes and reassess the client.
   3. Measure gastric output to determine excessive acid production.
   4. Determine whether the NG tube is patent and draining.

6. The nurse is planning care for a client scheduled for esophagogastroduodenoscopy and a barium swallow. What will the nurse plan as part of the client's care?

   1. Anticipating the client will receive a clear liquid diet in the evening and then receive nothing by mouth (NPO status) 6 to 12 hours before the test.
   2. Discussing with the client the NG tube and the importance of gastric drainage for 24 hours after the test.
   3. Explaining to the client that they will receive nothing by mouth (NPO status) for 24 hours after the test to make sure the stomach can tolerate food.
   4. Discussing the general anesthesia and explaining to the client that they will wake up in the recovery room.

7. A client was prescribed omeprazole several weeks ago. In evaluating the outcome of the client taking the medication, what would indicate that the medication has been effective?
   1. Heartburn pain has lessened.
   2. Blood pressure has decreased.
   3. Unable to eat spicy foods.
   4. Chronic pain has diminished.

8. A client is receiving medications through a nasogastric (NG) feeding tube. After the NG tube was inserted, the placement in the stomach was confirmed with an x-ray. What is the appropriate nursing action prior to administering a medication in the NG tube?
   1. Administer the medication and follow with a normal saline flush.
   2. Place the end of the NG tube in a glass of water and observe for bubbling.
   3. Insert 10 mL of air into the NG tube while auscultating the upper abdomen.
   4. Aspirate gastric contents and measure the pH of the gastric contents.

9. A client has a history of gastric ulcer. The nurse is monitoring the client for potential complications. What are the most common complications of gastric ulcers? **Select all that apply**.
   1. Perforation.
   2. Hemorrhage.
   3. Infection.
   4. Pyloric obstruction.
   5. Hemoptysis.

10. A 90-year-old client who resides in an assisted living center calls the nurse and reports having several diarrhea stools and vomiting everything that is eaten. The client reports that the nausea, vomiting, and diarrhea have been occurring over the past 24 hours. What vital sign change would the nurse be **most** concerned about?
    1. Temperature 99°F (37.2°C).
    2. Oxygen saturation 95% on room air.
    3. Blood pressure 95/68 mm Hg.
    4. Pulse 68 beats/min.

11. A client has a history of heartburn and acid reflux. The client is admitted to the hospital after vomiting 250 mL of bright red blood. Upon admission, the client states feeling a little dizzy, which is causing nausea. The following is the admission flowsheet.

| Health History | Nurses' Notes | Flow Sheet | Laboratory Results |

1030

Vital Signs:
- Temperature: 98.6°F (37°C)
- BP: 100/72 mm Hg
- Heart rate: 112 bpm and regular
- Respirations: 20 breaths/min
- SpO2: 96% on room air

Intake:
- NPO
- IV of 1000 mL of normal saline, infusing at 150 mL/hr

Output:
- 250 mL bright red blood
- 200 mL voiding, urine dark yellow

Complete the following sentences by choosing the most likely options for the missing information from the drop-down lists of options provided.

Based on a probable diagnosis of peptic ulcer disease, the client is experiencing _____1_____, as evidenced by _____2_____, _____2_____, and _____2_____. The three major complications of peptic ulcer disease are _____3_____, _____3_____, and _____3_____.

OPTIONS FOR 1	OPTIONS FOR 2	OPTIONS FOR 3
Respiratory distress	Melena	Infection
GI bleeding	Hypotension	Hemorrhage
Dumping syndrome	Hematochezia	Obstruction
Irritable bowel syndrome	Tachycardia	Perforation
Angina	Dizziness	Respiratory distress
Ulcerative colitis	Indigestion	Fluid overload
	Hematemesis	

12. A nurse is caring for a client who is newly admitted to the hospital.

| Health History | Nurses' Notes | Provider Orders | Laboratory Results |

1100 : Client is lying in bed with knees flexed and reporting severe abdominal pain (an 8 out of 10 scale). Client had several episodes of nausea and vomiting prior to admission.
On assessment, client shows facial grimacing, appears anxious, and is pale. Boardlike abdominal distention noted with diminished bowel sounds in all four quadrants.

- Temperature: 100.2°F (37.9°C)
- BP: 106/78 mm Hg
- Heart rate: 100 bpm and regular
- Respirations: 20 breaths/min
- SpO2: 96% on room air

The nurse is reviewing the client's assessment data to prepare the client's plan of care.

Complete the diagram by dragging from the choices below to specify what condition the client is most likely experiencing, two actions the nurse should take to address that condition, and two parameters the nurse should monitor to assess the client's progress.

Action to Take		Parameter to Monitor
Action to Take	Condition Most Likely Experiencing	Parameter to Monitor

Actions to Take	Potential Conditions	Parameters to Monitor
Maintain NPO status	Irritable bowel syndrome	Vital signs
Offer frequently clear liquids	Peptic ulcer disease	Intake and output
Place in supine position	Peritonitis	Bowel sounds
Administer antibiotics	Diverticulitis	Pain level
Start intravenous therapy		

⚡ Answers to Practice & Next Generation NCLEX (NGN) Questions

1. 1
Client Needs: Physiological Integrity/Physiological Adaptation
Clinical Judgment/Cognitive Skill: Take Action
Item Type: Multiple choice
Rationale & Test Taking Strategy: Note the **key** word, "best," for this priority test item. Coffee-ground material is characteristic of old blood. Bright red bleeding would indicate hemorrhage. This is a normal occurrence on the third postoperative day and should be correlated with the vital signs. The tube is in the correct position because it is draining gastric secretions. There is no indication to notify anyone or to irrigate the NG tube.

2. 3
Client Needs: Physiological Integrity/Physiological Adaptation
Clinical Judgment/Cognitive Skill: Recognize Cues
Item Type: Multiple Choice
Rationale & Test Taking Strategy: This is only the day after surgery; therefore, the area around the stoma has not had time to heal. There will be some capillary bleeding. The stoma should be pinkish-red and moist, and often there is some swelling present. There may be slight edema, but it should not be pitting around the peristomal area. There should be no sloughing around the stoma or discoloration of the stoma.

3. 1
Client Needs: Physiological Integrity/Physiological Adaptation
Clinical Judgment/Cognitive Skill: Analyze Cues
Item Type: Multiple Choice
Rationale & Test Taking Strategy: Note the **key** word, "immediate," for this priority test item about intestinal perforation. Intestinal perforation is characterized by increasing distention and a boardlike abdomen. There is frequently increasing pain with fever and guarding of the abdomen. Peritonitis occurs rapidly. The nurse should maintain the client NPO (nothing by mouth), keep the client on bed rest, and immediately notify the health care provider. Decreasing hemoglobin and hematocrit and decreasing blood pressure are associated with hemorrhage rather than perforation. Remember to select an answer that reflects what the question is specifically asking.

4. 4
Client Needs: Physiological Integrity/Pharmacological Therapies
Clinical Judgment/Cognitive Skill: Analyze Cues
Item Type: Multiple choice
Rationale & Test Taking Strategy: To answer this test item requires an understanding of each medication's action. Metoclopramide is a gastrointestinal stimulant and should not be given in situations where an intestinal obstruction is suspected. Hydroxyzine is an antiemetic as well as an antianxiety medication. Cimetidine is an antiulcer medication that decreases gastric acid production. Cephalexin is an antibiotic that may be used as a prophylaxis before intestinal surgery.

5. 4
Client Needs: Physiological Integrity/Physiological Adaptation
Clinical Judgment/Cognitive Skill: Prioritize Hypotheses
Item Type: Multiple Choice
Rationale & Test Taking Strategy: Note the **key** word, "priority," for caring for an immediate postoperative client who is reporting nausea. It is most important to maintain patency and drainage of the NG tube postoperatively. The NG tube should not be repositioned on this client. The tube should not be irrigated until patency is determined. The NG tube should not be clamped, especially when the client is reporting nausea. The gastric output is most often measured at the end of the shift, even if it appears to be excessive. Measuring the output would not be a priority over evaluating for patency.

6. 1
Client Needs: Physiological Integrity/Reduction of Risk Potential
Clinical Judgment/Cognitive Skill: Generate Solutions
Item Type: Multiple Choice
Rationale & Test Taking Strategy: Consider what the routine orders are prior to an oral diagnostic test. NPO status before a barium swallow and an EGD and a clear liquid diet the evening before the procedures are routine orders for these tests. There is no general anesthesia. The client can eat or drink as tolerated after the procedure, and there is no routine placement of nasogastric tubes.

7. 1
Client Needs: Physiological Integrity/Pharmacological Therapies
Clinical Judgment/Cognitive Skill: Evaluate Outcomes
Item Type: Multiple Choice
Rationale & Test Taking Strategy: To answer this test item, you need to know what the medication and its action involves. Omeprazole is a proton pump inhibitor prescribed to decrease the amount of stomach acid and is used to treat symptoms of gastro-esophageal reflux disorder, such as heartburn. It is also used to promote healing of erosive esophagitis. Common side effects include headache, abdominal pain, diarrhea, nausea, vomiting, gas (flatulence), dizziness, and upper respiratory infection. Omeprazole does not affect blood pressure. It is not indicated for the management of chronic pain and can have an adverse effect of abdominal pain. Clients should not be eating spicy foods while taking omeprazole to heal a stomach ulcer.

8. 4
Client Needs: Physiological Integrity/Reduction of Risk Potential
Clinical Judgment/Cognitive Skill: Generate Solutions
Item Type: Multiple Choice
Rationale & Test Taking Strategy: Consider that the NG tube has confirmed placement by x-ray. To administer the medication safely, it is of paramount importance that the nurse determine that the NG tube is in the stomach by measuring the pH of aspirated stomach contents, which provides an immediate confirmation of gastric placement. This verification of placement is always done even if the initial x-ray confirms placement. When the end of the NG tube is placed in a glass of water and bubbling occurs, this might indicate the possibility of the tube being in the airway; however, it is not an accurate method to determine placement in the stomach. Forcing air through the NG tube and auscultating the abdomen for the sound of the air is an unreliable method to determine tube placement.

9. **1, 2, 3, 4**
Client Needs: Physiological Integrity/Physiological Adaptation
Clinical Judgment/Cognitive Skill: Analyze CuesItem Type: Select All That Apply
Rationale & Test Taking Strategy: The test item is asking for *common* complications, which could be serious or not so serious. The most serious complication of a gastric ulcer is hemorrhage. Other complications include perforation, infection (peritonitis), and pyloric obstruction (due to scarring, edema, and inflammation at the gastric outlet), which can be serious. Hematemesis can occur with massive bleeding, not hemoptysis, which is the coughing-up of blood from the lungs.

10. **3**
Client Needs: Physiological Integrity/Physiological Adaptation
Clinical Judgment/Cognitive Skill: Analyze Cues
Item Type: Multiple Choice
Rationale & Test Taking Strategy: Note the **key** word, "most," significant vital sign change. The low blood pressure reading is of most concern, because older adults are at risk for dehydration from fluid loss related to vomiting and diarrhea. This low blood pressure can lead to safety issues related to orthostatic hypotension and subsequent falling in the older adult. The older adult would have an increased pulse and decreased blood pressure as signs of dehydration. The slightly elevated temperature can also occur with dehydration; however, it is usually a more significant finding in younger adults. Oxygen saturation is within normal limits.

11. A client has a history of heartburn and acid reflux. The client is admitted to the hospital after vomiting 250 mL of bright red blood. Upon admission, the client states they feel a little dizzy, which is causing nausea. The following is the admission flowsheet.

Health History	Nurses' Notes	Flow Sheet	Laboratory Results

1030

Vital Signs:
- Temperature: 98.6°F (37°C)
- BP: 100/72 mm Hg
- Heart rate: 112 bpm and regular
- Respirations: 20 breaths/min
- SpO2: 96% on room air

Intake:
- NPO
- IV of 1000 mL of normal saline, infusing at 150 mL/hr

Output:
- 250 mL bright red blood
- 200 mL voiding, urine dark yellow

Complete the following sentences by choosing the most likely options for the missing information from the drop-down lists of options provided.

Based on a probable diagnosis of peptic ulcer disease (PUD), the client is experiencing *GI bleeding*, as evidenced by *hematemesis*, *hypotension*, and *dizziness*. The three major complications of PUD are *hemorrhage*, *perforation*, and *obstruction*.
Client Needs: Physiological Integrity/Physiological Adaptation
Clinical Judgment/Cognitive Skill: Analyze Cues
Item type: Drop-Down Rationale
Rationale & Test Taking Strategy: The client is admitted because the bright red hematemesis is indicative of acute gastrointestinal (GI) bleeding. If the GI bleeding is massive, then fluid is lost and signs of hypotension, tachycardia, and restlessness can indicate hypovolemic shock. Coffee-ground emesis is associated with blood sitting in the stomach and GI tract. Melena (black or dark, tarry stool) indicates the presence of digested blood, which means the source of the bleeding is in the upper GI tract. Hematochezia is the passage of fresh blood either in or with the stool. The three major complications of peptic ulcer disease include *hemorrhage* (ulcer erodes blood vessels, leading to bleeding in the stomach and possible hypovolemic shock if bleeding is massive), *perforation* (erosion of the ulcer through the stomach or intestinal walls, leading to peritonitis), and *obstruction* (due to scarring and loss of musculature at the pylorus and narrowing of the stomach outlet characterized by persistent vomiting).

12. A nurse is caring for a client who is newly admitted to the hospital.

Health History	Nurses' Notes	Provider Orders	Laboratory Results

1100 : Client is lying in bed with knees flexed and reporting severe abdominal pain (an 8 out of 10 scale). Client had several episodes of nausea and vomiting prior to admission.
On assessment, client shows facial grimacing, appears anxious, and is pale. Boardlike abdominal distention noted with diminished bowel sounds in all four quadrants.

- Temperature: 100.2°F (37.9°C)
- BP: 106/78 mm Hg
- Heart rate: 100 bpm and regular
- Respirations: 20 breaths/min
- SpO2: 96% on room air

The nurse is reviewing the client's assessment data to prepare the client's plan of care.
Complete the diagram by dragging from the choices below to specify what condition the client is most likely experiencing, two actions the nurse should take to address that condition, and two parameters the nurse should monitor to assess the client's progress.

Actions to Take Start intra- venous therapy		Parameters to Monitor Vital signs
Actions to Take Administer antibiotics	Potential Conditions Peritonitis	Parameters to Monitor Pain level

Actions to Take	Potential Conditions	Parameters to Monitor
Maintain NPO status	Irritable bowel syndrome	Vital signs
Offer clear liquids frequently	Peptic ulcer disease	Intake and output
Place in supine position	Peritonitis	Bowel sounds
Administer antibiotics	Diverticulitis	Pain level
Start IV therapy		

Client Needs: Physiological Integrity/Physiological Adaptation
Clinical Judgment/Cognitive Skill: Recognize Cues, Analyze Cues, Generate Solutions, Take Action
Item Type: Bow-Tie
Rationale & Test Taking Strategy: Peritonitis can be life-threatening and often fatal if not diagnosed and treated immediately. It is an acute inflammation and infection of the visceral/parietal peritoneum and lining of the abdominal cavity. The cardinal signs of peritonitis are abdominal pain, tenderness, and distention often noted as a rigid and boardlike abdomen. Bowel sounds often disappear with the progression of the inflammation. When diagnosis and treatment of peritonitis are delayed, blood vessel dilation continues with shifting of fluid. The body responds to the infection by shunting extra blood to the area of inflammation (hyperemia). This shift of fluid can result in a significant decrease in circulatory volume and hypovolemic shock. Because of this, the immediate nursing actions are to start intravenous therapy, administer antibiotics, and place the client in a position of comfort, usually semi-Fowler. This position aids in ventilation and localizes the purulent abdominal infection in the lower abdomen or pelvis, not allowing it to extend upward toward the heart and lungs. Two important parameters to monitor are vital signs (watching for hypovolemia) and pain level.

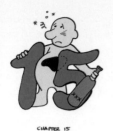

Hepatic and Biliary: Care of Adult Clients

CHAPTER 15
HEPATIC

PHYSIOLOGY OF THE HEPATIC AND BILIARY SYSTEM

Functions of the Liver

A. Synthesis of absorbed nutrients.
   1. Serum glucose regulation.
   2. Lipid (fat) metabolism.
   3. Protein metabolism.
B. Synthesis of prothrombin for normal clotting mechanisms. Vitamin K is necessary for adequate prothrombin production.
C. Vitamin and mineral storage.
   1. Produces and stores vitamins A and D.
   2. Vitamin B_{12} and iron are stored in the liver.
D. Drug metabolism: barbiturates, amphetamines, and alcohol are metabolized by the liver.
E. Production of bile and bile salts.
   1. Bile is continuously formed in the liver.
   2. Bilirubin, a bile pigment, is excreted by the liver.
      a. The spleen removes and breaks down the hemoglobin in worn-out red blood cells. This results in the production of bilirubin.
      b. Bilirubin is carried from the spleen to the liver for excretion.
      c. Bilirubin is conjugated in the liver (made water soluble) and secreted into the bile.

System Assessment: Recognize Cues

A. History.
   1. History of liver, gallbladder, or jaundice problems.
   2. History of bleeding problems.
   3. History of reproductive problems.
   4. Medication intake, alcohol consumption.
   5. Recent association with anyone with jaundice.
B. Physical assessment.
   1. Inspection.
      a. Skin.
         (1) Presence of vascular angiomas, skin lesions, or petechiae.
         (2) Hydration status.
         (3) Color of the skin (jaundiced).
         (4) Presence of peripheral edema.
      b. Abdomen.
         (1) Evidence of jaundice.
         (2) Contour of the abdomen.
         (3) Presence of visible abdominal wall veins.
   2. Palpation of the abdomen.

a. Pain, tenderness, presence of distention.
      b. Hepatomegaly, splenomegaly.
C. Nutritional assessment.
   1. Weight gain or loss; dietary intake.
   2. Problems of anorexia, nausea, and vomiting.

Pathophysiology of Jaundice

A. Jaundice may begin so gradually that it is not noticed immediately.
B. Increased levels of bilirubin cause a yellowish discoloration of the skin. It may be first observed as a yellow color in the sclera of the eyes. Serum bilirubin levels must be three times normal level (2–3 mg/dL [34–51 μmol/L]) for jaundice to occur. The yellow discoloration is due to deposits of bilirubin in the skin and body tissue.
C. Types of jaundice.
   1. Hemolytic jaundice.
      a. Occurs with an increase in the breakdown of red blood cells, which causes an increase in the amount of unconjugated bilirubin in the blood.
      b. Causes of hemolytic jaundice.
         (1) Blood transfusion reactions.
         (2) Sickle cell crisis; hemolytic anemias.
         (3) Hemolytic disease of the newborn.
   2. Hepatocellular jaundice.
      a. Results from the inability of the liver to clear normal amounts of bilirubin from the blood.
      b. Causes of hepatocellular jaundice.
         (1) Hepatitis, cirrhosis.
         (2) Hepatocellular cancer.
   3. Obstructive jaundice.
      a. Results from an impediment to bile flow through the liver and the biliary system.
      b. Obstruction may be within the liver or it may be outside the liver.
      c. Causes of obstructive jaundice.
         (1) Hepatitis; cirrhosis.
         (2) Liver or pancreatic cancer.
         (3) Obstruction of the common bile duct by a stone.

DISORDERS OF THE HEPATIC SYSTEM

Hepatitis

Widespread inflammation of the liver tissue is called *hepatitis.*
A. Types of hepatitis (see Table 15.1; Fig. 15.1).

Table 15.1   TYPES OF HEPATITIS

Characteristics	Sources of Infection	Spread of Infection	Diagnostic Tests and Drug Therapy
Hepatitis A Virus (HAV)			
Incubation: 15–50 days (peak incidence 25–30 days) • Fecal-oral (primarily fecal contamination and oral ingestion) • Can be spread by sexual contact (i.e., anal sex)	• Crowded conditions (e.g., day care, nursing home) • Poor personal hygiene • Poor sanitation • Contaminated food, milk, water, shellfish • Clients with subclinical infections, infected food handlers, sexual contact, IV drug users	• Most infectious during 2 weeks before onset of symptoms • Infectious until 1–2 weeks after the start of symptoms • Disease and recovery uneventful • Vaccination available	• Anti-HAV immunoglobulin M (IgM)—indicates acute infection • Anti-HAV immunoglobulin G (IgG)—not routinely done • No drug therapy available
Hepatitis B Virus (HBV)			
Incubation: 60–150 days (average 90 days) • Percutaneous (parenteral) or permucosal exposure to blood or blood products • Sexual contact • Perinatal transmission	• Unprotected sexual intercourse with an infected partner • Contaminated needles, syringes, and blood products • Asymptomatic carriers • Tattoos or body piercings with contaminated needles • HBV-infected mother (perinatal transmission) • Contact with blood or open sores of an infected person	• Before and after symptoms appear • Infectious for 4–6 months • Carriers continue to be infectious for life • Vaccination available	• HBsAg (hepatitis B surface antigen)—marker of infectivity; positive in chronic carriers • Anti-HBs (hepatitis B surface antibody)—previous infection or immunization • HBeAg (hepatitis B e-antigen)—marker of high infectivity • Anti-HBe (hepatitis B e-antibody)—indicates previous infection • Drug therapy—nucleoside and nucleotide analogs; interferon
Hepatitis C Virus (HCV)			
Incubation: 14–180 days (average 56 days) • Percutaneous (parenteral) or mucosal exposure to blood or blood products • High-risk sexual contact • Perinatal contact	• Needles and syringes • Blood and blood products • Sexual activity with infected partners • Born to an HCV-infected mother	• Begins 1–2 weeks before symptoms appear • Continues during clinical course and throughout life for chronic carriers • Majority go on to develop chronic hepatitis C and remain infectious • No vaccination available	• Anti-HCV (antibody to HCV)—acute or chronic infection marker • Drug therapy—direct-acting antivirals (DAAs)
Hepatitis D Virus (HDV)			
Incubation: same as HBV • HBV must precede HDV • Chronic carriers of HBV always at risk • Uncommon in the United States	• Same as HBV • Coinfection only with HBV • Routes of transmission same as for HBV	• Blood infectious at all stages of HDV infection • No vaccination available	• Anti-HDV—indicates past or current infection • HDV Ag (hepatitis D-antigen)—marker present within a few days of infection • No drug therapy available
Hepatitis E Virus (HEV)			
Incubation: 14–60 days (average 40 days) • Fecal-oral route • Outbreaks associated with contaminated water supply in developing countries • Uncommon in United States	• Contaminated water, poor sanitation • Found in Asia, Africa, and Mexico	• Not known • May be similar to HAV • Self-limited, acute illness • No vaccination available	• Anti-HEV IgM and IgG—present 1 week–2 months after onset of illness • No drug therapy available

TEST ALERT Follow infection control guidelines; standard precautions include blood and body fluids.

HEPATITIS A & E

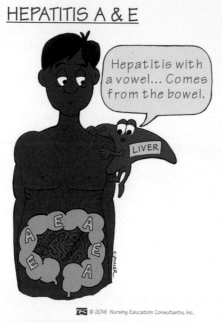

FIG. 15.1 Hepatitis with a Vowel Mnemonic. (From Zerwekh, J., Garneau, A., & Miller, C. J. [2017]. *Digital collection of the memory notebooks of nursing* [4th ed.]. Nursing Education Consultants.)

1. Toxic- and drug-induced hepatitis.
   a. Toxic: systemic poisons: carbon tetrachloride, gold compounds.
   b. Drug-induced: isoniazid (INH), chlorothiazide, methotrexate, methyldopa, acetaminophen.
2. Autoimmune hepatitis.
   a. Cause is unknown; associated with other autoimmune diseases.
   b. Requires different treatment than viral hepatitis; treated with corticosteroids and immunosuppressants.
B. The inflammatory process causes hepatic cell degeneration and necrosis.

> ❗ **NURSING PRIORITY** Follow infection control guidelines/protocols. Prevent transmission in the hospital, in addition to teaching the importance of personal hygiene.

Assessment: Recognize Cues

Regardless of the type of hepatitis, the clinical picture is similar.
A. Risk factors/etiology and sources/spread of disease (see Table 15.1).
B. Clinical manifestations: all clients experience inflammation of the liver tissue and exhibit similar symptoms.
   1. Anicteric phase.
      a. Anorexia, nausea, malaise, headache.
      b. Upper right quadrant discomfort.
      c. Low-grade fever; hepatomegaly.
   2. Icteric phase (jaundiced).
      a. Dark urine caused by increased excretion of bilirubin
      b. Pruritus due to accumulation of bile salts beneath the skin.
      c. Stools light and clay colored.
      d. Liver remains enlarged and tender.
   3. Posticteric phase (after jaundice).
      a. Malaise, easily fatigued.
      b. Hepatomegaly remains for several weeks.
   4. Anicteric hepatitis (absence of jaundice).
      a. Frequently occurs in children.
      b. Many clients with hepatitis A and hepatitis C (non-A, non-B) may not show clinical jaundice.
      c. Unexplained fever, general gastrointestinal (GI) disturbances.
      d. Anorexia and malaise.
   5. Onset of hepatitis A is more acute; symptoms are generally less severe.
   6. Onset of hepatitis B is more insidious; symptoms are more severe.
   7. Most cases of hepatitis C are asymptomatic or mild, but they tend to be persistent and lead to chronic liver disease.
C. Diagnostics (see Appendix 15.1).
   1. Antigen and antibody markers (see Table 15.1).
   2. Increased alanine aminotransferase (ALT), aspartate aminotransferase (AST), alkaline phosphatase, albumin, prothrombin time (PT)/international normalized ratio (INR), and serum bilirubin levels.

Analyze Cues and Prioritize Hypotheses

The most important problems are weight loss due to inflammation, especially with hepatitis A; fatigue due to infection; and decreased liver function resulting in diminished metabolic energy production.

Generate Solutions

Treatment
A. Prevention—routine immunizations for hepatitis A virus (HAV) and hepatitis B virus (HBV) for children.
B. Medications (see Table 15.1; Appendix 15.2).
C. HBV prevention—administer hepatitis B immune globulin (HBIG) for one-time or acute exposure.
D. Encourage good nutrition; no specific dietary modifications; client will probably not tolerate a high-fat diet.
E. Decreased activity; promote rest.

Nursing Interventions: Take Action

Goal: To control and prevent hepatitis.

A. Understand characteristics of transmission and preventive measures for hepatitis A.
   1. Good personal hygiene, especially handwashing.
   2. Participate in community activities for health education (e.g., environmental sanitation, food preparation, etc.).
   3. Identify individuals at increased risk for exposure: those with household contact, intimate sexual contact, day care centers, schools, travel to areas with increased rates of hepatitis A, and/or institutional contact with those with active disease.

4. Administer immune serum globulin (immunoglobulin G) within 2 weeks of exposure, if they do not have presence of anti-HAV antibodies (antibody to HAV).
5. Preexposure prophylaxis: hepatitis A vaccine (single dose).
6. Implement standard precautions.
7. Client should abstain from sexual activity during periods of communicability.

❗ OLDER ADULT PRIORITY Older adult clients are at higher risk for liver damage and complications of hepatitis.

B. Understand characteristics of transmission and preventive measures for hepatitis B.
   1. Identify individuals at increased risk for exposure: those with oral or percutaneous contact with hepatitis B surface antigen (HBsAg)-positive fluid and those who have had sexual contact with carriers within 4 weeks of the appearance of jaundice.
   2. Administration of hepatitis B vaccine.
   3. Postexposure prophylaxis: HBV vaccine series started and HBIG given within 24 hours of exposure.
C. Understand characteristics of transmission and preventive measures for hepatitis C.
   1. No vaccine for hepatitis C virus (HCV).
   2. Long-acting interferon is administered (pegylated interferon), along with antivirals (ribavirin).
D. Maintain strict contact-based standard precautions for hospitalized client with questionable diagnosis of hepatitis.

Goal: To promote healing and regeneration of liver tissue.
A. Bed rest with bathroom privileges initially; progressive activity according to liver function test results.
B. Promote psychological and emotional rest.
   1. Strict bed rest may increase anxiety.
   2. Frequently, young adults are concerned about body image; encourage verbalization and emphasize temporary nature of symptoms.
   3. Maintain communication and frequent contact.
C. Promote nutritional intake.
   1. Anorexia and decreased taste for food potentiate nutritional deficits.
   2. Small, frequent feedings of favorite foods, good oral hygiene, and food served in a pleasant atmosphere.
D. Encourage increased fluid intake.

🔅 Home Care

A. Continued need for adequate rest and nutrition until liver function test results are normal.
B. Avoid alcohol and over-the-counter (OTC) medications, especially those containing acetaminophen and phenothiazine.

TEST ALERT Evaluate client's use of OTC medications for potential interactions that may affect therapeutic treatment.

C. Clients with hepatitis B should avoid intimate and sexual contact until antibodies to the HBsAg are present and the client is no longer contagious.
D. If possible, client should have own bathroom.
E. Client and family must understand importance of personal hygiene and good handwashing.
F. Client should not donate blood.

📋 Hepatic Cirrhosis

Hepatic cirrhosis **is a chronic, progressive disease of the liver characterized by degeneration and destruction of liver cells.**
A. Liver regeneration is disorganized and results in the formation of scar tissue, which in time will exceed the amount of normal liver tissue.
B. Alcoholic cirrhosis (previously called Laennec): also called portal or nutritional cirrhosis; associated with alcohol abuse; accumulation of fat in liver cells leading to widespread inflammation and destruction of liver cells, which results in widespread scar formation.
C. Complications of cirrhosis.
   1. Portal hypertension.
      a. Esophageal varices form from collateral vessels in the lower esophagus and bleed easily.
      b. Hemorrhoids.
      c. Splenomegaly.
   2. Edema results from:
      a. Impaired liver synthesis of protein, resulting in decreased colloid osmotic pressure (hypoalbuminemia).
      b. Portal hypertension; malnutrition.
         (1) Ascites: accumulation of serous fluid in the peritoneal cavity.
      c. With increased pressure in the liver, excessive protein and water leak out of the liver into the abdomen.
      d. The presence of hypoalbuminemia results in decreased colloid osmotic pressure, which facilitates movement of fluid and protein into the abdominal cavity.
      e. Hyperaldosteronism causes increased amounts of sodium and water to be retained.
   3. Hepatic encephalopathy (coma) results from the inability of the liver to detoxify ammonia.
      a. Ammonia is a by-product of protein metabolism.
      b. Large quantities of ammonia remain in the systemic circulation and cross the blood-brain barrier, producing toxic neurologic effects.
   4. Hepatorenal syndrome: characterized by functional kidney failure with advancing azotemia, oliguria, intractable ascites.

TEST ALERT Identify changes in mental status.

Assessment: Recognize Cues
A. Risk factors/etiology.
   1. Excessive, prolonged alcohol consumption.
   2. Nutritional deficiencies.

3. Typically, these occur in a combination of alcoholism and nutritional deficiency, leading to a poorer prognosis.
4. Predisposing chronic hepatic and biliary infections.
B. Clinical manifestations (Fig. 15.2).
   1. Portal-systemic encephalopathy (Fig. 15.3).
      a. Level of concentration: ask client to repeat a series of numbers; if client has encephalopathy, he or she will be unable to repeat a four- to six-digit sequence.
      b. Memory: determine client's ability to recall recent events (yesterday or past week) and remote events (last year).
      c. Asterixis (flapping tremors): clients with asterixis are unable to hold the hands out in front of them when asked; a flapping of the hands will occur.
      d. Fetor hepaticus: musty, sweet odor to breath due to inability of liver to degrade digestive products.
C. Diagnostics—low albumin level and elevated PT/INR, AST, ALT, ammonia level, lactic dehydrogenase (see Appendix 15.1).

Analyze Cues and Prioritize Hypotheses

The most important problems are third spacing (ascites, fluid overload), potential for hemorrhage due to portal hypertension and esophageal varices, acute confusion due to elevated ammonia, pruritus due to increased bilirubin and jaundice.

> ❗ **NURSING PRIORITY** Clients with liver inflammation or cirrhosis should avoid large doses of vitamins and minerals. Vitamin A, iron, and copper can worsen liver damage.

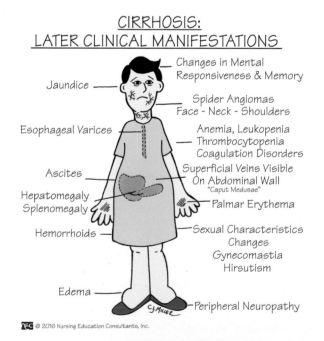

CIRRHOSIS: LATER CLINICAL MANIFESTATIONS

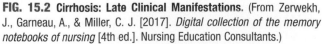

FIG. 15.2 Cirrhosis: Late Clinical Manifestations. (From Zerwekh, J., Garneau, A., & Miller, C. J. [2017]. *Digital collection of the memory notebooks of nursing* [4th ed.]. Nursing Education Consultants.)

HEPATIC ENCEPHALOPATHY
HEPATIC COMA

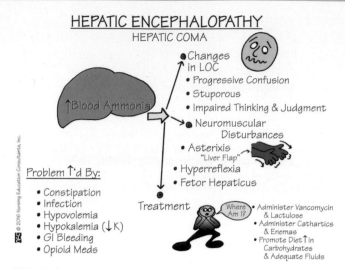

FIG. 15.3 Hepatic Encephalopathy. (From Zerwekh, J., Garneau, A., & Miller, C. J. [2017]. *Digital collection of the memory notebooks of nursing* [4th ed.]. Nursing Education Consultants.)

Generate Solutions

Treatment

A. Cirrhosis.
   1. Rest.
   2. Dietary modification: increase calories and carbohydrates; protein and fat may be consumed as tolerated.
   3. Vitamin supplement, especially vitamin B complex.
   4. Abstinence from alcohol.
B. Ascites.
   1. Intravenous (IV) albumin or other volume replacement after a high-volume paracentesis.
   2. Sodium restriction in diet.
   3. Fluid restriction for cases of severe ascites.
   4. Diuretics, usually a combination of a potassium sparing and a loop diuretic.
   5. Paracentesis for temporary relief.
   6. Nonsurgical procedures to decrease portal hypertension by shunting portal blood flow: transjugular intrahepatic portosystemic shunt (TIPS).
   7. Peritoneovenous shunt (LeVeen shunt): a surgical procedure for reinfusion of ascitic fluid into venous system; rarely used due to high rate of complications.
C. Esophageal varices.
   1. Blood transfusions to restore volume from bleeding varices; vitamin K to correct coagulation abnormalities; proton pump inhibitors to decrease gastric acidity.
   2. Administration of IV vasopressin produces vasoconstriction of the splanchnic arterial bed, decreases portal blood flow and portal hypertension; somatostatin analog therapy may also be administered.
   3. Endoscopic sclerotherapy: injection of a sclerosing agent directly into esophageal varices; bleeding may recur because there has been no reduction in portal hypertension.
   4. Endoscopic variceal ligation (EVL) or banding of the varices: often used in combination with sclerotherapy.

5. Balloon tamponade: mechanical compression of bleeding varices via esophageal gastric balloon tamponade (Minnesota tube; Linton-Nachlas tube; Sengstaken-Blakemore tube).

6. Shunting surgical procedures: decrease portal hypertension by shunting portal blood flow; usually performed after second major bleeding episode.

7. Management to prevent bleeding: beta-adrenergic blockers (propranolol), repeated sclerotherapy, endoscopic ligation, portosystemic shunts.

D. Decrease portal systemic encephalopathy.

1. Restriction of dietary protein intake.

2. Neomycin: decreases the normal flora in the intestines to reduce bacterial activity on protein.

3. Lactulose: used to reduce the amount of ammonia in the blood of clients with liver disease by drawing ammonia from the blood into the colon where it is removed from the body. May also be used to treat constipation because it pulls water into the colon to facilitate movement of waste through the GI system.

4. Control of GI hemorrhage to decrease protein available in the intestine.

Nursing Interventions: Take Action

Goal: To promote health in the client with cirrhosis.

A. Proper diet: increased protein as tolerated, adequate carbohydrates, vitamin supplements.

B. Adequate rest.

TEST ALERT Monitor client's hydration and nutritional status.

C. Avoid potential hepatotoxic OTC drugs (aspirin and acetaminophen).

D. Check all body secretions for frank or occult blood.

E. Abstinence from alcohol.

F. Attention and care should be given to the alcoholic client without being judgmental or moralizing.

G. Client should understand symptoms indicative of complications and when to seek medical advice.

H. Regular medical checkups.

Goal: To maintain homeostasis and promote liver function.

A. Rest and activity schedule based on clinical manifestations and laboratory data.

B. Measures to prevent complications of immobility.

C. Assist client to maintain self-esteem.

1. Maintain positive, accepting atmosphere in the delivery of care.

2. Encourage ventilation of feelings regarding disease.

D. Assist in activities of daily living, as necessary, to prevent undue fatigue.

E. Promote nutritional intake.

1. Good oral hygiene; between-meal nourishment.

2. Provide food preferences when possible.

3. Administer antiemetic before meals, if necessary.

4. Iron and vitamin supplements, especially vitamin B complex.

5. Nasogastric or parenteral feeding, if client is unable to maintain adequate intake.

F. Decrease discomfort of pruritus caused by jaundice: cool rather than warm baths; avoid excessive soap.

G. Maintain proper skin care to prevent breakdown.

H. Evaluate serum electrolyte levels, especially potassium and sodium levels, because of the use of diuretics to decrease ascites and edema.

I. Monitor temperature closely because of increased susceptibility to infection.

J. Assess for bleeding tendencies and prevent trauma to the mucous membranes.

K. Measure abdominal girth to determine whether it is increasing from ascitic fluid (Fig. 15.4).

Goal: If esophageal varices are present, decrease risk for active bleeding by implementing the following measures.

A. Soft, nonirritating foods.

B. Discourage straining at stool.

C. Decrease esophageal reflux.

D. No salicylate compounds (aspirin).

E. Evaluate sources of active bleeding.

1. Monitor vital signs.

2. Assess for melena and hematemesis.

Goal: To decrease bleeding from esophageal and gastric varices.

A. Gastric lavage with iced saline solution.

B. Assess and prevent complications associated with sclerotherapy.

1. Client is sedated and the throat is anesthetized before the procedure.

2. By means of endoscopy, the health care provider injects the sclerosing agent into the varices.

3. Bleeding from the varices should stop within minutes.

4. Client may experience chest discomfort for 2 to 3 days; administer an analgesic.

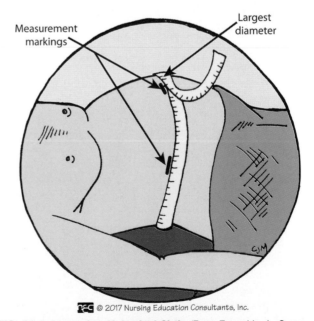

@ 2017 Nursing Education Consultants, Inc.

FIG. 15.4 Measuring Abdominal Girth. (From Zerwekh, J., Garneau, A., & Miller, C. J. [2017]. *Review course for the NCLEX.* Nursing Education Consultants.)

5. Esophageal perforation and ulceration are complications associated with treatment; observe client for development of severe chest pain.

6. Observe for return of active bleeding and *notify registered nurse (RN) immediately of any bright red vomitus or significant changes in vital signs.*

Goal: To provide safe care while the client has an esophageal tamponade balloon.

A. Constant observation is required while the balloon is inflated.

B. The client is to receive *absolutely* nothing by mouth; unable to swallow saliva; provide frequent oral and nasal hygiene.

C. Constant tension/traction is applied to maintain the pressure against the esophageal sphincter by the gastric balloon. The gastric balloon is *not* to be deflated while tension is present and the esophageal balloon is inflated. Label each lumen to identify balloon.

D. Deflate balloons as per agency policy to prevent tissue necrosis.

E. Keep the head of the bed elevated to decrease gastric regurgitation and nausea.

F. Keep scissors at the bedside in case the esophageal balloon moves into the oropharynx area and causes obstruction of the trachea. If this should occur, the lumen to the esophageal balloon should be cut to immediately deflate the balloon and relieve the obstruction.

Goal: To assess for and prevent complications associated with ascites.

A. Decrease sodium intake.

B. Administer diuretics, potassium supplements.

C. Daily measurements of abdominal girth.

D. Maintain semi-Fowler position to decrease pressure on the diaphragm.

E. Assess weight daily.

F. Monitor pulse oximetry for indications of respiratory distress.

Goal: To assess for and prevent complications of hepatic encephalopathy.

A. Frequent assessment of responsiveness.

B. Assess for changes in level of orientation and motor abnormalities (asterixis).

C. Provide and maintain a safe environment

D. Decrease production of ammonia.

1. Increase carbohydrates and fluids.

2. Decrease activity because ammonia is a by-product of metabolism.

3. GI bleeding will increase ammonia levels because of the breakdown of red blood cells.

4. Lactulose is used to promote excretion of ammonia in the stool; therapy must be titrated as diarrhea may occur.

5. Nonabsorbable intestinal antibiotics (see Appendix 14.2) will decrease protein breakdown.

E. Prompt treatment of hypokalemia.

Goal: To provide appropriate preoperative and postoperative care if surgical procedure is indicated.

A. Client is at increased risk for postoperative complications.

1. Hemorrhage, electrolyte imbalance.

2. Seizures, delirium.

B. Surgical procedures do not alter course of progressive hepatic disease.

Cancer of the Liver

Metastatic cancer of the liver **is more common than** *primary cancer of the liver.*

A. Liver is a common site for metastases because of increased rate of blood flow and capillary network.

B. Metastases are found in the liver in approximately one-half of all clients with late-stage cancer.

C. Prognosis is poor.

Assessment: Recognize Cues

A. Risk factors/etiology: malignancy elsewhere in the body.

B. Clinical manifestations.

1. Anorexia, weight loss, fatigue, anemia, peripheral edema, nausea, vomiting.

2. Right upper quadrant pain, ascites, jaundice.

C. Diagnostics—computed tomography (CT) or magnetic resonance imaging (MRI), fine needle biopsy (see Appendix 15.1).

Analyze Cues and Prioritize Hypotheses

The most important problems are the risk of metastasis to other organs, managing chemotherapy and/or radiation therapy side effects, and palliative care.

Generate Solutions

Treatment

Treatment is primarily palliative.

A. Surgical excision of tumor, if it is localized.

B. Chemotherapy: poor response.

C. Radiofrequency ablation (RFA) uses electrical energy to create heat to burn tumor (percutaneous approach).

D. Cryosurgery (cryoablation) uses liquid nitrogen to freeze liver tissue; not used for metastatic disease.

E. Percutaneous ethanol injection (PEI) or percutaneous acetic acid injection (PAI) used to treat unresectable liver cancer.

F. Chemoembolization, sometimes called transarterial chemoembolization (TACE), uses an embolic agent mixed with other meds to reduce the blood supply to the tumor.

G. Systemic chemotherapy not used; however, sorafenib (Nexavar) is used to treat metastatic liver cancer because it inhibits new blood vessel growth in tumors.

Nursing Interventions: Take Action

Focused on maintaining comfort; nursing care is the same as that for the client with advanced cirrhosis.

Acute Liver Failure

Acute liver failure **is a rapid onset of severe liver dysfunction in clients without a previous history of liver disease.**

Assessment: Recognize Cues

A. Risk factors/etiology.
   1. Use of acetaminophen with excess alcohol consumption.
   2. Drugs that have a toxic effect on the liver (isoniazid, sulfa-containing drugs, and nonsteroidal anti-inflammatory drugs [NSAIDs]).
   3. Viral hepatitis (HBV); less commonly with HAV.
B. Clinical manifestations.
   1. Changes in mentation—often first sign.
   2. Jaundice.
   3. Coagulation abnormalities.
   4. Encephalopathy.
C. Diagnostics (elevated bilirubin, liver function studies [enzymes]; see Appendix 15.1).
D. Complications.
   1. Kidney failure.
   2. Cerebral edema.

Analyze Cues and Prioritize Hypotheses

The most important problem is that the condition may progress rapidly, leading to a life-threatening clinical syndrome.

Generate Solutions

Treatment

A. Liver transplant, especially with clients who have severe encephalopathy.

Nursing Interventions: Take Action

Goal: To monitor for worsening of symptoms and complications.
A. Early transfer to intensive care unit.
B. Maintain adequate fluid balance to protect kidney function.
C. Monitor for cerebral edema; frequent neurologic checks.
D. Position head of bed elevated 30 degrees.
E. Avoid stimulating client and any straining or Valsalva maneuvers that may increase intracranial pressure.
Goal: To prepare client for liver transplant. (See next section.)

Liver Transplantation

Liver transplantation **is a therapeutic option for clients with end-stage liver disease; not recommended for widespread malignant disease.**

Assessment: Recognize Cues

A. Rigorous prescreening process.
B. Rejection less common than with kidney transplants.
C. Complications: transplant rejection, infection, bleeding.

Analyze Cues and Prioritize Hypotheses

The most important problems are transplant rejection, infection, bleeding, and the necessity to adhere to lifelong immunosuppressive therapy.

Generate Solutions

Treatment

A. Live liver transplant: portion of liver is donated.
B. Split liver transplant: donor liver is divided and given to two recipients.

Nursing Interventions: Take Action

Goal: To monitor for postoperative complications.
A. Assess neurologic status, monitor for hemorrhage and common respiratory problems of pneumonia, atelectasis, and pleural effusion.
B. Monitor IV fluids, nasogastric tube drainage, Jackson-Pratt drain, and T-tube drainage.
C. Administer antibiotics and analgesics.
D. Critical to monitor for infection the first 2 months after surgery; fever may be the only sign.
Goal: To provide nursing care of the immunocompromised client. (See Chapter 6.)

DISORDERS OF THE BILIARY TRACT

Cholelithiasis and Cholecystitis

Cholelithiasis **is the presence of stones in the gallbladder; this is the most common form of biliary disease.** *Cholecystitis* **is an inflammation of the gallbladder, which is frequently associated with stones; this condition may be acute or chronic.**

Assessment: Recognize Cues

A. Risk factors/etiology.
   1. Cholelithiasis (Fig. 15.5).

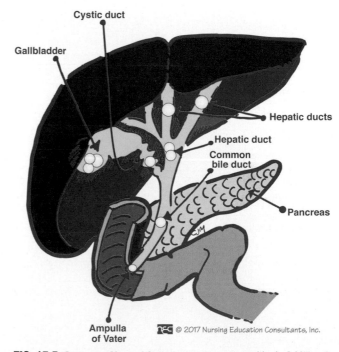

Cystic duct
Gallbladder
Hepatic ducts
Hepatic duct
Common bile duct
Pancreas
Ampulla of Vater

© 2017 Nursing Education Consultants, Inc.

FIG. 15.5 Common Sites of Gallstones. (From Zerwekh, J., & Miller, C. J. [2017]. *Review course for the NCLEX.* Nursing Education Consultants.)

a. Supersaturation of bile with cholesterol causes precipitate to occur.

b. Conditions upsetting cholesterol and bile balance include infection and disturbances of cholesterol metabolism.

c. Increased incidence in females, especially during pregnancy.

d. Increased incidence after age 40; obesity.

2. Cholecystitis (Fig. 15.6).

a. Associated with stone formation.

b. *Escherichia coli* is common bacteria involved.

c. May also be associated with neoplasms, anesthesia, or adhesions.

> ❗ **OLDER ADULT PRIORITY** Incidence of gallstone increases with age. Older adults are more likely to go from asymptomatic gallstones to serious complications of gallstones without biliary colic.

B. Clinical manifestations.

1. Cholelithiasis: severity of symptoms depends on the mobility of the stone and whether obstruction occurs.

a. Epigastric distress; feeling of fullness.

b. Abdominal distention.

c. Vague pain in the right upper quadrant after consumption of meals high in fat.

2. Obstruction of cystic ducts by stones; precipitating biliary colic.

a. Severe abdominal pain radiating to the back and shoulder.

b. Nausea, vomiting, tachycardia, diaphoresis.

c. Pain occurs 3 to 6 hours after consumption of a heavy meal, especially if high in fat.

d. Jaundice may occur with obstruction of bile flow.

e. Urine may become very dark and stools may be clay colored.

3. Cholecystitis.

a. Abdominal guarding, rigidity, rebound tenderness.

b. Fever.

c. Pain exacerbated by deep breathing.

d. Onset may be sudden with severe pain.

C. Diagnostics—ultrasound, CT, **hepatobiliary scintigraphy** (HIDA) scan, slightly elevated liver function studies (see Appendix 15.1).

Analyze Cues and Prioritize Hypotheses

The most important problems are pain due to inflammation and/or gallstones and weight loss due to nausea and anorexia.

Generate Solutions

Treatment

A. Cholecystectomy for cholelithiasis: surgical removal of the stones (see Fig. 15.7).

B. Laparoscopic cholecystectomy (see Fig. 15.7).

> ❗ **NURSING PRIORITY** Common postoperative problem of referred pain to the shoulder due to carbon dioxide (CO_2) that was not released or absorbed by body, which can irritate the phrenic nerve and diaphragm, causing difficulty breathing.

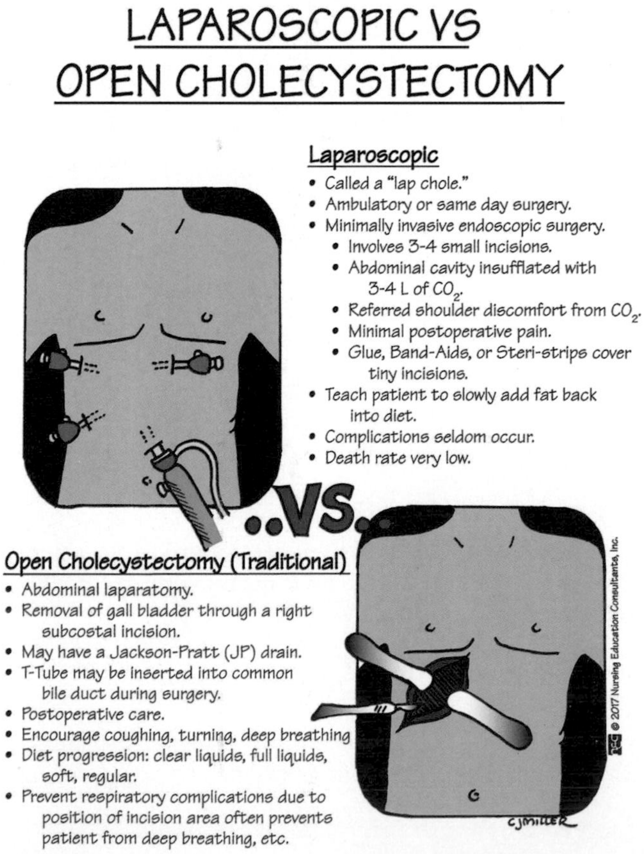

CHOLECYSTITIS

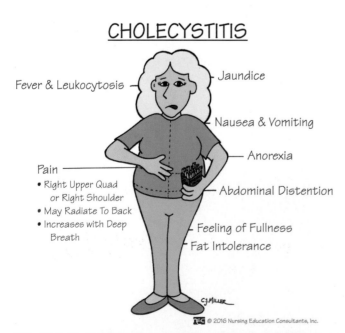

Fever & Leukocytosis

Jaundice

Nausea & Vomiting

Anorexia

Pain
- Right Upper Quad or Right Shoulder
- May Radiate To Back
- Increases with Deep Breath

Abdominal Distention

Feeling of Fullness

Fat Intolerance

© 2016 Nursing Education Consultants, Inc.

FIG. 15.6 Cholecystitis. (From Zerwekh, J., Garneau, A., & Miller, C. J. [2017]. *Digital collection of the memory notebooks of nursing* [4th ed.]. Nursing Education Consultants.)

LAPAROSCOPIC VS OPEN CHOLECYSTECTOMY

Laparoscopic
- Called a "lap chole."
- Ambulatory or same day surgery.
- Minimally invasive endoscopic surgery.
  - Involves 3-4 small incisions.
  - Abdominal cavity insufflated with 3-4 L of CO_2.
  - Referred shoulder discomfort from CO_2.
  - Minimal postoperative pain.
  - Glue, Band-Aids, or Steri-strips cover tiny incisions.
- Teach patient to slowly add fat back into diet.
- Complications seldom occur.
- Death rate very low.

...VS...

Open Cholecystectomy (Traditional)
- Abdominal laparotomy.
- Removal of gall bladder through a right subcostal incision.
- May have a Jackson-Pratt (JP) drain.
- T-Tube may be inserted into common bile duct during surgery.
- Postoperative care.
- Encourage coughing, turning, deep breathing
- Diet progression: clear liquids, full liquids, soft, regular.
- Prevent respiratory complications due to position of incision area often prevents patient from deep breathing, etc.

© 2017 Nursing Education Consultants, Inc.

FIG. 15.7 Laparoscopic versus Open Cholecystectomy. (From Zerwekh, J., Garneau, A., & Miller, C. J. [2017]. *Digital collection of the memory notebooks of nursing* [4th ed.]. Nursing Education Consultants.)

C. Cholecystitis.
   1. Anticholinergics to decrease secretions and promote relaxation of the gallbladder.
   2. Analgesics: hydromorphone or morphine.
   3. Antibiotics for potential infection, if indicated.
   4. Atropine and dicyclomine will relieve spasms and decrease pain.
   5. Ketorolac may be used to decrease spasms and pain in older adults.
D. Decrease dietary fat intake.

Nursing Interventions: Take Action

Goal: To decrease pain and inflammatory response.
A. Low-fat liquid diet during acute attack.
B. Low-fat solids added, as tolerated.
C. IV fluids and gastric decompression if nausea and vomiting are severe.
D. Antibiotics and analgesics.
E. Assess for indications of infection.
Goal: To provide appropriate preoperative nursing care if surgery is indicated.
Goal: To maintain homeostasis and prevent complications after laparoscopic cholecystectomy.
A. Client usually discharged after recovering from anesthesia.
B. Remove the bandages from the three to four puncture sites the day after surgery and shower, leaving the Steri-Strips intact, which will fall off in 7 to 10 days.
C. Teach client to report:
   1. Redness, swelling, bleeding, or bad-smelling drainage from wound site.
   2. Lack of a bowel movement or passing gas for 3 days or watery diarrhea for more than 3 days.
   3. Any bile-colored drainage or pus from any surgical site; severe abdominal pain that is not relieved by medication or is getting worse.
   4. Nausea, vomiting, chills, or fever greater than 101°F (38.3°C).
   5. Light-colored stool, dark urine, or yellow tint to the eyes or skin.
D. May resume normal activities gradually and return to work usually 1 week after surgery.
E. Follow a low-fat diet for several weeks, slowly introducing foods with fat content.
Goal: To maintain homeostasis and prevent complications after open cholecystectomy.
A. General postoperative care for clients having abdominal surgery.
B. Evaluate tolerance to diet and progress diet gradually to low-fat solids.
C. Penrose drain may be in place; client will frequently have large amounts of serosanguineous drainage; change dressing as indicated.
D. Modified left lateral recumbent position to facilitate the movement of CO_2 gas pocket away from the diaphragm.

PLACEMENT OF A T-TUBE

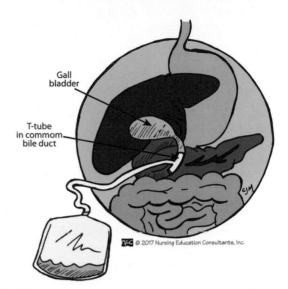

FIG. 15.8 Placement of a T tube. (From Zerwekh, J., Garneau, A., & Miller, C. J. [2017]. *Digital collection of the memory notebooks of nursing* [4th ed.]. Nursing Education Consultants.)

E. T tube may be used to maintain patency of bile duct and to facilitate bile drainage until edema subsides (Fig. 15.8).
   1. Maintain tube to gravity drainage.
   2. Observe amount and color of bile drainage.
   3. Do not irrigate or clamp tube; do not raise tube above the level of the gallbladder.
   4. Observe for bile drainage around the tube.
   5. Observe and record drainage (bloody initially, then greenish-brown).
   6. Drainage is usually around 500 mL/day for several days after surgery; will gradually decrease and the health care provider will remove the tube.
   7. Drains and/or tubes are typically not placed or used after a laparoscopic cholecystectomy.
F. Monitor urine and stool for changes in color.
Goal: To assist client to understand implications of disease process and measures to maintain health after an open cholecystectomy.
A. Dietary teaching regarding low-fat diet.
B. Weight reduction, if appropriate.
C. Avoid heavy lifting for 4 to 6 weeks.
D. Understand symptoms indicating bile obstruction (i.e., stool and urine changes) and advise health care provider accordingly.
E. *Report severe pain, increased distention, or leakage of bile from puncture sites to the RN.*

Appendix 15.1 DIAGNOSTICS OF THE HEPATIC AND BILIARY SYSTEM

LABORATORY TESTS	NORMAL	NURSING IMPLICATIONS
Serum Laboratory Tests		
Bilirubin		
Direct	0.1–0.3 mg/dL (1.7–5.1 µmol/L)	1. A rise in the serum level of bilirubin will occur if there is excessive destruction of red blood cells or if the liver is unable to excrete normal amounts of bilirubin.
Indirect	0.1–1.0 mg/dL (1.7–17.1 µmol/L)	
Total	0.2–1.3 mg/dL (5–21 µmol/L)	
Protein Studies		
Total serum protein	6.0–8.0 g/dL (60–80 g/L)	1. Proteins are responsible for maintaining the colloid oncotic pressure in the serum.
Serum albumin	3.5–5.0 g/dL (35–50 g/L)	2. Synthesis of protein and normal serum protein levels are affected by various liver impairments.
Serum globulin	2.0–3.5 g/dL (20–35 g/L)	
Serum Enzymes (Liver Function Studies)		
Lactic dehydrogenase (LDH)	140–280 units/L (0.83–2.5 µkat/L)	1. Elevated in heart failure, hemolytic disorders, hepatitis, liver damage.
LDH_5 Aspartate aminotransferase (AST)	10–26 units (0.10–0.26 µkat/L)	1. LDH_5 isoenzyme elevated in hepatitis. 2. Elevated in liver disease, acute hepatitis, myocardial infarction, pulmonary infarction.
Alanine aminotransferase (ALT)	10–40 unit/L (0.17–0.68 µkat/L)	1. Elevated in liver disease, shock.
Alkaline phosphatase (ALP)	38–126 units/L (0.65–2.14 µkat/L)	1. Primary sources of ALP in body are bone and liver. Abnormally high readings may be associated with either liver or bone disease and must be correlated with presenting clinical symptoms.
Serum blood ammonia	30–70 mcg/dL (21.42–50 µmol/L)	1. Increasing blood ammonia is indicative of the inability of the liver to convert ammonia to urea.
Hepatitis antigens and antibodies	Negative for antigens	1. Antigens indicate hepatitis (hepatitis B surface antigen [HBsAg] elevated in hepatitis B). Antibodies indicate exposure, current disease, or hepatitis B immunization.

Appendix 15.1 DIAGNOSTICS OF THE HEPATIC AND BILIARY SYSTEM—cont'd

LABORATORY TESTS	NORMAL	NURSING IMPLICATIONS

Biopsy

Liver Biopsy
Percutaneous needle aspiration of liver tissue

1. Informed consent procedure.
2. Client's status is NPO for 6 hr before procedure.
3. Blood coagulation study results should be available on the chart before biopsy procedure.
4. Immediately before needle insertion, have client take a deep breath, exhale completely, and hold breath. This immobilizes the chest wall and decreases the risk for penetration of the diaphragm with the needle.
5. Keep client on bed rest for 12–14 hr. Client should be positioned on the right side for 2 hr postprocedure to apply pressure and decrease risk for hemorrhage.
6. Assess for complications of pneumothorax and hemorrhage immediately after biopsy; assess for right upper abdominal pain or referred shoulder pain; observe for development of bile peritonitis.

TEST ALERT Monitor status of client after a procedure: position the client on right side with a pillow under the costal margin to facilitate compression of the liver.

Paracentesis

Abdominal Paracentesis
Needle puncture of the abdomen to remove ascites fluid, obtain fluid for analysis, or initiate peritoneal dialysis (kidney client)

1. Informed consent procedure.
2. Obtain weight and vital signs prior to procedure.
3. Have client void prior to procedure to prevent injury to the bladder.
4. Position the client in bed with head of bed elevated.
5. After the procedure, apply a dressing to the site and monitor for leakage.
6. Weigh client after procedure and document both weights before and after procedure (client should have weight loss).
7. Maintain bed rest per protocol.

Cholangiography

Percutaneous Transhepatic Cholangiography (PTC)
IV injection of radiopaque dye to visualize the biliary duct system

1. Client's status is NPO for 8 hr before the test.
2. Assess for sensitivity to iodine.
3. Administer prophylactic IV antibiotic 1 hr prior to surgery.
4. Evaluate for iodine reaction after the test.
5. Client should drink large amounts of fluid after test to increase excretion of dye.

Nuclear Imaging Scans (Scintigraphy)

Hepatobiliary Scintigraphy (HIDA)
Shows size, shape, and position of biliary system. Radionuclide (Tc–99 m) injected IV; client positioned under a camera or counter to record distribution of tracer

1. Explain to client that traces of radionuclide pose minimal danger.
2. Needs to lie flat during scanning procedure.

Ultrasound

Gallbladder Ultrasound

Uses high-frequency sound waves to examine the gallbladder; provides information about presence of tumors and patency of vessels and detects gallstones

Hepatobiliary ultrasound: detects abscesses, cysts, tumors, and cirrhosis

1. Client is NPO for 8–12 hr because gas can reduce quality of images and food can cause gallbladder contraction.
2. Explain to client that a conductive gel (lubricant) will be applied to the skin and a transducer placed on the area.

Endoscopy

Endoscopic Retrograde Cholangiopancreatography (ERCP)

Fiber-optic endoscope and fluoroscopy inserted orally, descended into duodenum, then into common bile duct and pancreatic ducts, where contrast medium is injected for visualization of the structures

1. Client is NPO for 8 hr before procedure.
2. Explain that sedative will be given before and during procedure.
3. Check for allergy to contrast medium.
4. Informed consent must be signed.
5. Check vital signs—monitor for perforation or infection; pancreatitis is most common complication.
6. Check for return of gag reflex before giving fluids.

IV, Intravenous; *NPO*, nothing by mouth.

Appendix 15.2   HEPATITIS DRUG THERAPIES

Acute Viral Hepatitis: No specific drug therapy, only supportive therapy with antiemetics but not phenothiazines. Preventive immunizations (see Chapter 2).

MEDICATION	SIDE EFFECTS	NURSING IMPLICATIONS
Chronic Hepatitis B Therapies: Do not eradicate the virus; produce a decrease in viral load, liver enzymes, and rates of disease progression and drug resistance.		
Immune Modulators Pegylated interferon (long acting): SubQ a-interferon: SubQ *Nucleoside and Nucleotide Analogs* Entecavir: PO Tenofovir: PO	Flulike symptoms: aches, fatigue, headache, nausea, anorexia, fever; insomnia, hair thinning, diarrhea, weight loss, severe depression Possible nephrotoxicity	*Interferon Alpha* 1. Monitor and teach to anticipate flulike symptoms. 2. Monitor for severe depression. 3. Teach client to avoid crowds and people with infections. *Nucleoside and Nucleotide Analogs* 1. Monitor kidney function. 2. Relapse rate is often high following discontinuation of treatment. 3. Monitor laboratory work for potential nephrotoxicity and lactic acidosis.
Chronic Hepatitis C Therapies: In the past the first-line therapies used were pegylated interferon, a-interferon along with ribavirin. Currently, direct-acting antivirals are used: protease inhibitors, NS5A inhibitors, NS5B polymerase inhibitors.		
Protease Inhibitors, Second Generation Grazoprevir: PO Simprevir: PO Paritaprevir: PO *NS5A Inhibitors* Daclatasvir Elbasvir *NS5B Inhibitors* Sofosbuvir Ribavirin: PO	Possible nephrotoxicity and hepatoxicity, rash, itching, nausea, headache Headache, fatigue, nausea Hemolytic anemia, anorexia, cough, dyspnea, insomnia, pruritus, rash, teratogenicity, conjunctivitis	*Protease Inhibitors, Second Generation* 1. Monitor CBC and chemistry panel. 2. Monitor liver and kidney function. *NS5A and NS5B Inhibitors* 1. Monitor liver enzymes, especially ALT elevation. 2. Do not administer amiodarone with daclatasvir/sofosbuvir combination; can lead to bradycardia and chest pain. *Ribavirin* 1. Frequent rest periods. 2. Small, frequent, light meals.

ALT, Alanine aminotransferase; *CBC*, complete blood count; *PO*, by mouth; *subQ*, subcutaneous.

⚡ **Practice & Next Generation NCLEX (NGN) Questions**

Hepatic and Biliary: Care of Adult Clients

More questions on
evolve

1. A client had a paracentesis 2 hours ago. What would be an effective outcome from the procedure?
   1. Reduced pain
   2. Increased blood pressure
   3. Increased respiratory rate
   4. Decreased weight

2. A client with ascites calls the nurse and is tachypneic. The nurse auscultates bilateral crackles in the lower lobes. What would be a **priority** nursing action to help alleviate the symptoms?
   1. Place the client in high-Fowler position.
   2. Call the health care provider.
   3. Increase IV infusion rate.
   4. Initiate oxygen therapy.

3. What physiologic characteristics would the nurse find while checking the skin of a client with cirrhosis of the liver?
   1. Spider angiomas on the chest, yellow-tinted skin color, bruises
   2. Cyanosis, red- to pink-colored extremities, glassy eyes
   3. Dusky blue color, fruity breath, yellow-tinted skin color
   4. Yellow-tinted skin color, varicose veins, glassy eyes

4. A client being treated for ascites is placed on a strict low-sodium diet. Considering the diet, what foods would the nurse encourage the client to select?
   1. Pasta and milk
   2. Whole wheat bread
   3. Slices of apple
   4. Peanut butter on crackers

5. The nurse is caring for a client with advanced liver disease. What would the nurse expect to find while assessing this client?
   1. Client has difficulty maintaining normal blood pressure.
   2. Urine output is significantly decreased.
   3. Stools are black and tarry.
   4. Client has a large abdomen with excessive free fluid.

6. The client is returning to their room following a laparoscopic cholecystectomy. What is the **best** position for this client?
   1. Modified left lateral recumbent position with knees flexed
   2. Semi-Fowler to promote breathing
   3. Prone to decrease problems with aspiration
   4. Supine to decrease stress on the suture line

7. In report, the nurse is told that one of the assigned clients has advanced liver disease and has a high level of serum ammonia. What would the nurse expect to find with this client?
   1. Increased breathing problems
   2. Altered level of consciousness
   3. Fragile skin and easy bruising
   4. Yellowish skin discoloration

8. A client with advanced cirrhosis is diagnosed with esophageal varices. What would cause the nurse the **most** concern regarding complications associated with the varices?
   1. Difficulty swallowing
   2. Coughing up bright red blood
   3. Decreased gag reflex
   4. Anorexia and dyspepsia

9. A client is preparing to have a HIDA scan. What information about the HIDA does the nurse need to explain to the client? **Select all that apply**.
   1. Uses a radioactive isotope that is injected intravenously
   2. Will need to have a small high-fat meal prior to the test
   3. Requires less than 10 minutes to complete the scan
   4. Measures the amount of bile flow into the biliary tract
   5. Expect a small device to roll over the body

10. The nurse is making a home visit to a client with HAV. Before assessing the client, the nurse will gather the equipment and perform what action next?
    1. Wipe the bedside table with alcohol preps.
    2. Place the supplies on a clean, convenient work area.
    3. Spread paper towels on the work area and wash hands.
    4. Put on a gown and gloves.

11. The clinic nurse is reviewing the nurses' notes and laboratory results of a young adult who has been diagnosed with hepatitis A.

Health History	Nurses' Notes	Provider Orders	Laboratory Results

1400 : The client is a 20-year-old college student who reports to the clinic with mild jaundice. The client reports flulike symptoms of headache, low-grade fever, nausea, loss of appetite, and malaise over the past week. The client reports taking acetaminophen for the fever, which was effective. Approximately 2 weeks ago, the client traveled to Mexico with friends over spring break holiday. The client is anxious about the yellow color of the eyes and yellow tint to the skin.

LABORATORY TEST	RESULT	REFERENCE RANGE
HBsAg	Negative	Negative
HBsAB	Positive	Positive: previous exposure or immunization Negative: no exposure
Alanine Transaminase (ALT)	314 U/L	4–36 U/L (4–36 U/L)
Aspartate Transaminase (AST)	288 U/L	0–35 U/L (0–35 U/L)
Total Bilirubin	2.8/dL	0.3–1.0 mg/dL
Anti-HAV IgM	Positive	Negative
Anti-HCV antibody	Negative	Negative

For each health teaching information about hepatitis A listed below, use an X to specify whether the information would be appropriate health teaching to reinforce with the client at this time.

POTENTIAL HEALTH TEACHING	APPROPRIATE HEALTH TEACHING
Encourage close contacts to obtain hepatitis B vaccine.	
Avoid sexual contact with others.	
Wash hands frequently, especially before and after toileting.	
Avoid preparing foods while infectious.	
Avoid sharing toothbrushes.	
Explain that jaundice in the sclera may be permanent.	
Limit fluid intake.	
Use separate bath and hand towels with friends or family.	

12. A 62-year-old client reports to the acute care clinic complaining of nausea and vomiting for the past couple days and abdominal distention and lower-extremity edema.

Health History	Nurses' Notes	Provider Orders	Laboratory Results

1100 : Client is oriented to time, place, and person and reports insomnia, fatigue, and some right-sided abdominal discomfort. The client has been a heavy alcohol drinker for the past 30 years and has a history of type 2 diabetes diagnosed 20 years ago. Past history reveals client has been hospitalized for upper gastrointestinal bleeding and currently drinks less than three drinks per day. Abdomen is distended (ascites) with active bowel sounds. Client's skin and sclera are slightly jaundiced. Vital signs are stable. Client reports gaining 5 lbs over the past 2 days.

POTENTIAL NURSING ACTIONS	INDICATED	NON-ESSENTIAL	CONTRA-INDICATED
Obtain a daily weight			
Assess neurologic status q2h			
Maintain supine position			
Administer hydrocodone/acetaminophen for moderate to severe pain			
Ambulate client in hall hourly			
Monitor for alcohol withdrawal			

For each potential nursing action listed below, use an X to specify whether the action would be Indicated (appropriate or necessary), Non-Essential (makes no difference or not necessary), or Contraindicated (could be harmful) for the client's care at this time.

⚡ Answers to Practice & Next Generation NCLEX (NGN) Questions

1. 4
Client Needs: Physiological Integrity/Physiological Adaptation
Clinical Judgment/Cognitive Skill: Evaluate Outcomes
Item Type: Multiple Choice
Rationale & Test Taking Strategy: Ask yourself what happens during a paracentesis. Peritoneal fluid (ascites) is removed from the abdomen via a slender needle or catheter. The body weight should decrease due to the loss of ascites fluid and this loss should make it more comfortable for the client and improve ventilation. The client should have vital signs and weight measured before and after the paracentesis procedure. The client's pulse and respiratory rate should diminish if elevated prior to the procedure due to the relief of pressure from the fluid on the diaphragm and the weight of the ascites fluid. Abdominal discomfort should be minimal from the actual procedure and typically the ascites does not cause pain.

2. 4
Client Needs: Physiological Integrity/Physiological Adaptation
Clinical Judgment/Cognitive Skill: Prioritize Hypotheses
Item Type: Multiple Choice
Rationale & Test Taking Strategy: Note the **key** word, "priority," for a nursing action to alleviate tachypnea. The priority for the client is to alleviate the dyspnea by providing supplemental oxygen and positioning the client in low Fowler (30-degree elevation), which should alleviate some of the pressure of the ascites fluid on the diaphragm and lungs. Normally, clients with tachypnea would be positioned in high Fowler; however, the nurse needs to consider the enlarged abdominal area due to the ascitic fluid. Increasing the intravenous rate will contribute to fluid overload, which would not be indicated for this client. If the oxygen therapy and positioning do not assist in reducing the dyspnea and tachypnea, then the health care provider should be called.

3. 1
Client Needs: Physiological Integrity/Physiological Adaptation
Clinical Judgment/Cognitive Skill: Recognize Cues
Item Type: Multiple Choice
Rationale & Test Taking Strategy: To answer this test item, you need to know the signs and symptoms of cirrhosis. Recall how cirrhosis affects many body systems and this test item focuses on the skin. Keep in mind that all the items in the options need to be correct for the option to be the answer. The client with liver disease will have problems with bruising, petechiae, and spider angiomas. There is a characteristic yellowing or jaundice color of the skin due to the increased bilirubin level. There should not be a problem with hypoxia or changes in level of consciousness until the final stages of the disease. Fruity breath is associated with diabetic ketoacidosis. Glassy eyes is not a skin problem; however, the appearance is found with clients who are intoxicated.

4. 3
Client Needs: Physiological Integrity/Basic Care and Comfort
Clinical Judgment/Cognitive Skill: Take Action
Item Type: Multiple Choice
Rationale & Test Taking Strategy: In nutrition test items, look for foods that are similar because often the different food is the correct answer. In this test item, three of the options have a bread group (pasta, whole wheat bread, and crackers), which is high in sodium. Fresh fruits and vegetables have the lowest sodium content. The client should avoid breads, pastries, dairy products, and all processed meats because they are high in sodium.

5. 4
Client Needs: Physiological Integrity/Physiological Adaptation
Clinical Judgment/Cognitive Skill: Recognize Cues
Item Type: Multiple Choice
Rationale & Test Taking Strategy: Think about the symptoms of advanced liver disease, which most often is due to cirrhosis. The client with liver disease has a problem with portal hypertension that causes the problem of ascites—a collection of fluid in the peritoneal cavity. Melena or bloody stool may occur with bleeding problems, along with esophageal varices. There is usually no problem with urinary output or maintaining normal blood pressure levels.

6. 2
Client Needs: Physiological Integrity/Physiological Adaptation
Clinical Judgment/Cognitive Skill: Take Action
Item Type: Multiple Choice
Rationale & Test Taking Strategy: Note the **key** word, "best" position for the client following a laparoscopic cholecystectomy. Postoperative laparoscopic cholecystectomy clients frequently have diaphragm irritation from the carbon dioxide (CO_2). Semi-Fowler position will promote the movement of the CO_2 from the area of the diaphragm to decrease the irritation as well as promote breathing and reduce strain on the sutures. A modified left lateral recumbent position with knees flexed does not address the client's breathing. Having the client lay prone or supine does not promote breathing.

7. 2
Client Needs: Physiological Integrity/Physiological Adaptation
Clinical Judgment/Cognitive Skill: Analyze Cues
Item Type: Multiple Choice
Rationale & Test Taking Strategy: To answer this test item, it requires you to understand what the effect of an elevated serum ammonia does to the body. The increased serum ammonia will cross the blood-brain barrier and cause problems such as altered or decreased levels of consciousness. The other options are common in clients with liver problems but are not due to an elevated ammonia level.

8. 2
Client Needs: Physiological Integrity/Physiological Adaptation
Clinical Judgment/Cognitive Skill: Analyze Cues
Item Type: Multiple Choice
Rationale & Test Taking Strategy: Note the **key** word, "most," related to complications associated with esophageal varices. Bleeding from esophageal varices, which are dilated, distorted, and engorged veins, is a complication of cirrhosis. They are the result of portal hypertension and congestion. When the varices rupture, the client will cough up bright red blood (hematemesis). The client usually does not have problems with swallowing or with the gag reflex. Anorexia and dyspepsia are common problems with cirrhosis but not with esophageal varices.

9. **1, 4**
Client Needs: Physiological Integrity/Reduction of Risk Potential
Clinical Judgment/Cognitive Skill: Take Action
Item Type: Select All That Apply
Rationale & Test Taking Strategy: A HIDA scan is ordered to visualize and determine patency of the biliary system. Clients need to be in NPO (nothing by mouth) status before the procedure and will receive a radioactive isotope (tracer) that is injected intravenously. The radioactive tracer is given about 20 minutes before a large camera is positioned very close to the body. Hepatobiliary imaging is usually completed within 1 to 4 hours after administration of the radioactive isotope. When there is decreased bile flow, it indicates a biliary obstruction.

10. **3**
Client Needs: Safe and Effective Care Environment/ Safety and Infection Control
Clinical Judgment/Cognitive Skill: Prioritize Hypotheses
Item Type: Multiple Choice
Rationale & Test Taking Strategy: Note the **key** word, "next," which asks what the nurse should do after gathering equipment during a home care visit. Think about standard precautions. Hepatitis A is transmitted via fecal contamination and oral ingestion. It is important to maintain standard precautions before and after client contact. The use of standard precautions should prevent transmission of HAV to the health care worker. Paper towels are used to create a clean area surface and hand hygiene is important. Notice that hand hygiene is only in the option that is the answer. Alcohol preps are not effective. The mask is not appropriate because hepatitis is not spread by respiratory secretions.

11. The clinic nurse is reviewing the nurses' notes and laboratory results of a young adult who has been diagnosed with hepatitis A.

Health History	Nurses' Notes	Vital signs	Laboratory Results

1400 : The client is a 20-year-old college student who reports to the clinic with mild jaundice. The client reports flulike symptoms of headache, low-grade fever, nausea, loss of appetite, and malaise over the past week. The client reports taking acetaminophen for the fever, which was effective. Approximately 2 weeks ago, the client traveled to Mexico with friends over spring break holiday. The client is anxious about the yellow color of the eyes and yellow tint to the skin.

LABORATORY TEST	RESULT	REFERENCE RANGE
HBsAg	Negative	Negative
HBsAB	Positive	Positive: previous exposure or immunization Negative: no exposure
Alanine transaminase (ALT)	314 U/L	4–36 U/L
Aspartate transaminase (AST)	288 U/L	0–35 U/L
Total bilirubin	2.8/dL (μmol/L)	0.3–1.0 mg/dL (5.1–17.1 μmol/L)
Anti-HAV IgM	Positive	Negative
Anti-HCV antibody	Negative	Negative

For each health teaching information about hepatitis A listed below, use an X to specify whether the information would be appropriate health teaching to reinforce with the client at this time.

POTENTIAL HEALTH TEACHING	APPROPRIATE HEALTH TEACHING
Encourage close contacts to obtain hepatitis B vaccine.	
Avoid sexual contact with others.	X
Wash hands frequently, especially before and after toileting.	X
Avoid preparing foods while infectious.	X
Avoid sharing toothbrushes.	X
Explain that jaundice in the sclera may be permanent.	
Limit fluid intake.	
Use separate bath and hand towels from friends or family.	X

Client Needs: Physiological Integrity/Physiological Adaptation
Clinical Judgment/Cognitive Skill: Generate Solutions
Item type: Matrix Multiple Choice
Rationale & Test Taking Strategy: Hepatitis A infections are caused by the hepatitis A virus (HAV). It is important for the nurse to reinforce teaching the client ways to prevent the spread of the infection because the primary transmission route is fecal-oral; however, transmission of HAV can occur from any sexual activity with an infected person and is not limited to fecal-oral contact. Poor sanitation and contaminated water or food (e.g., shellfish) are contributing factors. The client is most infectious 2 weeks before onset of symptoms and unlikely to be infectious after the first week following the onset of jaundice. Fluid intake should be encouraged.

Rest is an essential intervention to assist the liver to repair and heal. Proper handwashing is important in the prevention of HAV transmission. The client should avoid preparing foods while infectious and sharing toothbrushes. It is best to have the client have their own bathroom; however, if this is not possible, the client should use separate bath and hand towels. HBV vaccine is given for its prevention. As the liver heals and repairs, the jaundice should resolve.

12. A 62-year-old client reports to the acute care clinic complaining of nausea and vomiting for the past couple days and abdominal distention and lower-extremity edema.

| Health History | Nurses' Notes | Vital signs | Laboratory Results |

1100 : Client is oriented to time, place, and person and reports insomnia, fatigue, and some right-sided abdominal discomfort. The client has been a heavy alcohol drinker for the past 30 years and has a history of type 2 diabetes diagnosed 20 years ago. Past history reveals client has been hospitalized for upper gastrointestinal bleeding and currently drinks less than 3 drinks per day. Abdomen is distended (ascites) with active bowel sounds. Client's skin and sclera are slightly jaundiced. Vital signs are stable. Client reports gaining 5 lbs over the past 2 days.

For each potential nursing action listed below, use an X to specify whether the action would be Indicated (appropriate or necessary), Non-Essential (makes no difference or not necessary), or Contraindicated (could be harmful) for the client's care at this time.

POTENTIAL NURSING ACTIONS	INDICATED	NON-ESSENTIAL	CONTRA-INDICATED
Obtain a daily weight.	X		
Assess neurologic status q2h.	X		
Maintain supine position.			X
Administer hydrocodone/ acetaminophen for moderate to severe pain.			X
Ambulate client in hall hourly.		X	
Monitor for alcohol withdrawal.	X		

Client Needs: Physiological Integrity/Physiological Adaptation
Clinical Judgment/Cognitive Skill: Generate Solutions
Item type: Matrix Multiple Choice
Rationale & Test Taking Strategy: The client with cirrhosis should have daily weights to monitor for fluid retention. The neurologic status should be assessed q2h to monitor for deteriorating signs, such as confusion, which could indicate hepatic encephalopathy. Monitoring for alcohol withdrawal is an indicated nursing action, as the client reports drinking daily. Hydrocodone/acetaminophen should be questioned, if not contraindicated, because acetaminophen can be toxic for clients with liver disease. Because of the ascites, clients often experience dyspnea and should be placed in semi-Fowler or high-Fowler position to obtain maximal respiratory efficiency. Ambulating hourly is nonessential, as these clients are often too ill and remain on bedrest.

Neurology: Care of Adult Clients

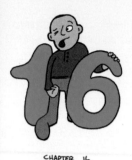

CHAPTER 16
NEUROLOGY

PHYSIOLOGY OF THE NERVOUS SYSTEM

A. Central nervous system (CNS): consists of brain and spinal cord (Fig. 16.1).
B. Peripheral nervous system:
1. Consists of the 12 cranial and 31 spinal nerves and the autonomic nervous system (ANS) (Fig. 16.2).
2. ANS response (Fig. 16.3; Table 16.1).
C. Neuron: the functional cell of the nervous system.
D. Supporting cells (neuroglia cells) provide support, nourishment, and protection to the neuron.
E. Myelin sheath—dense membrane or insulator around the axon.
F. Nerve regeneration: entire neuron is unable to undergo complete regeneration.
G. Meninges: protective membranes that cover the brain and spinal cord.
1. Pia mater: a delicate vascular connective tissue.
2. Arachnoid: a delicate nonvascular, waterproof membrane that contains cerebrospinal fluid (CSF).
3. Dura mater: a tough white fibrous outer layer of protection.
H. CSF.
1. Serves to cushion and protect the brain and spinal cord; brain literally floats in CSF.
2. CSF is clear, colorless, watery fluid.
I. Cerebrum: the largest portion of the brain; separated into hemispheres; the cerebral cortex is the surface layer of each hemisphere.
1. Frontal—controls higher cognitive function, memory retention, voluntary eye movements, voluntary motor movement, and expressive speech (Broca area).
2. Parietal—controls and interprets spatial information.
3. Temporal—contains Wernicke area, which is responsible for receptive speech and for integration of somatic, visual, and auditory data.
4. Occipital: interprets vision.
J. Cerebellum: works with cerebrum to coordinate muscle movement; maintains balance.
K. Brainstem: consists of the midbrain, pons, and the medulla.
1. Midbrain: responsible for motor coordination and visual and auditory relay centers.
2. Pons: helps to regulate respiration.
3. Medulla: Has vital centers concerned with respiratory, vasomotor, and cardiac function.

L. Diencephalon: part of the brain located between the cerebrum and midbrain.
1. Thalamus: relays sensory messages; pain gateway.
2. Hypothalamus.
a. Regulation of visceral activities, including body temperature, fluid and electrolyte regulation, motility and secretions of the gastrointestinal (GI) tract, arterial blood pressure.
b. Regulation of endocrine glands via influence on the pituitary gland.
c. Neurosecretion of antidiuretic hormone, which is stored in the pituitary gland.
M. Spinal cord.
1. Ascending (afferent) tracts: sensory pathways.
2. Descending (efferent) tracts: motor pathways.
3. Intervertebral disks lie between the vertebrae to provide flexibility to the spinal column.
4. Nucleus pulposus is the fibrocartilaginous portion of the intravertebral disk; acts as shock absorber for the spinal cord.

System Assessment: Recognize Cues

A. History.
1. Neurologic history.
a. Avoid suggesting symptoms to the client.
b. How the problems first presented and the overall course of the illness are important.
c. Mental status must be assessed before the history data from the client can be assumed to be accurate.

> **! NURSING PRIORITY** In the older adult client, assess orientation and mental status before continuing assessment of neurologic function (Box 16.1).

2. Medical history.
3. Family history: presence of hereditary or congenital problems.
4. Personal history: activities of daily living (ADLs); any change in routine.
5. History and symptoms of current problem.
a. Paralysis or paresthesia; syncope.
b. Headache, dizziness; speech problems.
c. Visual problems; changes in personality.
d. Memory loss; nausea, vomiting.

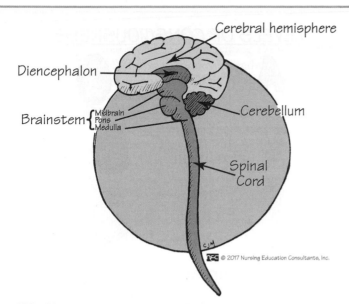

FIG. 16.1 Major Division of the Central Nervous System. (From Zerwekh, J., Garneau, A., & Miller, C. J. [2017]. *Digital collection of the memory notebooks of nursing* [4th ed.]. Nursing Education Consultants.)

LEVELS OF SPINAL NERVES

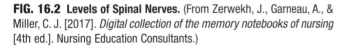

FIG. 16.2 Levels of Spinal Nerves. (From Zerwekh, J., Garneau, A., & Miller, C. J. [2017]. *Digital collection of the memory notebooks of nursing* [4th ed.]. Nursing Education Consultants.)

B. Physical assessment.
1. General observation of client.
   a. Posture, gait, coordination; perform Romberg test (have client stand with feet together, arms at sides; stand next to client to prevent falls; ask client to close eyes and continue to stand still). Positive if client loses balance and starts to fall.
   b. Position of rest for the infant or young child.
   c. Personal hygiene, grooming.
   d. Evaluate speech and ability to communicate.
      (1) Pace of speech: rapid, slow, halting.
      (2) Clarity: slurred or distinct.

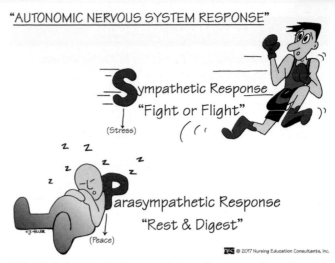

FIG. 16.3 Autonomic Nervous System Response. (From Zerwekh, J., Garneau, A., & Miller, C. J. [2017]. *Digital collection of the memory notebooks of nursing* [4th ed.]. Nursing Education Consultants.)

Table 16.1 AUTONOMIC NERVOUS SYSTEM

Area Affected	Sympathetic	Parasympathetic
Pupil	Dilates	Constricts
Bronchi	Dilates	Constricts
Heart	Increases rate and contractility	Decreases rate and contractility
Gastrointestinal	Inhibits peristalsis	Stimulates peristalsis
	Stimulates sphincter	Inhibits sphincters
Bladder	Relaxes bladder muscle	Contracts bladder muscle
	Constricts sphincter	Relaxes sphincter
Adrenal glands	Increases secretion of epinephrine and norepinephrine	

(3) Tone: high pitched, rough.
(4) Vocabulary: appropriate choice of words.
2. Mental status (must take into consideration the client's culture and educational background) (Box 16.2).

❗ NURSING PRIORITY Level of consciousness and mental status are critical assessment data for the client with neurologic deficits.

   a. Level of consciousness (Fig. 16.4).
      (1) Oriented to person, place, time, and situation (in order of importance).
      (2) Appropriate response to verbal and tactile stimuli.
      (3) Memory; problem-solving abilities.
   b. Mood.
   c. Thought content and intellectual capacity.

3. Interstitial edema occurs when CSF builds up due to an increase in CSF production or decrease in CSF absorption.
D. Regardless of the cause, increased ICP will result in progressive neurologic deterioration; the specific deficiencies seen are determined by the area and extent of compression of brain tissue.
E. If the infant's cranial suture lines are open, increased ICP will cause separation of the suture lines and an increase in the circumference of the head.

> **! NURSING PRIORITY** There is no single set of symptoms for all clients with increased ICP; symptoms depend on the cause and on how rapidly increased ICP develops. Vigilant assessment of the client is required!

Assessment: Recognize Cues

A. Risk factors/etiology.
1. Cerebral edema caused by some untoward event or trauma, including toxic exposure, blunt trauma, and fluid and electrolyte imbalance.
2. Brain tumors.
3. Intracranial hemorrhage caused by intracerebral, epidural, or subdural bleeding (closed head injuries or ruptured blood vessels).
4. Subarachnoid hemorrhage, hydrocephalus.
5. Cerebral embolism, resulting in necrosis and edema of areas supplied by the involved vessel.
6. Cerebral thrombosis, resulting in ischemia of the area and leading to edema and congestion of affected area.
7. Encephalitis/meningitis.
B. Clinical manifestations (bedside neurologic checks) (Fig. 16.7).

> **TEST ALERT** Provide care for client experiencing increased ICP (Box 16.3).

1. Assess for *changes* in level of consciousness because change is the cardinal indicator of increased ICP.
   a. Any alteration in level of consciousness (early sign for both adults and children)—irritability, restlessness, confusion, lethargy, and difficulty in arousing—may be significant.

> **! NURSING PRIORITY** The first sign of a change in the level of ICP is a change in level of consciousness; this may progress to a decrease in level of consciousness.

   b. Inappropriate verbal and motor response; delayed or sluggish responses.
   c. As the client loses consciousness, hearing is the last sense to be lost.
2. Changes in vital signs.
   a. Increase in systolic blood pressure with widening pulse pressure.
   b. Decrease in pulse rate.

   c. Alteration in respiratory pattern (Cheyne-Stokes respiration, hyperventilation).
   d. Assess temperature with regard to overall problems; temperature usually increases.

> **! NURSING PRIORITY** Cushing triad: increasing systolic pressure, with widening pulse pressure, decreased pulse rate, and altered respirations. Increased ICP is well established when this occurs. It is considered a neurologic emergency!

3. Pupillary response: normal pupils should be round, midline, equal in size, and equally briskly reactive to light and should accommodate to distance. Abnormal findings include:
   a. Ipsilateral: pupillary changes occurring on the same side as a cerebral lesion.
   b. Contralateral: pupillary changes occurring on the side opposite a cerebral lesion.
   c. Unilateral dilation of pupils.
   d. Sluggish or no pupillary response to light and poor or absent accommodation.
4. Motor and sensory function: normal is indicated by the ability to move all extremities with equal strength. Abnormal findings include:
   a. Unilateral or bilateral weakness or paralysis.
   b. Failure to withdraw from painful stimuli.
   c. Posturing: decorticate, decerebrate, flaccid, or opisthotonos.
   d. Seizure activity; ataxia.
5. Headache.
   a. Constant with increasing intensity.
   b. Exacerbated by movement.
   c. Photophobia.
6. Vomiting: projectile vomiting without prior nausea.
7. Infants.
   a. Tense, bulging fontanel(s).
   b. Separated cranial sutures.
   c. Increasing frontal-occipital circumference.
   d. High-pitched cry.
C. Diagnostics (see Appendix 16.1).
D. Complications.
1. CSF leaks, especially in client with basilar skull fracture; risk for meningitis.
2. Herniation: shifting of the intracranial contents from one compartment to another; involves herniation through the tentorium cerebelli; affects area that controls vital functions.
3. Permanent brain damage or death.

Analyze Cues and Prioritize Hypotheses

The most important problems are impaired cognition, mobility, and sensory perception due to the increased pressure on the brain causing inadequate brain tissue perfusion.

Generate Solutions

Treatment

A. Treatment of the underlying cause of increasing pressure.

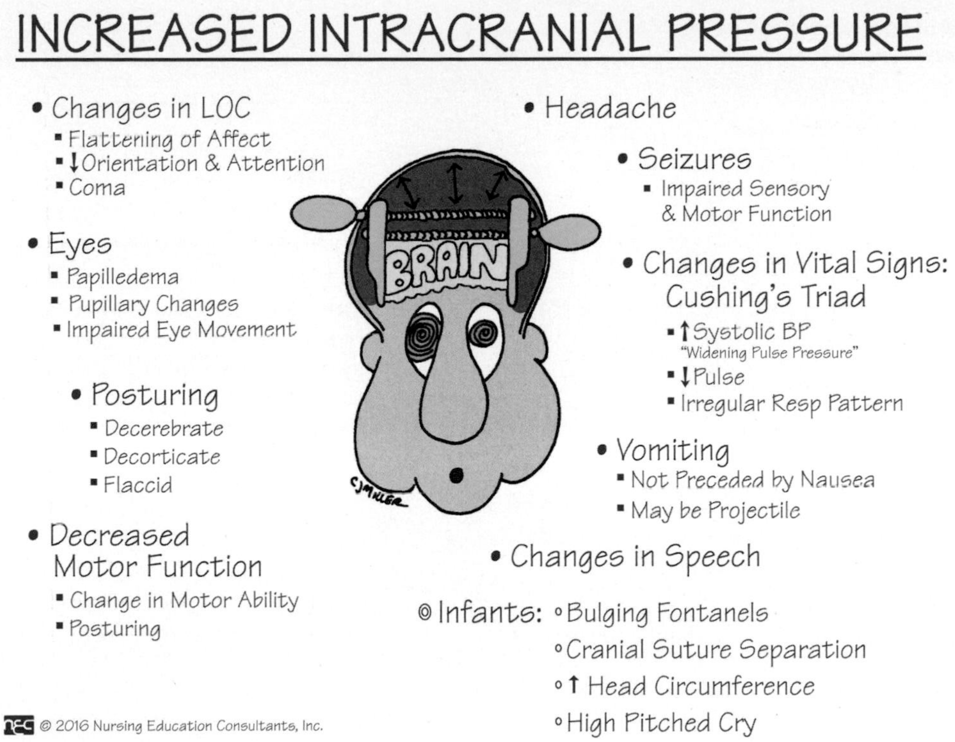

INCREASED INTRACRANIAL PRESSURE

- Changes in LOC
  - Flattening of Affect
  - ↓Orientation & Attention
  - Coma

- Eyes
  - Papilledema
  - Pupillary Changes
  - Impaired Eye Movement

- Posturing
  - Decerebrate
  - Decorticate
  - Flaccid

- Decreased Motor Function
  - Change in Motor Ability
  - Posturing

- Headache

- Seizures
  - Impaired Sensory & Motor Function

- Changes in Vital Signs: Cushing's Triad
  - ↑Systolic BP "Widening Pulse Pressure"
  - ↓Pulse
  - Irregular Resp Pattern

- Vomiting
  - Not Preceded by Nausea
  - May be Projectile

- Changes in Speech

- Infants: ○ Bulging Fontanels
  - ○ Cranial Suture Separation
  - ○ ↑ Head Circumference
  - ○ High Pitched Cry

© 2016 Nursing Education Consultants, Inc.

FIG. 16.7 Increased Intracranial Pressure. (From Zerwekh, J., Garneau, A., & Miller, C. J. [2017]. *Digital collection of the memory notebooks of nursing* [4th ed.]. Nursing Education Consultants.)

B. Neurologic checks every hour or as ordered.
1. May involve correlation of several variables including level of consciousness, vital signs, speech, facial symmetry, grasp strength, leg strength, and pupil responses.
2. Careful comparison with previous assessment is critical to detect incremental changes.
C. Intravenous (IV) and oral fluids to maintain normal fluid volume status if mean arterial pressure (MAP) is low to normal. Often, normal saline solution is fluid of choice; 5% dextrose in water potentiates cerebral edema.
D. Medications.
1. Osmotic diuretic, hypertonic saline.
2. Corticosteroids (vasogenic edema).
3. Anticonvulsants, antihypertensives.
E. Maintain adequate ventilation; prevent hypoxia and hypercapnia.
F. Placement of ventriculostomy drain or ventriculoperitoneal shunt.

Nursing Interventions: Take Action

Goal: To identify and decrease problem of increased ICP.
A. Neurologic checks, as indicated by client's status (Table 16.2).
B. Maintain head of bed (HOB) in semi-Fowler position (15–30 degrees) to promote venous drainage and respiratory function.

❗ NURSING PRIORITY Change client's position. If the client with increased ICP develops hypovolemic shock, do not place client in Trendelenburg position.

C. Change client's position slowly; avoid extreme hip flexion and extreme rotation or flexion of neck. Maintain the head and spinal column in midline position.
D. Monitor urine specific gravity.
E. Evaluate intake and output.
1. In response to diuretics.
2. As correlated with changes in daily weight.
F. Suction only as necessary.
G. Sedatives and narcotics can depress respiration; use with caution because they mask symptoms of increasing ICP.
H. Client should avoid strenuous coughing, Valsalva maneuver, and isometric muscle exercises.
I. Avoid straining with stools (increases intrathoracic pressure sporadically).
J. In infants, measure frontal-occipital circumference to evaluate increase in size of the head.
K. Control hyperthermia.
Goal: To maintain respiratory function.

❗ NURSING PRIORITY An obstructed airway is one of the most common problems in the unconscious client; position to maintain patent airway or use airway adjuncts.

A. Prevent respiratory problems of immobility.
B. Evaluate patency of airway frequently; as level of consciousness decreases, client is at increased risk for accumulating secretions and airway obstruction by the tongue.
C. Monitor O_2 saturation, arterial blood gases (ABGs); maintain $Paco_2$ levels as prescribed.
D. Maintain airway; suction only when needed. Limit suction to less than 10 seconds for adults; hyperoxygenate pre- and post-suctioning.

Table 16.2 GLASGOW COMA SCALE (GCS)

Category of Response	Appropriate Stimulus	Response	Score
Eyes open	Approach bedside Verbal command Pain	Spontaneous response Opening of eyes to name or command Lack of opening of eyes to previous stimuli but opening to pain Lack of opening of eyes to any stimulus Untestable	4 3 2 1 U
Best verbal response	Verbal questioning with maximum arousal	Appropriate orientation, conversant, correct identification of self, place, year, and month Confusion; conversant but disoriented in one or more spheres Inappropriate or disorganized use of words (e.g., cursing), lack of sustained conversation Incomprehensible words, sounds (e.g., moaning) Lack of sound, even with painful stimuli Untestable	5 4 3 2 1 U
Best motor response	Verbal command (e.g., "raise your arm, hold up two fingers")	Obedience in response to command	6
	Pain: (pressure on proximal nailbed—peripheral; trapezius pinch—central)	Localization of pain, lack of obedience but presence of attempts to remove offending stimulus Flexion withdrawal,[a] flexion of arm in response to pain without abnormal flexion posture Abnormal flexion, flexing of arm at elbow and pronation, making a fist Abnormal extension, extension of arm at elbow, usually with adduction and internal rotation of arm at shoulder Lack of response Untestable	5 4 3 2 1 U

[a]Added to the original scale by many centers.

From Harding, M., Kwong, J., & Roberts, D., Hagler, D., & Reinisch, C. [2023]. *Lewis's Medical-surgical nursing: Assessment and management of clinical problems* [12th ed.]. Mosby.

E. Client may require intubation and respiratory support from a ventilator.

Goal: To protect client from injury.

A. Maintain seizure precautions.

B. Restrain client only if absolutely necessary; struggling against restraints increases ICP.

C. Do not clean the ears or nasal passages of a client with a head injury or a client who has had neurosurgery. Check for evidence of a CSF leak: CSF placed on a white absorbent paper or white gauze pad can be distinguished from other fluids by the "halo" sign, a clear or yellowish ring surrounding a spot of blood. *Notify registered nurse (RN) if there is evidence of a CSF leak—presence of a halo sign.*

D. Aspiration is a major problem in the unconscious client; place the client in semi-Fowler position for tube feeding after ensuring correct tube placement.

E. Maintain quiet, nonstimulating environment.

F. Inspect eyes and prevent corneal ulceration.

1. Protective closing of eyes, if eyes remain open.

2. Irrigation with normal saline solution or methylcellulose drops to restore moisture.

Goal: To maintain psychological equilibrium.

A. Neurologic checks should be done on a continual basis to detect potential problems.

B. Encourage verbalization of fears regarding condition.

C. Give simple explanation of procedures to client and family.

D. Altered states of consciousness will cause increased anxiety and confusion; maintain reality orientation.

E. If unconscious, continue to talk to client; describe procedures and treatments; always assume client can hear.

F. Assist parents and family to work through feelings of guilt and anger.

Goal: To prevent complications of immobility. (See Chapter 3.)

Goal: To maintain elimination.

A. Urinary incontinence: may use condom catheter or indwelling bladder catheter.

B. Keep perineal area clean; prevent excoriation.

C. Monitor bowel function; evaluate for fecal impaction.

TEST ALERT Notify primary health care provider when client demonstrates signs of potential complications; interpret what data for a client need to be reported immediately.

Home Care

A. Teach client and family signs of increased ICP.

B. Call the doctor if any of the following are observed:
1. Changes in vision.
2. Increased drainage from incision area or clear drainage in the ears.
3. Abrupt changes in sleeping patterns or irritability.
4. Headache not responding to medication.
5. Changes in coordination; disorientation.
6. Slurred speech; unusual behavior.
7. Seizure activity; vomiting.
C. Review care of surgical incision, wounds, or drains.

Brain Tumors

Brain tumors **may be primary (originate from tissue within the brain) or secondary (metastasized from other areas of the body).**
A. Supratentorial: tumors occurring above the tentorium, primarily the cerebrum.
B. Infratentorial: tumors occurring below the tentorium, primarily in the cerebellum or the brainstem.
C. Regardless of the origin, site, or presence of malignancy, problems of increased ICP occur because of the limited area in the brain to accommodate an increase in the intracranial contents.

Assessment: Recognize Cues

A. Clinical manifestations: symptoms correlate with the location and growth rate of the tumor.
1. Headache.
   a. Recurrent. May vomit on arising and then feel better.
   b. More severe in the morning; affected by position.
   c. Headache in infant may be identified by persistent, irritated crying and head rolling.
2. Vomiting: with or without nausea; can be projectile.
3. Papilledema (edema of the optic disc).
4. Seizures (focal or generalized).
5. Dizziness and vertigo.
6. Mental status changes: lethargy and drowsiness, confusion, disorientation, personality changes.
7. Focal weakness: hemiparesis.
8. Sensory disturbances: language, coordination, visual.
9. Head tilt: child may tilt the head because of damage to extraocular muscles; may be first indication of a decrease in visual acuity.
10. Changes in vital signs indicative of increasing ICP (Cushing triad—severe systolic hypertension with widening pulse pressure and bradycardia).
11. Cranial enlargement in the infant younger than 18 months.
B. Diagnostics—skull x-rays, magnetic resonance imaging (MRI), and computed tomography (CT) scan (see Appendix 16.1).
C. Complications.
1. Meningitis, brainstem herniation, diabetes insipidus, and syndrome of inappropriate antidiuretic hormone (SIADH) secretion.
2. Residual effects may include seizures, dysarthria, dysphasia, disequilibrium, and permanent brain damage.

Box 16.3 INCREASING INTRACRANIAL PRESSURE

Adult
- Early: Restless, irritable, lethargic
- Intermediate: Unequal pupil response, projectile vomiting, vital signs changes
- Late: Decreased level of consciousness, decreased reflexes, hypoventilation, dilated pupils, posturing

Infant/Child
- Early: Poor feeding, tense fontanel, headache, nausea and vomiting, increased pitch of cry, unsteady gait
- Intermediate (younger than 18 months): Increased head circumference, altered consciousness, bulging fontanel; shrill cry, severe headache, blurred vision, stiff neck
- Late: Same as adult

Analyze Cues and Prioritize Hypotheses

The most important problems are identification of the type of brain tumor and neurologic deficits that occur as the tumor grows.

Generate Solutions

Treatment
A. Medical.
1. Corticosteroids, antiemetics.
2. Anticonvulsants.
3. Complementary and alternative medicine.
4. Chemotherapy: oral, IV, intrathecal, implanted.
B. Radiation: x-rays, gamma knife, stereotactic radiosurgery, brachytherapy.
C. Surgical intervention: craniotomy/craniectomy, biopsy, shunt placement, reservoir placement, laser removal.

Nursing Interventions: Take Action

Goal: To provide appropriate preoperative nursing interventions.
A. General preoperative care with exceptions, as noted.
B. Prepare client and family for appearance of the client after surgery, location of waiting room, contact information.
C. Encourage verbalization regarding concerns about surgery.
D. Skin preparation is usually done in the operating room.

Goal: To monitor changes in ICP after craniotomy (see Box 16.3).
A. Obtain frequent vital signs, neurologic checks, and cranial nerve assessments.
B. Carefully evaluate level of consciousness; increasing lethargy or irritability may be indicative of increasing ICP.
C. Discourage coughing (elevates ICP).

Goal: To prevent postoperative complications.
A. Monitor respiratory status.
1. Monitor breath sounds, respiratory pattern, O_2 saturation, ABGs as ordered.
2. HOB elevation (unless contraindicated) and turn q2 hours, deep breathe.

3. Suction as necessary. Suction increases ICP; hyper-oxygenate and limit suction to less than 10 seconds.

B. Evaluate dressing.
   1. Location and amount of drainage.
   2. Clarify with surgeon whether the nurse or the surgeon will change dressing.
   3. Evaluate for CSF leak through the incision and *report any drainage or CSF leak to RN*.

C. Maintain semi-Fowler position and monitor for signs and symptoms of meningitis, if there is a CSF leak from ears or nose.

D. Postoperative positioning for client who has had infratentorial surgery is as follows:
   1. Bed generally kept flat with gradual HOB elevation (as prescribed).
   2. Position client on either side; avoid supine position.
   3. Maintain head and neck in midline.

E. Keep nothing by mouth (NPO) for 24 hours.

F. Postoperative position for client who has had supratentorial surgery: semi- to low-Fowler position.

G. Trendelenburg position is contraindicated for clients who have had either infratentorial or supratentorial surgery.

H. Do not position craniectomy client on the operative side.

I. Maintain fluid and electrolyte balance.

J. After client is awake and the swallow and gag reflexes have returned, begin offering clear liquids by mouth.

K. Closely monitor intake and output, electrolytes, and osmolarity levels.

L. Evaluate changes in temperature: may be due to respiratory complications (infection) or to alteration in the function of the hypothalamus.

M. Provide appropriate postoperative pain relief.
   1. Administer short-acting opioids, acetaminophen.
   2. Maintain quiet, dim atmosphere.
   3. Avoid sudden movements.

N. Prevent complications of immobility.

O. Maintain seizure precautions.

Home Care

See home care for client with increasing ICP.

Stroke

Stroke, **or brain attack, is the disruption of the blood supply to an area of the brain, resulting in tissue necrosis and sudden loss of brain function. Stroke is the leading cause of adult disability in the United States.**

A. Transient ischemic attack (TIA).
   1. Brief episode of neurologic dysfunction; usually resolves within 60 minutes.
   2. Considered a warning sign of an impending stroke.
   3. Teach client to seek immediate treatment for any stroke symptoms. Cannot predict whether symptoms are TIA or stroke. Time is crucial!

B. Types of stroke.
   1. Ischemic stroke.

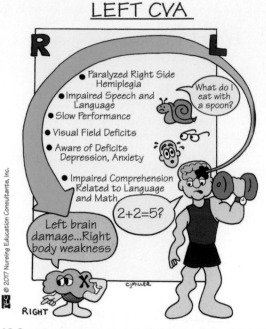

FIG. 16.8 Left Cerebrovascular Accident. (From Zerwekh, J., Garneau, A., & Miller, C. J. [2017]. *Digital collection of the memory notebooks of nursing* [4th ed.]. Nursing Education Consultants.)

a. Thrombotic stroke: formation of a clot that results in the narrowing of a vessel lumen and eventual occlusion.
   (1) Associated with hypertension and diabetes.
   (2) Produces ischemia of the cerebral tissue distal to occlusion and edema to the surrounding areas.

b. Embolic stroke: occlusion of a cerebral artery by an embolus.
   (1) Common site of origin is the endocardium.
   (2) May affect any age group; sudden onset of symptoms.

2. Hemorrhagic stroke.
   a. Bleeding into brain tissue, subarachnoid space, or ventricles.
   b. Resultant clot compresses brain tissue.
   c. Abrupt onset of symptoms; headache, focal neurologic deficits.
   d. The area of edema resulting from tissue damage may precipitate more damage than the vascular damage itself.

C. Neuromuscular deficits.
   1. Damage to the left side of the brain will result in paralysis of the right side of the body (Figs. 16.8 and 16.9).
   2. Both upper and lower extremities of the involved side are weakened or paralyzed.
   3. With a stroke, the client has neurologic deficits related to mobility, sensation, and cognition.

Assessment: Recognize Cues

A. Risk factors/etiology (see Box 16.4).

B. Rapid assessment and diagnosis of stroke is critical!

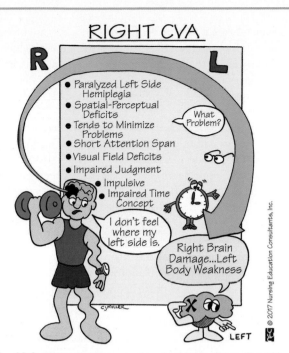

FIG. 16.9 Right Cerebrovascular Accident. (From Zerwekh, J., Garneau, A., & Miller, C. J. [2017]. *Digital collection of the memory notebooks of nursing* [4th ed.]. Nursing Education Consultants.)

1. Evaluate airway, breathing, circulation (ABCs), neurologic assessment, time of symptom onset within 10 minutes, or arrival to emergency department.
   a. FAST assessment (Fig. 16.10).
   b. National Institutes of Health Stroke Scale (NIHSS)—standard tool for assessing neurologic status after an acute stroke.
2. Noncontrast CT scan within 25 minutes of arrival (rule out hemorrhagic stroke).

C. Clinical manifestations.
1. TIA.
   a. Visual defects: blurred vision, diplopia, blindness of one eye, tunnel vision.
   b. Transient hemiparesis, gait problems, ataxia.
   c. Slurred speech; confusion.
   d. Transient numbness of an extremity.
2. Stroke symptoms may occur suddenly with an embolism, more gradually with hemorrhage or thrombosis; manifestations vary according to which cerebral vessels are involved.
   a. Hemiplegia: loss of voluntary movement; damage to the right side of the brain will result in left-sided weakness and paralysis and unilateral body neglect (unaware of paralyzed left side and neglects or ignores it).
   b. Aphasia: defect in using and interpreting the symbols of language; may include written, printed, or spoken words; most common with left brain damage.
   c. May be unaware of the affected side; neglect syndrome ensues.
   d. Cranial nerve impairment: chewing, gag reflex, dysphagia, impaired tongue movement, facial

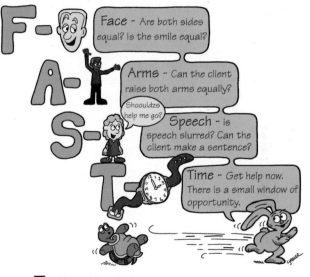

FIG. 16.10 FAST Recognition of Stroke. (From Zerwekh, J., Garneau, A., & Miller, C. J. [2017]. *Digital collection of the memory notebooks of nursing* [4th ed.]. Nursing Education Consultants.)

droop, ptosis, pupillary changes, abnormal eye movements.
   e. May be incontinent initially.
   f. Agnosia: a perceptual defect that causes a disturbance in interpreting sensory information; client may not be able to recognize previously familiar objects.
   g. Cognitive impairment of memory, judgment, proprioception (awareness of one's body position).
   h. Hypotonia (flaccidity) for days to weeks, followed by hypertonia (spasticity).
   i. Visual defects.

    j. Apraxia: can move the affected limb but is unable to carry out learned movements.

    k. Increased ICP; drowsiness to coma.

    l. Gait disturbances.

D. Diagnostics—noncontrast CT scan, MRI, cerebral angiogram, electroencephalogram (EEG) (see Appendix 16.1).

Analyze Cues and Prioritize Hypotheses

The most important problems are inadequate brain tissue perfusion leading to potential increased ICP, decreased mobility, aphasia, dysarthria, altered sensory perception.

Generate Solutions

Treatment

Immediate treatment (differs depending on whether thrombotic or hemorrhagic stroke).

A. Prevent stroke.

    1. Aspirin, platelet inhibitors.

    2. Antihypertensives, anticoagulants if appropriate.

    3. Smoking cessation.

B. Ischemic stroke.

    1. IV recombinant tissue plasminogen activator (tPA) to fibrinolyse clot and reestablish blood flow.

    2. No antiplatelet therapy for 24 to 48 hours following tPA infusion.

C. Hemorrhagic stroke.

    1. Manage blood pressure.

    2. Prepare for surgery—possible craniotomy for aneurysm repair.

    3. Administer nimodipine to reduce risk of arterial spasm from a subarachnoid hemorrhage.

    4. Monitor blood pressure, heart rate, and loss of consciousness (LOC).

D. Surgical interventions.

    1. Carotid endarterectomy or carotid angioplasty and stent placement.

    2. Craniotomy for evacuation of hematoma, aneurysm clipping.

E. Specific therapies to resolve physical, speech, or occupational complications, including use of assistive devices.

Nursing Interventions: Take Action

Goal: To prevent stroke through client education (see Box 16.4).

A. Identification of individuals with reversible risk factors and measures to reduce them.

B. Appropriate medical attention for control of chronic conditions conducive to the development of stroke.

C. Teach high-risk clients early signs of TIA/stroke and to seek medical attention immediately if they occur.

Goal: To maintain patent airway and adequate cerebral oxygenation.

A. Place client in side-lying position with head elevated; keep NPO until swallow evaluation.

B. Assess for symptoms of hypoxia; administer oxygen or assist with endotracheal intubation and mechanical ventilation as necessary.

C. Maintain patent airway; if client unconscious, use oropharyngeal airway to prevent airway obstruction by the tongue.

D. Client is prone to obstructed airway and pulmonary infection; have client cough and deep-breathe every 2 hours.

Goal: To assess for and implement measures to decrease ICP (see nursing goals for increased ICP).

Goal: To maintain adequate nutritional intake.

A. Swallow evaluation prior to initiating oral feedings; dysphagia is common after stroke.

B. Administer oral feedings with caution; check for presence of gag and swallowing reflexes before feeding.

C. Place food on the unaffected side of the mouth.

D. Select foods that are easy to control in the mouth (thick liquids) and easy to swallow; thin liquids often promote coughing because client is unable to control them.

E. Maintain high-Fowler position for feeding.

F. Maintain privacy and unrushed atmosphere.

G. Use assistive devices as necessary (e.g., rocker knife, curved fork, plate guards).

H. If client is unable to tolerate oral intake, enteral feedings may be initiated.

> **TEST ALERT** Identify potential for aspiration; assess client's ability to eat.

Goal: To preserve function of the musculoskeletal system.

A. Passive range of motion (ROM) on affected side; active ROM on unaffected side.

B. Collaborate with physical and occupational therapy to promote best outcomes.

C. Prevent foot drop: passive exercises; high-topped tennis shoes; ambulation as soon as possible.

D. Legs should be maintained in a neutral position; prevent external rotation of affected hip by placing a trochanter roll or rolled pillow at the thigh.

E. Reposition every 2 hours but limit the period of time spent on the affected side.

> **! NURSING PRIORITY** Protect the client's affected side: do not give injections on that side, watch for pressure areas when positioning, have client spend less time on affected side than in other positions.

F. Assess for adduction and internal rotation of the affected arm; maintain arm in a neutral (slightly flexed) position with each joint slightly higher than the preceding one.

G. Restraints should be avoided because they often increase agitation.

H. Maintain joints in position of normal function to prevent flexion contractures.

I. Assist client out of bed on the unaffected side; this allows client to provide some stabilization and balance with the good side (Fig. 16.11).

> **TEST ALERT** Mobility: Assist client to ambulate, perform active and passive ROM exercises, assess for complications of immobility, prevent deep vein thrombosis (DVT), prevent skin breakdown, and encourage independence.

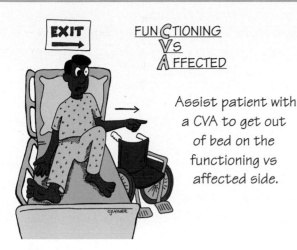

EXIT →

FUNCTIONING
Vs
AFFECTED

Assist patient with a CVA to get out of bed on the functioning vs affected side.

© 2017 Nursing Education Consultants, Inc.

FIG. 16.11 Cerebrovascular Accident—Functioning versus Affected Side. (From Zerwekh, J., Garneau, A., & Miller, C. J. [2017]. *Digital collection of the memory notebooks of nursing* [4th ed.]. Nursing Education Consultants.)

Goal: To maintain homeostasis.

A. Monitor vital signs, cardiac rhythms, and heart and lung sounds.
B. Monitor hydration status.
 1. Assess skin turgor.
 2. Monitor intake and output (I&O) and daily weight.
 3. Assess for the development of peripheral edema.
C. Determine previous bowel patterns and promote normal elimination.
 1. Avoid use of urinary catheter, if possible; if catheter is necessary, remove as soon as possible.
 2. Offer bedpan or urinal every 2 hours; helps establish a schedule.
 3. Allow client to sit upright (bedside commode or toilet) to facilitate passage of stool.
 4. Prevent constipation: provide increased bulk in diet, stool softeners, etc.
 5. Provide privacy and decrease emotional trauma related to incontinence.

TEST ALERT Assess and manage a client with an alteration in elimination. Establish a toileting schedule; the client who has had a stroke will need assistance in reestablishing a normal bowel and bladder routine.

D. Prevent problems of skin breakdown through proper positioning, good skin hygiene, and adequate nutrition.
E. Assist client to identify problems of vision.
F. Maintain psychological homeostasis.
 1. Client may be very anxious because of a lack of understanding of what has happened and the inability to communicate.
 2. Speak slowly and clearly and explain what has happened.
 3. Assess client's communication abilities and identify methods to promote communication.

Home Care

A. Encourage independence in ADLs.
B. Identify clothing that is easy to get in and out of.
C. Active participation in ROM; have client do own ROM on affected side.
D. Physical, occupational, and speech therapy for retraining of lost function.
E. Assist client to maintain sense of balance when in the sitting position; client will frequently fall to the affected side
F. Encourage participation in carrying out daily personal hygiene.
G. Teach client safe transfer from bed to wheelchair and provide assistance as needed (see Fig. 16.11).
H. Bowel and bladder training program.
 1. To promote bladder tone, encourage urination (with or without assistance) every 2 hours rather than allowing the client to void when feeling the urge.
 2. Teach client to perform Kegel exercises regularly.
 3. Advise client to avoid caffeine intake.
 4. Increased bulk in diet will help avoid constipation.
 5. Increase fluids to 2000 mL/day as tolerated.
 6. Administer stool softeners PRN (as needed).
 7. Establish regular daily time for bowel movements.
I. Encourage social interaction.
 1. Speech therapy (see Appendix 16.3).
 2. Frequent and meaningful verbal stimuli.
 3. Allow client plenty of time to respond.
 4. Speak slowly and clearly; do not give too many directions at one time. Use short sentences.
 5. Do not "talk down to" client or treat client as a child (elder speak).
 6. Client's mental status may be normal; do not assume it is impaired.
 7. Nonverbal clients do not lose their hearing ability.
J. Evaluate family support and the need for home health services.

TEST ALERT Assist family to manage care of a client with long-term care needs; determine needs of family regarding ability to provide home care after discharge.

Myasthenia Gravis

Myasthenia gravis (MG) **is a sporadic neuromuscular disease characterized by fatigue and fluctuating muscle weakness. It is most often caused by an autoimmune attack on acetylcholine receptors at the neuromuscular junction. Nerve impulses are not transmitted, and muscles do not contract.**

Assessment: Recognize Cues

A. Risk factors/etiology.
 1. Autoimmune disease.
 2. Tends to affect women at a younger age than men.

B. Clinical manifestations.
  1. Primary problem is fluctuating skeletal muscle weakness and fatigue. Muscular fatigue increases with activity; worse at the end of the day.
    a. Ptosis (drooping of the eyelids) and diplopia (double vision) are frequently the first symptoms.
    b. Impairment of facial mobility and expression.
    c. Impairment of chewing and swallowing.
    d. Speech impairment; voice weakens after long conversations.
    e. No sensory deficit, loss of reflexes, or muscular atrophy.
    f. Poor bowel and bladder control.
  2. Course is variable.
    a. May stabilize, short-term remission, or severe progression.
    b. Exacerbations may occur; precipitated by stress (physical or emotional).
  3. *Myasthenic crisis:* an acute exacerbation of muscle weakness that may require intubation and mechanical ventilation to support respiratory effort.
    a. Severe respiratory distress and hypoxia.
    b. Increased pulse and blood pressure.
    c. Decreased or absent cough or swallow reflex.
  4. *Cholinergic crisis:* a toxic response to the anticholinesterase medications; anticholinesterase medications must be withheld—this response is rare with proper dosing of pyridostigmine.
    a. Nausea, vomiting, and diarrhea.
    b. Weakness with difficulty in swallowing, chewing, and speaking.
    c. Increased secretions and saliva.
    d. Muscle fasciculation; constricted pupils.
C. Diagnostics (see Appendix 16.1).
  1. Electromyography (EMG): shows a decreasing response of muscles to stimuli.
  2. Tensilon test.
    a. Used for diagnosing MG.
    b. Used to differentiate cholinergic crisis from myasthenic crisis.
    c. IV injection of edrophonium causes immediate, although short-lived, relief of muscle weakness.

Analyze Cues and Prioritize Hypotheses

The most important problems are fatigue and skeletal muscle weakness that increases with activity and worsens by the end of the day and potential for inadequate ventilatory process.

Generate Solutions

Treatment
A. Anticholinesterase (cholinergic) medications (see Appendix 16.2).
  1. Neostigmine.
  2. Pyridostigmine.
B. Corticosteroids.
C. Plasma electrophoresis (plasmapheresis): separation of plasma to remove autoantibodies from the bloodstream.
D. Immunosuppressive therapy.
E. Surgical removal of the thymus (thymectomy).

Nursing Interventions: Take Action

Client may be hospitalized for acute myasthenic crisis, cholinergic crisis, or for respiratory tract infection.
Goal: To maintain respiratory function.
A. Assess for increasing problems of difficulty breathing. Measure forced vital capacity frequently to assess respiratory status.
B. Determine client's medication schedule.
C. Assess ability to swallow; prevent problems of aspiration.

> **! NURSING PRIORITY** Identify clients at high risk for aspiration; do not give the client experiencing a myasthenic crisis anything to eat or drink.

D. Evaluate effectiveness of cough reflex.
E. Be prepared to intubate or provide ventilatory assistance.
Goal: To distinguish between a myasthenic crisis and a cholinergic crisis.
A. Maintain adequate ventilatory support during crisis.
B. Assist in administration of Tensilon test to differentiate crisis.
  1. Myasthenic crisis: client's condition will improve.
  2. Cholinergic crisis: client's condition will temporarily worsen.
C. If myasthenic crisis occurs, neostigmine may be administered.
D. If cholinergic crisis occurs, atropine may be administered and cholinergic medications may be reevaluated.
E. Avoid use of sedatives and tranquilizers, which can cause respiratory depression.
F. Provide psychological support during crisis.

Home Care

A. Teach client importance of taking medication on a regular basis; peak effect of the medication should coincide with mealtimes.
B. If ptosis becomes severe, client may need to wear an eye patch to protect cornea (alternate eye patches if problem is bilateral).
C. Emotional upset, severe fatigue, infections, and exposure to extreme temperatures may precipitate a myasthenic crisis.

Multiple Sclerosis

Multiple sclerosis (MS) is characterized by multiple areas of demyelination from inflammatory scarring of the myelin sheath surrounding neurons in the brain and spinal cord (CNS).
A. The progression of the disease results in destruction of the myelin, and the nerve fibers become involved.
  1. Loss of the myelin sheath causes decreased impulse conduction, destruction of the nerve axon, and disruption of the impulse conduction.
  2. Demyelination occurs in irregular scattered patches throughout the CNS.
B. The condition is chronic, with unpredictable remissions and exacerbations.

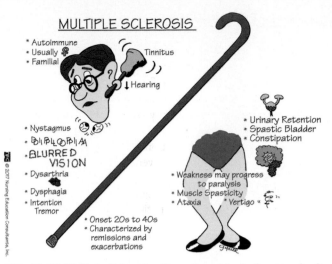

MULTIPLE SCLEROSIS

* Autoimmune
* Usually ♀
* Familial

Tinnitus

↓Hearing

* Nystagmus
* DIPLOPIA
* BLURRED VISION
* Dysarthria
* Dysphagia
* Intention Tremor

* Urinary Retention
* Spastic Bladder
* Constipation

* Weakness may progress to paralysis
* Muscle Spasticity
* Ataxia * Vertigo

* Onset 20s to 40s
* Characterized by remissions and exacerbations

FIG. 16.12 Multiple Sclerosis. (From Zerwekh, J., Garneau, A., & Miller, C. J. [2017]. *Digital collection of the memory notebooks of nursing* [4th ed.]. Nursing Education Consultants.)

Assessment: Recognize Cues

A. Risk factors/etiology: cause is unknown.
   1. More common in women; onset usually 20 to 50 years of age.
   2. More common in cooler climates.
B. Clinical manifestations (Fig. 16.12).
   1. Signs and symptoms vary from person to person, as well as within the same individual, depending on the area of involvement.
   2. Psychosocial.
      a. Intellectual functioning remains intact, but short-term memory, attention, and information processing may become difficult.
      b. Emotional lability: increased excitability and inappropriate euphoria.
      c. Emotional effects of the chronic illness and changes in body image.
C. Diagnostics: no definitive diagnostic test. MRI may show plaques. Elevated IgG levels in CSF.

Analyze Cues and Prioritize Hypotheses

The most important problems are impaired immunity due to autoimmune process and prescribed drug therapy, impaired mobility (muscle spasticity, intention tremors, fatigue), visual and cognitive problems.

Generate Solutions

Treatment

A. No cure; medical treatment is directed toward slowing of the disease process and relief of symptoms.
B. Medications to decrease edema and inflammation of the nerve sites.
   1. Anti-inflammatory agents.
   2. Immunomodulator agents: interferons, fingolimod.
   3. Adrenocorticotropic hormone for acute exacerbations.
   4. Natalizumab, an IV monoclonal antibody.
   5. Glatiramer acetate, a synthetic protein similar to myelin.

Nursing Interventions: Take Action

Client may be hospitalized for diagnostic workup or for treatment of acute exacerbation and complications.

Goal: To maintain homeostasis and prevent complications during an acute exacerbation of disease symptoms.
A. Maintain adequate respiratory function.
   1. Prevent respiratory tract infection.
   2. Good pulmonary hygiene.
   3. Prevent aspiration; sitting position for eating.
   4. Evaluate adequacy of cough reflex.
B. Maintain urinary tract function.
   1. Prevent urinary tract infection.
   2. Increase fluid intake, at least 2000 mL/24 hours.
   3. Evaluate voiding: assess for retention and incontinence.
C. Maintain nutrition.
   1. Evaluate coughing and swallowing reflexes.
   2. Provide food that is easy to chew.
   3. If client is experiencing difficulty swallowing, observe client closely during fluid intake.

Goal: To prevent complications of immobility. (See Chapter 3.)

Goal: To promote psychological well-being.
A. Focus on remaining capabilities.
B. Encourage independence and assist client to gain control over environment.
C. If impotence is a problem, initiate sexual counseling.
D. Assist client to work through the grieving process.
E. Identify community resources available.

Home Care

A. Reinforce teaching about medical regimen and side effects of the medications.
B. Physical therapy to maintain muscle function and decrease spasticity.
C. Measures to maintain voiding; may need to perform self-catheterization.
D. Safety measures because of decreased sensation.
   1. Check bath water temperature.
   2. Wear protective clothing in the winter.
   3. Avoid heating pads and clothing that is constrictive.
E. Client should understand that relapses are frequently associated with an increase in physiologic and psychological stress. Avoid triggers, if possible.

TEST ALERT Determine client's ability to care for self; plan with family to assist client to meet self-care needs.

Guillain-Barré Syndrome

Guillain-Barré syndrome is an acute, rapidly progressing motor neuropathy involving segmental demyelination of nerve roots in the spinal cord and medulla. Demyelination causes inflammation, leading to edema, nerve root compression, decreased nerve conduction, and rapidly ascending paralysis. Both sensory and motor impairment occur.

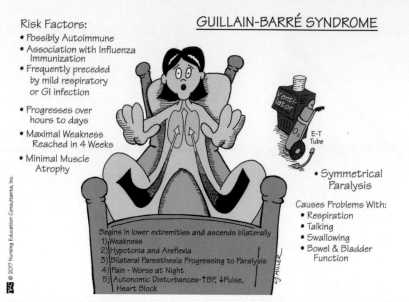

Risk Factors:
- Possibly Autoimmune
- Association with Influenza Immunization
- Frequently preceded by mild respiratory or GI infection
- Progresses over hours to days
- Maximal Weakness Reached in 4 Weeks
- Minimal Muscle Atrophy

GUILLAIN-BARRÉ SYNDROME

- Symmetrical Paralysis

Causes Problems With:
- Respiration
- Talking
- Swallowing
- Bowel & Bladder Function

Begins in lower extremities and ascends bilaterally
1) Weakness
2) Hypotonia and Areflexia
3) Bilateral Paresthesia Progressing to Paralysis
4) Pain - Worse at Night
5) Autonomic Disturbances-↑BP, ↓Pulse, Heart Block

FIG. 16.13 Guillain-Barré Syndrome. (From Zerwekh, J., Garneau, A., & Miller, C. J. [2017]. *Digital collection of the memory notebooks of nursing* [4th ed.]. Nursing Education Consultants.)

Assessment: Recognize Cues

A. Clinical manifestations (Fig. 16.13).
   1. Paresthesias and weakness are often first symptoms.
   2. Progressive weakness and paralysis typically begin in the lower extremities and ascend bilaterally.
   3. Paralysis decreases as the client begins recovery; most often, there are no residual effects.

> **! NURSING PRIORITY** Of the neuromuscular disorders, Guillain-Barré syndrome is the most rapidly developing and progressive condition. It is potentially fatal if unrecognized.

B. Diagnostics (see Appendix 16.1).
   1. Elevated protein concentration in CSF.
   2. EMG and nerve conduction studies.

Analyze Cues and Prioritize Hypotheses

The most important problems are ventilatory failure and diminished gas exchange due to impaired respiratory movements.

Generate Solutions

Treatment (Supportive)
A. Respiratory support, possibly mechanical ventilation.
B. Immunosuppressives and immunoglobulins (IV immunoglobulin G [IVIG]).
C. Plasmapheresis: plasma exchange.

Nursing Interventions: Take Action

Goal: To evaluate progress of paralysis and initiate actions to prevent complications.
A. Evaluate rate of progress of paralysis; carefully *assess changes in respiratory pattern and report to RN.*
B. If ascent of paralysis is rapid, prepare for endotracheal intubation and respiratory assistance.
C. Frequent evaluation of cough and swallow reflexes.

1. Remain with client while client is eating; have suction equipment available.
2. Maintain NPO if gag reflex is impaired.
3. Enteral feedings may be required; gastric emptying is delayed; monitor residual volumes.
D. Prevent complications of immobility during period of paralysis.
E. Assess for involvement of ANS.
   1. Orthostatic hypotension.
   2. Hypertension.
   3. Cardiac dysrhythmias.
   4. Urinary retention and paralytic ileus.

Goal: To prevent complications of hypoxia if respiratory muscles become involved.

Goal: To maintain psychological homeostasis.
A. Simple explanation of procedures.
B. Complete recovery is anticipated.
C. Provide psychological support during period of assisted ventilation.
D. Keep client and family aware of progress of disease.

📋 Amyotrophic Lateral Sclerosis

Amyotrophic lateral sclerosis (ALS), also known as Lou Gehrig disease, is a progressive, invariably fatal degeneration of motor neurons. Causes are unknown, and there is no cure.

Assessment: Recognize Cues

A. Clinical manifestations.
   1. Twitching, cramping, fatigue, and muscle weakness may be early symptoms.
   2. May initially complain of "clumsiness."
   3. Dysarthria and dysphagia.
   4. Muscle spasticity, hyperreflexia, fasciculations.
   5. Muscle weakness progresses until all body is involved. Inability to breathe, speak, swallow.

PARKINSON'S DISEASE

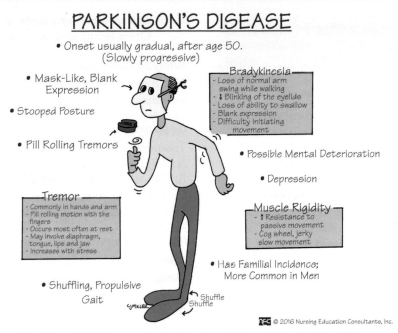

- Onset usually gradual, after age 50.
  (Slowly progressive)

- Mask-Like, Blank Expression
- Stooped Posture
- Pill Rolling Tremors

Bradykinesia
- Loss of normal arm swing while walking
- ↓ Blinking of the eyelids
- Loss of ability to swallow
- Blank expression
- Difficulty initiating movement

- Possible Mental Deterioration
- Depression

Tremor
- Commonly in hands and arm
- Pill rolling motion with the fingers
- Occurs most often at rest
- May involve diaphragm, tongue, lips and jaw
- Increases with stress

Muscle Rigidity
- ↑ Resistance to passive movement
- Cog wheel, jerky slow movement

- Has Familial Incidence; More Common in Men

- Shuffling, Propulsive Gait

Shuffle
Shuffle

© 2016 Nursing Education Consultants, Inc.

FIG. 16.14 Parkinson Disease. (From Zerwekh, J., Garneau, A., & Miller, C. J. [2017]. *Digital collection of the memory notebooks of nursing* [4th ed.]. Nursing Education Consultants.)

6. Intellectual functioning and all five senses are usually unaffected.
7. Death generally from respiratory infection.

B. Diagnostics: EMG, nerve conduction studies, muscle biopsy.

Analyze Cues and Prioritize Hypotheses

The most important problems are progressive muscle weakness and wasting that leads to paralysis, and ultimately the respiratory muscles are affected.

Generate Solutions

Treatment

A. Riluzole slows progression; protects motor neurons from degeneration and death.

B. Supportive care.

Nursing Interventions: Take Action

Goal: To provide ongoing assessment in assisting client to deal with progressive symptoms.

A. Promote independence in ADLs.
   1. Conserve energy; space activities.
   2. Physical, occupational, speech therapy.
   3. Use of support devices to prolong independence in ambulation and ADLs.

B. Promote nutrition.
   1. Small, frequent feedings.
   2. Have client sit upright with head slightly flexed forward while eating.
   3. Keep suction equipment easily available during meals.

C. Encourage family and client to talk about losses and the difficult choices they face.

D. Assist family and client to identify need for advanced directives and to complete them.

E. Palliative/hospice care.

Parkinson Disease

Parkinson disease is a progressive neurodegenerative disorder with gradual onset that causes destruction and degeneration of dopamine-releasing nerve cells in the basal ganglia; results in damage to the extrapyramidal system, causing difficulty controlling or initiating voluntary movement.

Assessment: Recognize Cues

A. Risk factors/etiology.
   1. More common in men.
   2. Exact cause unknown; genetic and environmental factors play a role.

B. Clinical manifestations (Fig. 16.14).

C. Diagnostics: no specific diagnostic test.

Analyze Cues and Prioritize Hypotheses

The most important problems are muscle rigidity, resting tremors, and postural/gait changes that lead to decreased mobility, self-care deficits, and safety concerns.

Generate Solutions

Treatment

A. Medication to enhance dopamine secretion (see Appendix 16.2).
   1. Anticholinergic medications to decrease effects of acetylcholine.
   2. Clients frequently become tolerant to medications and require adjustments in types of medications and medication schedules.

B. Physical/occupational therapy

C. Surgical therapy: aim is to decrease symptoms.
   1. Ablation (destruction of tissue).
   2. Deep brain stimulation (DBS).

2. Ophthalmic ointment and eye patches may be required at night.

E. As function returns, active facial exercises may be performed.

Goal: To assist client to maintain a positive self-image.

A. Changes in physical appearance may be dramatic.

B. Tell client that the condition is usually self-limiting with minimal, if any, residual effects.

C. Client may require counseling if change in facial appearance is permanent.

Seizure Disorders

A *seizure* is a paroxysmal, uncontrolled electrical discharge of neurons in the brain that interrupts normal function. *Epilepsy* is a disease marked by a continuing predisposition to recurrent seizures, with neurobiologic, cognitive, psychological, and social consequences. Incidence is higher in young children and older adults.

Assessment: Recognize Cues

A. Types of seizures (Box 16.5; Fig. 16.15).

B. Clinical manifestations.

Box 16.5   CLASSIFICATION OF SEIZURES

Simple focal seizures (remains conscious throughout seizure)
- Rarely last longer than 1 min.
- Confined to a specific area (hand, arm, leg); client may experience unusual sensations.
- Client may experience unusual feelings (anger, sadness, joy) and/or see, hear, taste, or smell things that are not real.

Complex focal seizures (may have LOC)
- May lose consciousness for 1–3 min.
- May produce automatisms (lip smacking, grimacing, repetitive hand movements).
- Client may be unaware of environment and wonder what is happening at the beginning of the seizure.
- In the period after the seizure, client may experience amnesia and confusion.

Generalized seizures (bilaterally symmetric and without local onset)
- No warning or aura, as client loses consciousness for a few seconds to several minutes.
- Absence (formally called petit mal): Characterized by a short period of time when the client is in an altered level of consciousness. Staring, blinking period (followed by resumption of normal activity) is characteristic. May occur more than 100 times per day; may go unnoticed; in general, onset is in childhood between the ages of 4 and 12 years; rarely continues past adolescence.
- Tonic-clonic seizures: May last 2–5 min. Full recovery may take several hours; client may be confused, amnesic, and irritable during this recovery period.
  - **Tonic phase:** LOC with stiffening and rigidity of muscles. Apnea and cyanosis are common during this period; phase generally lasts for approximately 1 min.
  - **Clonic phase:** Hyperventilation, with rapid jerking movements. Tongue biting, incontinence, and heavy salivation may occur during this period (Fig. 16.11).

---

1. Prodromal phase: sensations or behaviors that precede a seizure.
2. Aural phase: sensory warning that is similar each time a seizure occurs.
3. Ictal phase: first symptoms to end of seizure activity.
4. Postictal phase: recovery period.

C. Complications: status epilepticus (continuous seizure activity)—**a neurologic emergency!** *Any continuous seizure activity should be reported immediately to the RN.*

D. Diagnostics—EEG, CT scan, MRI.

Analyze Cues and Prioritize Hypotheses

The most important problems are prevention of injury and adherence to taking antiepileptic medication regularly.

Generate Solutions

Treatment

A. Antiepileptic medication.

B. Surgery for clients unresponsive to drug therapy.

Nursing Interventions: Take Action

Goal: To protect client from injury (seizure precautions).

A. Monitor client's compliance with taking antiepileptic medications as prescribed.

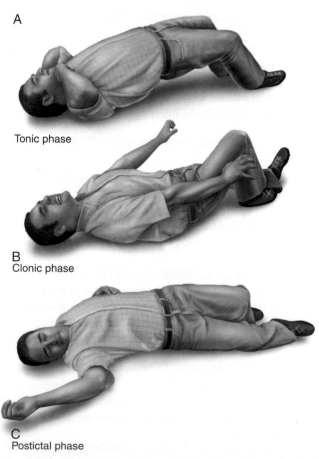

A
Tonic phase

B
Clonic phase

C
Postictal phase

FIG. 16.15 Tonic-Clonic Seizure Activity. (From Black, J. M., & Hawks, J. H. [2000]. *Medical surgical nursing. Clinical management for positive outcomes* [8th ed.]. Saunders.)

B. Make environment safe by removing potentially unsafe objects.

C. Keep suction, bag-valve-mask resuscitator, and airway equipment at bedside.

D. Pad side rails to prevent injury during seizures.

Goal: To assess client during seizure.

A. Identify any activities that occurred immediately before the seizure.

B. Was the client aware a seizure was going to occur? If so, how did client know?

C. Describe types of movements that occurred and the body area affected (e.g., jaw clenched, tongue biting).

D. Presence of incontinence.

E. Period of apnea and cyanosis.

F. Presence of automatisms (lip smacking, grimacing, chewing).

G. Duration of seizure.

H. Changes in level of consciousness.

I. Condition of client after seizure: oriented, level of activity, any residual paralysis or muscle weakness.

> **TEST ALERT** Report characteristics of a client's seizure; assess changes in client's neurologic status.

Goal: To maintain patent airway and protect client during seizure.

A. Remain with the client who is having a seizure; note the time the seizure began and how long it lasted.

B. Turn client to the side to protect airway.

C. Do not attempt to force anything into the client's mouth if the jaws are clenched shut.

D. If the jaws are not clenched, place an airway in the client's mouth. This protects the tongue and also provides a method of suctioning the airway, should the client vomit.

E. Protect the client from injury (risk for falling out of bed or striking self on bedrails, etc.).

F. Loosen any constrictive clothing.

G. Do not restrain client during seizure activity; allow seizure movements to occur but protect client from injury.

H. Evaluate respiratory status; if vomiting occurs, be prepared to suction the client to clear the airway and prevent aspiration.

I. Maintain calm atmosphere and provide for privacy after the seizure activity.

J. Reorient client.

> **! NURSING PRIORITY** Airway management and ventilation cannot be performed on a client who is experiencing a tonic-clonic seizure. After the seizure is over, evaluate the airway and initiate ventilations as necessary.

Home Care

A. Identify activities/events that precipitate the seizure activity.

B. Avoid alcohol intake, fatigue, and loss of sleep.

C. Take medications as directed.

D. Counseling for the family and for the client to assist them in maintaining positive coping mechanisms.

E. Wear medical alert bracelet or have identification card.

Head Injury

Head injury is any injury or trauma to the scalp, skull, or brain. Serious head injuries are called *traumatic brain injury (TBI)*.

A. Classification.

1. Penetrating head injury: dura is pierced, as in stabbing or shooting.

2. Closed head injury: blunt trauma, acceleration (whiplash), or deceleration (collision); most common head injury in civilian life.

3. Children and infants are more capable of absorbing direct impact because of the pliability of the skull.

4. Coup-contrecoup injury: damage to the site of impact (coup) and damage on the side opposite the site of impact (contrecoup) when brain "bounces" freely inside skull (Fig. 16.16).

5. Primary injury to the brain occurs by compression and/or tearing and shearing stresses on vessels and nerves.

6. Secondary injury occurs from cerebral bleeding, hypoxia, hypotension, ischemia, and cerebral edema in response to the primary injury and frequently precipitates an increase in ICP.

B. Types of head injuries.

1. Concussion: most common brain injury; injury (jolt) to brain or body shakes the brain, causing temporary interference in brain function.

   a. Usually from blunt trauma due to contact sports or falls.

   b. May cause brief LOC, headache, sensitivity to light/noise, difficulty concentrating, sleep difficulties, emotional lability.

   c. Generally short term but symptoms may persist for weeks to months: postconcussive syndrome.

2. Contusion (a bruise on the brain).

   a. Multiple areas of petechial hemorrhages.

   b. Headache, pupillary changes, dizziness, unilateral weakness.

   c. Blood supply is altered in the area of injury; swelling, ischemia, and increased ICP.

   d. May last several hours to weeks.

3. Intracranial hemorrhage.

   a. Epidural hematoma: a blood vessel (often a meningeal artery) in the dura mater is damaged; a hematoma rapidly forms between the dura and the skull, precipitating an increase in ICP.

      (1) Momentary LOC, then free of symptoms (lucid period), and then lethargy and coma—seldom evident in children.

      (2) Symptoms of increasing ICP may develop within minutes after the lucid interval.

B. Calcium channel blocker, nimodipine to reduce risk of vasospasm.

C. Anticonvulsants; analgesics for headache

D. Fluids to maintain systolic blood pressure.

E. Stool softeners.

F. May require ventricular drainage for hydrocephalus.

Nursing Interventions: Take Action

Goal: To prevent further increase in ICP and possible rupture.

A. Bed rest; bathroom privileges may be permitted.

B. Constant monitoring of condition to identify occurrence of bleeding or vasospasm as evidenced by symptoms of *increasing ICP or new or changing neurologic deficits and report immediately to RN.*

C. Client should avoid straining, sneezing, pulling up in bed, and acute flexion of the neck.

D. Elevate HOB 30 to 45 degrees to promote venous return.

E. Quiet, darkened, nonstimulating environment: disconnect telephone; limit visitors; promote relaxation.

F. Administer analgesics cautiously; the client should continue to be easily aroused so that neurologic checks can be performed.

G. No hot or cold beverages or food, no caffeine, no smoking.

H. DVT prophylaxis.

I. Maintain seizure precautions.

> **⚠ NURSING PRIORITY** If the client survives the rupture of the aneurysm and rebleeding occurs, it is most likely to occur within the next 24 to 48 hours.

Goal: To assess for and implement nursing measures to decrease ICP (see nursing goals for increased ICP).

Goal: To provide appropriate preoperative nursing interventions (see nursing goals for brain tumor).

Goal: To maintain homeostasis and monitor changes in ICP after craniotomy.

📋 Spinal Cord Injury

Spinal cord injury (SCI) is damage to the spinal cord housed inside the spinal column and is generally a result of trauma. The degree of injury is classified as complete, resulting in loss of both sensory and motor function below the level of injury, or incomplete, with some sensation or motor function below the level of injury.

A. Risk factors.
   1. Young, adult men are at highest risk.
   2. Also an increased risk in older adults, when falls become more common.
   3. Most common causes include motor vehicle crashes, falls, violence, and sports injuries.

B. Initially after the injury, the nerve fibers swell and circulation to the spinal cord is decreased; hemorrhage and edema occur, causing an increase in the ischemic process,

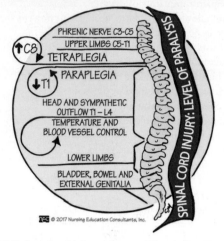

FIG. 16.17 Spinal Cord Injury: Areas of Paralysis. (From Zerwekh, J., Garneau, A., & Miller, C. J. [2017]. *Digital collection of the memory notebooks of nursing* [4th ed.]. Nursing Education Consultants.)

which progresses to necrotic destruction of the spinal cord.

C. Consequences of SCI depend on the extent of damage, as well as the level of cord injury (Fig. 16.17).
   1. The higher the lesion, the more severe the sequelae.
      a. Clients with lesions at C or higher require ventilatory support.
      b. Lesions between T1 and T8 often allow use of the hands.
      c. Lesions below T8 often allow upper body control.
   2. Complete transection (complete cord dissolution, complete lesion): immediate loss of all sensation and voluntary movement below the level of injury; minimal, if any, return of function.
   3. Cord edema peaks in approximately 2 to 3 days and subsides within approximately 7 days after the injury.
   4. Spinal shock: decreased reflexes, loss of sensation, flaccid paralysis below level of injury. Resolves in days to weeks; return of reflexes and development of spasticity.
   5. Neurogenic shock: disruption of sympathetic nervous system causes hypotension due to peripheral vasodilation and bradycardia. Hypothermia can occur due to vasodilation. Most common in cervical and high thoracic injury (T6 and above).
   6. Autonomic dysreflexia can occur in clients with an injury at T6 or higher following resolution of spinal shock.
      a. A noxious stimulus below the level of injury triggers the sympathetic nervous system, which causes a release of catecholamines (epinephrine, norepinephrine).
      b. Most common stimuli causing the response are a full bladder or bowel, urinary tract infection, pressure ulcers, and skin stimulation.

    c. Severe hypertension (systolic may be greater than 300), nausea, pounding headache, bradycardia, restlessness, piloerection, flushing and sweating above the level of injury, and blurred vision are the most common body responses.

7. Bladder dysfunction will occur as a result of the injury; normal bladder control is dependent on the sensory and motor pathways and the lower motor neurons being intact.

8. Long-term rehabilitation potential depends on the amount of damage done to the cord, which may not be evident until several weeks after the injury.

Assessment: Recognize Cues

A. Clinical manifestations: depend on level of SCI (see Fig. 16.17).
1. Cervical injury, especially at C5 and above, will cause respiratory compromise.
2. Depending on degree of injury, the degree of paralysis and amount of sensory loss below the level of injury will vary.
3. Monitor for spinal shock and neurogenic shock.

B. Diagnostics—CT scan, MRI (see Appendix 16.1).

C. Complications.
1. Respiratory stasis; pulmonary edema and emboli.
2. Cardiovascular compromise from neurogenic shock; autonomic dysreflexia.
3. Skin breakdown resulting in localized and systemic infections.
4. Immobility issues causing renal and GI compromise.
5. Psychological, social, and body image issues.

Analyze Cues and Prioritize Hypotheses

The most important problems are potential for respiratory distress or failure, cardiovascular instability, decreased mobility and sensory perception due to spinal cord damage and edema.

Generate Solutions

Treatment

A. Emergency intervention required; manage airway, breathing, and circulation.

B. Immobilization of the vertebral column in cervical fracture.
1. Cervical tongs (Crutchfield, Gardner-Wells) for cervical immobility.
2. Halo vest/jacket traction to promote mobility.
3. Sterno-occipital mandibular immobilizer (SOMI) brace worn with cervical fusion.

C. Spinal surgery to decompress spinal cord and stabilize spine.

D. Respiratory support as necessary.

Nursing Interventions: Take Action

Goal: To maintain stability of the vertebral column and prevent further cord damage.

A. Emergency care and treatment.

1. Suspect SCI if there is any evidence of direct trauma to the head or neck area (contact sports, diving accidents, motor vehicle accidents).
2. Immobilize client and institute spinal precautions; maintain body alignment and do not allow the neck to flex.
3. Airway, status of breathing, and circulation are the primary concerns initially after injury.
4. Neurogenic shock may occur within the first 24 hours; observe for decreased blood pressure, severe bradycardia.

> **! NURSING PRIORITY** Do not hyperextend the neck in a client with a suspected cervical injury. Airway should be opened by the jaw-lift method. Improper handling of the client often results in extension of the damaged area.

5. Maintain cervical spinal precautions and body alignment; do not remove cervical collar or spinal board until area of injury is identified.
6. Maintain patent airway at all times.

B. Maintain stability of the vertebral column as indicated by the level of injury.
1. Prescribe and maintain bed rest on firm mattress with supportive devices (sandbags, skin traction, etc.); maintain alignment in the supine position; logroll without any flexion or twisting.
2. Maintain cervical traction: tongs are inserted into the skull with traction and weights applied; do not remove weights; to turn: logroll, specialty bed, or turning frame to maintain spinal alignment.
3. Halo vest/jacket traction: maintains cervical immobility but allows client to be mobile.
    a. If bolts or screws come loose, keep the client immobilized and call the health care provider.
    b. Clean pin sites according to facility policy; observe for infection.
    c. Monitor skin under vest and provide skin care.
    d. Roll client onto side at the edge of the bed and allow client to push up from the mattress to a sitting position. *Never* use the halo vest frame to assist the client to turn or sit up.
    e. Correct size of wrench should be kept at bedside to remove the anterior bolts in case of emergency.
    f. Assist client to maintain balance when standing; the traction is heavy for a person who is weak and the client is at increased risk for falling.
4. Maintain extremities in neutral, functional position.

> **TEST ALERT** Apply, maintain, or remove orthopedic devices (e.g., traction, splints, braces, casts).

Goal: To identify level of damage and changes in neurologic status.

A. Assess respiratory function: symmetric chest expansion, bilateral breath sounds, presence of retractions, or dyspnea.

B. Motor and sensory evaluation.

1. Ability to move extremities; strength of extremities.
2. Sensory examination, including touch and pain.
3. Presence of deep tendon reflexes.
C. Ongoing assessment and status of:
   1. Bladder, gastric, bowel function.
   2. Psychological adjustment to the injury.
D. Evaluate history of how injury occurred; obtain information regarding how client was transported.
E. Determine status of pain.

Goal: To maintain respiratory function.
A. Frequent assessment of respiratory function during the first 48 hours.
   1. Determine development of hypoxia.
   2. Auscultate breath sounds.
   3. Observe breathing pattern for use of sternocleidomastoid and intercostal muscles for respiration.
   4. Evaluate ABG values and pulse oximetry.
B. Maintain adequate respiratory function, as indicated.
   1. Chest physiotherapy.
   2. Incentive spirometry.
   3. Changing position within limits of injury.
   4. Assess for complications of atelectasis, pulmonary emboli, and pneumonia.
   5. Nasopharyngeal or endotracheal suctioning based on airway and level of injury.

Goal: To maintain cardiovascular stability.
A. Assess for spinal shock.
   1. Monitor vital signs and evaluate changes.
   2. Vagal stimulation, hypothermia, and hypoxia may precipitate spinal shock.
   3. Assess deep tendon reflexes and muscle strength as resolution of shock occurs.
B. Assess for neurogenic shock.
   1. Monitor blood pressure, heart rate.
   2. May require fluids to increase blood pressure; atropine to increase heart rate.
   3. Monitor body temperature and maintain normothermia.
   4. Apply antiembolism stockings or elastic wraps to the legs to facilitate venous return. (Lack of muscle tone and loss of sympathetic tone in the peripheral vessels result in decreases in both venous tone and venous return, which predispose client to DVT.)
C. Assess for development of autonomic dysreflexia if it occurs:
   1. Elevate HOB and check the client's blood pressure.
   2. Assess for sources of stimuli: distended bladder (check urinary tubing), fecal impaction, constipation, tight clothing.
   3. Relieve the stimuli and dysreflexia will subside.
   4. Maintain cardiovascular support during period of hypertension.
   5. A hypertensive crisis from dysreflexia will require immediate intervention.
D. Evaluate cardiovascular responses when turning or suctioning client.

Goal: To maintain adequate fluid and nutritional status.
A. During the first 48 hours, evaluate GI function frequently; decrease in function may necessitate use of a nasogastric tube to decrease distention.
B. Prevent complications of nausea and vomiting.
C. Evaluate bowel sounds and client's ability to tolerate oral fluids.
D. Increase protein and calories in diet; may need to decrease calcium intake.
E. Evaluate for presence of paralytic ileus.
F. Increase fiber in diet to promote bowel function.

Goal: To prevent complications of immobility.

Goal: To promote bowel and bladder function.
A. Urine is retained as a result of the loss of autonomic and reflexive control of the bladder.
   1. Intermittent catheterization or indwelling catheter may be used initially to prevent bladder distention.
   2. Perform nursing interventions to prevent urinary tract infection; avoid urinary catheterization, if possible.
B. Determine type of bladder dysfunction based on level of injury.
C. Assess client's awareness of bladder function.
D. Initiate measures to institute bladder control.
   1. Establish a schedule for voiding; have client attempt to void every 2 hours.
   2. Use the Credé method (pressure applied over symphysis pubis) in adults for manual expression of urine.
   3. May be necessary to teach client self-catheterization.
   4. Record output and evaluate for presence of residual urine.
E. Evaluate bowel functioning.
   1. Incontinence and paralytic ileus frequently occur with spinal shock.
   2. Incontinence and impaction are common later.
F. Initiate measures to promote bowel control (after spinal shock is resolved).
   1. Identify client's bowel habits before injury.
   2. Maintain sufficient fluid intake and adequate bulk in the diet.
   3. Establish specific time each day for bowel evacuation.
   4. Assess client's awareness of need to defecate.
   5. Teach client effective use of the Valsalva maneuver to induce defecation.
   6. Induce defecation by digital stimulation, suppository, or, as a last resort, enema.

Goal: To maintain psychological equilibrium.
A. Provide simple explanations of all procedures.
B. Anticipate outbursts of anger and hostility as client begins to work through the grieving process and adjusts to changes in body image.
C. Anticipate and accept periods of depression in client.
D. Encourage independence whenever possible; allow client to participate in decisions regarding care and to gain control over environment.

E. Encourage family involvement in identifying appropriate diversional activities.

F. Avoid sympathy and emphasize client's potential.

G. Initiate frank, open discussion regarding sexual functioning.

H. Assist client and family to identify community resources.

I. Assist client to set realistic short-term goals.

Appendix 16.1 NEUROLOGIC SYSTEM DIAGNOSTICS

Skull and Spine X-ray Studies

Simple x-ray films are obtained to determine fractures, calcifications, etc.

Electroencephalography (EEG)

A graphic recording of the electrical activity of the brain to assess cerebral activity; useful for diagnosing seizure disorders; used as a screening procedure for coma; also serves as an indicator for brain death. May also be used to assess sleep disorders, metabolic disorders, and encephalitis.

Nursing Implications

1. Explain to client that procedure is painless and there is no danger of electrical shock.
2. Determine from health care provider if any medications should be withheld before test, especially tranquilizers and sedatives.
3. Caffeinated foods, beverages, or other stimulants may be prohibited before examination.
4. Client's hair should be clean before the examination; after the examination, assist client to wash electrode paste out of hair.

Carotid Doppler Ultrasonography

A noninvasive ultrasound scan to estimate blood flow in carotid and cerebral vessels to assess for stenosis. No preparation is necessary.

Magnetic Resonance Imaging (MRI)

Uses magnetic energy to align hydrogen molecules in the body and create detailed images of body tissues including brain, spinal cord, and spinal column.

Nursing Implications

1. Procedure will take approximately 1 hour; client must lie still during that time.
2. All metal objects should be removed from the client (dental bridges, hearing aids, hair clips, jewelry, buckles, medicine patches with foil backing).
3. Screen for implanted medical devices; may not be MRI compatible.
4. Contrast medium may be used: assess for allergy to shellfish, iodine, or contrast dye. Ensure adequate hydration.
5. Poor candidates for MRI include the following:
   a. Clients who are confused, hemodynamically unstable, or require life-supporting equipment.
   b. Clients with implanted medical devices, pins, clips, or joint replacements.
   c. Pregnant clients: if required can be done; preferably after first trimester.
   d. Obese clients: may not fit in scanner.

Computerized Axial Tomography (CAT)/ Computed Tomography (CT) Scan

Computer-assisted x-ray examination of thin cross-sections of the brain to identify hemorrhage, tumor, edema, infarctions, and hydrocephalus. Machine is large, donut-shaped tube with table through the middle.

Nursing Implications

1. Explain appearance of scanner to client and explain importance of remaining absolutely still during the procedure.
2. Remove all objects from client's hair; for 4 to 6 hours before test, client receives fluids only.
3. Dye may be injected via venipuncture; assess for iodine allergy and advise the client that they may experience a flushing or warm sensation when the dye is injected.
4. Contrast dye may discolor urine for about 24 hours.
5. Dye may be injected into spinal cord for assessment of intervertebral disks and bone density.

Brain Scan

A scanner traces the uptake of radioactive dye in the brain tissue. The dye is concentrated in the damaged tissue; it will take approximately 2 hours after dye is injected for the scan to be completed.

Nursing Implications

1. Determine whether medications need to be withheld before procedure.
2. Client will be asked to change positions during the test to visualize the brain from different angles.
3. The client should not experience any pain.

Caloric Testing

Test is performed at bedside by introducing cold or warm water (or air) into the external auditory canal. It is contraindicated in the client with a ruptured tympanic membrane and is not done on the client who is awake. If cranial nerve VIII is stimulated, nystagmus rotates toward the irrigated ear. If no nystagmus occurs, a pathologic condition is present.

Lumbar Puncture

A needle is inserted into the lumbar area at the L3–L4 or L4–L5 level (in subarachnoid space); spinal pressure is measured and spinal fluid withdrawn; contraindicated in presence of increased ICP. Normal spinal fluid values: opening pressure, 60 to 150 mm water; specific gravity, 1.007; pH, 7.35; clear/colorless fluid; protein concentration, 15 to 45 mg/dL (0.15–0.45 g/L); glucose concentration, 45 to 75 mg/dL (2.5–4.2 mmol/L); no microorganisms present; no blood.

Continued

Appendix 16.2   MEDICATIONS—cont'd

℞

Antiparkinsonism Agents

MEDICATIONS	SIDE EFFECTS	NURSING IMPLICATIONS
Dopamine Replacements: Assist to restore normal transmission of nerve impulses.		
Levodopa: PO (rarely used alone) Carbidopa/levodopa: PO	*Early:* Anorexia, nausea and vomiting, abdominal discomfort, orthostatic hypotension *Long-term:* Abnormal, involuntary movements, especially involving the face, mouth, and neck; behavioral disturbances involving confusion, agitation, and euphoria	1. Administer PO preparations with meals to decrease GI distress. (High-protein meals reduce levodopa absorption.) 2. Almost all clients will experience some side effects, which are dose related; dosage gradually increased according to client's tolerance and response. 3. Dose is titrated to achieve optimal effect. 4. Teach the client to not stop taking the medication abruptly.
Dopamine Agonists: Mimic dopamine by blocking dopamine receptors.		
Apomorphine: subQ Bromocriptine: PO Pramipexole: PO Ropinirole: PO Apomorphine Rotigotine: transdermal patch	Orthostatic hypotension, constipation, dry mouth, drowsiness, chest pain, peripheral edema, sleep disorders	1. Dose is adjusted gradually. 2. Teach client to move from sitting to standing position slowly. 3. Can cause compulsive behavior (gambling, binge eating, sexual urges).
Antiviral Agent (Dopamine Releaser): Promotes release of dopamine; may help reduce levodopa-induced dyskinesias.		
Amantadine hydrochloride: PO	Orthostatic hypotension, dyspnea, dizziness, drowsiness, blurred vision, constipation, urinary retention (side effects are dose related)	1. Less effective than levodopa; produces a more rapid clinical response.

CNS, Central nervous system; *GI,* gastrointestinal; *GU,* genitourinary; *IM,* intramuscular; *IV,* intravenous; *PO,* by mouth (orally); *subQ,* subcutaneous.

Appendix 16.3   APHASIA

℞

Aphasia is the inability to comprehend or use language. Aphasia may be receptive, expressive, or global. Dysphasia is a term also used to describe impaired communication. Approximately 90% of people are left-brain dominant; the left side of the brain controls communication. That is why, for most people, damage to the left side of the brain from stroke or injury causes aphasia. Clients with aphasia are often frustrated and irritable. Emotional lability is common. Accept the behavior in a manner that prevents embarrassment for the client.

TYPES OF APHASIA	NURSING IMPLICATIONS
Wernicke (fluent or receptive aphasia; left temporal lobe damage): Cannot understand oral or written communication. Client cannot interpret or comprehend speech or read. May be able to talk but the language is meaningless. *Broca (expressive aphasia, left frontal lobe damage):* Inability to speak or to write. However, the client can comprehend incoming speech and can read and is aware of the deficit and may become frustrated and angry. *Mixed:* Most aphasia involves both the sensory and motor aspects of speech. Rarely is aphasia only sensory or only motor. *Global aphasia:* All communication and receptive function is lost. *Dysarthria:* A disturbance in the muscular control of speech. Does not affect the meaning of communication or comprehension, just the mechanics of speech—pronunciation, articulation, and phonation.	1. Stand in front of the client; speak clearly and slowly. 2. Do not shout or speak loudly; the client can hear. 3. Be patient; give the client time to respond; do not press the client for immediate answers. 4. Use nonverbal communications such as touch, smiles, and gestures. 5. Assist the client with motor aphasia to practice repeating simple words such as *yes, no,* and *please.* 6. Listen carefully, try to understand, and try to communicate; this conveys to the client that you care. 7. Involve family members in practice and assist them to identify ways they can support the client.

TEST ALERT Assist client to communicate effectively.

⚡ Practice & Next Generation NCLEX (NGN) Questions

Neurology: Care of Adult Clients

More questions on
ⓔvolve

1. The nurse is caring for a client who is in the recovery room following a craniotomy. What nursing assessment data would be **most** important for the nurse to report?
   1. A pulse rate decrease from 90 to 70 beats/min.
   2. A decrease in blood pressure from 140/90 to 120/80.
   3. Orientation change from alert and oriented to lethargic and confused.
   4. Decrease in bilateral breath sounds at the base of the lungs.

2. A client is experiencing signs and symptoms of increased intracranial pressure (ICP). Which response would be a characteristic change in the client's pupils with increased ICP?
   1. Reactive to light and pinpoint.
   2. Dilated and reactive to light.
   3. One is larger than the other.
   4. Fixed and pinpoint.

3. A client is experiencing autonomic dysreflexia. What is the **first** nursing action for this client?
   1. Change the urinary catheter.
   2. Sit the client up in bed.
   3. Check for fecal impaction.
   4. Administer dopamine.

4. A client has a tonic-clonic (formerly grand mal) seizure. What nursing action is the **highest** priority?
   1. Loosen or remove constricting clothing and protect the client from injuring themself.
   2. Maintain a patent airway by turning the client on the side and suctioning, if necessary.
   3. Remain with the client and administer anticonvulsant medications as ordered by the health care provider.
   4. Describe and record events before the onset of the seizure, during the seizure, and after the seizure.

5. The nurse is assessing a newly diagnosed client with myasthenia gravis. Which assessment finding would the nurse identify as characteristic of the condition?
   1. Tremor.
   2. Neuromuscular rigidity.
   3. Ptosis.
   4. Paresthesia of the lower extremities.

Questions 6 to 11 relate to the following case study.

6. A client is admitted to the emergency department. The client has a history of type 2 diabetes, hypertension, and breast cancer, which was treated with chemotherapy and radiation therapy 10 years ago following a left radical mastectomy. **Highlight the assessment findings that require follow-up by the nurse.**

Health History	Nurses' Notes	Provider Orders	Laboratory Results

1300 : A 57-year-old client appears weak and has slurred speech while answering questions. The client has some facial drooping and significant swelling and difficulty in raising the left arm.

- Temperature: 98°F (37°C)
- BP: 148/98 mm Hg
- Heart rate: 76 bpm and regular
- Respirations: 20 breaths/min
- SpO2: 95% on room air

LABORATORY

TEST	RESULT	REFERENCE RANGE
Glucose	62 mg/dL	70–100 mg/dL
A1c	6.9%	Less than 5.7% (normal) Less than 7% (client with diabetes)

7. The nurse is planning the care for the client in the scenario in question 11.

   For each client finding, use an X to specify whether the finding is consistent with the disease process of transient ischemic attack (TIA) or stroke. Each finding may support more than one disease process.

CLIENT FINDING	TIA	STROKE
Slurred speech		
Double vision		
Sudden weakness in the extremity		
Symptoms resolve within 1–24 hours		
No residual deficit remains after 24 hours		
Facial drooping		
Headache		

---

8. The following is an updated nurses' note.

Health History	Nurses' Notes	Provider Orders	Laboratory Results

1300 : A 57-year-old client appears weak and has slurred speech while answering questions. The client has some facial drooping and significant swelling and difficulty in raising the left arm.

- Temperature: 98°F (37°C)
- BP: 148/98 mm Hg
- Heart rate: 76 bpm and regular
- Respirations: 20 breaths/min
- SpO2: 95% on 4L/min of oxygen via nasal cannula

1310 : IV therapy initiated.

1330 : Client returns from noncontrast CT scan and is increasingly more restless.

- Temperature: 98°F (37°C)
- BP: 188/80 mm Hg
- Heart rate: 56 bpm, full and bounding pulse
- Respirations: 30 breaths/min, irregular
- SpO2: 93% on 4L/min of oxygen via nasal cannula

1335 : IRecombinant tissue plasminogen activator is administered.

Complete the following sentences by choosing the most likely options for the missing information from the lists of options provided.

The client is experiencing signs of _____1_____ as evidenced by _____2_____, _____2_____, _____2_____, and _____2_____.

OPTIONS FOR 1	OPTIONS FOR 2
Stroke	Increasing BP
Hemorrhage	Decreased respirations
Hydrocephalus	Bradycardia
Increased IOP	Widening pulse pressure
Transient ischemic attack	Increased pulse deficit
Shock	Rapid, irregular respirations

9. The client is admitted to the neurologic unit.

Use an X to identify the nursing actions listed below that are Indicated (appropriate or necessary), Contraindicated (could be harmful), or Non-Essential (makes no difference or not necessary) for the client's care at this time.

NURSING ACTION	INDICATED	CONTRAINDICATED	NON-ESSENTIAL
Place in Trendelenburg position			
Rotate client's head to the right			
Reduce stimuli in the room; low room lights			
Continuous pulse oximeter monitoring			
Encourage Valsalva maneuver			
Elevate HOB 20–30 degrees			
Frequent neuro checks			
Push fluids			
Monitor for seizure activity			
Determine favorite foods			

10. Two days later the client has stabilized, following the prescribed treatment. The vital signs have returned to normal. Indications of increased intracranial pressure have resolved. The client has slowly begun to eat and is having difficulty with swallowing and chewing food. What are nursing interventions to address the client's dysphagia? **Select all that apply**.
    1. Reinforce the information from the speech therapist to improve the client's swallowing.
    2. Place client in low Fowler position for meals and taking oral medication.
    3. Make sure the client tilts the head and neck backward when trying to swallow.
    4. Have client swallow a small sip of water before eating or taking an oral medication.
    5. Allow client to choose soft foods that are easily swallowed.
    6. Encourage ingesting foods of a different texture at the same time.
    7. Instruct the client to take small bites of food.
    8. Inspect mouth for food trapped in cheek pockets

11. The client is being discharged and the nurse is evaluating the current assessment findings to determine what client outcomes have improved.

    For each body system/function, select the current assessment finding that indicates the client's conditions have improved. More than one client finding may be selected for each body system/function. Each category must have at least one response.

BODY SYSTEM/ FUNCTION	CURRENT ASSESSMENT FINDING
Neurologic	☐ Alert and oriented × 3 ☐ PERRLA
Endocrine	☐ FBS 99 mg/dL ☐ A1c 7.2%
Cardiovascular	☐ BP 142/88 ☐ Pulse 78 beats/min, regular
Gastrointestinal	☐ Choking and coughing when taking oral medication ☐ Swallows a sip of water without difficulty

⚡ Answers to Practice & Next Generation NCLEX (NGN) Questions

1. 3
Client Needs: Physiological Integrity/Physiological Adaptation
Clinical Judgment/Cognitive Skill: Prioritize Hypotheses
Item Type: Multiple Choice
Rationale & Test Taking Strategy: Note the **key** word, "most," important assessment data to report following a craniotomy. The first sign of increased intracranial pressure is a change in level of consciousness. *This should be reported to the registered nurse or health care provider.* The change in blood pressure and pulse rate should be monitored, but they are not indicative of significant problems. With a decrease in breath sounds, the client's lungs should be auscultated and oxygen therapy delivered as prescribed.

2. 3
Client Needs: Physiological Integrity/Physiological Adaptation
Clinical Judgment/Cognitive Skill: Recognize Cues
Item Type: Multiple Choice
Rationale & Test Taking Strategy: With increased ICP, one pupil may be larger and have a decreased or sluggish reaction as compared to the other pupil. The dilation frequently occurs ipsilaterally, or on the same side as the lesion. As increased ICP becomes more severe, there is pressure on the optic nerve and both pupils will dilate with no reaction to direct light stimulus. Certain medications and illicit drug substances may cause pinpoint or dilated pupils.

3. 2
Client Needs: Physiological Integrity/Physiological Adaptation
Clinical Judgment/Cognitive Skill: Take Action
Item Type: Multiple Choice
Rationale & Test Taking Strategy: Note the **key** word, "first" action when a client experiences autonomic dysreflexia. The priority is to have the client sit upright, which is the easiest and quickest nursing action to take that will assist with lowering blood pressure. Often, blockage of a urinary catheter, urinary tract infection, or a full bladder or bowel distention can precipitate autonomic dysreflexia, along with tight clothing around the chest, abdomen, or an extremity; pain or contact with a hard or sharp object; and environmental temperature changes. Dopamine is an inotropic agent used to treat severe hypotension, so it would not be indicated because the client is experiencing severe hypertension during an autonomic dysreflexia episode.

4. 2
Client Needs: Physiological Integrity/Physiological Adaptation
Clinical Judgment/Cognitive Skill: Prioritize Hypotheses
Item Type: Multiple Choice
Rationale & Test Taking Strategy: Note the **key** word, "highest priority" nursing action during a tonic-clonic seizure. The priority after a tonic-clonic seizure is to maintain a patent airway. The question is asking for a nursing intervention after the seizure is over. Clothing should be loosened when the seizure begins. Medications can be given later and charting can also be done at a later time. The nurse needs to remain with the client, and the events of the seizure need to be recorded, but the priority of this question is the airway.

5. 3
Client Needs: Physiological Integrity/Physiological Adaptation
Clinical Judgment/Cognitive Skill: Recognize Cues
Item Type: Multiple Choice

Rationale & Test Taking Strategy: The primary problem of myasthenia gravis is skeletal muscle fatigue with sustained muscle contraction; symptoms are predominantly bilateral. Other signs, which are frequently the first symptoms, include ptosis (drooping of the eyelids) and diplopia (double vision). Fatigue increases with activity. Impairment of facial mobility and expression, difficulty chewing and swallowing, speech impairment (dysarthria), and poor bowel and bladder control also occur. There is no paresthesia of the lower extremities. Tremor and neuromuscular rigidity are seen often in Parkinson disease.

Questions 6-11 relate to the following unfolding case scenario.

6. A client is admitted to the emergency department. The client has a history of type 2 diabetes, hypertension, and breast cancer, which was treated with chemotherapy and radiation therapy 10 years ago following a left radical mastectomy. **Highlight the assessment findings that require follow-up by the nurse.**

Health History	Nurses' Notes	Provider Orders	Laboratory Results

1300 : A 57-year-old client appears weak and has slurred speech while answering questions. The client has some facial drooping and significant swelling and difficulty in raising the left arm.

- Temperature: 98°F (37°C)
- BP: 148/98 mm Hg
- Heart rate: 76 bpm and regular
- Respirations: 20 breaths/min
- SpO2: 95% on room air

LABORATORY
TEST	RESULT	REFERENCE RANGE
Glucose	62 mg/dL (8.0 mmol/L) L	70–100 mg/dL (3.9–5.6 mmol/L)
A1c	6.9%	Less than 5.7% (normal) Less than 7% (client with diabetes)

Client Needs: Physiological Integrity/Physiological Adaptation
Clinical Judgment/Cognitive Skill: Recognize Cues
Item type: Highlight in Text
Rationale & Test Taking Strategy: The nurse needs to follow up on the client's symptoms of slurred speech, facial drooping, and left arm weakness, which may indicate a stroke or transient ischemic attack (TIA). The elevated blood pressure could be an underlying issue causing the symptoms. The blood sugar is low and needs monitoring because the client is a type 2 diabetic and hypoglycemia symptoms can be like a stroke or TIA (i.e., weakness, confusion, headache, dizziness, loss of balance or coordination). The left arm swelling (lymphedema) is probably from the mastectomy. The weakness or difficulty raising the arm could be due to the left mastectomy and it could also be a symptom of a stroke or TIA.

7. The nurse is planning the care for the client in the scenario in question 11.

For each client finding, use an X to specify whether the finding is consistent with the disease process of TIA or stroke. Each finding may support more than one disease process.

CLIENT FINDING	TIA	STROKE
Slurred speech	X	X
Double vision	X	X
Sudden weakness in the extremity	X	X
Symptoms resolve within 1–24 hours	X	
No residual deficit remains after 24 hours	X	
Facial drooping	X	X
Headache	X	X

Client Needs: Physiological Integrity/Physiological Adaptation
Clinical Judgment/Cognitive Skill: Analyze Cues
Item type: Matrix Multiple Response
Rationale & Test Taking Strategy: The client who has a TIA experiences temporary neurologic dysfunction due to a brief interruption in cerebral blood flow. The symptoms of TIA are like a stroke; however, symptoms of a TIA resolve within 30 to 60 minutes and may last as long as 24 hours without residual deficit. A client with a stroke and a TIA typically has these five common symptoms that occur suddenly: (1) confusion or trouble speaking or understanding others; (2) numbness or weakness of the face, arm, or leg; (3) trouble seeing in one or both eyes; (4) dizziness, trouble walking, or loss of balance or coordination; and (5) severe headache with no known cause.

8. The following is an updated nurses' note.

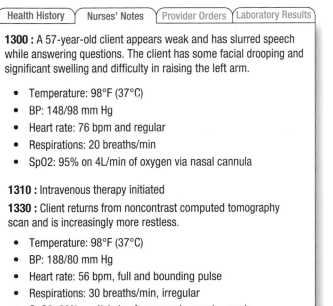

| Health History | Nurses' Notes | Provider Orders | Laboratory Results |

1300 : A 57-year-old client appears weak and has slurred speech while answering questions. The client has some facial drooping and significant swelling and difficulty in raising the left arm.

- Temperature: 98°F (37°C)
- BP: 148/98 mm Hg
- Heart rate: 76 bpm and regular
- Respirations: 20 breaths/min
- SpO2: 95% on 4L/min of oxygen via nasal cannula

1310 : Intravenous therapy initiated

1330 : Client returns from noncontrast computed tomography scan and is increasingly more restless.

- Temperature: 98°F (37°C)
- BP: 188/80 mm Hg
- Heart rate: 56 bpm, full and bounding pulse
- Respirations: 30 breaths/min, irregular
- SpO2: 93% on 4L/min of oxygen via nasal cannula

1335 : Recombinant tissue plasminogen activator is administered.

Complete the following sentences by choosing the most likely options for the missing information from the drop-down lists of options provided.
The client is experiencing signs of *increased intracranial pressure* as evidenced by *increasing blood pressure, widening pulse pressure, bradycardia,* and *rapid, irregular respirations.*

Client Needs: Physiological Integrity/Physiological Adaptation
Clinical Judgment/Cognitive Skill: Prioritize Hypotheses
Item type: Drop-Down Rationale
Rationale & Test Taking Strategy: The client is most at risk for the complication of increased intracranial pressure (ICP) resulting from edema during the first 72 hours after the onset of the stroke. Increased ICP is evidenced by Cushing triad, which is a rising systolic blood pressure, widening pulse pressure (systolic and diastolic readings are further apart), and bradycardia. Other signs are rapid, irregular respirations, changing level of consciousness, increased restlessness, and pupillary change.

9. The client is admitted to the neurological unit.

Use an X to identify the nursing actions listed below that are Indicated (appropriate or necessary), Contraindicated (could be harmful), or Non-Essential (makes no difference or not necessary) for the client's care at this time.

NURSING ACTION	INDICATED	CONTRA-INDICATED	NON-ESSENTIAL
Place in Trendelenburg position.		X	
Rotate client's head to the right.		X	
Reduce stimuli in the room; low room lights.	X		
Do continuous pulse oximeter monitoring.	X		
Encourage Valsalva maneuver.		X	
Elevate the head of the bed 20–30 degrees.	X		
Do frequent neuro checks.	X		
Push fluids.		X	
Monitor for seizure activity.	X		
Determine favorite foods.			X

Client Needs: Physiological Integrity/Physiological Adaptation
Clinical Judgment/Cognitive Skill: Generate Solutions
Item type: Matrix Multiple Choice
Rationale & Test Taking Strategy: The nurse needs to perform frequent "neuro checks" on this client to gather data regarding any neurologic deficits. The client should be positioned with the head of the bed elevated, usually 20 to 30 degrees. It is important to maintain the head in a midline, neutral position to promote venous drainage

from the brain. The nurse should avoid sudden and acute hip or neck flexion during positioning. Trendelenburg position is contraindicated along with increasing fluids, as this may cause increased intracranial pressure. Oxygen therapy is ordered to prevent hypoxia for the client that has an oxygen saturation (SpO2) less than 95% or per agency or primary health care provider protocol. Reducing stimuli and lowering lights are indicated measures for the client experiencing a stroke, along with monitoring for seizure activity. It is not an essential nursing measure to determine the client's favorite foods at this time.

10. **1, 4, 5, 7, 8**
Client Needs: Physiological Integrity/Physiological Adaptation
Clinical Judgment/Cognitive Skill: Take Action
Item type: Extended Multiple Response: Select All That Apply
Rationale & Test Taking Strategy: The client with dysphagia is referred to a speech therapist for assessment of swallowing problems and the development of a plan to improve swallowing. The nurse needs to assess the client's ability to swallow before offering food by asking the client to take a small sip of water and encouraging small bites of food. The client should be positioned in high-Fowler position, as this position uses gravity to assist in swallowing. It is helpful to turn the head to the unaffected side while eating. Providing soft foods initially because they are easier to swallow is an appropriate intervention. The client should avoid putting foods of different textures in the mouth at the same time. The nurse should inspect the client's mouth for food trapped in cheek pockets, along with providing scrupulous oral hygiene after a meal. The nurse should show patience when feeding the client and provide directions for swallowing as needed. Meals should be unrushed and not stressful for the client to assist with addressing the altered swallowing problem.

11. The client is being discharged and the nurse is evaluating the current assessment findings to determine what client outcomes have improved.

For each body system/function below, select the current assessment findings that indicate the client's conditions have improved. More than one client finding may be selected for each body system/function. Each category must have at least one response.

BODY SYSTEM/ FUNCTION	CURRENT ASSESSMENT FINDING
Neurological	☐ Alert and oriented x 3 ☐ PERRLA
Endocrine	☐ FBS 99 mg/dL ☐ A1c 7.2%
Cardiovascular	☐ BP 142/88 ☐ Pulse 78 beats/min, regular
Gastrointestinal	☐ Choking and coughing when taking oral medication ☐ Swallows a sip of water without difficulty

Client Needs: Physiological Integrity/Physiological Adaptation
Clinical Judgment/Cognitive Skill: Evaluate Outcomes
Item type: Extended Multiple Response: Multiple Response Grouping
Rationale & Test Taking Strategy: The client's neurological status is stable as evidenced by the client being alert and oriented x 3 (person, place, and time) and the pupils are PERRLA, which means pupils are equal, round, and reactive to light and accommodation. The blood sugar no longer indicates hypoglycemia; however, the A1c is elevated (above 7% for client with diabetes) from the admission value. Swallowing a sip of water without difficulty indicates a small improvement due to the techniques suggested by the speech therapist. However, the client is still experiencing dysphagia, as noted by choking and coughing when taking oral medication.

CHAPTER SEVENTEEN

Musculoskeletal: Care of Adult Clients

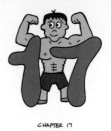

CHAPTER 17
MUSCULO SKELETAL

PHYSIOLOGY OF THE MUSCULOSKELETAL AND CONNECTIVE TISSUE

Bones

A. Bone function.
1. Bones support framework to allow weight bearing.
2. Bones provide protection for underlying organs.
3. Bones act as a lever, allowing movement through the attachment of tendons and muscles.
4. Bones contain hematopoietic tissue for red and white blood cell (WBC) production.
5. Bones are storage units for inorganic minerals like calcium and phosphorus.

B. Bone structure.
1. Periosteum: dense fibrous membrane covering the bone.
2. Diaphysis: main shaft of the bone; marrow is in the center.
3. Epiphysis: the widened area found at the end of a long bone.
4. Epiphyseal plate (growth zone): a cartilage area in children that provides for longitudinal growth of the bone.

C. Bone maintenance and healing.
1. Bone remodeling: removal of old bone by osteoclasts (resorption); deposition of new bone by osteoblasts (ossification).
   a. Weight-bearing stress stimulates local bone resorption and formation; during states of immobility when weight bearing is prevented, calcium is lost from the bone.
   b. Vitamin D promotes absorption of calcium.
2. Bone healing (Fig. 17.1).

> **TEST ALERT** Identify pathophysiology related to an acute or chronic condition (e.g., signs and symptoms).

Connective Tissue: Joints and Cartilage

A. Joints.
1. A joint is a point where bones meet and facilitate body movement, which depends on cartilage for movement and flexibility. Cartilage not only covers bone for smooth movement but also acts as a shock-absorbing pad and connector.
2. Synovial fluid is secreted and serves to decrease friction by lubricating the joint.

B. Articular cartilage is rigid, connective, avascular tissue that covers the end of each bone.
C. Ligaments and tendons are tough, fibrous connective tissues that provide stability while continuing to permit movement.
1. Tendons attach muscles to the bone.
2. Ligaments attach bones to joints.

Skeletal Muscle

A. Function: skeletal muscles move bones through contraction and relaxation; muscles also store protein for energy and metabolism.
B. Energy is consumed when skeletal muscles contract in response to a stimulus.
1. Lactic acid, a by-product of muscle metabolism, accumulates if the amount of oxygen available to the cell is not sufficient.
2. Muscle fatigue results from:
   a. Increased work of the muscle, with inadequate oxygen supply.
   b. Depletion of glycogen and energy stores.
C. Muscle contraction.
1. Flexion: bending at a joint.
2. Extension: straightening of a joint.
3. Abduction: action moving away from the body.
4. Adduction: action moving toward the body.
5. Hypertrophy (increase in muscle mass) will occur if muscle is exercised repeatedly.
6. Atrophy (decrease in muscle mass) will occur with muscle disuse.

System Assessment: Recognize Cues

A. History.
1. History of musculoskeletal injuries, musculoskeletal surgeries, neuromuscular disabilities, inflammatory and metabolic conditions directly or indirectly affecting the musculoskeletal system.
2. Familial predisposition to orthopedic problems.
3. Level of normal activity, occupation, exercise, recreation.
4. Existence of other chronic health problems.

B. Physical assessment.
1. Initial inspection for gross deformities, asymmetry, and edema.
2. Nutritional status: appropriateness of client's weight and body frame; 24-hr diet recall, dietary supplements.

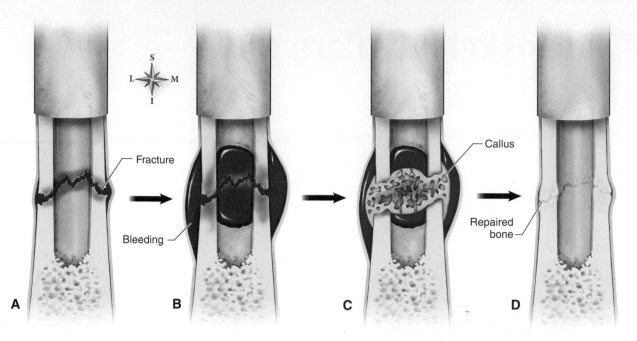

FIG. 17.1 Bone Repair. (From Patton K, Thibodeau G. [2024]. *The human body in health and disease.* [8th ed.]. Elsevier.)

3. Joints.
   a. Movement: active and passive; examine active movement first; compare movement and range of motion (ROM) on one side of the body with movement and ROM on the opposite side.
   b. Inflammation and tenderness: with or without movement.
   c. Presence of joint deformities and dislocations.
   d. Palpate joints for crepitus.
4. Evaluate limb length and circumference if hypertrophy or inconsistency in bone length is evident.
5. Evaluate client's spinal alignment, posture, and gait.
6. Evaluate skeletal muscle.
   a. Bilateral muscle strength.
   b. Coordination of movement.
   c. Presence of atrophy or hypertrophy.
   d. Presence of involuntary muscle movement.
7. Assess peripheral pulses and peripheral circulation.
8. Assess for presence and characteristics of pain.
   a. Specify type of pain and exact location.
   b. Identify precipitating and/or alleviating factors (most musculoskeletal pain is relieved by rest).
   c. Ask about back pain and/or injury.
9. Sensory changes: assess for decreased sensation in extremities.
10. Body mechanics (Box 17.1).
11. Changes in the older adult (Box 17.2).

TEST ALERT Orthopedic questions may be based on concepts of immobility, nursing assessment of an extremity, compromised circulation, and/or general perioperative care. Pay close attention to the direction of the question.

Box 17.1 BODY MECHANICS

The wider the base of support, the greater the stability.
- Position feet wide apart.

The lower the center of gravity, the greater the stability.
- Flex the knees; let the strong muscles of the legs do the work.
- Position close to client.

Face the client; keep back, pelvis, and knees aligned; avoid twisting.

Balance activity between arms and legs.
- Avoid bending to lift; this decreases strain on the back.

Encourage client to assist.
- Pivoting, turning, rolling, and leverage require less work.

Person with heaviest load should coordinate team efforts.

Obtain assistance for a lift with heavy or difficult transfers or moves.
- Use a gait belt for all client transfers.

Teach client proper body mechanics.

DISORDERS OF MUSCULOSKELETAL AND CONNECTIVE TISSUE

Intervertebral Disc Disease

Intervertebral disc disease affects the cartilage discs located between the vertebrae of the spinal column. Problems may involve deterioration, herniation, or dysfunction of the intervertebral discs. Any section of the cervical, thoracic, or lumbar spine can be affected by this disease.

Assessment: Recognize Cues

A. Risk factors/etiology.
   1. Disease causing structural deterioration.

| Box 17.2   OLDER ADULT CARE FOCUS |

Musculoskeletal Changes
- Decreased bone density leads to more frequent fractures.
- Decrease in subcutaneous tissue results in less soft tissue over bony prominences.
- Degenerative changes in the musculoskeletal system alter posture and gait.
- Degenerative changes in cartilage and ligaments result in joint stiffness and pain.
- Range of motion of extremities decreases; older adult may need increased assistance with activities of daily living.
- Slowed movement and decreased muscle strength lead to decreased response time.
- Loss of height from disc compression, posture changes, kyphosis, and "dowagers hump."

2. Obesity.
3. Injury or stress to an area of the spinal column causing a tear or weakening of the annulus fibrosus portion of an intervertebral disc, allowing herniation of the disc. (The most common area for this type of injury is in the lumbar spine.)
4. Occupations that involve heavy lifting or extended periods of sitting or driving.

B. Clinical manifestations (lumbar disc).
1. Low back pain, commonly radiating down one buttock and posterior thigh.
2. Coughing, straining, sneezing, bending, twisting, and lifting exacerbate the pain.
3. Lying supine and raising the leg in an extended position will precipitate the pain.

C. Diagnostics – x-ray, magnetic resonance imaging (MRI), computed tomography (CT) scan (Appendix 17.1).

Analyze Cues and Prioritize Hypotheses
The most important problems involve relief of pain and promotion of safety because of possible alterations in mobility.

Generate Solutions
Treatment
A. Medical (conservative).
1. Analgesics, muscle relaxants, antiseizure drugs, nonsteroidal anti-inflammatory drugs (NSAIDs), antidepressants, and/or epidural corticosteroid injections.
2. Weight reduction, if appropriate.
3. Ice may be used for the first 48 hrs after injury; then moist heat is a better analgesic.
4. Activity modification, good body mechanics, back brace.
5. Physical and/or ultrasound therapy, transcutaneous electrical nerve stimulation (TENS), and massage.
6. Back-strengthening exercises once the pain subsides.
7. Alternative treatment: acupuncture or acupressure.

B. Surgical.
1. Laminectomy: removal of the herniated portion of the disc; surgery may include fusion, which involves bone grafts to stop movement between the vertebrae.
2. Microdiscectomy.
3. Intradiscal electrothermoplasty (IDET).
4. Artificial disc replacement.
5. Spinal fusion with or without instrumentation.

Nursing Interventions: Take Action (for the nonsurgical client)
Goal: To relieve pain by means of conservative measures and prevent recurrence of the problem.
A. Decrease muscle spasm/pain with analgesics, muscle relaxants, decreased activity, and cold or hot applications.
B. Begin ambulation slowly and avoid having client bend, stoop, twist, sit, or lift.
C. Instruct the client and family regarding the principles of appropriate body mechanics: how to turn and reposition in bed and how to get out of bed.
D. The client will need a firm mattress; sleeping in the prone position, especially with a pillow, should be avoided.
E. Instruct the client and family regarding lower back (core strengthening) exercises.
F. Encourage correct posture; instruct client to avoid prolonged standing.
G. Client should sit in straight-backed chairs; avoid prolonged periods of sitting or standing.
H. Semireclining position with forward flexion of lumbar spine (recliner) may be position of comfort.

Nursing Interventions: Take Action (for the surgical client – laminectomy and/or spinal surgery)
Preoperative Goal: To prepare client for laminectomy and/or spinal surgery.
A. Perform preoperative nursing interventions, including education, as appropriate.
B. Have client practice logrolling.
C. Have client practice voiding from supine position.
D. Discuss with client postoperative pain and anticipated methods to decrease pain.
E. Evaluate bowel and bladder function.
F. Identify specific characteristics of pain to be included in database for comparison with pain after surgery.
G. Establish a baseline neurologic assessment for postoperative reference.

Postoperative Goal: Promote comfort and pain relief and maintain spinal alignment after laminectomy and/or spinal surgery.
A. Keep the bed in flat position.
B. Logroll client when turning.
C. Keep pillows between the legs when client is positioned on their side.
D. The client who has had microdisc surgery will have fewer limitations on mobility. Often, the client may assume a position of comfort.
E. Assist with application of back brace, if ordered.

Postoperative Goal: To maintain homeostasis and assess for complications after laminectomy and/or spinal surgery.

A. Evaluate incision area for possible leakage of spinal fluid and bleeding; notify health care provider of clear fluid leaking from incisional area and severe headache associated with the loss of spinal fluid.

B. Analgesics may be given via a patient-controlled analgesia pump or epidural catheter.

C. Assess pain and determine whether there is any pain radiation.

TEST ALERT Assess client's need for pain management and intervene as needed using pharmacologic and nonpharmacologic comfort measures.

D. Perform neurovascular checks of extremities.

E. Normal bladder function returns in 24 to 48 hrs; assess current status of voiding. Assess for urinary retention and loss of sphincter control. *Need to notify registered nurse (RN) or surgeon immediately; it may be an indication of cord compression.*

⚠ NURSING PRIORITY The client who has undergone laminectomy and/or spinal surgery frequently has trouble voiding; this may be because of edema in the area of surgery that interferes with normal bladder sensation. Palpate the suprapubic area to make sure the bladder is not full.

F. Ambulate as soon as indicated (frequently on first postoperative day if no fusion was done).

G. If fusion was performed, may need to apply body brace before ambulation.

H. The client who has undergone microlaminectomy experiences less pain, is frequently out of bed on the day of surgery, and has fewer complications.

I. Paralytic ileus and constipation are common complications; assess for decreased bowel sounds and abdominal distention.

TEST ALERT Identify factors that interfere with elimination.

📋 Fractures

A fracture is a disruption or break in the continuity of the bone

A. Traumatic fractures are the most common type of fracture and occur as a result of physical force to a bone or stress greater than the tensile strength of the bone.

B. Pathologic fractures occur as a result of a disease process, rather than excessive traumatic force, such as osteosarcoma, osteoporosis.

C. Classification of fractures (Fig. 17.2).
   1. Type:
      a. Complete: fracture line extends through the entire bone; the periosteum is disrupted on both sides of the bone.
      b. Incomplete: fracture line extends only partially through the bone, often the result of bending or

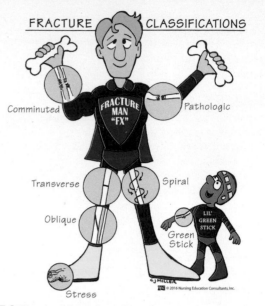

FIG. 17.2 Types of Fractures. (From Zerwekh J, Miller CJ. [2017]. *NCLEX review course.* Chandler, AZ: Nursing Education Consultants, Inc.)

crushing forces applied to a bone (hairline-type fractures).
      c. Comminuted: fracture with multiple bone fragments; more common in adults.
      d. Greenstick: A nondisplaced fracture in which the periosteum is intact across the fracture and the bone is still in alignment; more common in children.
      e. Impacted: complete fracture in which bone fragments are driven into each other.
   2. Classified according to location on the bone: proximal, middle, or distal.
   3. Stable versus unstable fracture.
      a. Stable: a portion of the periosteum usually remains intact; frequently transverse, spiral, or greenstick fractures.
      b. Unstable: bones are displaced at the time of injury, with poor approximation; frequently comminuted or impacted.
      c. Simple, closed fracture: does not produce a break in the skin.
      d. Complex, open, or compound fracture: involves an open wound through which the bone has protruded. (See Fig. 17.2 for more information on types of fractures.)

⚠ NURSING PRIORITY Age, displacement of the fracture, the site of the fracture, nutritional level, medications, and blood supply to the area of injury are factors influencing the time required for the fracture to heal. Be familiar with the terms used to describe fractures.

Assessment: Recognize Cues

A. Clinical manifestations.
   1. Edema, swelling of soft tissue around the injured site.

2. Pain: immediate, severe.
3. Abnormal positioning of extremity; deformity.
4. Loss of normal function.
5. False movement: movement occurs at the fracture site; bone should not move except at joints.
6. Crepitus: palpable or audible crunching as the ends of the bones rub together.
7. Discoloration of the skin around the affected area.
8. Sensation may be impaired if there is nerve damage.
B. Diagnostics – x-ray (Appendix 17.1).

Fracture Complications

A. Infection (osteomyelitis): especially in injuries resulting in an open fracture and soft tissue injury.
B. **Compartment syndrome:** muscle, nerves, and vessels are restricted within a confined space (myofascial compartment) within an extremity.
   1. Etiology.
      a. Decreased compartment size from cast, splints, tight bandages, tight surgical closure.
      b. Increase in compartment contents caused by hemorrhage and/or edema.
   2. Clinical manifestations of compartment syndrome.

> **TEST ALERT** Manage a client with alteration in hemodynamics, tissue perfusion, and hemostasis (cerebral, cardiac, peripheral).

      a. Muscle ischemia occurs as a result of compression of structures in the compartment.
      b. Arterial compression may not occur; pulses may still be present.
      c. May cause permanent damage if pressure not relieved immediately.
      d. Client reports excessive or significant increase in pain unrelieved by analgesics.
      e. Loss of movement and sensation distal to injury.
      f. Skin is pale and cool to the touch distal to the injury.
      g. Capillary refill greater than 3 secs.
      h. Occurrence of compartment syndrome may be decreased by elevation of the extremity and application of ice packs after initial injury.
      i. Treatment is directed toward immediate release of pressure: if the client has a cast, the cast may be "bivalved" – the cast is split in half, and the halves are secured around the extremity by a wrap, such as an elastic bandage.
      j. Volkmann ischemic contracture: compartment syndrome in the arms that compromises circulation; occurs most often as a result of short arm cast used to immobilize a fracture of the humerus.
      k. Can result in permanent damage in a short time period (6-8 hrs).
      l. Paresthesia is frequently the first sign; pulselessness is a late sign.
      m. Blisters may be associated with twisting-type fractures or compartmental syndrome.
C. Venous stasis and thrombus formation are related to immobility. Preventive measures may be initiated, such

as use of low doses of a low-molecular-weight heparin (enoxaparin). Monitor for pulmonary embolism.
D. Fat embolism.
   1. Associated with fractures or surgery on long bones (especially the femur); primarily occurs in adults.
   2. Clinical manifestations generally occur within 12 to 48 hrs of injury.
   3. Fat embolism produces symptoms of acute respiratory distress and hypoxia.
   4. Early immobilization of fractures, especially of long bones, is the best prevention of fat emboli.
E. Chronic complications.
   1. Improper healing: delayed union, nonunion, or angulation (bone heals at a distorted angle).
   2. Avascular necrosis: disrupted blood supply to bone, leading to death of bone tissue.

Analyze Cues and Prioritize Hypotheses

The most important problems are acute pain, muscle spasm, edema, potential for neurovascular compromise (compartment syndrome), and infection.

Generate Solutions

Treatment
A. Immediate immobilization of suspected fracture area.

> **⚠ NURSING PRIORITY** With an open or compound fracture, splint the extremity and cover the wound with a sterile dressing.

B. Fracture reduction.
   1. Closed reduction: nonsurgical, manual realignment of the bones; then injured extremity is usually placed in a cast for continued immobilization until healing occurs.
   2. Open reduction and internal fixation (ORIF): surgical correction of alignment.
C. Traction (Fig. 17.3).
   1. Purposes.
      a. Immobilization of fractures until surgical correction is done; immobilization or alignment of fracture until sufficient healing occurs to permit casting.
      b. Decrease, prevent, or correct bone or joint deformities associated with muscle diseases and bone injury.
      c. Prevent or reduce muscle spasm.
   2. Types.
      a. Skeletal: wire or metal pin is inserted into or through the bone.
      b. Skin: force of pull is applied directly to the skin and indirectly to the bone.
D. Cast application to maintain immobility of affected area.
   1. Cast applied to immobilize joints above and below the injured area.
   2. Short or long arm or leg cast.
   3. Body jacket cast for spinal injuries.
   4. Hip spica cast for femoral fractures.

EXAMPLES OF COMMON TYPES OF TRACTION

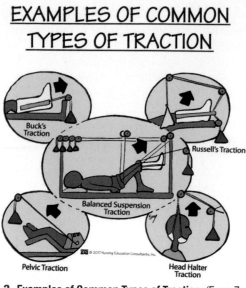

FIG. 17.3 Examples of Common Types of Traction. (From Zerwekh J, Miller CJ. [2017]. *NCLEX review course.* Chandler, AZ: Nursing Education Consultants, Inc.)

E. Fixation devices.
1. External fixation: application of a rigid external device consisting of pins placed through the bone and held in place by a metal frame; requires meticulous care of pin insertion sites (Fig. 17.4).
2. Internal fixation: done through an open incision; hardware (pins, plates, rods, screws) is placed in the bone.
3. Both methods may be used to treat a fracture.

Specific Fractures

Assessment: Recognize Cues

A. Colles fracture.
1. Fracture of the distal radius.
2. Primary complication is compartment syndrome.

B. Fractured pelvis.
1. Frequently occurs in older adults and is associated with falls.
2. May cause serious intraabdominal injuries (hemorrhage) and urinary tract injury.
3. Bed rest is prescribed for clients with stable fractures.
4. Combination of traction, cast, and surgical intervention may be used for the client with a complex fracture.
5. Turn client only on specific orders.

C. Femoral shaft fracture.
1. Common injury in young adults and children.
2. Treatment.
   a. Immobility is achieved by means of a hip spica cast in older children.
   b. 90- to 90-degree traction (Fig. 17.3): balanced skeletal traction for fractured femur.
   c. Older child and adult.
      (1) Internal fixation (adults).
      (2) Balanced skeletal traction for 8 to 12 weeks.

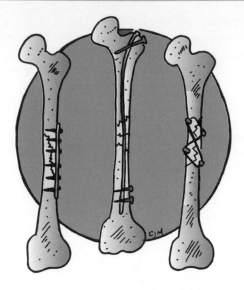

© 2017 Nursing Education Consultants, Inc.

FIG. 17.4 Internal Fixation Devices. Internal fixation devices can be pins, plates, intramedullary rods, or metal and bioabsorbable screws. (From Zerwekh J, Garneau A, Miller CJ. [2017]. *Digital collection of the memory notebooks of nursing images.* [4th ed]. Chandler, AZ: Nursing Education Consultants, Inc.)

     (3) Immobilization by application of a hip spica cast alone or after balanced skeletal traction.

D. Characteristics of bones in children affecting fracture and fracture healing.
1. Presence of epiphyseal plate; if epiphyseal plate is damaged in the fracture, this may affect the growth of long bones.
2. Bones are more porous and allow for greater flexibility.

E. Rib fractures.
1. Usually heal in 3 to 6 weeks with no residual impairment.
2. Painful respirations cause client's breathing to be shallower and coughing to be restrained; this precipitates buildup of secretions and decreased ventilation, leading to atelectasis and pneumonia.
3. Chest taping or strapping is not usually done, because it decreases thoracic excursion.
4. Multiple rib fractures may precipitate the development of a pneumothorax or a tension pneumothorax (see Chapter 11).

F. Mandible fracture.
1. Wiring of jaws (intermaxillary fixation) is treatment.
2. Postoperative problems: airway obstruction and aspiration of vomitus.
   a. Wire cutters near the client at all times in case of emergency (cardiac or respiratory arrest).
   b. Suction client if vomiting.
   c. Cutting wires may complicate problem.
3. Tracheostomy set at bedside.
4. Oral hygiene and use of pad/pencil or picture board for postoperative communication.
5. Discharge teaching: oral care, techniques for handling secretions, how and when to use wire cutters, diet (problems with constipation and flatus caused by low-bulk, high-carbohydrate liquid supplements).

Fracture Immobilization – Splinting

Nursing Interventions: Take Action

Goal: To immobilize a fractured extremity and to provide emergency care before transporting client.

A. Evaluate circulation distal to injury.

> ❗ **NURSING PRIORITY** Identify orthopedic situations that can cause compromised circulation and neurologic damage; intervene and obtain assistance.

B. Splint and immobilize extremity before transfer.
C. If pulses are not present or if the extremity must be realigned to apply splint for transfer, apply just enough traction to support and immobilize the fractured extremity in a position of proper alignment. Once the traction is initiated, do not release it until the extremity has been properly splinted.

> **TEST ALERT** Do not apply traction to compound fractures; traction may cause more damage to tissue and vessels.

D. Elevate the affected extremity, if possible, to decrease edema.

Fracture Immobilization – Casts

Nursing Interventions: Take Action

Goal: Maintain immobilization and prevent complications.
A. Plaster cast: allow cast to dry adequately before moving the client or handling the cast.
   1. Encourage drying of cast by using fans and maintaining adequate circulation.
   2. Avoid handling wet cast to prevent indentions in the cast, which may precipitate pressure areas inside the cast; support cast on plastic covered pillows while drying.
   3. Reposition client every 2 hrs to increase drying on all cast surfaces.
   4. "Petaling" a cast is done to cover the rough edges and prevent crumbling of a plaster cast; edges are covered with small strips of waterproof adhesive.
   5. Try not to get the cast wet; after the cast is dry and the initial edema is resolved, may use low setting on hair dryer after exposure to water.

> ❗ **NURSING PRIORITY** Teach client: DO NOT get plaster cast wet, remove any type of padding, insert any objects inside cast, bear weight on new cast for 48 hrs (if weight-bearing type), or cover cast with plastic for long periods of time.

B. Synthetic casts (fiberglass, polyester cotton knit) are lighter and require a minimal amount of drying time.
   1. Frequently used for upper body cast.
   2. Preferable for infants and children.
   3. Cast does not crumble around the edges and does not soil as easily.
   4. Cast dries rapidly if it gets damp, and it does not disintegrate in water; some synthetic casts can be immersed for bathing.
C. Continue to assess for compromised circulation and compartment syndrome.
D. Body jacket cast and hip spica cast.
   1. Evaluate for abdominal discomfort caused by cast compression of mesenteric artery against duodenum (cast syndrome).
   2. Relief of abdominal pressure can be achieved by means of nasogastric tube and suction or cast removal and reapplication.
   3. Evaluate for pressure areas over iliac crest.
E. Elevate casted extremity, especially during the first 24 hrs after application.
F. Apply ice packs over the area of injury (keeping cast dry) during the first 24 hrs.
G. Encourage movement and exercise of unaffected joints.
H. Assess for infection underneath the cast.
   1. Unpleasant (foul) odor and/or drainage (especially purulent) emanating from inside of cast.
   2. Generalized body temperature elevation.
   3. Increased warmth over outside of the cast (hot spot).
I. Teach client how to use an assistive device for immobility – crutches, cane, or walker (Appendix 17.3).

Fracture Immobilization – Traction

Nursing Interventions: Take Action

Goal: To maintain immobilization and prevent complications (Fig. 17.5).
A. Assume that traction is continuous unless the doctor orders otherwise.
B. Carefully assess for skin breakdown, especially on the underside of the client.

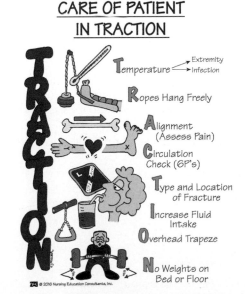

FIG. 17.5 Care of a Patient in Traction. (From Zerwekh J, Garneau A, Miller CJ. [2017]. *Digital collection of the memory notebooks of nursing images.* [4th ed]. Chandler, AZ: Nursing Education Consultants, Inc.)

C. Do not change or remove traction weight on a client with continuous traction.

D. The traction ropes and weights should hang free from any obstructions.

E. Traction applied in one direction requires an equal countertraction to be effective.
   1. Do not let the client's feet touch the end of the bed; this will cause the countertraction to be lost.
   2. Do not allow the traction weights to rest on anything at the end of the bed; this negates the pull of the traction.

F. Carefully assess the pin sites in clients with skeletal traction. Osteomyelitis is a serious complication of skeletal traction.

> **TEST ALERT** Recognize conditions that increase risk for insufficient vascular perfusion; monitor effective functioning of therapeutic devices; prevent complications of immobility. Most clients with fractures will experience some level of immobility.

Goal: To prevent complications of immobility (see Chapter 3).

Fracture Immobilization – External or Internal Fixation Devices

Goal: To maintain immobilization and prevent complications from external or internal fixation.

A. Inspect exposed skin and pin sites for infection.

B. Cleanse around pin sites using sterile technique.

C. Apply antibiotic ointment to pin sites as ordered.

D. Perform wound care on incisional area or area of trauma.

E. Observe carefully for development of infection.

F. Evaluate for circulatory and neurosensory impairment.

Home Care

A. Teach client what not to do.
   1. Do not bear weight on the affected extremity until instructed to do so.
   2. Do not allow the cast to get wet if it is the type that cannot get wet (discuss alternatives to tub baths).
   3. Do not insert any objects into the cast or remove any padding.
   4. Do not move or manipulate pins on an external fixator device.

B. Client should report symptoms associated with swelling or an increase in pain, especially pain unrelieved by analgesics.

C. Assess pin sites for evidence of infection.

Fractured Hip

Fractured hips **are common in older adults, with the majority resulting from a fall. Incidence in women older than 65 years of age is increased because of loss of postural stability and loss of bone mass.**

Assessment: Recognize Cues

A. Clinical manifestations.
   1. External rotation and adduction of the affected extremity.
   2. Shortening of the length of the affected extremity.
   3. Severe pain, tenderness, and muscle spasms.

B. Diagnostics – x-ray.

Analyze Cues and Prioritize Hypotheses

The most important problems are acute pain, muscle spasm, edema, potential for neurovascular compromise (compartment syndrome), and infection.

Generate Solutions

Treatment

A. Initially, a splint is positioned to immobilize fracture and decrease muscle spasms. Buck's traction is no longer recommended for preoperative immobilization.

B. Surgical repair (fixed or sliding nail plates, replacement prostheses, or hip joint replacement) as soon as client's condition allows (permits earlier mobility and prevents complications of immobility).

Nursing Interventions: Take Action (after surgery)

Goal: To monitor and prevent complications (Box 17.3).

A. Circulatory and neurologic checks distal to area of injury.

B. Position to prevent flexion, adduction, and internal rotation, which cause dislocation of the prosthesis.

> **TEST ALERT** Position client to prevent complications.

   1. Do not adduct the affected leg past the neutral position.
   2. Maintain the affected leg in an abducted position with an abduction pillow or pillows between the legs.
   3. Avoid flexion of the hip of more than 90 degrees, such as bending down to pick up something or tie shoes.

> **Box 17.3 OLDER ADULT CARE FOCUS**
>
> **Musculoskeletal Nursing Implications**
> - Older adults have difficulty maintaining immobility after fractures; therefore, fractures are frequently repaired with surgical intervention (open reduction and internal fixation [ORIF]).
> - Older adults heal more slowly, so use of extremity and weight bearing may be delayed.
> - Complications of immobility occur more frequently; mobilize hospitalized clients as early as possible.
> - Do not rely on fever as the primary indication of infection; decreasing mental status is more common.
> - Contractures are more common in older adults.
> - Encourage older adults to use assistive devices such as canes and walkers.

4. Prevent internal or external rotation by using sandbags, pillows, and trochanter rolls at the thigh.
5. Extreme external rotation accompanied by severe pain is indicative of hip prosthesis displacement.
C. Check health care provider's order regarding positioning and turning.
D. Evaluate blood loss.
1. Check the operative site for signs of hemorrhage.
2. Measure the diameter of both thighs to evaluate the presence of internal bleeding in the affected extremity.

> **❗ NURSING PRIORITY** The client is especially prone to complications of immobility (thromboembolism after hip fracture); use nursing interventions to minimize complications.

📋 Total Hip Arthroplasty (total hip replacement)

Total hip arthroplasty (THA) or replacement may be done because of a pathologic fracture or a disease process such as arthritis with the goal to provide relief of pain and improve function.

Assessment: Recognize Cues

A. History of osteoarthritis, rheumatoid arthritis (RA), connective tissue disease, or trauma.
B. Slow loss of cartilage leads to loss of motion, chronic pain.

Nursing Interventions: Take Action

Goal: To provide preoperative care and preoperative and postoperative instructions.
A. Encourage client to practice using either crutches or a walker, whichever is anticipated to be used after surgery.
B. Encourage client to practice moving from bed to a chair in the manner that will be necessary after surgery.
C. Help the client begin practicing the postoperative exercises so they will understand and be able to do them correctly after surgery.
D. Client should discontinue use of platelet antiaggregant medications, such as NSAIDs; clopidogrel; anticoagulants, such as warfarin; and over-the-counter drugs and supplements, such as oral ginkgo, green tea, and ginseng, for 7 days before surgery.
1. Assess the client for other medications that may promote hemorrhage during or after surgery.

Goal: To provide postoperative care and prevent complications (Fig. 17.6).
A. Supine position with head slightly elevated, maintain abduction of affected leg.
B. Quadriceps exercises.
C. Neurologic and circulation checks.
D. Client is mobilized on first or second postoperative day to prevent complications of immobility; may use antiembolism stockings and/or sequential compression devices on lower extremities to prevent venous stasis.
E. Low-molecular-weight heparin (Appendix 12-2) may be given to prevent thrombophlebitis.
F. Keep client's heels off the bed to prevent skin breakdown.
G. Legs should not be crossed.

> **❗ NURSING PRIORITY** After surgery, do not allow the repaired hip to flex greater than 90 degrees; avoid adduction and internal rotation of extremity. Excessive flexion and adduction may dislocate the hip prosthesis.

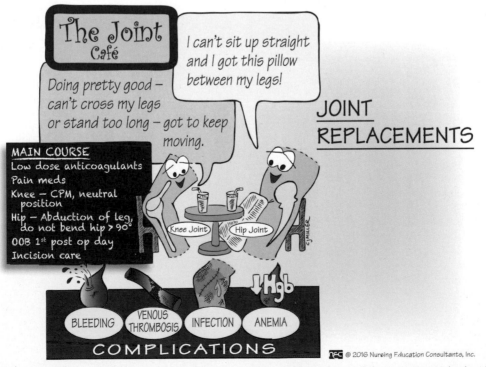

FIG. 17.6 Joint Replacement. (From Zerwekh J, Garneau A, Miller CJ. [2017]. *Digital collection of the memory notebooks of nursing.* [4th ed.]. Chandler, AZ: Nursing Education Consultants, Inc.)

H. Look for signs of possible hip dislocation.
   1. Increased hip pain.
   2. Shortening of affected leg.
   3. External leg rotation.
   4. If symptoms of possible hip dislocation are observed, contact the surgeon immediately.

Total Knee Arthroplasty (total knee replacement)

Total knee arthroplasty (TKA) is the replacement or reconstruction of the knee joint to relieve pain and improve joint stability after severe destruction or deterioration of the knee joint.

Assessment: Recognize Cues

A. Slow loss of cartilage leads to loss of motion, chronic unremitting pain, and instability (Box 17.4).
B. Presence of osteoporosis may necessitate bone grafting to augment defects.

Nursing Interventions: Take Action

Goal: To provide preoperative care by planning for postdischarge transitions of care.
Goal: To provide postoperative care and prevent complications.
A. Frequent neurovascular checks.
B. Compression dressing may be used immediately after the operation to immobilize knee.
C. Emphasis on physical therapy.
   1. Quadricep exercises first postoperative day, progressing to straight leg raises and gentle ROM to increase muscle strength and obtain 90-degree knee flexion.

Box 17.4   OLDER ADULT CARE FOCUS

Protecting Joints

- If pain lasts longer than 1 hr after exercise, change the exercises that involve that joint.
- Plan activity and work that conserve energy; do important tasks first.
- Alternate activities; do not do all heavy tasks at one time.
- Minimize stress on joints; sit rather than stand, avoid prolonged repetitive movements, move around frequently, and avoid stairs or prolonged grasping.
- Use largest muscles rather than smaller ones; use shoulders or arms rather than hands to push open doors; pick up items without stooping or bending; use leg muscles; women should carry purses on their shoulders rather than in their hands.
- Painful, acutely swollen inflamed joints should not be exercised beyond basic range of motion.
- Regular exercise can be done even when joints are slightly painful and stiff; swimming and bike riding maintain mobility without weight bearing.
- Expect changes in mental status after surgery.
- There may be a role change in the family as a result of the client's decreased mobility.

---

2. Continuous passive motion (CPM) machine to promote joint mobility.
3. Full weight bearing on extremity is started before discharge.

Osteoporosis

Osteoporosis is a chronic, progressive metabolic bone disease that involves an imbalance between new bone formation and bone resorption.

A. Primary osteoporosis is the most common type; occurs most often in women after menopause because low levels of estrogen are associated with an increase in bone resorption. Osteoporosis can occur in men and is considered underdiagnosed; as many as one in four men over 50 years of age will have an osteoporosis-related fracture.
B. Bone loss occurs predominantly in the vertebral bodies of the spine, the femoral neck in the hip, and the distal radius of the arm. Bone mass declines, leaving the bones brittle and weak.

Assessment: Recognize Cues

A. Risk factors/etiology (Fig. 17.7).
   1. Age/sex/ethnicity: incidence increases in white and Asian women after 50 years of age.
   2. Endocrine disorders of the thyroid and parathyroid glands.
   3. Nutritional deficits: insufficient intake of dietary calcium and/or vitamin D.
B. Clinical manifestations.
   1. May be asymptomatic until x-ray films demonstrate skeletal weakening or a fracture occurs. Bone loss of 25% to 40% must occur before osteoporosis can be identified on standard x-ray films.
   2. Spinal deformity and "Dowagers hump."
      a. Results from repeated pathologic, spinal vertebral fractures.
      b. Gradual loss of height (Fig. 17.8).
      c. Increase in spinal curvature (kyphosis).
   3. Spinal fractures may occur spontaneously or as a result of minimal trauma.
   4. Chronic low thoracic and midline back pain.
   5. Height loss may precipitate thoracic problems, decrease in abdominal capacity, and decrease in exercise tolerance.
   6. Hip fractures and vertebral collapse are the most debilitating problems.
C. Diagnostics (Appendix 17.1).
   1. Serum laboratory values of calcium, vitamin D, phosphorus, and alkaline phosphatase may be normal or low.
   2. Bone mineral density (BMD) measurements through quantitative ultrasound (QUS) and dual energy x-ray absorptiometry (DEXA or DXA).
      a. DXA results are reported as T-scores.
      b. T-score between +1 and −1 is normal; T-score between −1 and −2.5 indicates osteopenia; T score of −2.5 or lower indicates osteoporosis.

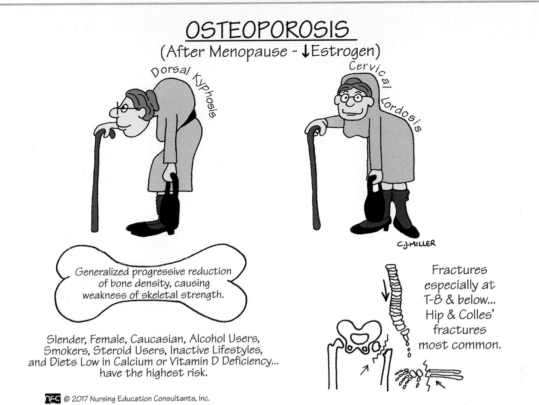

FIG. 17.7 Osteoporosis. (From Zerwekh J, Garneau A, Miller CJ. [2017]. *Digital collection of the memory notebooks of nursing images.* [4th ed]. Chandler, AZ: Nursing Education Consultants, Inc.)

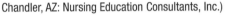

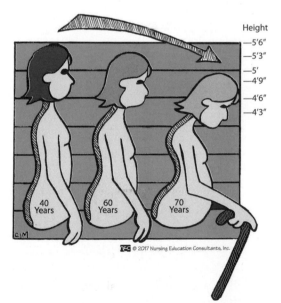

FIG. 17.8 Progression of Osteoporosis. (From Zerwekh J, Garneau AJ, Miller CJ. [2017]. *Digital collection of the memory notebooks of nursing.* [4th ed.]. Chandler, AZ: Nursing Education Consultants, Inc.)

D. Complications.
  1. Complications include bone fractures occurring in the vertebral bodies, distal radius, or hip.

Analyze Cues and Prioritize Hypotheses

The most important problems are the potential for fractures and possible falls.

Generate Solutions

Treatment

A. Dietary: increased intake of protein, calcium, and vitamin D.
B. Medications.
  1. Calcium supplements: daily intake of calcium should be approximately 1000 mg for men and women and 1200 mg for postmenopausal women over the age of 70.
  2. Vitamin D supplements (800-1000 IU recommended daily for men and postmenopausal women over age 50) to enhance utilization of calcium; spending 20 mins daily in the sun will provide adequate vitamin D.
  3. Antiresorptive medications, such as bisphosphonates and calcitonin to facilitate increased bone density (Appendix 17.2).
C. Exercise: activities that put moderate stress on bones by working them against gravity (walking, racquet sports, jogging).
  1. Swimming and yoga may not be as beneficial because of decreased stress on bone mass.
  2. Walking for 30 mins three to five times a week is the most effective exercise in preventing osteoporosis.
  3. Weight-bearing exercise decreases the development of osteoporosis and possibly increases new bone formation.
D. Compression fractures of the vertebrae usually heal without surgical intervention.

Nursing Interventions: Take Action

Goal: To decrease pain and promote activities to diminish progression of disease.
A. Pain relief.
   1. Initial bed rest, firm mattress.
   2. Narcotic analgesics initially, followed by NSAIDs.
B. Assess bowel and bladder function; client will be prone to constipation and paralytic ileus if vertebrae are involved.
C. Regular daily exercise; encourage outdoor exercises (increases utilization of vitamin D).
D. Increased calcium and vitamin D intake and hormone replacement therapy.

Home Care

A. Decrease falls and injury by maintaining safe home environment.
B. The client should understand the need to continue taking medications, even if they do not make the client feel better. It is important for the client to understand that the calcium and vitamin D supplements are necessary to prevent further bone loss.
C. Do not exercise if pain occurs.
D. Avoid heavy lifting, stooping, and bending. Review and demonstrate good body mechanics with the client.

Osteomyelitis

Osteomyelitis **is an infection of the bone, bone marrow, and surrounding soft tissue. The most common causative organism is** *Staphylococcus aureus.*

Assessment: Recognize Cues

A. Clinical manifestations.
   1. Acute.
      a. Tenderness, swelling, and warmth in affected area.
      b. Drainage from infected site.
      c. Systemic symptoms: fever, chills, nausea, and night sweats.
      d. Constant pain in affected area; worsens with activity.
      e. Circulatory impairment.
   2. Chronic: present longer than 1 month; failed to respond to initial course of antibiotic therapy.
      a. Drainage from wound or sinus tract.
      b. Recurrent episodes of bone pain.
      c. Diminished systemic signs: low-grade fever; local signs of infection more common.
      d. Remission and exacerbation of problem.
B. Diagnostics (Appendix 17.1).
   1. Bone or tissue biopsy.
   2. Wound and/or blood culture.
   3. Elevated WBC count, sedimentation rate, and C-reactive protein.
   4. X-rays and radionuclide bone scan, MRI, and CT.

Analyze Cues and Prioritize Hypotheses

The most important problems are potential loss of mobility, bone pain, and possible systemic infection.

Generate Solutions

Treatment
A. Intensive intravenous (IV) antibiotics; oral antibiotic therapy for 6 to 8 weeks.
B. Immobilization of affected area.
C. Surgical debridement may be necessary.
D. Hyperbaric oxygen therapy to stimulate circulation and healing.

Nursing Interventions: Take Action

Goal: To decrease pain, promote comfort, and decrease spread of infection.
A. Administer analgesics and provide nonpharmacologic pain relieving interventions.
B. Maintain correct body alignment.
   1. Move affected extremity gently and with support.
   2. Prevent contractures, especially of affected extremity.
C. If there is an open wound, maintain wound (contact) precautions (Chapter 6).
D. Client is usually discharged on antibiotic therapy and instructed on the importance of keeping all follow-up care appointments.

TEST ALERT Assess and document wound response to antibiotic therapy and wound care management.

Amputation

An *amputation* **is the removal of part of an extremity at various anatomic locations.**

Assessment: Recognize Cues

A. Indications for amputation.
   1. Peripheral vascular disease, especially vascular disease of lower extremities.
   2. Severe trauma or congenital disorders.
   3. Acute or widespread infections (e.g., gas gangrene).
   4. Malignant tumors.
B. Diagnostic tests: dependent on underlying problem.

Analyze Cues and Prioritize Hypotheses

The most important problems are the potential for the residual limb to have decreased perfusion, acute pain (phantom limb pain), decreased mobility, decreased self-esteem and body image change, and deficits in activities of daily living (ADLs).

Generate Solutions

Treatment
A. Underlying condition is identified.
B. Diagnostic tests to determine viability of the limb.

Nursing Interventions: Take Action

Goal: To prevent further loss of circulation to the extremity and to promote psychological stability, comfort, and the optimal level of mobility.
A. Monitor circulation before surgery.

B. Provide preoperative care regarding upper-extremity exercises to promote arm strength for postoperative activities such as crutch walking and gait training.

C. Discuss the phenomenon of phantom limb pain and its management in the postoperative period.

> **TEST ALERT** Identify and prevent complications of immobility; use positioning to prevent contractures; provide support for client with unexpected alteration in body image; help client ambulate and move with assistive devices; promote wound healing; and assist client with use of prosthesis.

Goal: To manage pain control and residual limb wound care postoperatively.

A. In the immediate postoperative period (24 hrs), the residual limb may be elevated using one pillow to decrease edema and promote comfort. After the first 24 hrs, the joint above the amputation site is kept in an extended position.

B. During the immediate postoperative period, frequently monitor vital signs and evaluate residual limb dressing for bleeding; have a surgical tourniquet available should postoperative hemorrhaging occur.

> **TEST ALERT** Postoperative hemorrhaging requires immediate intervention and notification of the health care provider.

C. Administer analgesics for postoperative pain, including phantom limb pain.

D. Prevent flexion contractures, which delay the rehabilitative course of care.
  1. Avoid 45- to 90-degree flexion of residual limb. In cases involving lower limbs, do not allow client to sit in a chair for more than 1 hr during the immediate postoperative period.
  2. Have client lie on their abdomen for 30 mins three or four times per day and position the hip in extension while prone.

E. Postoperative dressing changes on residual limb are done using sterile technique to prevent infection.

F. A rigid compression dressing (plaster molded over dressing) may be applied to prevent injury and to decrease swelling. In children, after an amputation, the placement of a temporary prosthesis immediately after surgery may promote functioning and psychological adaptation.
  1. Controlling the edema will enhance healing and promote comfort.
  2. Changes of the rigid dressing are necessary; as the residual limb heals, it also shrinks.

G. The compression dressing may be changed three or four times before a permanent prosthesis is fitted. The compression dressing may be formed so that it can attach to a prosthesis.

H. If the client is not fitted with a rigid compression dressing, the residual limb will be shaped with a compression bandage.

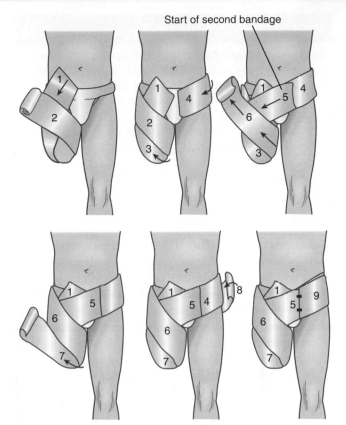

Start of second bandage

FIG. 17.9 Bandaging for Above-the-Knee and Below-the-Knee Amputation. (From Ignatavicius DD, Workman ML. [2021]. *Medical-surgical nursing: patient-centered collaborative care.* [10th ed.]. Saunders.)

  1. Ace bandage elastic wrapping is often used for compression of this type (Fig. 17.9).
  2. It should be worn at all times except during physical therapy and bathing.

Goal: To help the client understand measures for residual limb care after the wound has healed.

A. Continually assess for skin breakdown; visually inspect the residual limb for redness, abrasions, or blistering.

B. The residual limb should be washed daily, carefully rinsed, and dried; residual soap and moisture contribute to skin breakdown.

C. Do not apply anything to the residual limb (alcohol increases skin dryness and cracking; lotions keep skin soft and hinder use of prosthesis).

Home Care

A. Client should put the prosthesis on when they get up and should wear it all day. The residual limb tends to swell if the prosthesis is not applied. The more the client wears the prosthesis, the less swelling will be experienced and the more comfortable and proficient the client will become in using the prosthesis.

B. Using a lower limb prosthesis requires 40% to 60% more energy for walking (Box 17.5).

C. Refer to community health nurse for instruction on ambulation, transfer techniques, prone positioning, and proper residual limb care.

a. Primarily involves weight-bearing joints; occurs as a result of mechanical stress.
b. May also involve joints in the fingers and vertebral column.
2. Symptoms occurring in the joint.
a. Pain, swelling, tenderness.
b. Crepitation: a grating sound or feeling with movement.
c. Instability, stiffness, and immobility.
3. Pain occurs on motion and with weight bearing.
4. Pain increases in severity with activity.
5. Heberden nodes: bony nodules on the distal finger joints.
C. Diagnostics – CT scan, MRI, bone scan (Appendix 17.1).

Analyze Cues and Prioritize Hypotheses

The most important problems are persistent pain due to joint edema, cartilage deterioration from inflammation, and the potential for immobility.

Generate Solutions

Treatment

A. Medications for pain relief: salicylates (aspirin), acetaminophen, NSAIDs (ibuprofen), COX-2 inhibitors.
1. Intraarticular injection of corticosteroids, methotrexate, DMARDs, and hyaluronic acid.
B. Activity balanced with adequate rest.
C. Weight reduction, if appropriate.
D. Physical therapy and exercise.
E. Surgical intervention with joint replacement.
F. Complementary and alternative therapies include acupuncture, oral intake of glucosamine and chondroitin, application of topical analgesics.

Nursing Interventions: Take Action

Goal: To relieve pain, prevent further stress on the joint, and maintain function.

A. Acutely inflamed joint should be immobilized with splint or brace.
B. Plan ADLs to prevent stress on involved joints and provide adequate rest periods.
C. Heat compresses can be used for relief of pain; cold compresses may be used if joint is inflamed.
D. It is important to maintain regular exercise program; decrease activity in acutely inflamed, painful joints.

> **! NURSING PRIORITY** More than 4000 mg daily of acetaminophen increases risk for liver damage in adults. Clients taking large doses (300-500 mg/kg/day) of aspirin (acetylsalicylic acid) should be closely monitored for signs and symptoms of salicylism (toxicity). Aspirin poisoning is an acute medical emergency and is potentially lethal.

Goal: To help client understand measures to maintain health (see Box 17.4).

A. Identify activities requiring increased stress on involved joints.

B. Maintain regular exercise program (e.g., walking, swimming) to promote muscle strength and joint mobility.
C. Encourage independence in ADLs.
Goal: To maintain psychological equilibrium and promote positive self-esteem.

Gout

Gout **is a recurring arthritic condition causing the accumulation of uric acid crystals in one or more joints. Uric acid crystals may be found in articular, periarticular, and subcutaneous tissues. Hyperuricemia is a diagnostic finding secondary to a defect in the metabolism of uric acid.**

Assessment: Recognize Cues

A. Clinical manifestations.
1. Intense pain and inflammation of one or more small joints, especially those in the large toe.
2. Characterized by remissions and exacerbations of acute joint pain.
3. Onset is generally rapid with swollen, inflamed, painful joints and typically occurs at night.
4. Presence of tophi or uric acid crystals in the area around the large toe, joints of the fingers, along tendons, and in skin and cartilage.
B. Diagnostics: serum uric acid level greater than 6 mg/dL (356.91 µmol/L).
C. Complications.
1. Uric acid kidney stones.

Analyze Cues and Prioritize Hypotheses

The most important problems are relief of joint pain, increasing fluids (to promote excretion of uric acid), and managing diet.

Generate Solutions

Treatment

A. Medications.
1. Antigout, such as colchicine, allopurinol (Appendix 17.2).
2. NSAIDs for pain and to assist in preventing attacks.
B. Decrease amount of purine in diet (Chapter 2).

Nursing Interventions: Take Action

Goal: To prevent acute attack, promote comfort, and maintain joint mobility.

A. Medications should be given early in the attack to decrease the severity of the attack.
B. Protect affected joint: immobilize, no weight bearing.
C. Cold packs may decrease pain.
D. Decreased amount of purine in diet by avoiding foods such as shellfish, lentils, red wine, asparagus, spinach, beef, chicken, and pork.
E. Encourage high fluid intake to increase excretion of uric acid and to prevent the development of uric acid stones.
F. Help client identify activities and aspects of lifestyle that precipitate attacks, such as decreasing alcohol consumption.

Lyme Disease

Lyme disease is the most common vector-borne disease in the United States. An inflammatory response to bacteria *Borrelia burgdorferi*; if not treated, causes chronic arthritic pain and swelling in the large joints, carditis, and nervous system problems.

Assessment: Recognize Cues

A. Risk factors/etiology.
   1. Caused by the bacterium *B. burgdorferi* and transmitted by the bite of an infected deer tick.
   2. Residence or recreation in wooded areas of Northeastern United States from Maine to Maryland and the upper Midwestern states of Minnesota and Wisconsin.
B. Clinical manifestations (Fig. 17.10).
   1. *Erythema migrans* (EM), a skin lesion ("bull's-eye rash"), anywhere on the body. EM is an expanding area of redness with a bright red border and central clearing around what appears to be a small red papule appearing after the removal of a tick.
   2. Acute flulike symptoms, such as low-grade fever, chills, headache, stiff neck, fatigue, swollen lymph nodes, and migratory joint and muscle pain.
   3. Symptoms usually occur in a week but may be delayed for up to 30 days.
C. Diagnostics
   1. Serum enzyme immunoassay (EIA) followed by immunoblot (Western blot) (Appendix 17.1).
   2. Complete blood count (CBC) and erythrocyte sedimentation rate (ESR) are usually normal.
D. Complications (if untreated).
   1. Chronic arthritis pain and joint swelling.
   2. Carditis.
   3. Central nervous system problems such as severe headaches or poor motor coordination.
   4. Posttreatment Lyme disease syndrome occurs in approximately 10% to 20% of persons treated with antibiotics for Lyme disease; they experience lingering fatigue or joint and muscle pain.

Analyze Cues and Prioritize Hypotheses

The most important problems are early recognition of the symptoms (bull's-eye rash) and treatment with antibiotic therapy.

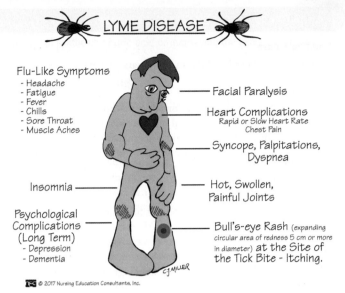

FIG. 17.10 Lyme Disease. (From Zerwekh J, Garneau AJ, Miller CJ. [2017]. *Digital collection of the memory notebooks of nursing.* [4th ed.]. Chandler, AZ: Nursing Education Consultants, Inc.)

Generate Solutions

Treatment

A. Medications
   1. Antibiotics: doxycycline, cefuroxime, and amoxicillin. (Erythromycin is used in clients allergic to penicillin.) (Appendix 6.2.)
   2. NSAIDs for pain.

Nursing Interventions: Take Action

Goal: To prevent tick bites and seek early treatment.

A. Teach people living in endemic areas of measures to prevent tick bites: inspect body thoroughly after walking in wooded areas, wear light-colored clothing, and remove ticks early using tweezers.
B. Avoid folk solutions such as painting the tick with nail polish or petroleum jelly.
C. Wash bitten area with soap and water and apply antiseptic.
D. Teach client to see a health care provider immediately if flulike symptoms or bull's-eye rash appear within 2 to 30 days after removal of tick.

Appendix 17.1 DIAGNOSTIC STUDIES

Serum Diagnostics

Anti-CCP

Measures the presence of antibodies to cyclic citrulline protein; these antibodies are specific diagnostic markers for RA. This diagnostic test can provide early detection of RA.

Antinuclear Antibody

Measures the presence of antibodies that destroy the nucleus of body tissue cells (i.e., those seen in connective tissue diseases); a positive test result is associated with systemic lupus erythematosus.

Complement

Essential body protein to measure immune and inflammatory reactions; usually depleted in RA.

Alkaline Phosphatase

Enzyme produced by osteoblasts; elevated levels found in osteoporosis, healing fractures, bone cancer, osteomalacia.

Aldolase

Elevated levels in muscular dystrophy (MD).

Continued

Appendix 17.2 MEDICATIONS—cont'd

MEDICATIONS	SIDE EFFECTS	NURSING IMPLICATIONS
Methotrexate: PO, IV, IM	Toxic effects: hepatotoxicity, bone marrow suppression Nausea, vomiting, stomatitis Teratogenesis	1. Caution women of childbearing age to avoid pregnancy; use birth control during and 3 months after treatment. 2. Monitor CBC and liver enzymes regularly. 3. Avoid alcohol during therapy. 4. Administer with food.
Hydroxychloroquine: PO	Toxic effects: retinopathy, skeletal muscle myopathy, or neuropathy Headache, anorexia, dizziness	1. Recommend eye examinations every 3 months. 2. Not recommended for children. 3. Therapeutic effect may take 3-6 months.
Leflunomide: PO	Toxic effects: hepatotoxicity, diarrhea, teratogenesis	1. Not recommended for women who may become pregnant. 2. May slow the progression of joint damage caused by rheumatoid arthritis and improves physical function.

Biologic Therapy: Disease-modifying antirheumatic drugs (DMARDs): Agents that bind to tumor necrosis factor (TNF) to decrease inflammatory and immune responses; used in cases of severe arthritis.

Etanercept: subQ Adalimumab; subQ Certolizumab pegol: subQ Golimumab: subQ Infliximab: IV	Increased risk for infections, injection site reactions, heart failure, headache, nausea, dizziness	1. Use cautiously in clients with heart disease. 2. Rotate injection sites at least 1 inch apart. 3. Advise clients that injection site reaction generally decreases with continued therapy. 4. Do not administer to clients with chronic or localized infections. 5. Have client report signs of infection, bruising, or bleeding. 6. Assess client for infections; administer tuberculosis skin test and chest x-ray prior to starting.
Abatacept: IV	Not recommended for combined use with other TNF inhibitors	1. Indicated for clients who do not respond to TNF inhibitors or other DMARDs.
Tocilizumab: IV Anakinra: IV Rituximab: IV	Increased risk for infections, GI perforation, liver injury, hematologic effects	1. Used for patients with moderate-to-severe RA who have not responded to other DMARDs. 2. Do not combine with other immunosuppressants.

CBC, Complete blood count; *CNS,* central nervous system; *GI,* gastrointestinal; *HF,* congestive heart failure; *IM,* intramuscular; *IV,* intravenous; *PO,* by mouth (orally); *RA,* rheumatoid arthritis; *subQ,* subcutaneous; *TNF,* tumor necrosis factor.

Appendix 17.3   ASSISTIVE DEVICES FOR IMMOBILITY

Crutches

Measuring a Client (Fig. 17.11)
- Measurement may be taken with client supine or standing.
- Supine: measure the distance from the client's axilla to a point 6 inches (15 cm) lateral to the heel.
- Standing: measure the distance from the client's axilla to a point 4 to 6 inches (10-15 cm) to the side and 4 to 6 inches (10-15 cm) in front of the foot.
- Adjust hand bars so that client's elbows are flexed approximately 30 degrees.
- If client was measured while supine, assist client to stand with crutches. Check the distance between client's axilla and arm pieces. You should be able to put three of your fingers between client's axilla and the crutch bar.

Four-Point Alternate Gait
- The four-point alternate gait is used by clients who can bear partial weight on both feet (e.g., clients with arthritis or cerebral palsy). It is a particularly safe gait in that there are three points of support on the floor at all times.

- This gait provides a normal walking pattern and makes some use of the muscles of the lower extremities.

Three-Point Alternate Gait
- For the three-point alternate gait, the client must be able to bear the total body weight on one foot; the affected foot or leg is either partially or totally non-weight bearing.
- In this gait, both crutches are moved forward together with the affected leg while the weight is being borne by the client's hands on the crutches. The unaffected leg is then advanced forward.

Crutch Walking
- Up stairs: Unaffected leg moves up first, followed by the crutches and the affected leg.
- Down stairs: Crutches and affected leg move down first, body weight is transferred to the crutches, and the unaffected leg is moved down.

TEST ALERT Assess client's use of assistive devices, evaluate correct use, and help client ambulate with an assistive device.

Canes (Fig. 17.12)

- The cane is used on the side opposite the affected leg.
- The cane and the affected leg move together.

Walkers

- The client takes a step, lifts the walker and moves it forward, then takes another step.

- Gain balance before moving walker forward again; balance provides stability and equal weight bearing.

> **! NURSING PRIORITY** *Safety* is an important priority for the client who uses an assistive device for ambulation. Make sure the client demonstrates correct use of the device.

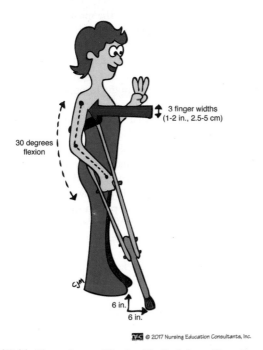

FIG. 17.11 Measuring a Client with Crutches. (From Zerwekh J, Garneau A, Miller CJ. [2017]. *Digital collection of the memory notebooks of nursing*. [4th ed.]. Chandler, AZ: Nursing Education Consultants, Inc.)

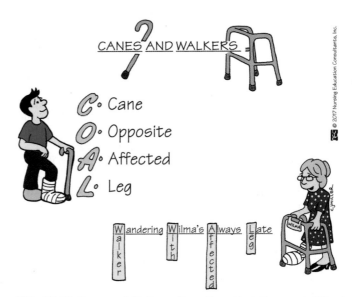

FIG. 17.12 Canes and Walkers. (From Zerwekh J, Garneau A, Miller CJ. [2017]. *Digital collection of the memory notebooks of nursing*. [4th ed.]. Chandler, AZ: Nursing Education Consultants, Inc.)

⚡ Answers to Practice & Next Generation NCLEX (NGN) Questions

1. 2, 4, 6
Client Needs: Physiological Integrity/Reduction of Risk Potential
Clinical Judgment/Cognitive Skill: Take Action
Item Type: Select All That Apply
Rationale & Test Taking Strategy: Recall that most scans require either a contrast dye or radioisotope. The procedure will include an IV injection of a radioisotope that is given 2 hours before the procedure. Ensure client empties bladder before the procedure. The procedure takes about 1 hour. The client will lie supine during the procedure. Fluid intake should be increased after the procedure to promote excretion of radioisotope. Food or fluids are not limited before the scan, and no biopsy of the bone will be taken. Bone scans are used less often today because of the availability of more sophisticated equipment, such as magnetic resonance imaging.

2. 2
Client Needs: Physiological Integrity/Physiological Adaptation
Clinical Judgment/Cognitive Skill: Generate Solutions
Item Type: Multiple Choice
Rationale & Test Taking Strategy: Client should lie on the abdomen for 30 minutes three or four times a day and position the hip in extension while prone. Also, to prevent flexion contractures, client should avoid sitting in a chair for more than an hour. The residual limb is wrapped from distal to proximal. Ice packs are not used on the residual limb after surgery because the cold restricts blood flow. Anti-inflammatory medications may be used for pain relief but not to prevent edema.

3. 1
Client Needs: Physiological Integrity/Physiological Adaptation
Clinical Judgment/Cognitive Skill: Prioritize Hypotheses
Item Type: Multiple Choice
Rationale & Test Taking Strategy: Note the **key** word, "priority," assessment information related to a fractured hip. Circulation and neurosensory status distal to the fracture are always priorities for clients with fractures. The amount of swelling is important, but the primary concern regarding swelling is circulatory and neurosensory deficits. The amount of bone healing cannot be assessed. There is concern regarding pain, but circulatory and neurologic checks are the priority actions.

4. 1
Client Needs: Physiological Integrity/Physiological Adaptation
Clinical Judgment/Cognitive Skill: Analyze Cues
Item Type: Multiple Choice
Rationale & Test Taking Strategy: The movement and sensation should be evaluated before surgery to serve as a baseline for comparison during the postoperative recovery period. Movement of the legs and assessment of sensation should be unchanged compared with the preoperative status. Radiating leg pain is diagnostic of the condition and assessing it before surgery is not as beneficial as determining movement and sensation.

5. 2, 3, 5, 6
Client Needs: Physiological Integrity/Physiological Adaptation
Clinical Judgment/Cognitive Skill: Prioritize Hypotheses
Item Type: Select All That Apply
Rationale & Test Taking Strategy: Note the **key** word, "priority," concerns for a client with a mandibular fracture. First, ask yourself where the mandible is. Two potential life-threatening problems in the immediate postoperative period are airway obstruction and aspiration of vomitus. Because the client cannot open the jaws, it is essential that an airway is maintained. Place the client on the side with the head slightly elevated immediately after surgery. The wire cutter or scissors may be used to cut the wires or elastic bands in case of an emergency. Although pain is an important consideration for any postoperative client, it is not a life-threatening priority, nor are the client's inability to speak or bleeding.

6. 4
Client Needs: Physiological Integrity/Physiological Adaptation
Clinical Judgment/Cognitive Skill: Prioritize Hypotheses
Item Type: Multiple Choice
Rationale & Test Taking Strategy: Note the **key** word, "best," nursing intervention to address phantom limb pain, which is the persistent altered sensory perception in the amputated body part that is unpleasant or painful. Phantom limb pain should be carefully assessed, and medication should be administered. The pain is expected, and it will probably go away eventually; however, this does not assist the client to currently manage the pain. Exercise will not relieve or prevent phantom limb pain. It is not therapeutic to remind the client that the limb has been removed and thus it cannot be hurting.

7. 2
Client Needs: Physiological Integrity/Pharmacological Therapies
Clinical Judgment/Cognitive Skill: Prioritize Hypotheses
Item Type: Multiple Choice
Rationale & Test Taking Strategy: Note the **key** word, "most" important information about methotrexate that the client needs to know. Laboratory work will need to be done periodically during administration to monitor for the development of anemia, leukopenia, thrombocytopenia, and/or hepatic toxicity. Hirsutism and menstrual changes occur with long-term corticosteroid use. Methotrexate should be given 1 hour before or 2 hours after meals to prevent vomiting when given by mouth (PO). Antiemetics are given concurrently with the medication.

8. 2
Client Needs: Physiological Integrity/Physiological Adaptation
Clinical Judgment/Cognitive Skill: Evaluate Outcomes
Item Type: Multiple Choice
Rationale & Test Taking Strategy: Note the **key** word, "not." Review the statements; three will be accurate or true and the one that is incorrect will be the answer. Clients with total hip replacement should not bring their operative leg across midline, which may result in a prosthesis dislocation. Clients should maintain abduction (pillow between legs) and use elevated toilet seats. Crossing the legs is adduction, which is contraindicated for this client.

9. 1
Client Needs: Physiological Integrity/Pharmacological Therapies
Clinical Judgment/Cognitive Skill: Take Action
Item Type: Multiple Choice
Rationale & Test Taking Strategy: For the medication to be adequately absorbed, there must be no food in the stomach. A large glass of water should be used to take the medication to make sure it does not lodge in the esophagus. The client should not lie down for 30 minutes after taking the medication because any gastric reflux of

the medication can be very irritating to the esophagus. Orthostatic hypotension is not a side effect, and the medication should not be taken at bedtime.

10. **4**
Client Needs: Physiological Integrity/Basic Care and Comfort
Clinical Judgment/Cognitive Skill: Take Action
Item Type: Multiple choice
Rationale & Test Taking Strategy: Note the **key** words, "most" and "safest." The safest and best technique is figure-eight wrapping because it prevents restriction of blood flow due to how it is applied. It is important to decrease the tightness of the bandages while wrapping in a distal-to-proximal direction. Once the bandage is wrapped, then anchor the bandage to the highest joint, such as above the knee for BKAs. For wrapping a residual limb to be effective, the nurse needs to reapply the bandages every 4 to 6 hours or more often if they become loose. The other bandage wrapping techniques are not appropriate for wrapping a stump on the residual limb.

11. The following is the nurses' notes of a client being seen at a clinic.

| Health History | Nurses' Notes | Provider Notes | Laboratory Results |

1800: A 50-year-old client presents to the clinic with complaints of joint pain, which have interfered with the daily walking of her dog. Client reports morning stiffness and some painful, red bumps on her hands. The client is obese and has been on a low-calorie diet to lose weight since she was diagnosed with type 2 diabetes.

- Temperature: 99.8°F (37.7°C)
- BP: 142/88 mm Hg
- Heart rate: 74 bpm and regular
- Respirations: 18 breaths/min
- SpO2: 98% on room air

For each client finding, use an X to specify whether the finding is consistent with the disease process of rheumatoid arthritis or osteoarthritis. Each finding may support more than one disease process.

CLIENT FINDING	RHEUMATOID ARTHRITIS	OSTEOARTHRITIS
Unilateral joint pain		X
Affects primarily the upper extremities	X	
Morning stiffness	X	X
Heberden and Bouchard nodes on hands		X
Obesity		X
Low grade fever	X	
Joint deformity – Boutonniere and swan neck	X	
Joint pain improves with activity	X	

Client Needs: Physiological Integrity/Physiological Adaptation
Clinical Judgment/Cognitive Skill: Analyze Cues
Item Type: Matrix Multiple Response
Rationale & Test Taking Strategy: Osteoarthritis (OA) is the progressive deterioration and loss of articular (joint) cartilage and bone in one or more joints. OA is a nonsystemic condition characterized by joint pain, which may be unilateral or involve a single joint, usually affecting weight-bearing joints (e.g., spine, hips, and knees). With OA there is transient stiffness in the morning and after sitting that tends to lessen 10 to 15 minutes after joint movement. Joint pain is relieved after rest or sleep and worsens with activity. Although OA is not typically a bilateral, symmetric disease, Heberden and Bouchard large bony nodes appear on both hands, especially in women. The nodes may be painful and red. Rheumatoid arthritis (RA) is a chronic, progressive, systemic (may affect other areas of the body besides the joints), inflammatory autoimmune disease process that affects primarily the synovial joints and usually affects the upper extremities first. Clients with RA have morning stiffness, which may last several hours, and the joint pain improves with activity. Boutonniere deformity and swan-neck deformity are common joint deformities of the hand in RA.

12. A 62-year-old client is scheduled for a below-the-knee amputation of the left leg due to a necrotic diabetic foot ulcer. The client has poorly controlled type 2 diabetes, history of sleep apnea, and hypertension and smokes two packs/day. Following surgery, the client has a rigid plaster dressing and immediate prosthetic fitting.

Select the anticipated orders from each of the following categories.

CATEGORY	ORDERS
Monitoring	☐ Insert a urinary catheter and monitor hourly output ☐ Elevate the residual limb for 24 to 48 hours ☐ Empty wound drainage system every 1 to 2 hours
Medications	☐ Analgesic ☐ Antibiotic ☐ Diuretic
Physical therapy	☐ Muscle-strengthening exercises ☐ Rewrap the residual limb every 1 to 2 days ☐ Limit range-of-motion exercises

Client Needs: Physiological Integrity/Physiological Adaptation
Clinical Judgment/Cognitive Skill: Generate Solutions
Item Type: Extended multiple response: Multiple Response Grouping
Rationale & Test Taking Strategy: Clients with diabetes, especially poorly controlled, are more susceptible to injury and tissue failure (i.e., necrotic skin ulcers), which leads to compromised healing. The client with a below-the-knee amputation (BKA) will need to have the residual limb elevated for 24 to 48 hours to prevent edema and hemorrhage. Following this early postoperative period, the client should lie prone for 20 to 30 minutes every 3 to 4 hours to prevent hip contracture until the client is able to be up and about at regular intervals. The residual limb should be extended. Clients with BKA are better able to begin early walking

and weight-bearing exercises than those whose limb has been amputated above the knee. The residual limb should be rewrapped several times a day with an elastic bandage applied in a figure-eight manner. Usually, the rigid dressing is removable to monitor for bleeding and drainage. Pain medication and prophylactic antibiotics would be ordered. The client will have a wound drainage system, which needs monitoring every 1 to 2 hours following surgery and range-of-motion exercises are performed regularly to prevent complications of immobility and loss of function. Diuretics and monitoring urine output are not key priorities for this client.

CHAPTER EIGHTEEN

Reproductive Care of Adult Clients

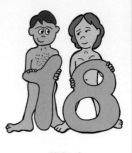

CHAPTER 18
REPRODUCTIVE

PHYSIOLOGY OF THE REPRODUCTIVE SYSTEM

Male Reproductive System

A. Penis: serves both reproductive and urinary function.
B. Scrotum: a double pouch of skin that protects the testes and sperm by maintaining temperature lower than that of the body.
C. Testes (gonads): sperm formation and production of testosterone occur here.
D. Epididymis: a tubular, coiled segment of the spermatic duct that stores spermatozoa until they are mature and then transports sperm from the testis to the vas deferens.
E. Prostate gland: produces a slightly alkalotic substance that provides both nourishment and mobility for spermatozoa.
F. Semen.
   1. Alkaline pH: 7.2 to 7.4.
   2. Average volume of ejaculate: 2.5 to 4 mL; may vary from 1 to 10 mL.
   3. Sterility: sperm count less than 20 million/mL (normal sperm count ~100 million/mL).

Female Reproductive System

A. Vagina: a thin-walled, muscular membranous canal that has the ability to dilate and contract to facilitate giving birth and the act of intercourse.
B. Cervix: lower portion of the uterus that protrudes into the vagina.
   1. Provides an alkaline environment to shelter sperm from the acidic vagina.
   2. Cervical mucus pH increases (alkaline) and becomes clear and more viscous at ovulation, similar to egg-white consistency.
C. Uterus: a hollow, pear-shaped, muscular pelvic organ; endometrium is the inner mucosal lining; undergoes cyclic changes as a result of hormonal levels.
D. Fallopian tubes: act to extract an ovum from the ovaries each month; if fertilization occurs, this takes place in the outer third of the fallopian tube.
E. Ovaries: located behind and below the fallopian tubes; produce ova, estrogen, and progesterone.
F. Breasts: function as an organ of sexual stimulation; nipple acts as a conduit for the flow of milk during breastfeeding.
G. Menstrual cycle (Box 18.1).

H. Menopause – time when menstruation stops; most often after age 45.
   1. Occurs when a woman has no menstrual period for 12 months and is no longer able to become pregnant.
   2. Common symptoms (Fig. 18.1).
   3. Hormone replacement therapy (Appendix 18.1).

System Assessment: Recognize Cues

A. Female assessment.
   1. Obtain history data related to sexual activity, sexually transmitted infections (STIs), pregnancies, surgeries, menstrual cycle, breast abnormalities, urinary symptoms, or pain.
      a. Assess for vulvar discharge, erythema, growths, or pain.
      b. Assess breasts for lumps/masses, nipple abnormalities, or changes in the skin.
      c. Pelvic examination with Pap smear should be performed at least yearly.
      d. Breast self-examination (BSE) should be performed by patient monthly, beginning at onset of puberty.
      e. Mammogram should be performed yearly beginning at 30 years of age or earlier if considered high risk.
         (1) Women between 40 and 44 years of age at average risk have the option to start screening with a mammogram every year.
         (2) Women 45 to 54 at average risk should get mammograms every year.
         (3) Women 55 and older at average risk can switch to a mammogram every other year, or they can choose to continue yearly mammograms. Screening should continue as long as a woman is in good health and is expected to live at least 10 more years.
B. Male assessment.
   1. Obtain history data related to sexual activity, STIs, erectile dysfunction (ED), urinary symptoms, surgeries, or pain.
   2. Assess penis, scrotum, and testicles for growths, masses, or ulcers.
      a. Testicular self-examination should be performed by the patient monthly beginning with onset of puberty.

467

Box 18.1 FEMALE REPRODUCTIVE CYCLE

Ovarian Cycle

- *Follicular phase:* first 14 days of a 28-day cycle
  - Follicle-stimulating hormone (FSH) and luteinizing hormone (LH) stimulate the maturation of ova in preparation for fertilization.
  - Estrogen peaks when ovulation occurs, typically about 14 days before the next menstrual period.
  - Body temperature drops and then rises by 0.5°-1°F around the time of ovulation.
- *Luteal phase:* days 15 to 28 of a 28-day cycle
  - LH and progesterone are the primary hormones released.
  - The uterus prepares for possible implantation of a fertilized ovum.
  - If fertilization and implantation do not occur, the endometrial lining of the uterus will degrade and be shed during menstruation, and the cycle begins again.

Menstrual Cycle

- Phase I: Menstrual Phase
  - 2-5 days of bleeding.
  - Endometrium sloughs away as menstrual flow begins.
  - Decreased secretion of progesterone and estrogen.
  - New follicle starts to mature.
- Phase II: Proliferative Phase
  - Lasts about 9 days.
  - Follicle grows and egg matures.
  - Estrogen increases and stimulates the endometrium to return to normal state and begin to thicken.
- Phase III: Ovulatory Phase
  - Ovulation (follicle ruptures and releases the egg) occurs 14 days before menses.
  - If pregnancy does not occur, the thickened tissue on the endometrium of the uterus is sloughed off because of the drop in progesterone and estrogen leading to the menstrual "period" or menses.
- Phase IV: Secretory Phase
  - Days 15 to 28
  - Corpus luteum secretes progesterone.
  - Endometrium continues to thicken in response to estrogen and progesterone.
  - Uterus prepares to receive fertilized ovum.

  b. Digital rectal examination (DRE) and prostate-specific antigen (PSA) should be performed yearly beginning at 50 years of age or earlier if considered high risk.

DISORDERS OF THE MALE REPRODUCTIVE SYSTEM

Prostate Disorders

Benign prostatic hyperplasia (BPH) **or hypertrophy: enlargement of prostate gland tissue.**

Cancer of the prostate: **a malignancy of the prostate gland.**

Both conditions encroach on the urethra and decrease the diameter of the bladder opening. Both can eventually cause bladder obstruction.

MENOPAUSE

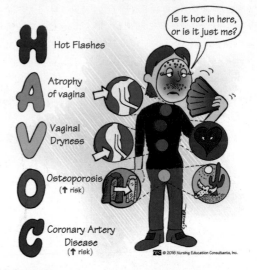

FIG. 18.1 Menopause. (From Zerwekh J, Garneau A, Miller CJ. [2017]. *Digital collection of the memory notebooks of nursing.* [4th ed.]. Chandler, AZ: Nursing Education Consultants, Inc.)

Assessment: Recognize Cues

A. Risk factors/etiology.
   1. BPH: very common in men older than 50 years.
   2. Prostatic carcinoma: rarely found in men younger than 60 years; usually found in the posterior lobe of the prostate gland.
B. Clinical manifestations.
   1. Common to both disorders.
      a. Bladder outlet obstruction.
         (1) Urinary hesitancy, frequency, urgency, and dribbling.
         (2) Nocturia, hematuria, urinary retention, and a sensation of incomplete emptying of the bladder.
         (3) Urinary retention may cause overflow urinary incontinence and dribbling after voiding.
      b. Acute retention may cause hydroureter and pressure in the kidney.
      c. Increased incidence of urinary tract infection (UTI) caused by residual urine.
   2. Prostatic cancer.
      a. Tumor grows slowly and is confined to capsule; therefore, prostate may appear normal, thus delaying the diagnosis.
      b. On DRE, asymmetric prostatic enlargement; prostate is described as "stony hard" and fixed.
      c. Obstruction is rare unless BPH is also present.
      d. Pain in the lumbosacral area may be presenting symptom as a result of metastasis.
C. Diagnostics.
   1. DRE.
   2. Cystoscopy and bladder scan.
   3. Urinalysis with culture and sensitivity.
   4. Transrectal and/or transabdominal ultrasound.

5. To rule out or diagnose cancer.
   a. Prostate-specific antigen (normal PSA 0-4 mcg/L or ng/mL).
   b. Tumor markers for diagnosis, staging, and monitoring progress.
   c. Needle biopsy of prostate; definitive test for diagnosing cancer.

D. Complications.
   1. BPH.
      a. Preoperative.
         (1) UTI, hematuria.
         (2) Acute urinary retention.
         (3) Hydroureter (distention of the ureter) and hydronephrosis (enlargement of kidney caused by postrenal obstruction) with resultant kidney failure.
         (4) Bladder stones.
      b. Postoperative.
         (1) Hemorrhage: especially in the first 24 hrs.
         (2) Urinary incontinence, bladder spasms.
         (3) Retrograde ejaculation: semen is passed back into the bladder rather than out through the penis. This causes milky or cloudy urine.
         (4) Infection.

> **!** **NURSING PRIORITY** Assess all male clients older than 50 years for symptoms of BPH. BPH occurs in 80% of men older than 80 years.

   2. Prostatic cancer.
      a. Preoperative.
         (1) Complications are similar to BPH.
         (2) Cancer may spread via the perineal lymphatic system to the regional lymph nodes. May metastasize to the pelvic bones, bladder, lungs, and liver.
      b. Postoperative.
         (1) Increased problems with deep venous thrombosis caused by lithotomy position during open perineal resection.
         (2) Change in sexual functioning: impotence and failure to ejaculate.
         (3) Urinary incontinence/dribbling.

Analyze Cues and Prioritize Hypotheses

The most important problems are urinary retention resulting from bladder outlet obstruction, overflow urinary incontinence, possible sexual dysfunction, and decreased self-esteem because of BPH. For prostate cancer, the potential for metastasis increases with delayed/inadequate treatment.

Generate Solutions

Treatment
A. Medical.
   1. BPH: 5-alpha-reductase inhibitors and alpha-adrenergic blockers to shrink prostatic tissue (Appendix 18.1).

   2. "Watchful waiting" when there are mild symptoms may include decreasing caffeine intake, avoiding decongestants and anticholinergics, and restricting fluid intake.
   3. Prostate cancer: radiation, hormonal therapy, and chemotherapy for malignancy.
B. Surgical: size of prostate, presence of malignancy, and general health dictate the type of surgery.
   1. Transurethral resection of the prostate (TURP): removal of prostatic tissue via a resectoscope, which is passed through the urethra (Fig. 18.2).
   2. Transurethral incision of the prostate (TUIP): making transurethral slits or incisions into prostate to relieve obstruction; effective with minimally enlarged prostate (BPH); indicated for clients who are poor surgical candidates.
   3. Transurethral microwave therapy (TUMT) and transurethral needle ablation (TUNA): microwaves are delivered directly to the prostate; heat causes necrosis of tissue; both procedures are done on an outpatient basis.
   4. Internal radiation therapy (brachytherapy) involves the placement of tiny radioactive "seeds" into the prostate for treatment of cancer.
   5. Hormone therapy (antiandrogen medications – leuprorelin): depriving the cancer cells of testosterone may help slow the growth of prostatic cancer.
   6. Cryotherapy (cryoablation): liquid nitrogen is applied to the prostate via a transrectal ultrasound probe; dead cells are absorbed by the body.
   7. Prostatectomy: removal of the prostate via suprapubic, retropubic, or perineal approach; may be done by incision or laparoscopically; most often for removal of malignancy; robotic-assisted surgery used most frequently (less bleeding and pain and faster recovery).

Nursing Interventions: Take Action

Goal: To promote elimination, treat UTI, and provide client education (Box 18.2).

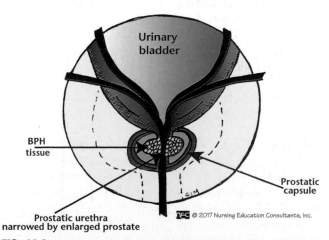

FIG. 18.2 Benign Prostatic Hypertrophy. (From Zerwekh J, Garneau A, Miller CJ. [2017]. *Digital collection of the memory notebooks of nursing.* [4th ed.]. Chandler, AZ: Nursing Education Consultants, Inc.)

Benign Prostatic Hypertrophy
General

- All men older than 50 years of age should be assessed for urinary retention and adequacy of bladder emptying.
- Increased problem with urinary stasis; increased straining to urinate; increased incidence of infections.

After surgery

- Closely evaluate for presence of infection, especially urinary tract and respiratory.
- Assess fluid balance; confusion and agitation may be symptoms of fluid overload.
- Help the client ambulate as soon as possible – increased risk for pooling of blood in pelvic cavity and pulmonary emboli from immobility.
- Client is at increased risk for falls.
- Determine psychological response to physical stress (confusion, disorientation); orient to surroundings frequently.

A. Evaluate adequacy of voiding and presence of urinary retention and infection.

B. Teach client to avoid bladder distention, which results in loss of muscle tone.
   1. Do not postpone the urge to void; it is important to prevent overdistention of the bladder, which further complicates the problem.
   2. Avoid drinking a large amount of fluid in a short period.
   3. Avoid alcohol and caffeine products because of their diuretic effect.

C. Encourage annual DRE of the prostate for all men older than 50 years, or earlier if at high risk.

D. Examination is recommended every 6 months for clients who have BPH or who have had a prostatectomy.

Goal: To maintain closed irrigation after surgery in the client who has undergone TURP or suprapubic prostatectomy (Fig. 18.3).

A. Continuous bladder irrigation (CBI) with sterile, antibacterial isotonic irrigating solution (also referred to as a Murphy drip or closed bladder irrigation).
   1. CBI is done with a triple-lumen catheter: one lumen for inflating the balloon (30-50 mL water), one for maintaining outflow of urine, and one for the instillation of the continuous irrigating solution.
   2. Provides continuous irrigation to prevent bleeding and to flush the bladder of tissue and clots after TURP.
   3. If clots occur, the catheter may be irrigated, or the rate of flow may be increased until the drainage outflow clears.
   4. Calculate intake and output carefully; amount of bladder irrigation fluid must be subtracted from total output to determine client's true urinary output.
   5. Monitor/titrate CBI so the outflow is light pink without clots; notify surgeon of any increase in bleeding.

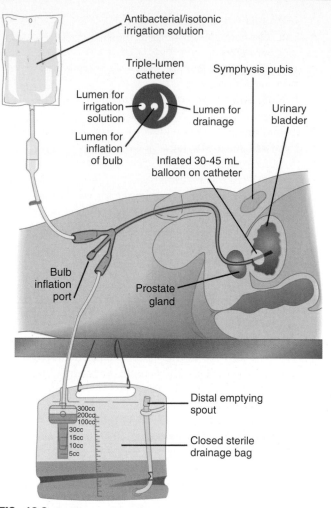

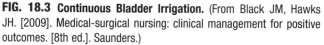

FIG. 18.3 Continuous Bladder Irrigation. (From Black JM, Hawks JH. [2009]. Medical-surgical nursing: clinical management for positive outcomes. [8th ed.]. Saunders.)

   6. If catheter is occluded and does not drain properly, turn off the CBI until catheter patency is reestablished. *Notify registered nurse (RN) immediately.*

B. Blood clots and tissue are normal for the first 24 hrs after TURP.

C. If client has excessive bleeding, the health care provider may increase the size of the balloon on the indwelling catheter and put traction on the catheter to compress the area of bleeding.

D. Client should void within 6 hrs of catheter removal.

> **❗ NURSING PRIORITY** Maintain CBI for the client who has undergone TURP; prevent overdistention of the bladder. If client complains of pain, check the urinary drainage and make sure it is patent. Obstruction most commonly occurs in the first 24 hrs because of clots in the bladder. Monitor for irrigation fluid being overabsorbed with signs and symptoms of headache, dizziness, shortness of breath, hypertension, bradycardia, and change in the level of consciousness. *Notify RN or surgeon immediately.*

E. Bladder spasms: belladonna and opium suppositories or antispasmodics are administered as needed; spasms often occur because of the presence of clots in the catheter; check the catheter for patency.

F. The sensation of a full bladder is common while irrigation is occurring. Client may require frequent explanation regarding the irrigation. Advise the client to avoid bearing down in an attempt to void.

Goal: To provide postoperative care (Fig. 18.4).

A. After client is ambulatory, encourage walking rather than sitting or lying for prolonged periods.

B. Teach client exercises to control urinary stream and maintain continence.
   1. Have client contract perineal muscles (Kegel exercises) by squeezing buttocks together.
   2. Instruct client to practice starting and stopping the stream several times while voiding.

C. Provide an opportunity for open discussion of sexual concerns. Retrograde ejaculation or ED may occur as a result of nerve damage during surgery.

D. Dribbling after voiding is a common problem that often subsides within a few weeks.

E. Teach client to avoid straining during bowel movement; encourage diet high in fiber and administer stool softeners as needed.

F. Discuss with client the importance of maintaining a high fluid intake to prevent UTIs.

G. Encourage client to minimize use of caffeine-containing products, which may cause bladder spasms.

Goal: To provide postoperative care for a client after radical open prostatectomy.

A. Maintain adequate pain control, frequently with patient-controlled analgesia.

B. As a result of the surgical position and postoperative immobility, client is at high risk for venous thromboembolism (VTE).
   1. Monitor sequential compression devices.
   2. Apply antiembolism stockings.
   3. Administer low-dose prophylactic anticoagulant therapy.
   4. Monitor prothrombin time/international normalized ratio (PT/INR) while client is on anticoagulants. Instruct client/family regarding bleeding precautions.

TEST ALERT Identify symptoms of VTE.

C. Perineal prostatectomy and total prostatectomy for cancer frequently result in ED and urinary incontinence caused by damage to the pudendal nerves.

D. Emphasize importance of not straining against catheter to relieve bladder pressure.

E. Evaluate for urinary retention.

! NURSING PRIORITY Explain procedure to client and family. It is important to clarify for the client the information the doctor gives them; however, it is the doctor's responsibility to advise the client regarding any complications they may experience with sexual functioning.

Home Care

A. Teach client how to care for catheter and relieve obstruction if discharged with urinary catheter in place.

B. Avoid use of suppositories and enemas.

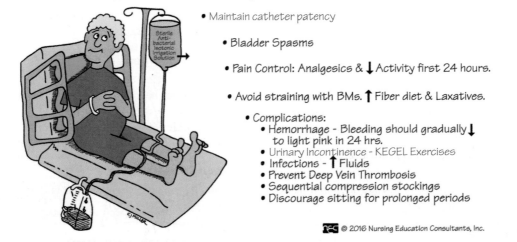

TURP
(Transurethral Resection of the Prostate)

• Continuous or Intermittent Bladder Irrigation (CBI)
  (Usually discontinued after 24 hrs, if no clots.)   Murphy Drip

• Close observation of drainage system—
  (↑ Bladder distention causes pain & bleeding.)

• Maintain catheter patency

• Bladder Spasms

• Pain Control: Analgesics & ↓ Activity first 24 hours.

• Avoid straining with BMs. ↑ Fiber diet & Laxatives.

• Complications:
  • Hemorrhage - Bleeding should gradually ↓ to light pink in 24 hrs.
  • Urinary Incontinence - KEGEL Exercises
  • Infections - ↑ Fluids
  • Prevent Deep Vein Thrombosis
  • Sequential compression stockings
  • Discourage sitting for prolonged periods

© 2016 Nursing Education Consultants, Inc.

FIG. 18.4 Transurethral Resection of the Prostate. (From Zerwekh J, Garneau A, Miller CJ. [2017]. *Digital collection of the memory notebooks of nursing.* [4th ed.]. Chandler, AZ: Nursing Education Consultants, Inc.)

Nursing Interventions: Take Action

Goal: To prevent wound infection and pressure on the vaginal suture line after surgery.

A. Preoperative teaching.
B. Postoperative period.
   1. Prevent wound infection.
   2. Apply ice pack locally to relieve perineal discomfort and swelling.
   3. Indwelling catheter for 4 days after anterior colporrhaphy.
   4. Monitor for excessive vaginal bleeding.
   5. Teach Kegel exercises.
C. Frequent perineal care in addition to care after each voiding or defecation.

Home Care (postoperative)

A. Encourage use of stool softeners to prevent straining.
B. Prevent constipation.
C. Certain activities are restricted until area has healed: lifting objects heavier than 5 lb, intercourse, and prolonged standing, walking, and sitting.
D. Call the doctor if there is persistent pain or purulent, foul-smelling vaginal discharge.
E. Teach catheter care if client is discharged with urinary catheter.

Vaginal Inflammatory Conditions

Assessment: Recognize Cues

A. Common predisposing factors.
   1. Excessive douching.
   2. Oral contraceptives, steroids.
   3. Antibiotics: especially broad spectrum, which wipe out normal vaginal flora (vagina is protected by an acidic pH and the presence of *Döderlein bacilli*).
   4. Improper cleaning after voiding and defecating.
   5. Assess for recurrent chronic infection; there may be an underlying condition (prediabetic state, HIV infection) that should be further evaluated.
B. Bacterial vaginosis.
   1. Characteristics.
      a. Causative organisms: *E. coli*, *Haemophilus vaginalis*, and *Gardnerella vaginalis*.
      b. Profuse watery discharge, "fishy smell."
      c. Itching, redness, burning, and edema, which are exacerbated by voiding and defecation.
   2. Treatment: metronidazole.
   3. Complications: bacterial vaginosis may increase susceptibility to STIs and HIV infection if woman is exposed to either.
   4. Factors associated with bacterial vaginosis include multiple sex partners but may occur in non-sexually active women; associated with douching and smoking.
   5. Sexual partners do not have to be treated, as the infection is caused by a change in normal vaginal flora and not considered a STI.

C. Candidiasis.
   1. Characteristics.
      a. Organism: *Candida albicans* (fungus).
      b. Internal itching, beefy red irritation, and inflammation of vaginal epithelium.
      c. White, cheese-like, odorless discharge that clings to the vaginal mucosa.
      d. Occurs frequently and is difficult to cure.
      e. Increased risk in women with diabetes and women taking birth control pills, during pregnancy, and after treatment with antibiotics.
      f. Clients with recurrent candidiasis vaginitis should be offered HIV testing, especially if unresponsive to first-line treatment.
      g. Is not considered an STI.
   2. Treatment: metronidazole or tinidazole.
D. Trichomoniasis.
   1. Characteristics.
      a. Organism: *Trichomonas vaginalis* (protozoan).
      b. May be asymptomatic.
      c. Itching, burning, dyspareunia (painful intercourse).
      d. Frothy, green-yellow, copious, malodorous vaginal discharge; strawberry spot (petechiae) on cervix.
      e. Sexual partners must be treated also because of cross infection; men are usually asymptomatic.
   2. Treatment: antibacterial/antiprotozoal medication.
   3. Prevention: avoid extended time in synthetic or tight-fitting undergarments; use of condoms may reduce incidence of STIs.
E. Postmenopausal vaginitis (atrophic vaginitis).
   1. Characteristics.
      a. Lack of estrogen (this is also the cause).
      b. Itching and burning.
      c. Loss of vaginal tissue folds and epithelial covering.
   2. Treatment: estrogen vaginal cream or tablet insert.

Analyze Cues and Prioritize Hypotheses

The most important problems are infection (and cross infection with sexual partner), relief of vaginal discomfort, and potential for sterility if infection goes untreated.

Nursing Interventions: Take Action

Goal: To teach client to prevent infection by performing appropriate personal hygiene, decrease inflammation, and promote comfort.

A. Appropriate cleansing from front of vulva to back of perineal area.
B. Client should not douche; douching removes normal protective bacteria from vaginal cavity and introduces other bacteria.
C. If infection is chronic, it may be necessary to have sexual partner tested and treated; partner may be reinfecting the woman.
D. Discourage use of feminine hygiene sprays, as they cause increased irritation.
E. Discourage client from wearing constricting clothing and synthetic underwear (encourage use of cotton underwear).

Goal: To educate the woman regarding correct use of medication.

A. Vaginal tablets and creams are often used.
  1. Handwashing before and after insertion of suppository or application of cream.
  2. Remain recumbent for 30 mins after application to promote absorption and prevent loss of the medication from the vaginal area.
  3. Wear a perineal pad to prevent soiling of clothing with vaginal drainage.

Abnormal (dysfunctional) Uterine Bleeding

Bleeding that is excessive or abnormal in amount or frequency without regard to systemic conditions; occurs when the hormonal events responsible for balance of the client's cycle are interrupted.

Assessment: Recognize Cues

A. Amenorrhea.
  1. Absence of menses.
    a. Primary: no menstruation has occurred by age 16.
    b. Secondary: woman previously had menses.
  2. May be indicative of menopause.
  3. May be first indication of pregnancy.
  4. Occurs when woman has lost a critical percentage of fat (e.g., athletes, clients with anorexia).
B. Menorrhagia.
  1. Excessive vaginal bleeding.
  2. Single episode of heavy bleeding may indicate a spontaneous abortion.
  3. May be associated with an intrauterine device (IUD), hypothyroidism, uterine fibroids, or hormone imbalance.
C. Metrorrhagia.
  1. Vaginal bleeding between periods.
  2. May be normal menopause.
  3. Ectopic pregnancy.
  4. Breakthrough bleeding from oral contraceptives or IUD.
  5. Cervical polyps.

> **! NURSING PRIORITY** Vaginal bleeding after menopause or surgical hysterectomy is a symptom of a problem that needs to be evaluated.

Analyze Cues and Prioritize Hypotheses

The most important problems are excess bleeding, anemia, and potential for cancer of the reproductive tract.

Nursing Interventions: Take Action

Goal: To help client manage bleeding episodes.
A. Help determine cause of problem.
B. Report excessive bleeding, abdominal pain, fever.
C. Treatment.
  1. Dilation and curettage (D&C) for diagnostic purposes in older women.

2. Endometrial ablation (balloon thermotherapy).
3. Removal of fibroids.
  a. Often done on outpatient basis with either general, regional, or local anesthesia.
  b. Spotting and vaginal drainage are common for several days; if amount is more than a normal period or if it lasts longer than 2 weeks, client should call the doctor.
  c. Client should report any signs of infection: fever; foul, purulent discharge; increasing abdominal pain.
  d. NSAIDs are often used for pain control.
  e. Client should avoid sexual intercourse and use of tampons for about 2 weeks.
D. Assess and treat for anemia.
  1. Encourage diet high in iron.
  2. Administer iron preparations if required.

Endometriosis

Endometriosis **is the presence of endometrial tissue outside of the uterus. The tissue responds to hormonal stimulation by bleeding into areas within the pelvis, causing pain and adhesions.**

Assessment: Recognize Cues

A. Risk factors/etiology.
  1. Cause not fully understood.
  2. Most common in women in their late 20s and early 30s who have never been pregnant.
B. Clinical manifestations.
  1. Dysmenorrhea: deep seated aching pain in the lower abdomen, vagina, posterior pelvis, and back occurring 1 to 2 days before menses.
  2. Abnormal excessive uterine bleeding and dyspareunia; painful defecation.
C. Diagnostics.
  1. Laparoscopy.
  2. Ultrasonography.
D. Complications.
  1. Infertility, adhesions, bowel obstruction.

Analyze Cues and Prioritize Hypotheses

The most important problems are menstrual discomfort, excess menstrual bleeding, and potential for sterility.

Generate Solutions
Treatment
A. Medical.
  1. Androgenic agents may be given over a 6- to 8-month period.
  2. Oral contraceptives.
  3. Condition recedes during pregnancy.
B. Surgical.
  1. Laser treatment of endometrial tissue in the extra-uterine sites.
  2. Hysterectomy (usually carried out in women close to menopause).

Nursing Interventions: Take Action

Goal: To help client minimize the pain and discomfort associated with endometriosis.

A. Warm baths or moist heat packs may reduce discomfort.

B. Encourage client to explore alternative sexual positions that may minimize discomfort during intercourse.

C. Encourage client to discuss abstinence with partner if intercourse is painful.

Goal: To help client understand measures to maintain health.

A. Teach client about disease process; clarify any false ideas.

B. Provide emotional reassurance; discuss potential for infertility.

Pelvic Inflammatory Disease

Pelvic inflammatory disease (PID) **is an infectious condition of the pelvic cavity that involves the fallopian tubes, ovaries, and/or peritoneum.**

Assessment: Recognize Cues

A. Risk factors/etiology.
  1. Complication of gonorrhea and *C. trachomatis*.
  2. IUDs are correlated with an increased incidence of PID.
  3. Increased number of sexual partners.
  4. Increases risk for repeat cases after previous episode of PID.
B. Clinical manifestations.
  1. Lower abdominal pain that worsens over time.
  2. General malaise, fever, chills, nausea, and vomiting.
  3. Pain on urinating and with intercourse.
  4. Vaginal discharge that is heavy and purulent.
  5. Chronic PID: persistent pelvic pain, secondary dysmenorrhea, dysfunctional uterine bleeding, and periodic episodes of acute symptoms.
C. Diagnostics.
  1. Culture and sensitivity of drainage from the vagina or cervix.
  2. Ultrasonography, laparoscopy.
D. Complications.
  1. Sterility caused by adhesions and strictures within the fallopian tubes.
  2. Ectopic pregnancy.
  3. Pelvic abscess or peritonitis.
  4. Septic shock.

Analyze Cues and Prioritize Hypotheses

The most important problems are pelvic infection caused by sexually transmitted pathogens and, if not treated, the risk of sterility.

Generate Solutions

Treatment

A. Medical: broad-spectrum antibiotics, analgesics.

B. Surgical: incision and drainage of abscesses with or without a laparotomy.

Nursing Interventions: Take Action

Goal: To prevent the spread and extension of the infection.

A. Maintain semi-Fowler position to promote drainage of the pelvic cavity by gravity.

B. Strict medical asepsis when in contact with discharge; wound and skin precautions.

C. Encourage oral fluids and maintain adequate nutrition.

D. Client should avoid sexual activity during therapy and avoid douching at all times.

E. Strongly encourage sexual partner or partners to seek medical treatment.

Uterine Leiomyoma

Leiomyomas, **also called fibroids or myomas, are very commonly found in women. These are benign, slow-growing solid tumors of the uterine myometrium (muscle layer).**

Assessment: Recognize Cues

A. Risk factors/etiology.
  1. Peak incidence in early 40 s.
  2. More prevalent in black women.
B. Clinical manifestations.
  1. Heavy vaginal bleeding.
  2. Possible pain and dyspareunia (painful intercourse).
  3. Constipation and urinary frequency and/or retention.
C. Diagnostics.
  1. Low hematocrit.
  2. Test thyroid-stimulating hormone (TSH) to rule-out hypothyroidism.
  3. Transvaginal ultrasonography.
D. Complications.
  1. Hemorrhage.
  2. Postoperative infection.

Analyze Cues and Prioritize Hypotheses

The most important problems are prolonged or heavy bleeding as a result of fibroid growth (myoma).

Generate Solutions

Treatment

A. Uterine artery embolization, endometrial ablation, and hysterectomy are choices for women who no longer desire pregnancy.

B. Minimally invasive surgery (MIS) techniques, such as a myomectomy, to prevent removing the uterus. If not, a hysterectomy is the procedure of choice.

Nursing Interventions: Take Action

Goal: To provide self-management education.

A. Teach client about any activity restrictions, diet, sexual activity, wound care (if any), complications, the need for follow-up care, and the importance of reporting any of the following:
  1. Signs of infection at an incision site (redness, open areas, drainage that is thick or foul smelling.

2. Pain, tenderness, redness, or swelling in the calf muscles.

3. Pain or burning on urination.

B. With an *abdominal* hysterectomy, client may experience abdominal or shoulder discomfort because of the introduction of carbon dioxide gas during a *laparoscopic* procedure.

C. Teach patients who had a *vaginal* hysterectomy to promptly report to their surgeon excessive or increasing bleeding.

D. Teach client to report a fever over 100.4°F (38°C).

Cervical Cancer

Cancer of the uterine cervix, **which can invade the bladder, rectum, and other pelvic areas in an advanced stage.**

Assessment: Recognize Cues

A. Risk factors/etiology.
1. Multiple sex partners.
2. Early sexual activity.
3. History of STIs, herpes simplex virus type 2 (HSV-2).
4. Genital warts (human papillomavirus [HPV]-positive), abnormal Pap smears.

B. Clinical manifestations.
1. Clients are asymptomatic until late in disease stage.
2. Thin, watery drainage that becomes dark and foul smelling as the disease progresses.
3. Abnormal vaginal bleeding (spotting) or discharge.
4. Low back pain.
5. Painful sexual intercourse.

C. Diagnostics.
1. Pap smear.
   a. Initial Pap smear at age 21 or after first sexual intercourse.
   b. Pap smears are continued after menopause and hysterectomy.
   c. Research shows that testing for HPV may be better than the Pap test for cervical cancer screening.
2. Cervical biopsy.

!! NURSING PRIORITY If cancer of the cervix is identified before it becomes invasive (or in the in-situ stage), there is virtually a 100% cure rate.

Analyze Cues and Prioritize Hypotheses

The most important problems are the potential for metastasis of the cancer, loss of reproductive capacity, and impaired coping.

Generate Solutions

Treatment

A. Medical.
1. Prevention through regular screening and vaccination against HPV (Gardasil).
2. Radiation therapy, either internal (radium implant) or external for invasive cancer.

B. Surgical intervention. (Procedure depends on extent of the cancer.)
1. Conization (cryosurgery): used for carcinoma in situ.
2. Vaginal hysterectomy: removal of the uterus. Fallopian tubes and ovaries remain intact.
3. Hysterectomy: total abdominal hysterectomy with bilateral salpingo-oophorectomy (TAH-BSO); includes removal of fallopian tubes and ovaries.
4. Radical hysterectomy: a panhysterectomy plus a partial vaginectomy and removal of lymph nodes.
5. Pelvic exoneration: radical hysterectomy plus total vaginectomy, removal of bladder with urinary diversion, bowel resection, and colostomy.

Nursing Interventions: Take Action

Goal: Provide health teaching to help clients prevent and/or detect premalignant cervical dysplasia.

A. Warning signs of cancer.
B. Importance of yearly Pap smears.
C. Encourage verbalization of feelings related to the surgery and diagnosis of cancer.
D. Prevention with early immunization against HPV and safe sex education.
E. Prevention, early detection, and treatment of STIs.

Goal: To provide preoperative and postoperative teaching in preparation for a total abdominal hysterectomy.

A. General preoperative care.
B. After surgery, assess for complications, such as backache or decreased urine output, because these symptoms can indicate accidental ligation of the ureter.
C. Urinary retention may occur as a result of bladder atony and edema; explain to client the need for a urinary retention catheter.
D. Early ambulation is encouraged to prevent postoperative thrombophlebitis.
E. Determine whether hormone replacement therapy will be used and provide appropriate teaching.
F. If dyspareunia occurs, client should contact their health care provider.

Breast Cancer

The most common malignancy in females; second to lung cancer as a leading cause of cancer death in women in the United States.

Assessment: Recognize Cues

A. Risk factors/etiology.
1. Female gender.
2. The incidence of recurrence of breast cancer is significant.
3. Family history of breast cancer; however, 85% of women with breast cancer have a negative family history.
4. Inherited genetic abnormality *(BRCA1* gene).
5. Advancing age (postmenopausal).
6. Nulliparity or parity after the age of 30.
7. Early menses, late menopause.

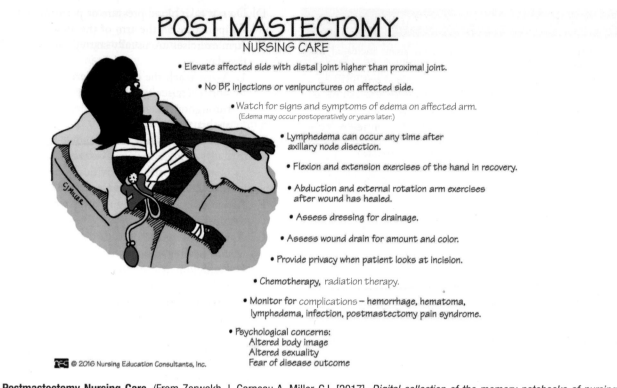

FIG. 18.6 Postmastectomy Nursing Care. (From Zerwekh J, Garneau A, Miller CJ. [2017]. *Digital collection of the memory notebooks of nursing.* [4th ed.]. Chandler, AZ: Nursing Education Consultants, Inc.)

the same or opposite sex; may also be transmitted via contaminated needles and in utero to a fetus.

2. One person can have more than one STI at a time.
3. All sexual partners need to be evaluated.

B. Nursing role is to recognize and provide factual information.
   1. Mode of transmission.
   2. Prevention of transmission.
   3. Importance of contacts being identified and treated.
   4. Information provided in an accepting, nonjudgmental manner.
   5. Oral contraceptives do not provide any protection.

C. Clients with STIs should be tested for HIV.

D. Hepatitis B and HPV are considered STIs.

> **! NURSING PRIORITY** Consider all oral, genital, and rectal lesions to contain pathologic organisms until otherwise documented.

📋 Syphilis

Syphilis **is caused by the spirochete** *Treponema pallidum,* **which is transmitted by direct contact with primary chancre lesion or body secretions (saliva, blood, vaginal discharge, semen) and transplacentally to the fetus.**

Assessment: Recognize Cues

A. Risk factors/etiology.
   1. Incubation period is 10 to 90 days, with an average of 20 to 30 days.

2. Highly infectious during the primary stage. Blood contains the spirochete during the secondary stage; usually noninfectious after 1 year during the latent stage; noninfectious in the late (tertiary) stage.

B. Clinical manifestations.
   1. Primary stage.
      a. Chancre: small, hard, painless lesion found on the penis, vulva, lips, vagina, or rectum.
      b. Usually heals spontaneously within 2 to 3 weeks with or without treatment.
      c. Highly contagious during this stage.
      d. Will progress without treatment.
   2. Secondary stage.
      a. Usually begins anywhere from 2 weeks to 6 months after the initial chancre has healed.
      b. May be asymptomatic or may have maculopapular rash on the palms of the hands and soles of the feet, sore throat, and headache; gray mucous patches in the mouth.
      c. Symptoms disappear within 2 to 6 weeks.
   3. Latent stage.
      a. Absence of clinical symptoms.
      b. Noninfectious after 1 year in the latent stage.
      c. Results of serologic tests for syphilis remain positive.
      d. Transmission can occur through blood contact.
      e. Majority of clients remain in this stage without further symptoms.
   4. Tertiary stage.
      a. Gummas: chronic, destructive lesions may develop in skin, bone, and liver.

b. Neurologic problems from mild personality changes to tremors and major psychoses.

5. Congenital syphilis.
   a. Maculopapular rash over face, genital region, palms, and soles.
   b. Snuffles: a mucopurulent nasal discharge indicative of some degree of respiratory obstruction.
   c. After the age of 2 years, Hutchinson teeth appear. These are notched central incisors with deformed molars and cusps.

C. Diagnostics.
   1. Serologic screening: Venereal Disease Research Laboratories (VDRL).
   2. Rapid plasma reagin test (PRP and RPR) may produce false-negative results in early stages.
   3. Fluorescent treponemal antibody absorption (FTA-ABS) test.
   4. *T. pallidum* particle agglutination (TP-PA) test.
   5. The FTA-ABs and TP-PA tests are used to confirm the diagnosis of syphilis. The VDRL and RPR tests are used for screening purposes.

Analyze Cues and Prioritize Hypotheses

The most important problems are transmission of infection to sexual partners, transplacental to fetus, and potential for long-term neurologic and cardiovascular complications if the infection is left untreated.

Generate Solutions

Treatment

A. Medical.
   1. Penicillin G or aqueous procaine penicillin G.
   2. May use tetracycline or doxycycline if allergic to penicillin.

Nursing Interventions: Take Action

Goal: To treat and prevent the spread of infection and educate client.

A. If a pregnant woman is treated before 18 weeks' gestation, the fetus will usually be born unaffected.

B. Education regarding means of transmission, prevention, and treatment.

C. Adequate case finding and treatment of contacts. All sexual contacts should be contacted and treated within 90 days.

D. Mandatory reporting to local public health authorities.

Gonorrhea

An STI that may also affect the rectum, pharynx, and eyes. Caused by the bacterium *Neisseria gonorrhoeae* and transmitted by direct contact with exudate via sexual contact or to the neonate during passage through the birth canal.

Assessment: Recognize Cues

A. Risk factors/etiology.
   1. Incubation period is 3 to 7 days.
   2. Contagious as long as organism is present.

B. Clinical manifestations.
   1. In men.
      a. Urethritis, epididymitis, dysuria, and purulent urethral discharge.
      b. Increased evidence of asymptomatic disease or a chronic carrier state in males.
   2. In women.
      a. Initial urethritis or cervicitis that is often mild enough to remain undetected by client.
      b. Vulvovaginitis, vaginal discharge, dysuria.
   3. Both men and women experience arthralgias – joint pain from disseminated gonococcal infection (DGI).
   4. Neonates may develop ophthalmia neonatorum if eyes not treated at birth. Permanent blindness occurs without treatment.

C. Diagnostics.
   1. Nucleic acid amplification test (NAAT).
   2. Positive Gram stain smear of discharge or secretions (not as sensitive as other tests).
   3. Positive culture.

D. Complications.
   1. In men: prostatitis, urethral stricture, urethritis, and sterility.
   2. In women: PID, Bartholin abscess, ectopic pregnancy, infertility.

Analyze Cues and Prioritize Hypotheses

The most important problems are transmission of infection to sexual partners, transplacental to the fetus, discomfort, urethral and vaginal discharge, and the potential for infertility.

Generate Solutions

Treatment

A. Medical.
   1. Dual antibiotic therapy: IM ceftriaxone plus oral azithromycin.

Nursing Interventions: Take Action

Goal: To treat and prevent the spread of infection and educate client.

A. Prophylactic antibiotic treatment to the eye in all newborns to prevent ophthalmia neonatorum.

B. Encourage follow-up cultures at 4 to 7 days after treatment and again at 6 months.

C. Teach importance of abstinence from sexual intercourse until cultures are negative.

D. Urge client to inform sexual partner so that they may be treated for infection. All sexual partners should also be treated within 60 days of diagnosis.

E. Importance of taking the full course of antibiotics.

Genital Herpes

Genital herpes is a highly contagious infection caused primarily by the herpes simplex virus 2 (HSV-2) and characterized by recurrent outbreaks. Subsequent outbreaks are usually less severe than the original outbreak of lesions.

Appendix 18.1 MEDICATIONS USED IN REPRODUCTIVE SYSTEM DISORDERS

R

MEDICATIONS	SIDE EFFECTS	NURSING IMPLICATIONS

Benign Prostatic Hyperplasia: Medications decrease the size of the prostate or relax smooth muscle, therefore decreasing pressure on the urinary tract.

Alpha Adrenergic Antagonists

MEDICATIONS	SIDE EFFECTS	NURSING IMPLICATIONS
Doxazosin: PO Tamsulosin: PO Terazosin: PO Silodosin: PO Alfuzosin: PO *Note: all generic names end in "osin."*	Dizziness, fatigue, orthostatic hypotension, headaches, retrograde ejaculation, nasal stuffiness	1. Advise client of possible problems of decreased blood pressure and orthostatic hypotension, especially 30 min to 2 hrs after first dose (first dose syncope). 2. Prostatic cancer should be ruled out before medications are started. 3. Medication should decrease problems of urination associated with BPH. 4. Monitor blood pressure closely if taking antihypertensive medications. 5. Assess for urinary hesitancy, incomplete emptying of the bladder, decreased urinary stream, and urgency before and throughout therapy. 6. Administer at same time each day, 30 mins after the same meal. 7. Avoid grapefruit products.

5α-Reductase Inhibitors

MEDICATIONS	SIDE EFFECTS	NURSING IMPLICATIONS
Finasteride: PO Dutasteride: PO Dutasteride plus tamsulosin: PO	Erectile dysfunction, decreased libido, decreased ejaculation volume	1. Client should take contraceptive precautions or not have sexual intercourse with women who could become pregnant. 2. Women who are or may become pregnant should not handle the tablets. 3. Client should not donate blood within 6 months after drug administration to avoid possibility of women receiving medication via blood transfusion.

Antifungal/Protozoal Medications: Used to treat vaginal fungal infections.

MEDICATIONS	SIDE EFFECTS	NURSING IMPLICATIONS
Clotrimazole: intravaginally (OTC) Miconazole: intravaginally Fluconazole: PO Terconazole: intravaginally Metronidazole: PO *Note: all generic names end in "azole."*	Nausea, vomiting, headache, vaginal irritation	1. Creams are not recommended to be used with tampons or diaphragms. 2. Not recommended for use during pregnancy or lactation. 3. Metronidazole is used to treat trichomoniasis and bacterial vaginosis (BV); instruct client *to avoid alcohol* because it can lead to serious side effects of throbbing headaches, nausea, excessive vomiting, hyperventilation, and tachycardia. 4. Suppositories or applicators are used to place medication in the vagina. 5. If client does not see improvement within 3 days, they should return to their health care provider. 6. Fluconazole can be given orally as a single dose for vaginal candidiasis.

Hormone Replacement Therapy: For treatment of symptoms of menopause.

MEDICATIONS	SIDE EFFECTS	NURSING IMPLICATIONS
Conjugated estrogen: PO, intravaginally Synthetic conjugated estrogen: PO, IV, IM, intravaginally Micronized estradiol: PO, IM, intravaginally Estradiol: transdermal patches Estradiol: vaginal tablets	Nausea, vomiting, breakthrough bleeding, weight gain, swollen tender breasts, increased blood pressure	1. Estrogen compounds should be given with progesterone combinations. 2. Important for menopausal women to continue with 1200 mg/day calcium intake, vitamin D supplementation, and weight-bearing exercises along with estrogen replacement to prevent osteoporosis. 3. Should not be used by women who have known or suspected breast cancer, undiagnosed vaginal bleeding, or possible pregnancy. 4. Used with precaution – or not at all – in women with clotting disorders or history of VTE/PE. 5. Report any unusual bleeding to primary care provider.

Appendix 18.1   MEDICATIONS USED IN REPRODUCTIVE SYSTEM DISORDERS—cont'd

MEDICATIONS	SIDE EFFECTS	NURSING IMPLICATIONS
Medroxyprogesterone acetate: PO, IM	Menses may become more irregular (breakthrough bleeding), skin reactions (hives, acne)	1. *Use:* for menopausal women who still have a uterus; significantly decreased risk for uterine cancer when used with estrogen therapy. Birth control injection given every 3 months, medroxyprogesterone. 2. Women should continue with increased calcium intake, vitamin D supplementation, and weight-bearing exercises to prevent osteoporosis; should have yearly Pap smears, mammograms, and cholesterol level tests.

Erectile Dysfunction Medications: Cause smooth muscle relaxation and an increase in blood flow into the corpus cavernosum of the penis, with engorgement and subsequent erection.

MEDICATIONS	SIDE EFFECTS	NURSING IMPLICATIONS
Sildenafil: PO Vardenafil: PO Tadalafil: PO Avanafil: PO *Note: all generic names end in "afil."*	Hypotension can be a serious side effect Headache, flushing, visual changes, priapism	1. Should not be taken concurrently with nitrates. 2. α blockers (used for treatment of BPH) are contraindicated in the client taking tadalafil and vardenafil; should be used with caution in client taking sildenafil. 3. If chest pain occurs after taking these medications, seek immediate medical care. 4. Primary differences in the medications are the onset and duration of action. 5. Priapism, painful erection, or erection lasting more than 4 hrs may require medical intervention to prevent penile damage.

❗ **NURSING PRIORITY** Always inquire if a client is taking an ED medication before treating chest pain with any nitrate medication.

BPH, benign prostatic hyperplasia; *ED,* erectile dysfunction; *HRT,* hormone replacement therapy; *IM,* intramuscular; *IV,* intravenous; *OTC,* over the counter; *PE,* pulmonary embolism; *PO,* by mouth (oral); *VTE,* venous thromboembolism.

Practice & Next Generation NCLEX (NGN) Questions
Reproductive Care of Adult Clients

1. It has been 48 hrs since a surgery for a left mastectomy. What would the nurse reinforce in the teaching plan for this client? **Select all that apply**.
   1. Massage the wound site with essentials oils once incision has healed.
   2. Avoid needle sticks in the left arm.
   3. Begin active exercises immediately, such as pendulum arm swings.
   4. Keep affected arm close to the body.
   5. Elevate the arm on pillows to prevent edema.
   6. Take blood pressure measurements from the right arm.

2. The nurse is preparing a female client for a pelvic examination. In planning the care for the client, what is important for the nurse to do before the examination?
   1. Make sure the client had a bowel prep and cleansing enema.
   2. Carefully document the menstrual cycle; client should not be in last third of cycle.
   3. Question the client regarding her last period and the possibility of pregnancy.
   4. Make sure the client voids before the procedure.

3. The nurse is caring for a client the first postoperative day after a left-sided mastectomy. What observations would cause the nurse the most concern?
   1. Temperature of 100.6°F (38.1°C), pulse of 110 beats/min.
   2. Moderate amount of serosanguineous drainage on dressing.
   3. Left forearm and hand swollen, palpable radial pulse.
   4. Urine output of 40 mL/hr, slight increase in blood glucose level.

4. An older adult client complains of vaginal itching and burning. What would be the **best** nursing management?
   1. Douche daily with a weak vinegar solution.
   2. Apply estrogen vaginal cream.
   3. Wash the perineal area well with soap and water.
   4. Encourage the use of a water-based lubricant during intercourse.

5. The night-shift nurse notes at the end of their shift that a client who had a mastectomy had a total of 90 mL of serosanguineous drainage from the incision over a 24-hr period. What is the **best** nursing action?
   1. Report amount of drainage to the surgeon.
   2. Start frequent blood pressure checks and observe for hemorrhage.
   3. Continue to monitor the drainage.
   4. Reinforce packing at the wound site.

6. A client is 1 day postoperative after a transurethral resection of the prostate (TURP) with continuous bladder irrigation (CBI). The nurse notes bright red urinary drainage. What are the **priority** nursing actions? **Select all that apply**.
   1. Determine how much fluid has infused with the CBI.
   2. Monitor hemoglobin and hematocrit.
   3. Document findings in the electronic health record.
   4. Irrigate the catheter according to protocol.
   5. Increase the rate of the bladder irrigation.
   6. Notify the surgeon.

7. The nurse is reinforcing the teaching to a client with pelvic inflammatory disease (PID). The nurse instructs the client to sleep with their head elevated about 45 degrees. What is the rationale behind instructing the client to sleep in this position?
   1. Assists to localize drainage in the lower abdomen
   2. Decreases abdominal muscle tension
   3. Makes coughing and deep breathing more effective
   4. Prevents scarring of the fallopian tubes

8. An older adult male client is admitted with benign prostatic hyperplasia (BPH). Which finding by the nurse will require immediate action?
   1. BP 178/98 mm Hg.
   2. Report of lower abdominal pain.
   3. Bladder ultrasound value of 850 mL.
   4. Heart rate of 100 beats/min.

9. What is important for the nurse to understand about a gonorrhea infection in a female client?
   1. May be asymptomatic.
   2. Temperature will be elevated.
   3. Irregular menses.
   4. Appearance of a chancre.

10. A female client has been receiving antibiotic therapy for the treatment of pelvic inflammatory disease (PID). What client outcome would identify that the intervention and treatment plan were effective?
    1. Diminished pelvic pain and tenderness.
    2. Decreased dysuria.
    3. Relief from nausea and vomiting.
    4. Improved libido.

11. A 78-year-old male is seen in the emergency department.

Health History	Nurses' Notes	Vital Signs	Laboratory Results

0830: Client reports that he has not had good urine flow for the past couple years, but now is having increasing difficulty urinating. About 18 hrs ago, the client reports his urinary stream was reduced to a dribble with severe pain in the lower abdomen. Abdomen is distended.

Health History	Nurses' Notes	Vital Signs	Laboratory Results

PSA level 3.2 ng/mL (Normal < 4.0 ng/mL)

Drag 1 condition and 1 client assessment finding to fill in each blank in the following sentence.

The client is at greatest risk for developing _____ because of _____, _____ and _____.

CONDITION	ASSESSMENT FINDING
Bladder stones	Difficulty urinating
Urinary tract infection	PSA level 3.2 ng/mL
Constipation	Dribbling urinary stream
Kidney damage	Prostate cancer
Acute urinary retention	Abdominal distention

---

12. The following is a postoperative nurses' note.

Health History	Nurses' Notes	Vital Signs	Laboratory Results

1300: A 52-year-old woman had a left mastectomy with axillary lymph nodes removed, breast reconstructive surgery, and is 2 days postoperative. Breast dressing is dry and intact. Jackson-Pratt drain in place with 15 mL of serosanguineous fluid. Client has begun arm exercises, ambulates in the hall, and is on a regular diet. Pain is 3 on a scale of 10 and is managed with PO acetaminophen and codeine.

For each potential complication listed below, drop down to select the potential nursing intervention that would be appropriate for the client at this time. Each complication may support more than one potential nursing intervention, but a least one option in each category needs to be selected.

POTENTIAL COMPLICATION	APPROPRIATE NURSING ACTION
Infection	
Hemorrhage	
Lymphedema	

NURSING ACTIONS FOR POTENTIAL INFECTION	NURSING ACTIONS FOR POTENTIAL HEMORRHAGE	NURSING ACTIONS FOR POTENTIAL LYMPHEDEMA
Irrigate breast drainage tubes. Monitor surgical site for swelling. Inspect wound dressings.	Assess vital signs hourly. Watch for signs of heaviness in the affected arm. Monitor hemoglobin and hematocrit.	Take BP on unaffected arm. Keep affected arm below heart level. Maintain semi-Fowler's position.

⚓ Answers to Practice & Next Generation NCLEX (NGN) Questions

1. **2, 4, 5, 6**
Client Needs: Physiological Integrity/Physiological Adaptation
Clinical Judgment/Cognitive Skill: Take Action
Item Type: Select All That Apply
Rationale & Rationale & Test Taking Strategy: Important teaching to include in the discharge plan of care for a mastectomy client includes the avoidance of needlesticks in the arm on the side of the mastectomy and avoidance of blood pressure measurements on this arm. This is to prevent any type of trauma that might lead to the development of lymphedema. Active exercises, such as pendulum swings and wall climbing, are started after the incision has healed. As the area heals, abduction and external rotation will help to improve the range of motion. The use of oils and lotions applied to the healed incision is not necessary.

2. **4**
Client Needs: Physiological Integrity/Reduction of Risk Potential
Clinical Judgment/Cognitive Skill: Generate Solutions
Item Type: Multiple Choice
Rationale & Test Taking Strategy: It is important for the bladder to be empty. This will promote comfort for the client and make it easier for the health care provider to examine the pelvic contents. A cleansing enema is not done. The client may be anywhere in her menstrual cycle; however, clients usually do not schedule an exam during their menstrual periods. Pregnancy is a consideration; however, an empty bladder is more important immediately before the examination.

3. **3**
Client Needs: Physiological Integrity/Physiological Adaptation
Clinical Judgment/Cognitive Skill: Analyze Cues
Item Type: Multiple Choice
Rationale & Test Taking Strategy: Recall the complications that can occur following a mastectomy. Look at all the options—are they expected? It is important to observe the arm on the affected side of the client who has had a mastectomy. If the lymph drainage in the arm has been compromised, there is an increased risk of swelling and edema on the affected arm. The arm should be protected from tests such as needlesticks or blood pressure assessment. The temperature and slight increase in blood glucose level are normal for the first postoperative day. An elevated pulse could relate to the client experiencing postoperative pain. A moderate amount of serosanguineous drainage on the dressing is expected on the first postoperative day. Urine output of 40 mL/hr is normal.

4. **2**
Client Needs: Physiological Integrity/Physiological Adaptation
Clinical Judgment/Cognitive Skill: Prioritize Hypotheses
Item Type: Multiple Choice
Rationale & Test Taking Strategy: Note the **key** word, "best." The itching and burning may be caused by drying of the vaginal walls. The estrogen cream will help to decrease this problem. The client should not douche, and soap may further irritate the area. A water-based lubricant may improve lubrication during sexual activity for the older adult but will not resolve the problem.

5. **3**
Client Needs: Physiological Integrity/Physiological Adaptation
Clinical Judgment/Cognitive Skill: Prioritize Hypotheses
Item Type: Multiple Choice

Rationale & Test Taking Strategy: Note the **key** word, "best." This is a nursing care priority test item. Up to 100 mL of serosanguineous fluid would be an acceptable amount of drainage over a 24-hour period in a client who has had a mastectomy. Drains are usually removed when there is less than 25 mL in a 24-hour period. There is no indication of hemorrhage or the need to perform frequent blood pressure checks. If the nurse observes a greater amount of fluid in the drains, then it would be important to notify the surgeon.

6. **4, 5, 6**
Client Needs: Physiological Integrity/Physiological Adaptation
Clinical Judgment/Cognitive Skill: Prioritize Hypotheses
Item Type: Select All That Apply
Rationale & Test Taking Strategy: Note the **key** word, "priority," which alerts you that this is a nursing care priority test item. Blood-tinged urine is normal for the first few days after surgery. If arterial bleeding occurs, the urinary drainage is bright red or ketchup-like with numerous clots. The nurse needs to notify the surgeon immediately and irrigate the catheter with normal saline solution per surgeon or hospital protocol. Additional surgical intervention may be needed to clear the bladder of clots and stop bleeding. Be sure to maintain the flow of the irrigant to keep the urine pink-tinged to clear. Although monitoring the hemoglobin and hematocrit, calculating intake and output, and documenting the findings on the electronic health record are indicated, they are not the priorities for the client who is hemorrhaging following TURP surgery.

7. **1**
Client Needs: Physiological Integrity/Physiological Adaptation
Clinical Judgment/Cognitive Skill: Analyze Cues
Item Type: Multiple choice
Rationale & Test Taking Strategy: Think about why positioning the client with PID would be important. The nurse reinforces the teaching to the client to maintain a semi-Fowler position to prevent or decrease movement of the contaminated or infected fluid to the upper abdomen and the area of the diaphragm. Coughing and deep breathing would be more effective in high-Fowler position. The position does not decrease abdominal muscle tension or prevent scarring of the fallopian tubes.

8. **3**
Client Needs: Physiological Integrity/Physiological Adaptation
Clinical Judgment/Cognitive Skill: Recognize Cues
Item Type: Multiple Choice
Rationale & Test Taking Strategy: Note the key word, "immediate." This is a nursing care priority test item. Go through each option and determine if it is normal or not and if it relates to benight prostatic hyperplasia (BPH). The high bladder scan/ultrasound value confirms the retention of a large volume of urine that will require urinary catheterization. The nurse is aware that an acute complication of BPH is urinary retention due to bladder outlet obstruction caused by the enlarged prostate gland. Acute urinary retention is a medical emergency that requires prompt bladder drainage. The elevated heart rate and blood pressure and the lower abdominal pain are indications of the discomfort caused by the full bladder and more than likely those symptoms will diminish as the bladder is catheterized.

9. **1**
Client Needs: Physiological Integrity/Physiological Adaptation
Clinical Judgment/Cognitive Skill: Analyze Cues
Item Type: Multiple Choice

Rationale & Test Taking Strategy: Because the site of a gonorrhea infection is often the cervix, the client may be asymptomatic. Women typically have more asymptomatic infections than men. The temperature is not elevated, and the menstrual period is not affected by the infection. A chancre is found in primary syphilis infections.

10. **1**
Client Needs: Physiological Integrity/Pharmacological Therapies
Clinical Judgment/Cognitive Skill: Evaluate Outcomes
Item Type: Multiple Choice
Rationale & Test Taking Strategy: The nurse would know that the treatment plan was effective when the client has relief of pain because the antibiotic therapy has decreased the inflammation and destroyed the microorganisms causing the PID. Dysuria is not a typical finding of PID but is found with a urinary bladder infection. Relief from nausea, vomiting, and malaise, along with an improved libido, may be secondary findings but are not indications of effective treatment.

11. A 78-year-old male is seen in the emergency department.

Health History	Nurses' Notes	Vital Signs	Laboratory Results

0830: Client reports that he has not had good urine flow for the past couple years, but now is having increasing difficulty urinating. About 18 hrs ago, the client reports his urinary stream was reduced to a dribble with severe pain in the lower abdomen. Abdomen is distended.

Health History	Nurses' Notes	Vital Signs	Laboratory Results

PSA level 3.2 ng/mL (Normal < 4.0 ng/mL)

Drag one condition and one client assessment finding to fill in each blank in the following sentence.

The client is at greatest risk for developing *acute urinary retention* due to *difficulty urinating, dribbling urinary stream,* and *abdominal distention.*

Client Needs: Physiological Integrity/Physiological Adaptation
Clinical Judgment/Cognitive Skill: Analyze Cues
Item Type: Drag-and-Drop Rationale
Rationale & Test Taking Strategy: The client is at risk for acute urinary retention as evidenced by difficulty urinating, dribbling urinary stream, and abdominal distention. More than likely, the client has benign prostatic hypertrophy (BPH) because the prostate-specific antigen (PSA) test was within the normal range. The PSA is elevated with prostate cancer. When the prostate enlarges, the client will begin to experience symptoms including frequency, nocturia, and urgency. As BPH progresses, there can be complete obstruction of urinary flow, which becomes an urgent problem requiring immediate urinary bladder catheterization.

12. The following is a postoperative nurses' note.

Health History	Nurses' Notes	Vital Signs	Laboratory Results

1300: A 52-year-old woman had a left mastectomy with axillary lymph nodes removed, breast reconstructive surgery, and is 2 days postoperative. Breast dressing is dry and intact. Jackson-Pratt drain in place with 15 mL of serosanguineous fluid. Client has begun arm exercises, ambulates in the hall, and is on a regular diet. Pain is 3 on a scale of 10 and is managed with PO acetaminophen and codeine.

For each potential complication listed below, drop down to select the potential nursing intervention that would be appropriate for the client at this time. Each complication may support more than one potential nursing intervention, but at least one option in each category needs to be selected.

POTENTIAL COMPLICATION	APPROPRIATE NURSING ACTION FOR EACH POTENTIAL COMPLICATION
Infection	Monitor surgical site for swelling. Inspect wound dressings
Hemorrhage	Assess vital signs hourly. Monitor hemoglobin and hematocrit.
Lymphedema	Take blood pressure on unaffected arm. Maintain semi-Fowler position.

Client Needs: Physiological Integrity/Physiological Adaptation
Clinical Judgment/Cognitive Skill: Take Action
Item Type: Drop Down in Table
Rationale & Test Taking Strategy: Postoperative care following a mastectomy includes monitoring for complications, which are infection, hemorrhage (breast tissue is very vascular), and lymphedema. The nurse should monitor vital signs for temperature elevation and laboratory studies for an elevated white blood cell count, inspect the dressings for purulent drainage, and watch for swelling at the incision site. Hemorrhage is monitored by checking vital signs and monitoring hemoglobin and hematocrit values. The nurse should position the client so that drainage tubes (Jackson-Pratt drains) or any collection device is not pulled or kinked. The client should have the head of the bed elevated at least 30 degrees with the affected arm elevated on a pillow while awake. Keeping the affected arm elevated will promote lymphatic fluid return after removal of lymph nodes and lymph channels. Symptoms of lymphedema such as sensations of heaviness, aching, fatigue, numbness, tingling, and/or swelling in the affected arm, as well as swelling in the upper chest, should be reported to the surgeon. When lymphedema occurs, it often becomes a chronic problem. The nurse should not take a blood pressure on the affected arm, draw blood, or administer injections. Skin care is important.

Generate Solutions

Treatment

A. Medical (Appendix 19.2).
  1. Broad-spectrum antibiotics, especially the sulfon-amides for lower UTIs; fluoroquinolones for upper UTIs (Appendix 6.2).
  2. Urinary analgesics, such as phenazopyridine.
  3. Antispasmodics, antipyretics.
B. Dietary.
  1. Encourage fluid intake of 3000 mL/day, unless contraindicated.
    a. Discourage consumption of carbonated beverages and foods or drinks containing baking powder or baking soda. Caffeine, alcohol, citrus fruits, and highly spiced foods can cause bladder irritation.
    b. Daily intake of cranberry juice or cranberry essence tablets is helpful for some clients, as it appears to decrease the ability of bacteria to adhere to the epithelial cells lining the urinary tract.

Nursing Interventions: Take Action

Goal: To provide relief of pain, urgency, dysuria, and fever.
A. Antibiotics need to be taken as scheduled, and the full course must be completed. Initially, therapy may be required for 1 to 3 days; if problem is recurrent, 10 to 14 days of therapy may be required. For pyelonephritis, antibiotics may be taken for 14 to 21 days; severe symptoms may require hospitalization.
B. Encourage consumption of 8 to 10 glasses of fluids daily (3000 mL).
C. Teach client importance of voiding every 2 to 3 hrs during the day to completely empty the bladder.
D. Sitz baths may be taken to decrease irritation of urethra.
Goal: To prevent recurrence of infection.
A. Avoid sitting in a bathtub with added bubble bath products or other bath oils and fragrances; a warm bath will decrease symptoms, but nothing should be added to the water.
B. Explain importance of cleansing the perineal area from front to back after voiding and after each bowel movement. Avoid use of perineal sprays and powders.
C. If intercourse seems to predispose to infection, encourage voiding immediately before and after intercourse. A female client with recurrent UTIs may need to temporarily stop using a diaphragm and spermicidal creams/jelly.
D. Teach importance of long-term therapy if recurrent infections are a problem.
E. Encourage and explain the need for follow-up care to prevent complications of chronic UTIs.
F. Caffeine, alcohol, citrus juices, and carbonated beverages should be avoided.
G. Maintain adequate fluid intake.
Goal: To reduce catheter-associated UTIs (CAUTIs).
A. Discontinue indwelling catheters as early as possible.
B. Review agency's protocol to reduce CAUTI infections, as required by The Joint Commission implementation of a National Patient Safety Goal (NPSG).

Urinary Calculi

Stones may form anywhere in the urinary tract; the most common location for stones is in the pelvis of the kidney. If the stones are small, they may be passed into the bladder.
A. Stones in the bladder may increase in size if urinary stasis and alkaline pH are present.
B. Types of urinary calculi.
  1. Calcium oxalate or phosphate stones: tend to be small; account for 40% to 50% of all upper urinary tract calculi.
  2. Struvite stones: contain bacteria and tend to be large; more common in women than men.
  3. Uric acid stones: occur most often in clients with primary or secondary problems of uric acid metabolism (gout); high incidence in men, particularly Jewish men.
  4. Cystine stones: autosomal recessive defect that leads to cystine crystals being stuck in urinary tract.

Assessment: Recognize Cues

Regardless of the type of stone formed, the clinical manifestations, diagnostics, and treatment are essentially the same.
A. Risk factors/etiology.
  1. Infection, urinary stasis, immobility.
  2. Hypercalcemia and hypercalciuria (hyperparathyroidism, renal tubular acidosis).
  3. Excessive intake of dietary proteins, which increases uric acid production.
  4. Excessive consumption of foods high in oxalate, such as spinach, soy products, and peanuts.
  5. Excessive consumption of sodium, which causes the kidneys to excrete more calcium.
  6. Low fluid intake.
  7. Majority of clients are between 20 and 55 years of age, with increased incidence when family history is present. Stones occur more often in the summer months and warmer climates.
  8. Increased incidence of family history with stone formation caused by inherited metabolic risk factors.
  9. Bariatric surgery, short bowel syndrome, or other conditions that decrease oxalate absorption in the gut.
B. Clinical manifestations.
  1. Sharp, sudden, severe abdominal or flank pain.
    a. May be described as "colic," either ureteral or kidney.
    b. Pain may be intermittent, depending on the movement of the stone; spasm in the ureter occurs as it attempts to move the stone toward the bladder.
    c. Pain may radiate around the flank area, down into the bladder, the genitalia, and the thigh.
  2. Hematuria may be present as a result of the traumatic effects of the stone on the ureter and the bladder.
  3. Oliguria or anuria suggest urinary obstruction and must be treated immediately.
  4. Nausea and vomiting are common.

5. Struvite stones are associated with fever and infection.
C. Diagnostics (Appendix 19.1).
D. Complications.
   1. Recurrent stone formation.
   2. Infection, kidney failure.

Analyze Cues and Prioritize Hypotheses

The most important problems are acute pain, impaired urinary system function, and lack of knowledge about contributing factors to stone formation.

Generate Solutions

Treatment
A. Medical.
   1. Increase fluid intake to 2000 mL/day to decrease urine concentration, unless contraindicated.
   2. Medications that prevent the absorption of calcium (thiazide diuretics and phosphates).
   3. Spasmolytic agents (anticholinergics).
   4. For uric acid stones, allopurinol.
   5. Opioids for pain relief.
   6. Dietary.
      a. Sodium may also be restricted, as it increases the excretion of calcium in the urine.
      b. Decrease in protein intake or an alkaline-ash diet for clients with uric acid stones.
      c. Decrease intake of cola, coffee, and tea, which tend to increase the risk for calculi formation.
      d. Maintain normal levels of calcium in diet (800-1000 mg) for calcium oxalate stones. Calcium binds with oxalate in the GI tract and prevents it from entering the blood and the urinary tract, where it contributes to the development of calcium oxalate stones.
      e. Decrease intake of oxalate sources such as spinach, black tea, and rhubarb for calcium oxalate stones (Table 2-4, Therapeutic Meal Plans).
B. Surgical.
   1. Nephrolithotomy: incision into the kidney and removal of the stone.
   2. Ureterolithotomy: incision into the ureter to locate a stone and remove it.
   3. Stenting: insertion of a small tube (stent) into ureter via ureteroscopy to dilate ureter to enlarge passageway for expulsion of stone or stone fragments or to temporarily bypass a stone that cannot be removed immediately.
C. Lithotripsy: cystoscopic, percutaneous ultrasonic, laser, or extracorporeal shock-wave lithotripsy (ESWL).
   1. For ESWL, client is anesthetized.
      a. Sound waves travel through the water and are directed to the stone. The force of the sound waves shatters the stone, and the remains are excreted in the urine.
      b. It is essential that the client remain absolutely motionless during the procedure, which lasts about 30 to 45 mins. Therefore, some form of sedation or analgesia is necessary during the procedure.

   c. Occasionally, a ureteral stent is placed after lithotripsy procedures to promote passage of stone fragments and left in place for 2 weeks.
   2. Hematuria is common after the procedure.
   3. Client must demonstrate the ability to urinate freely before discharge.

Nursing Interventions: Take Action

Goal: To relieve pain.
A. Administer analgesics as prescribed: morphine or hydromorphone.
B. Hot baths or moist heat applied to flank area.
C. Encourage increased fluid intake (2000 mL/day) to prevent dehydration, if not contraindicated.
D. Strain all urine and inspect for blood clots and passage of stone.
E. If stone is passed, it should be saved and sent to the laboratory for analysis to determine the type of stone so appropriate therapy can be maintained.

Goal: To promote understanding of health care regimen.
A. Dietary restrictions, depending on type of stone.
B. Discuss rationale, dose, frequency, and important information relating to medication administration.
C. Teach symptoms of recurring stone formation, such as hematuria, flank pain, and signs of infection.
D. Instruct client to continue high fluid intake (2000 mL/day).
E. Promote periodic medical follow-up visits to evaluate for symptoms of infection and recurring stone formation.

📋 Acute Kidney Injury

Acute kidney injury (AKI) **is a clinical syndrome with abrupt loss of kidney function that may occur over several hours or days, characterized by uremia. The most common causes are hypotension, prerenal hypovolemia, or exposure to a nephrotoxin.**

Phases of Acute Kidney Injury

A. Oliguric phase (Fig. 19.3).
   1. Urinary output decreases to less than 400 mL/24 hrs.
   2. Increase in blood urea nitrogen (BUN), creatinine, uric acid, potassium, and magnesium levels and presence of metabolic acidosis.
   3. Duration is 1 to 3 weeks; the longer it lasts, the less favorable the recovery.

> **🚫 OLDER ADULT PRIORITY** The older adult client loses the ability to concentrate urine; therefore, urinary output may not be significantly reduced in this stage of kidney injury.

   4. Nonoliguric acute kidney injury: urine output is greater than 400 mL/24 hrs, and urine is dilute.
B. Diuretic phase.
   1. Often has a sudden onset within 2 to 6 weeks after oliguric phase. Daily urine output is 1 to 3 L but may reach 5 L or more; urine is dilute.
   2. Hypovolemia and hypotension may occur as a result of massive fluid losses.

B. Maintain accurate intake and output record.

C. Determine weight daily (client may lose 0.2-0.3 kg/day during oliguric phase).

D. Assess fluid balance (hypervolemia or hypovolemia), urine specific gravity, pulmonary status, cardiac output, mental status changes (may indicate cerebral edema).

E. Assess status of electrolytes and kidney parameters: serum potassium, BUN, creatinine, phosphate levels; evaluate fluctuations of serum sodium levels and GFR.

F. Evaluate for hypertension or hypotension.

G. Support involved body systems.
   1. Cardiac dysrhythmias.
   2. Pulmonary function.

H. Avoid nephrotoxic medications, including nonsteroidal anti-inflammatory drugs (NSAIDs) and aminoglycosides.

Goal: To maintain nutrition.

A. Maintain dietary restrictions on sodium, potassium, and protein.

B. Encourage intake of carbohydrates and fats for energy source. Caloric needs are 30 to 35 kcal/kg.

C. Offer small frequent feedings; limit fluids.

D. Total parenteral or enteral nutrition may be necessary to promote healing if caloric intake cannot be maintained.

Goal: To prevent infection.

A. Avoid use of indwelling urinary catheter, if possible.

B. Assess for development of infectious processes (local or systemic). Client is at increased risk because of compromised immune system; may not have an elevated temperature.

C. Assess for and prevent UTI.

Goal: To prevent skin breakdown if incontinence occurs.

A. Frequent turning and positioning; inspect the skin for problem areas.

B. Beds and protective devices are used to prevent pressure areas.

C. Frequent range of motion exercises and activities to increase circulation.

Goal: To provide emotional support.

A. Always explain procedures.

B. Provide honest information regarding progress of condition.

C. May take 3 to 12 months for recovery.

D. Encourage client to express fears and concerns regarding condition.

Chronic Kidney Disease

Chronic kidney disease (CKD) **is a progressive, irreversible reduction in kidney function such that the kidneys are no longer able to maintain the body environment. The GFR gradually decreases as the nephrons are destroyed. The nephrons left intact are subjected to an increased workload, resulting in hypertrophy and inability to concentrate urine.**

Assessment: Recognize Cues

A. Risk factors/etiology.
   1. Chronic hypertension and poorly controlled diabetes account for about 70% of CKD cases.

   2. Chronic glomerulonephritis and pyelonephritis.
   3. Polycystic kidney disease.
   4. Kidney disease caused by nephrotoxic drugs or chemicals.
   5. SLE.
   6. More common in African Americans and Native Americans.
   7. Over 60 years of age.
   8. Family history of CKD.

B. Clinical manifestations (Fig. 19.4).
   1. GFR is less than 60 mL/min for longer than 3 months. A GFR less than 15 mL/min indicates kidney failure.
      a. Severe azotemia, metabolic acidosis.
      b. Hyperkalemia, hypernatremia, and hyperphosphatemia.
      c. Altered renin-angiotensin system.
   2. Urinary system: specific gravity of urine fixed at 1.010; proteinuria, casts, pyuria, hematuria; oliguria eventually leads to anuria less than 100 mL/24 hrs.
   3. Endocrine system.
      a. Hyperparathyroidism causes hypocalcemia and hyperphosphatemia, resulting in demineralization of the bones (renal osteodystrophy).
      b. Hypothyroidism.
   4. Hematologic system: anemia and bleeding, infection.
   5. Cardiovascular system: hypertension, CHF, uremic pericarditis, pericardial effusion, atherosclerotic heart disease.
   6. GI system: anorexia, nausea, vomiting, ammonia odor (uremic fetor) to the breath, GI bleeding, peptic ulcer disease, gastritis.
   7. Metabolic system: hyperglycemia, hyperlipidemia, gout, hypoproteinemia, carbohydrate intolerance.
   8. Neurologic system: general central nervous system depression and peripheral neuropathy, headaches, seizures, sleep disturbances.
   9. Musculoskeletal system: mineral and bone disorder (CKD-MBD), vascular calcification, osteomalacia.
   10. Integumentary system: yellow/gray discoloration, pruritus, uremic frost, ecchymosis.
   11. Psychological changes: emotional lability, withdrawal, depression, psychosis, personality and behavioral changes.
   12. Reproductive system: erectile dysfunction, amenorrhea.

C. Diagnostics (Appendix 19.1).
   1. Urinalysis for proteinuria or microalbuminuria.
   2. Elevated blood sugar and triglyceride levels.
   3. Increased serum potassium level.
   4. Decreased hemoglobin and hematocrit.

Analyze Cues and Prioritize Hypotheses

The most important problems are fluid overload, decreased cardiac function, weight loss, reduced bone density, hematologic abnormalities (bleeding, anemia), altered drug elimination caused by elevation in creatinine, and potential psychosocial alterations.

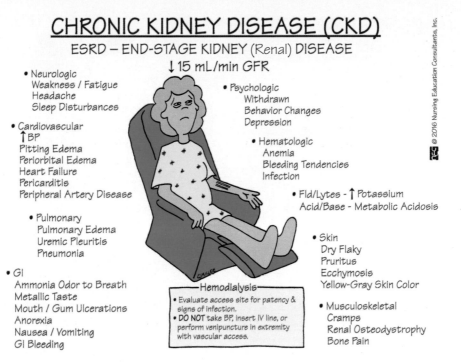

FIG. 19.4 Chronic Kidney Disease. (From Zerwekh J, Garneau A, Miller CJ. [2017]. *Digital collection of the memory notebooks of nursing.* [4th ed.]. Chandler, AZ: Nursing Education Consultants, Inc.)

Generate Solutions

Treatment

A. Medical.
1. Measures to reduce serum potassium level (see discussion under acute kidney injury).
2. Antihypertensives.
3. Diuretics: thiazide and loop diuretics may be used early in the course of disease.
4. Erythropoietin for treatment of anemia.
5. Phosphate binders and supplemental vitamin D for CKD-MBD.
B. Dietary.
1. Restricted protein intake; may vary from just a decrease in protein intake to a specific restriction of 20 to 40 g/day.
2. Fluid restriction: 600 to 1000 mL, adjusted according to urinary output and/or dialysis.
3. Sodium, potassium, and phosphate restriction: based on laboratory values.
C. Dialysis (Box 19.5).
D. Surgical: kidney transplantation - the primary limiting factor in the number of transplantations done is the availability of kidneys; the average wait is 18 months to 4 years; clients with blood types B and O have the longest wait.
1. Recipient criteria: candidates are evaluated on an individual basis as to how well they would benefit from transplantation.
2. Donor criteria: living related donors provide the best possible match with a 95% 1-year graft survival; when they are not available, cadaver donors are considered; these have a 90% 1-year graft survival.

Nursing Interventions: Take Action

Goal: To help the client maintain homeostasis in early CKD.

A. Evaluate adequacy of fluid balance.
1. Determine weight daily.
2. Control hypertension.
3. Discuss with the client how to monitor fluid intake and plan for the allocated amount to be distributed over the day.

TEST ALERT Monitor hydration status, identify signs of fluid and electrolyte imbalance, and identify interventions to correct any imbalance.

B. Encourage nutritional intake within dietary guidelines.
1. Relieve GI dysfunctions before serving meals.
2. Plan diet according to client's preferences, if possible.
3. Advise client that most salt substitutes contain potassium and should not be used.
C. Prevent constipation.
1. Include bran/fiber in diet.
2. Stool softeners.
D. Avoid use of sedatives and hypnotics; increased sensitivity to these medications is caused by decreased ability of kidney to metabolize and excrete them.
E. Monitor electrolyte balance, especially levels of potassium and calcium.

⚠ NURSING PRIORITY Hypocalcemia and hyperkalemia are critical problems and may cause fatal dysrhythmias.

F. Assess cardiovascular status to determine how effectively the client's cardiovascular system is compensating for

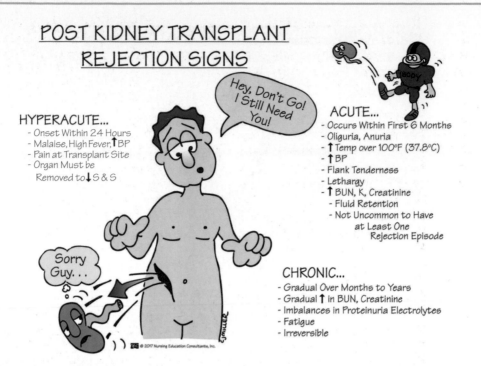

FIG. 19.5 Post-Kidney Transplant Rejection. (From Zerwekh J, Garneau A, Miller CJ. [2017]. *Digital collection of the memory notebooks of nursing.* [4th ed.]. Chandler, AZ: Nursing Education Consultants, Inc.)

the increased fluid load and increased workload from the chronic anemic state.

G. Assess client for bleeding tendencies initially related to a decrease in production of erythropoietin and decreased platelet adhesiveness. Encourage intake of folic acid (1 mg daily) for red blood cell production and integrity.

H. Evaluate client for pruritus and assist with measures to decrease skin irritation and itching.

I. Avoid products containing magnesium (antacids).

J. Assess client's activity tolerance in relation to anemia.

Goal: To provide emotional support and promote psychological equilibrium.

A. Encourage client to express concerns.

B. Recognize that the long-term management of a chronic disease may lead to anxiety and depression.

C. Encourage venting of feelings regarding lifestyle changes.

D. Encourage client and family members to seek out support groups, community resources, and other clients with kidney failure who are undergoing the same types of treatment.

Kidney Transplant

The transplantation of a kidney from a compatible-blood-typed deceased donor, blood relative, or a live donor. Transplanted kidney is usually placed extraperitoneally in the iliac fossa (usually right side to facilitate anastomosis and decrease occurrence of ileus), most commonly on the right lower side of the abdomen.

Assessment: Recognize Cues

A. Types of rejection (Fig. 19.5).

Analyze Cues and Prioritize Hypotheses

The most important problems are infection, the potential for rejection, and fluid and electrolyte imbalance.

Generate Solutions

Treatment

A. Immunosuppressant medications (Appendix 19.2).

B. Steroids (Appendix 6.2).

Nursing Interventions: Take Action

Goal: To provide preoperative care for client scheduled for kidney transplantation.

A. Maintain client's metabolic state as close to homeostasis as possible; continue with dialysis.

B. Tissue typing and antibody screening are conducted to determine histocompatibility of the donor and recipient.

C. Immunosuppressant drugs: may be started before surgery.

D. Conduct routine preoperative procedures, including labeling the arm with vascular access for dialysis, as the client may require dialysis in the immediate postoperative period.

Goal: To provide postoperative care for the kidney transplant recipient.

A. Immunosuppressant therapy is continued indefinitely; the most frequent combination of maintenance therapy consists of azathioprine, cyclosporine, and prednisone.

B. Assess for kidney graft function.

1. Maintain fluid and electrolyte balances because of early diuresis. Avoid dehydration.

2. Cadaveric transplant recipients may need dialysis because of acute tubular necrosis until the transplanted kidney begins to function.
3. *Report to RN any sudden decrease or change in urine output.*
C. Monitor for rejection.
D. Prevent and monitor for infection (UTI, pneumonia, and sepsis are biggest threats in the early posttransplantation period; fungal and viral infections are also common).
E. Atherosclerotic cardiovascular disease is common in transplant recipients. It is the leading cause of death in these clients.
F. Promote adaptation and psychological support for the client who has undergone successful transplantation.

Dialysis

Dialysis, **also called kidney replacement therapy (KRT), is the passage of particles (ions) from an area of high concentration to an area of low concentration across a semipermeable membrane.**

Assessment: Recognize Cues

A. Indications.
  1. GFR less than 15 mL/min.
  2. Fluid volume overload (e.g., pulmonary edema).
  3. Serum potassium level greater than 6 mEq/L (mmol/L).
  4. BUN level greater than 120 mg/dL (42.84 mmol/L).
  5. Uremia, uncontrolled hypertension, and metabolic acidosis.
  6. Severe bleeding from platelet dysfunction.
B. Complications.
  1. Peritoneal: possible bowel perforation from catheter insertion, infection, pain, hernias, pulmonary problems, protein loss, hyperglycemia in clients with diabetes.
  2. Hemodialysis: hypotension, muscle cramps, infection, disequilibrium syndrome, exsanguination.

Analyze Cues and Prioritize Hypotheses

The most important problems are infection during kidney replacement therapy and fluid and electrolyte imbalance.

Generate Solutions

▲Types of dialysis (Box 19.5). Note that dialysis solutions are high-alert medications.

Nursing Interventions: Take Action

Goal: To remove waste products of metabolism and excess fluid; to maintain a safe concentration of blood components.
A. Peritoneal dialysis.
  1. Prepare client for procedure: establish baseline criteria of laboratory values, weight, and vital signs; bowel and bladder should be empty.
  2. Provide support and information to the client when the peritoneal catheter is first inserted.
    a. Permanent peritoneal catheters are fitted with a device to keep them in place.

b. Temporary peritoneal catheters are inserted, and usually, a purse-string suture holds them in place; this usually occurs in the intensive care unit. *Remember the catheter is an open conduit to the peritoneal cavity.*
3. Type of peritoneal dialysis being used, and the physical stability of the client determine how long each cycle of dialysis will take.
4. Insufficient outflow (return of less than the amount of dialysate infused).
  a. Constipation is the primary cause of inflow and outflow problems.
  b. Check the tubing for patency and keep drainage bag below the level of the abdomen.
  c. Turn client from side to side or put client in semi-Fowler's position to increase abdominal pressure.

> **❗ NURSING PRIORITY** If dialysate is left in the peritoneal cavity too long, then hyperglycemia may occur, resulting from the high percentage of glucose in the dialysate fluid, which ensures hyperosmolarity. Heparin is sometimes added to the dialysate to prevent clotting of the catheter or tubing.

B. Hemodialysis.
  1. Vascular access site must be established; access may be temporary or permanent.

> **❗ NURSING PRIORITY** Do not take blood pressure, obtain blood samples, or infuse fluids or medications in the access site or the extremity that has a vascular access site. Report immediately any decrease or absence of pulsations or indications of decreased blood flow through the vascular access site.

2. Assess the patency of the pulses distal to the access site.

> **TEST ALERT** Provide care for client with a vascular access site before and after hemodialysis.

Goal: To maintain homeostasis after hemodialysis and monitor for complications.
A. Determine whether certain medications need to be withheld before dialysis (antihypertensives); in hospitalized clients, there are often standing orders for these situations.
B. Assess weight, blood pressure, peripheral edema, lung and heart sounds, and vascular access site before and after dialysis.
C. Most common side effects are hypotension, headache, muscle cramps, and bleeding from access site; monitor client for postural hypotension. If client has bleeding from the access site, apply pressure evenly and notify the dialysis unit.
D. Complications.
  1. Dialysis disequilibrium syndrome: cerebral edema and neurologic complications (headache, nausea, vomiting, seizures); may be minimized by slower dialysis.
  2. Sepsis, hepatitis B and C, blood loss, hypotension.

Goal: To provide emotional support and to promote psychological equilibrium.

A. Encourage client to express feelings of anger and depression. An increased rate of suicide exists among clients undergoing dialysis.

B. Encourage appropriate coping skills.

C. Clients undergoing chronic dialysis are in limbo; they know they are probably not going to get better and that they may or may not receive a transplant. Frequently, they have ambivalent feelings about dialysis; it maintains life but severely restricts lifestyle.

Kidney Tumors

Most kidney tumors are malignant and occur more frequently in men between the ages of 50 and 70 years. Most often, the tumor begins in the renal cortex, where it can actually become quite large before it begins to compress the adjacent kidney tissue. The most common areas of metastasis are the liver, lungs, and bone, especially the mediastinum.

Assessment: Recognize Cues

A. Clinical manifestations.
  1. Palpable abdominal mass.
  2. Hematuria, flank pain.
  3. Weight loss, weakness, anemia, hypertension.

B. Diagnostics - magnetic resonance imaging (MRI), computed tomography (CT) scan, kidney biopsy, renal scan.

Analyze Cues and Prioritize Hypotheses

The most important problems are the potential for metastasis of the cancer, loss of urinary tract function, the effect of treatment on sexuality, and impaired coping.

Generate Solutions

Treatment

A. Medical.
  1. Palliative radiation therapy.
  2. Biologic therapy with alpha interferon and interleukin 2.
  3. Cryoablation (freezing tumor) radiofrequency ablation (tumor destroyed by radiofrequency heat).
  4. Chemotherapy in metastatic disease.

B. Surgical: radical nephrectomy (includes kidney, adrenal gland, ureter, lymph nodes, and surrounding tissue); urinary diversion (Appendix 19.3).

Nursing Interventions: Take Action

Goal: To provide preoperative nursing care (Chapter 3).

A. Inform client that flank incision will be on affected side and that surgery will be performed in a hyperextended, side-lying position.

B. Often, client experiences postoperative muscle aches and discomfort as a result of surgical positioning.

C. Radiation, biologic therapy, or both after surgery.

Goal: To provide postoperative care.

A. Urinary output is important to assess; catheters should be labeled, and drainage should be recorded accurately.

B. Because of the level of the incision, respiratory complications are common; encourage coughing, deep breathing, and incentive spirometry every 2 hrs while client is awake.

C. Assess for abdominal distention and paralytic ileus.

D. Monitor for bleeding and unstable blood pressure after surgery; may be caused by removal of adrenal gland.

E. Provide adequate pain control.

Bladder Cancer

Most urothelial cancers occur in the bladder, which is why the term bladder cancer describes the condition. *Urothelial cancer* is also known as *transitional cell carcinoma (TCC)*.

Assessment: Recognize Cues

A. Clinical manifestations.
  1. Painless hematuria.
  2. Dysuria, frequency, urgency (occur when infection is present).

B. Diagnostics - MRI, CT scan, cystoscopy, gross or microscopic blood in urine.

Analyze Cues and Prioritize Hypotheses

The most important problems are the potential for metastasis of the cancer, loss of urinary tract function, the effect of treatment on sexuality, body image change (urinary diversion), and impaired coping.

Generate Solutions

Treatment

A. Medical.
  1. Radiation therapy.
  2. Intravesical immunotherapy.
  3. Chemotherapy in metastatic disease.

B. Surgical: transurethral resection of the bladder tumor; partial cystectomy; urinary diversion (Appendix 19.3).

Nursing Interventions: Take Action

Goal: To provide support for nonsurgical management.

A. Review safety measures when client receives an intravesical instillation.

B. Teach client about chemotherapy and radiation therapy effects.

Goal: To provide preoperative and postoperative nursing care (Chapter 3).

Goal: To provide self-management education about care of a urinary diversion.

A. Monitor for signs of infection.

B. Teach use of external pouching systems, technique for catheterizing a continent reservoir, medication, diet, and fluid therapy.

Appendix 19.1 DIAGNOSTICS OF THE URINARY-RENAL SYSTEM

LABORATORY TESTS	NORMAL	CLINICAL AND NURSING IMPLICATIONS
BUN level	6-20 mg/dL (2.1-7.14 mmol/L)	Common test used to diagnose kidney problems; may be affected by an increase in protein intake or tissue breakdown.
Creatinine level	0.6-1.3 mg/dL (53-115 μmol/L)	End product of protein and muscle catabolism; more accurate determinate of kidney function than the BUN level; values are higher in males. Elevated in kidney disease.
Calcium level	8.6-10.2 mg/dL (2.15-2.55 mmol/L)	Provides the matrix for bone and is important in muscle contraction, neurotransmission, and clotting; in chronic kidney failure, low levels of calcium lead to renal osteodystrophy.
Phosphorus level	2.4-4.4 mg/dL (0.78-1.42 mmol/L)	Phosphorus and calcium balances are inversely related; when phosphorus level is elevated, calcium level is decreased, which is seen in kidney disease.
Urinalysis	Color: Amber yellow Ketones: None Glucose: None pH: 4.6-8.0 (average 6) Specific gravity: (1.003-1.030)	Obtaining first-voided specimen in the morning is ideal. Presence of protein, WBC, RBC, glucose, bacteria, and hyaline casts indicate problems. Ensure specimen is examined within 1 hr of urinating. Dipstick urinalysis is initially performed to determine levels of nitrites and leukocyte esterase related to infections.
Urine culture and sensitivity		Colony count of at least 100,000 colonies/mL of urine indicates infection. Use sterile container for collection of urine. After cleaning, instruct client to start urination and then continue voiding in sterile container.
Urinary creatinine clearance	Males: 21-26 mg/kg/24 hrs Females: 16-22 mg/kg/24 hrs	Measure of GFR; 24-hr urine collection must be done; have client void and discard the first specimen and then begin timing the test; specimens should be kept cool or refrigerated. Decreased in kidney disease.
Urine specific gravity	Adults: 1.003-1.030 Children: 1.001-1.030	May be increased when the client is dehydrated and with glomerulonephritis. A decrease is associated with decreased tubular absorption. In kidney failure, it may be fixed at 1.010-1.012. Proteinuria will increase the specific gravity.
24-hr (composite) urine		Collection of all urine over a 24-hr period; measuring levels of calcium, phosphorous, magnesium, sodium, oxalate, citrate, sulfate, potassium, uric acid, and/or total volume. Specimen may be required to be on ice during collection.

Laboratory Diagnostics

PROCEDURE	CLINICAL AND NURSING IMPLICATIONS
KUB (kidneys, ureters, bladder) x-ray examination: a flat plate x-ray film of the abdomen and pelvis.	1. Bowel preparation may or may not be indicated.
Intravenous urography (IVP or excretory urogram): IV injection of radiopaque dye to visualize the urinary tract system.	1. Client's status is NPO for 8 hrs before procedure. 2. Cathartic or enema given the evening before procedure. 3. Radiocontrast medium may cause an allergic (hypersensitivity) reaction in iodine-sensitive clients. 4. Instruct client that they will need to lie still on table while serial x-ray films are taken. 5. Advise client that they may feel warm sensation and salty taste in mouth as dye is injected. 6. Evaluate for iodine reaction after test and encourage fluids after test to flush out the dye. 7. Be sure the older adult client is not dehydrated before the procedure; the contrast medium is nephrotoxic and can precipitate kidney failure. 8. Encourage fluids (if permitted or appropriate) after to flush out contrast media.
Retrograde pyelogram: An x-ray study of the urinary tract conducted during a cystoscopic examination; ureteral catheters are inserted into the renal pelvis, and dye is injected (retrograde) into the catheters.	1. Client's status is NPO for 8 hrs before test. 2. Assess for sensitivity to iodine. 3. Explain that there may be discomfort on insertion of the cystoscope. 4. General anesthesia may be indicated for procedure.

Continued

PROCEDURE	CLINICAL AND NURSING IMPLICATIONS
Renal arteriogram (angiogram): An IV injection of radiopaque dye into the renal artery (catheter is inserted into femoral artery) to visualize the renal blood vessels.	1. Client's status is NPO after midnight. 2. May have enema or cathartic the night before. 3. Preoperative medication is administered. 4. Client should be assessed for sensitivity to iodine before the procedure. 5. Evaluate venipuncture insertion site every 15-30 min after the procedure to assess for bleeding. 6. Assess pulses distal to the injection site to detect occluded blood flow. Compare pre- and postprocedure pulses. 7. Sandbag or pressure dressing may be applied to groin.
Renogram (renal scan): An IV injection of a radioactive nuclide (isotope) followed by use of a scanning device to detect radioactive emissions from the kidney(s); identifies kidney blood flow, tubular functions, and kidney excretion.	1. No specific activity or dietary restrictions. 2. Explain procedure to client.
Cystoscopy: A direct method to visualize the urethra and bladder by use of a tubular lighted scope (cystoscope). Scope may be inserted via the urethra or percutaneously.	1. Encourage fluids or administer fluids intravenously. 2. Explain lithotomy position that will be used. 3. Client may have general anesthesia or conscious sedation. 4. Preoperative medication is given. 5. Evaluate urine output after procedure; check for frequency, pink-tinged urine, and burning on urination (these are expected effects and will decrease with time). *Bright red blood in urine is not normal, and health care provider should be notified.* 6. Evaluate for orthostatic hypotension and thrombus formation after the procedure. 7. Provide warm sitz baths and mild analgesics to alleviate urethral discomfort.
Bladder scan: A portable ultrasound scanner used to estimate residual urine in the bladder.	1. No specific preparation. 2. After client voids, apply gel to the suprapubic area, and use scanner to visualize bladder and possible retained urine. 3. Make certain that the crosshairs on the aiming icon on the scanner are centered on or over the bladder; if crosshairs are offset, then the reading may not be accurate.

Urodynamic Studies

PROCEDURE	CLINICAL AND NURSING IMPLICATIONS
Cystometrogram (CMG): A procedure to determine the pressure exerted against the bladder wall by inserting a catheter and instilling water or saline solution; used to evaluate bladder capacity, bladder pressure, and voiding reflexes. **Urethral pressure profile or urethral pressure profilometry (UPP):** Evaluates for urinary incontinence and retention by recording variations of pressure in the urethra. **Urine stream testing:** Evaluates pelvic floor muscle strength.	1. Assess and evaluate for UTI after procedure. 2. Test is often indicated for clients having difficulty with urinary control (e.g., those with spinal cord traumatic injuries, stroke, etc.).
Kidney biopsy: A percutaneous needle biopsy to evaluate kidney disease by obtaining a specimen of kidney tissue for pathologic examination. Rarely done if client has only one kidney, uncontrolled hypertension, or a bleeding disorder.	1. Results of blood coagulation studies should be available on the chart before the biopsy procedure. 2. Results of IVP or ultrasound studies should be available before the biopsy. 3. Immediately after the procedure, pressure dressing is applied to biopsy site and checked frequently for bleeding. Right kidney is the usual biopsy site. 4. Assess for gross hematuria, flank pain, or a rise or fall in blood pressure. 5. Report pain radiating from the flank area to the abdomen. 6. Encourage intake of fluids: 3000 mL/day unless the client has kidney insufficiency. 7. Bed rest for 24 hrs. 8. Assess for complication of hemorrhage; may necessitate emergency surgical drainage or nephrectomy. 9. Avoid lifting heavy objects for 5-7 days. 10. Follow up with health care provider when anticoagulant drugs can be resumed.

Appendix 19.1 DIAGNOSTICS OF THE URINARY-RENAL SYSTEM—cont'd

PROCEDURE	CLINICAL AND NURSING IMPLICATIONS
Kidney ultrasound examination: A noninvasive procedure in which ultrasound waves are used, with the aid of a computer, to record images related to tissue density.	1. Encourage fluids, because test requires a full bladder. 2. Place in prone position. 3. Skin care to remove sonographic gel after procedure.

BUN, blood urea nitrogen; *GFR,* glomerular filtration rate; *IV,* intravenous; *IVP,* intravenous pyelogram; *KUB,* kidneys, ureters, and bladder; *NPO,* nothing by mouth; *UTI,* urinary tract infection.

Appendix 19.2 MEDICATIONS FOR THE URINARY SYSTEM

Urinary Medications

General Nursing Implications

- Encourage intake of 2000-3000 mL of fluid per day during treatment.
- Continue medication therapy until all medication has been taken.
- Most medications are better absorbed on an empty stomach; however, if GI distress occurs, they may be taken with food.
- Monitor intake and output and symptoms of increasing kidney problems.
- Check drug package insert for interactions with anticoagulants.

Urinary Tract Antiseptics: These drugs concentrate in the urine and are active against common urinary tract pathogens; they do not affect infections in blood or tissue.

MEDICATIONS	SIDE EFFECTS	NURSING IMPLICATIONS
Nitrofurantoin: PO, IM	GI upset, blood dyscrasia, and pulmonary reactions, peripheral neuropathy	1. Requires adequate kidney function to concentrate medication in urine. 2. Should not be administered to kidney transplant recipients. 3. Will turn the urine brownish orange. 4. Administer with meals or with milk.

Urinary Analgesics: Pain relievers typically used on urinary tract mucosa.

Phenazopyridine hydrochloride: PO Available OTC	Headache, GI disturbances	1. Contraindicated in kidney and liver dysfunction. 2. Advise client to report any yellow discoloration of skin or eyes. 3. Urine will turn orange. 4. Administer with caution in clients with impaired kidney function. 5. Can alter dipstick urine results.

Voiding Dysfunction: Drugs that assist with problems with voiding either related to inability to void or lack of voiding control.

Muscarinic Receptor Blockers: Suppress detrusor contractions and enhance bladder storage (drugs with anticholinergic activity).

Oxybutynin: PO, transdermal, topical gel	Drowsiness, dizziness, weakness, blurred vision, dry mouth, constipation	1. Contraindicated in glaucoma, myasthenia gravis, or GI obstruction. 2. Used cautiously in older adults. 3. Transdermal applications should rotate site and avoid reapplication to same site within 7 days. 4. Do not shower or bathe until 1 hr after applying topical gel.
Tolterodine: PO Solifenacin succinate: PO	Fatigue, headache, dry mouth, dry eyes, constipation	1. Grapefruit juice can increase blood levels. 2. May prolong QT interval, monitor for cardiac dysrhythmias.

α-Adrenergic Blockers: Reduce urethral sphincter resistance to urinary overflow.

Tamsulosin: PO	Headache, dizziness	1. Caution client about experiencing abnormal ejaculation. 2. Associated with increased incidence of rhinitis. 3. Avoid combining with hypotensive drugs.

Urinary Antispasmodics: Reduce bladder spasm.

Belladonna and opium (B&O): suppository	Drowsiness, dry mouth, urinary retention, rapid pulse	1. Considered a Schedule II drug. 2. Caution for clients with urinary retention issues such as BPH. 3. Contraindicated with glaucoma, hepatic or kidney disease, respiratory depression, alcohol use, or convulsive disorders.

Continued

Appendix 19.2   MEDICATIONS FOR THE URINARY SYSTEM—cont'd

℞

MEDICATIONS	SIDE EFFECTS	NURSING IMPLICATIONS
Glycoprotein Hormones: Stimulate bone marrow production of RBCs.		
Epoetin alfa: IV, subQ Darbepoetin alfa: IV, subQ	Hypertension, thromboembolic problems, headaches, GI disturbances	1. Closely evaluate hemodialysis access ports for clotting. 2. Evaluate client for adequate serum iron level, hematocrit, and blood pressure; adequate levels are required for medication to be effective. 3. Do not shake vial, because agitation can denature the protein. 4. *Use:* Maintain hemoglobin and hematocrit values in client with kidney failure and those who are HIV+ or on chemotherapy. For most clients, the hemoglobin should not exceed 10-11 gm/dL.

Immunosuppressive Medications

General Nursing Implications
• Avoid exposure to infection, wash hands frequently.
• Wear protective clothing; use sunscreen.
• Report any sore throat, fever, or other signs of infection to health care provider.
• Take medication at the same time each day to maintain consistent blood levels.
• No live virus vaccines or immunity-conferring agents should be administered while client is immunosuppressed.
• Depending on level of immunosuppression, client may need protective isolation.

Immunosuppressive Medications: Inhibit the immunologic response.

MEDICATIONS	ACTION	SIDE EFFECTS	NURSING IMPLICATIONS
Cytotoxic Drugs Azathioprine: PO, IV ▲ Methotrexate: PO, IV, IM subQ Cyclophosphamide: PO, IV, IM Mycophenolate mofetil: PO	Inhibits synthesis of T-cell DNA, RNA Blocks metabolism of purines Anti-inflammatory properties Used to suppress kidney transplant rejection and treat IBS and RA	Dose- and duration-dependent Bone marrow suppression: leukopenia, thrombocytopenia, anemia Nausea, vomiting, anorexia Alopecia, rash Hepatotoxicity	1. Interacts with allopurinol, causing an increase in azathioprine toxicity. 2. Avoid use in pregnancy. 3. Take with food or milk to decrease GI upset. 4. Should not be given to client with active infection. 5. Follow-up CBC should be done at least monthly while client is taking medication. 6. Closely monitor client for development of infections. 7. Many drug interactions, including prescribed.
Calcineurin Inhibitors Cyclosporine: PO, IV Tacrolimus: IV	Inhibits T-lymphocyte proliferation and function	Dose- and duration-dependent Infections, nephrotoxicity, hepatotoxicity, hypertension, hirsutism, gum hyperplasia, tremors, blood dyscrasias Side effects of tacrolimus are more toxic than cyclosporine	1. Monitor kidney function because nephrotoxicity occurs frequently. 2. Avoid use in pregnancy. 3. Use the pipette supplied by manufacturer to measure dose; mix with 4-8 oz (120-236 mL) of apple or orange juice. 4. Evaluate blood pressure and report elevations (especially occurs with heart transplants). 5. Monitor liver function studies and monitor BP in clients taking tacrolimus. 6. Good oral hygiene should be practiced to reduce gum problems. 7. Teach client that they should not stop taking the medication or change dosage without health care provider's order. 8. Serum blood levels and CBC are monitored at regular intervals. 9. Hirsutism that occurs is reversible. 10. Many drug interactions, including prescribed and OTC herbal medicines. Grapefruit juice can increase cyclosporine and tacrolimus levels.

Appendix 19.2 MEDICATIONS FOR THE URINARY SYSTEM—cont'd

MEDICATIONS	SIDE EFFECTS		NURSING IMPLICATIONS
Antibodies Muromonab-CD3: IV Basiliximab: IV	Monoclonal antibody that binds to CD3 receptors and inhibits T-cell function Basiliximab used for prophylaxis of acute organ rejection after kidney transplant	Fever, chills, dyspnea, chest pain bronchospasm, hypersensitivity reactions GI toxicity (diarrhea, nausea, abdominal pain)	1. More than 50% of clients experience a fever. 2. Have epinephrine and supportive emergency care available, because an allergic reaction can occur at any time during therapy. 3. Client may be premedicated with an IV glucocorticoid to minimize first dose reactions.
Glucocorticoids	See Appendix 6.2		
mTOR Inhibitors Sirolimus: PO Everolimus: PO	Suppresses lymphocyte proliferation; inhibits B cells from synthesizing antibodies	GI toxicity (diarrhea, nausea, vomiting, abdominal pain)	1. Has synergistic effect with cyclosporine and corticosteroids. 2. Avoid grapefruit and grapefruit juice. 3. Increases risk for infection. 4. Increases cholesterol and triglyceride levels. 5. Many drug interactions, including prescribed and OTC herbal medicines. 6. Avoid high fat foods, as they increase absorption.

CBC, complete blood count; *DNA*, deoxyribonucleic acid; *GI*, gastrointestinal; *Hgb*, hemoglobin; *HIV+*, human immunodeficiency virus-positive; *IBS*, irritable bowel syndrome; *IL-2*, interleukin 2; *IV*, intravenous; *PO*, by mouth (orally); *RA*, rheumatoid arthritis; *RNA*, ribonucleic acid; *subQ*, subcutaneously; *UTI*, urinary tract infection.

Appendix 19.3 URINARY DIVERSION

A urinary diversion is a means of diverting urinary output from the bladder to an external device or via a new avenue.

Temporary Urinary Diversion

Nephrostomy tubes (catheters): Insertion of catheters into the renal pelvis by surgical incision or percutaneous puncture. A small catheter is inserted into the renal pelvis and attached via connecting tubing to a closed-system drainage. Nephrostomy tubes may be temporary or permanent.

Nursing Implications
1. Provide routine nephrostomy tube care, with sterile dressing changes and tube flushing (if ordered).
2. Complications: Infection and secondary renal calculus formation; erosion of the duct by the catheter.

Ureteral catheters: Small, narrow catheters placed through the ureters into the renal pelvis; drain each renal pelvis individually. Often client also has a urinary retention catheter draining the urinary bladder. The catheter splints the ureters during healing and prevents edema from occluding the ureter.

Nursing Implications
1. Check frequently for placement of ureteral catheters; tension should be avoided.
2. Ureteral catheter should not be clamped or irrigated.
3. Maintain accurate intake and output records and label all catheters.

Incontinent Urinary Diversion

Ileal conduit (ileal loop): Transplantation of ureters into a segment of ileum or colon, which is then brought to the abdomen; a stoma

is then constructed. This type of urinary diversion is permanent (Fig. 19.6).

Nursing Implications
1. Stoma site is marked before surgery, because a device must be worn continuously.
2. Mucus is present in the urine after surgery when ileum segment is used; encourage a high fluid intake to "flush the ileal conduit."
3. Maintain meticulous skin care and changing of appliances.
4. Provide discharge instructions in regard to symptoms of obstruction, infection, and care of the ostomy; client needs information relating to purchase of supplies, ostomy clubs, follow-up visits, enterostomal therapists, and the importance of not irrigating the ileal conduit.

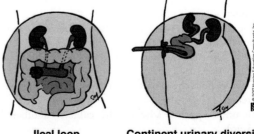

URINARY DIVERSIONS

Ileal loop   **Continent urinary diversion**

FIG. 19.6 Urinary Diversions. (From Zerwekh J, Garneau A, Miller CJ. [2017]. *Digital collection of the memory notebooks of nursing.* [4th ed.]. Chandler, AZ: Nursing Education Consultants, Inc.)

Continued

⚡ Practice & Next Generation NCLEX (NGN) Questions
Urinary Care of Adult Clients

More questions on
⊝volve

1. The client has had a right nephrostomy tube placed after a nephrolithotomy for removal of a kidney stone. When the client returns to the room, what is a **priority** nursing action?
   1. Irrigate the tube with 30 mL of normal saline solution four times a day.
   2. Clamp the tube if drainage is excessive.
   3. Advance the tube 1 in every 8 hrs.
   4. Ensure that the tube is draining freely.

2. A client with CKD has an internal arteriovenous fistula as the access site for hemodialysis on their left forearm. What action will the nurse take to protect this access site?
   1. Irrigate with heparin and normal saline solution every 8 hrs.
   2. Apply warm moist packs to the area after hemodialysis.
   3. Do not use the left arm to take blood pressure readings.
   4. Keep the arm elevated above the level of the heart.

3. The nurse is discussing the prevention of UTIs with a female client. What would be important to include in the discussion?
   1. Decrease fluid intake to decrease burning on urination.
   2. Take warm sitz baths with a mild bubble bath.
   3. Avoid spermicides with nonoxynol-9.
   4. Drink only acidic fluids such as orange juice.

4. At 0900, a 24-hr (composite) urine collection is started. What instructions will the nurse provide to the client?
   1. Place the first-voided specimen in the container and continue to collect the urine until 0900 the following day.
   2. Discard the first morning specimen, collect urine for the next 24 hrs, and make sure to void before the collection is completed at 0900 the following day.
   3. Discard the first morning specimen because it may contain concentrated abnormal components.
   4. Collect all urine from 0900 onward in separate containers that are labeled for time and amount of voiding.

5. A client returns from a percutaneous left kidney biopsy. What is a **priority** assessment finding after the procedure that needs to be reported to the health care provider?
   1. Dark, yellow urine.
   2. Increased bowel sounds.
   3. Nausea, vomiting, and anorexia.
   4. Bright red bleeding on dressing.

6. A client returns after having a cystoscopy performed under conscious sedation. The client does not have a urinary catheter in place and is voiding. What assessment findings require an immediate nursing action? **Select all that apply**.
   1. Gross hematuria.
   2. Severe abdominal pain.
   3. Blood clots in urine output.
   4. Temperature 99.2 °F (37.3°C)
   5. Urinary frequency.

7. What is the purpose of erythropoietin in the treatment of a client who has end-stage kidney disease?
   1. Promote blood clotting.
   2. Stimulate bone marrow to make red blood cells.
   3. Decrease the hemoglobin and hematocrit.
   4. Promote tubular secretion of sodium.

8. Which nursing observations indicate that a male client with a kidney stone is experiencing renal colic?
   1. Severe flank pain radiating toward the testicles.
   2. Stress incontinence with full bladder.
   3. Hematuria and severe burning on urination.
   4. Enuresis with hyperalbuminuria.

9. Which client is at the highest risk for developing CKD?
   1. Client with severe acute glomerulonephritis
   2. Client with placenta previa and hemorrhage at delivery
   3. Client with poorly controlled long-term hypertension
   4. Client who received IV aminoglycosides for an infection

10. A client has been prescribed nitrofurantoin for a urinary tract infection. What is important for the nurse to reinforce in the client's teaching plan about the medication?
    1. Take the medication on an empty stomach.
    2. May cause constipation and bloating.
    3. May make the urine a greenish color.
    4. Avoid spending time in the sunlight.

11. The nurse is admitting an older client with a UTI and possible kidney stone.

| Health History | Nurses' Notes | Vital Signs | Laboratory Results |

1500: An 83-year-old client is transferred from the nursing home to the hospital. Client is confused and screaming about severe pain in the lower back. Client reports nausea and vomiting for the past 3 hrs and discomfort when urinating. Client has a past history of stroke and hypertension, which is controlled with bumetanide and amlodipine.

- Temperature: 102.8°F (39.3°C)
- BP: 158/92 mm Hg
- Heart rate: 110 bpm and regular
- Respirations: 24 breaths/min
- SpO2: 96%

CLIENT FINDING	ACUTE PYELONEPHRITIS	CYSTITIS	URINARY CALCULI
Fever, chills			
Flank pain			
Urgency of urination			
Oliguria			
Nausea, vomiting			
Nocturia			
Dysuria			
Confusion			
Tachycardia			

For each client finding, use an X to specify whether the finding is consistent with the disease process of acute pyelonephritis, cystitis, or urinary calculi. Each finding may support more than one disease process.

12. A 75-year-old client has acute urinary retention after abdominal exploratory surgery. The nurse has an order for insertion of an indwelling urinary catheter and obtaining a urine specimen.

For each nursing action listed below, use an X to specify whether the action would be Indicated (appropriate or necessary), Non-Essential (makes no difference or not necessary), or Contraindicated (could be harmful), for *planning* the client's care at this time. Select only one response for each nursing action.

NURSING ACTIONS	INDICATED	NON-ESSENTIAL	CONTRAINDICATED
Use clean technique to insert the urinary catheter.			
Encourage fluids of 3000 mL/day.			
Keep the drainage bag below the level of the catheter or insertion site.			
Open the drainage system to collect the urine specimen.			
Empty the drainage bag by opening the drainage port at the bottom of the collection bag.			
Encourage a regular diet.			
Perform perineal care at least twice daily.			

Integumentary: Care of Adult Clients

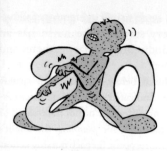

CHAPTER 20
INTEGUMENTARY

PHYSIOLOGY OF THE INTEGUMENTARY SYSTEM

A. Structure.
   1. Epidermis – outermost layer; contains the melanocytes and keratinocytes.
   2. Dermis – connective tissue below epidermis. Ridges in this layer form the fingerprints and footprints. Helps to maintain body temperature and regulate blood pressure (BP). Highly vascular.
   3. Hypodermis (subcutaneous) – located below dermis; anchors the muscles and bones to the skin; provides insulation, cushioning, temperature regulation.
   4. Nails.
   5. Hair.
   6. Glands.
      a. Sebaceous glands: produce sebum, an oily secretion that is deposited into the hair shaft.
      b. Apocrine glands: secrete an odorless fluid from the hair shaft, which, on contact with bacteria, produces a distinctive body odor. Concentrated in axilla and groin and become more active at puberty.
      c. Eccrine glands: sweat glands that are stimulated by elevated temperature and emotional stress.
B. Functions of the skin.
   1. Protection: barrier from the external environment is the primary function.
   2. Sensory: major receptor for general sensations such as touch, pain, hot, cold.
   3. Water balance.
      a. Water – 600 to 900 mL – is lost daily through insensible perspiration.
      b. Prevents loss of water and electrolytes from the internal environment.
   4. Regulates body temperature in response to external temperature.
   5. Involved in the activation of vitamin D.
   6. Delivery system for drugs.

System Assessment: Recognize Cues

A. Health history.
   1. History of rashes/lesions, hair loss, or changes in nails.
   2. Is any itching, burning, or discomfort associated with the problem?
   3. Contact with irritants, ultraviolet (UV) exposure, cold, unhygienic conditions, insect bites/stings.
   4. Current medications.
   5. Allergies to food, medications, insect stings, etc.
B. Physical assessment (Box 20.1).
   1. Inspection.
      a. Assess skin color.
         (1) Jaundice, cyanosis, erythema.
         (2) Vitiligo: loss of melanin, resulting in white, hypopigmented area.
         (3) Best areas to assess include the sclera, conjunctiva, nail beds, lips, and buccal mucosa.
      b. Assess vascularity.
         (1) Bruising, purpura, or petechiae.
         (2) Presence or absence of blanching with direct pressure.
      c. Assess lesions for:
         (1) Type, shape, color, size, distribution, grouping, and location.
         (2) Use a metric ruler to measure the size of the lesion.
         (3) Use appropriate specific terminology to describe and report type of lesion (Table 20.1).

Box 20.1 OLDER ADULT CARE FOCUS

Differences in Skin Assessment

Skin
- Increased wrinkling and sagging, redundant flesh around eyes, slowness of skin to flatten when pinched together (tenting)
- Dry, flaking skin: excoriation from scratching
- Thinning of skin
- Decreased rate of wound healing
- Increased incidence of bruising/skin tears
- Decreased sensation to touch, temperature, and pain
- Decreased subcutaneous fat, elastic fibers, and collagen stiffening

Hair
- Graying; dry, scaly scalp
- Thinning, baldness

Nails
- Thick, brittle, hardened nails with ridging and yellowing
- Prolonged return of blood with blanching
- Increased incidence of fungal infections

Table 20.1   COMMON DERMATOLOGIC LESIONS

Primary Lesions	Secondary Lesions
Macule: Flat, circumscribed area of color change in the skin without surface elevation; less than 1 cm in diameter (freckle, measles)	**Fissure:** Linear crack; may be dry or moist (athlete's foot, crack in corner of mouth)
Papule: Solid, elevated lesion; less than 1 cm in diameter (wart, elevated mole)	**Scale:** Excess epidermal cells caused by shedding (flaking of the skin)
Plaque: Circumscribed, solid lesion; greater than 1 cm in diameter (psoriasis, seborrheic keratosis)	**Scar:** Abnormal connective tissue that replaces normal skin (healed surgical incision)
Nodule: Raised solid lesion; larger and deeper than a papule	**Ulcer:** Loss of epidermis and dermis; crater-like; irregular shape (pressure ulcer, chancre)
Vesicle: Small elevation, usually filled with serous fluid or blood	**Atrophy:** Depression in skin resulting from thinning of the layers (aged skin, striae)
Bulla: Larger than a vesicle	**Excoriation:** Area where epidermis is missing, exposing the dermis (scabies, abrasion, scratch)
Pustule: Vesicle or bulla filled with pus (chickenpox, burn, herpes zoster [shingles])	**Petechiae:** Small red-to-purple spots on the skin caused by tiny hemorrhages in the dermal or submucosal layers
Wheal: Elevation of the skin caused by edema of the dermis (insect bite, urticaria, allergic reaction)	**Ecchymosis:** A blue-to-purple discoloration of the skin caused by leakage of blood into the subcutaneous tissue; usually as a result of tissue trauma
Cyst: Mass of fluid-filled tissue that extends to the subcutaneous tissue or dermis	

d. Assess for unusual odors, especially around lesions or in the intertriginous areas (axilla, overhanging abdominal folds, and groin).

e. Assess for chronic UV exposure and photoaging of skin – appearance of actinic (sun) keratoses (precancerous lesions), wrinkling, and telangiectasia.

(1) UVB – major factor of sunburn and nonmelanoma skin cancer.

(2) UVA – carcinogenic and causes accelerated aging effects.

f. Inspect hair (head and body for distribution) and nails (grooves, pitting, ridges, smoothness/thickness, and detachment from nail bed).

2. Palpation.

a. Determine temperature (use back of hand), tissue turgor (pinch under clavicle or back of hand), and mobility.

b. Evaluate moisture and texture.

C. Cultural considerations: assessment of color in dark skin is most easily determined in areas such as lips, mucous membranes, and nail beds.

D. Health promotion: sun exposure – use sun protection factor (SPF) 30 or higher if there is a history of skin cancer.

E. Diagnostics (see Appendix 20.1).

TEST ALERT Perform a risk assessment – evaluation of skin integrity.

BENIGN AND INFLAMMATORY DISORDERS

📋 Psoriasis

Psoriasis **is a chronic inflammatory autoimmune disorder characterized by rapid turnover of epidermal cells. Can be common in families.**

Assessment: Recognize Cues

A. Silvery scaling, plaques on the elbows, scalp, knees, palms, soles, trunk, and outside surface of the limbs.

B. If scales are scraped away, a dark red base of the lesion is seen, which will produce multiple bleeding points.

C. No cure; may improve, but then exacerbates throughout life.

D. Bilateral symmetry of symptoms is common.

Analyze Cues and Prioritize Hypotheses

The most important problems are body-image disturbance resulting from the appearance of the skin lesions and monitoring for infection as a complication of treatment measures.

Generate Solutions

Treatment

A. Medical.

1. Topical therapy.
   a. Coal tar preparation.
   b. Anthralin.
   c. Corticosteroids.
   d. Calcipotriene.
   e. Salicylic acid.
2. Photo chemotherapy.
   a. Psoralen, UVA (PUVA) therapy; must wear protective eyewear during treatment and for 24 hrs after therapy.
   b. UVB and narrow-band UVB radiation.
3. Systemic therapy: antimetabolites (methotrexate); less commonly used.
4. Biologic immunotherapy (adalimumab).

🏠 Home Care

A. Encourage verbalization regarding appearance.

B. Instruct client to use a soft brush to remove scales while bathing.

C. Assess client to determine factors that may trigger skin condition (e.g., emotional stress, trauma, seasonal changes).

D. Make sure client understands treatment and implications of care related to PUVA therapy and other treatments.

📋 Pressure Injury

A *pressure injury* (previously called a pressure ulcer; also known as decubitus ulcer, bedsore) is a localized injury to the skin and/or underlying tissue, usually over a bony prominence, resulting from pressure or pressure in combination with shear and/or friction.

> **TEST ALERT** Identify potential for skin breakdown: a pressure injury can and should be prevented. Identify clients at increased risk for ulcer development and begin preventive care as soon as possible. Do not wait for a reddened area to appear before preventive measures are initiated.

Assessment: Recognize Cues

A. Risk factors/etiology.
   1. Immobility/inactivity, shearing/friction/contractures.
   2. Inadequate nutrition.
   3. Fecal/urinary incontinence (maceration/excoriation).
   4. Decreased sensation/pain perception/circulation.
   5. Advancing age (loss of lean body mass; decreased elasticity of the skin; decreased venous and/or arterial blood flow).
   6. Equipment such as casts, restraints, traction devices, etc.
   7. Obesity, diabetes mellitus, low diastolic BP (less than 60 mm Hg).

B. Risk assessment instruments.
   1. Braden Scale.
      a. Scores six subscales: sensory perception, moisture, activity-mobility, nutrition, friction, and shear.
      b. Total score range is 6 to 23.
         (1) A score of 18 = at risk.
         (2) A score of 12 or less = high risk for development of a pressure ulcer.
      c. Most reliable and most often used assessment scale for pressure-ulcer risk.
   2. Pressure Ulcer Scale for Healing (PUSH tool).
      a. Developed by the National Pressure Ulcer Advisory Panel (NPUAP) as a quick, reliable tool to monitor the change in pressure-ulcer status over time.
      b. Ulcers are categorized according to size of the wound, exudate, and degree of tissue involvement.
      c. Monitor scoring over time: 0 = healed; 17 = not healed.

C. Clinical manifestations (Table 20.2).

Analyze Cues and Prioritize Hypotheses

The important problems include compromised tissue integrity and the potential for infection.

Generate Solutions

Treatment

A. Medical and surgical.
   1. Debridement: initial care is to remove moist, devitalized tissue.
      a. Surgical debridement: use of a scalpel or other instrument; used primarily when there is a large amount of nonviable tissue present.
      b. Mechanical debridement: wet-to-dry dressings, hydrotherapy, wound irrigation, and dextranomers (small beads poured over secreting wounds to absorb exudate).
      c. Enzymatic and autolytic debridement: use of enzymes or synthetic dressings that cover wound and self-digest devitalized tissue by the action of enzymes that are present in wound fluids.
   2. Wound cleansing: use normal saline solution for most cases.
      a. Use minimal mechanical force when cleansing to avoid trauma to the wound bed.
      b. Avoid the use of antiseptics (e.g., Dakin solution, iodine, hydrogen peroxide).
   3. Dressings: (should protect wound, be biocompatible, and hydrate).
      a. Moistened gauze.
      b. Film (transparent).
      c. Hydrocolloid (moisture and oxygen retaining).
      d. Alginate (absorbs exudate).
      e. Impregnated silver dressing (antimicrobial).
      f. Medicinal honey (lowers pH levels in wound, assists in autolytic debridement).
   4. Alternate therapies.
      a. Vacuum-assisted closure (VAC) – uses a wound-covering and vacuum device to remove fluids or infectious materials from the wound to enhance healing and promote the growth of granulation tissue.
      b. Electrical stimulation – uses a low-voltage current to stimulate blood supply and promote granulation formation.
      c. Hyperbaric oxygen therapy (HBO) – uses oxygen delivery at high pressure to force concentrated oxygen into the tissue to maximize tissue healing.
      d. Skin substitutes – use of laboratory engineered products. Used as a covering for the wound that is healing or awaiting grafting.
      e. Topical growth factors – facilitate wound healing by stimulating cell development and growth.

> ❗ **NURSING PRIORITY** Keep the pressure injury tissue moist and the surrounding intact skin dry.

Table 20.2   STAGES OF PRESSURE INJURY

Definition	*Diagram*

Stage 1: Nonblanchable erythema of intact skin

Intact skin with a localized area of nonblanchable erythema, which may appear different in darkly pigmented skin. Presence of blanchable erythema or changes in sensation, temperature, or firmness may precede visual changes. Color changes do not include purple or maroon discoloration; these may indicate deep-tissue pressure injury.

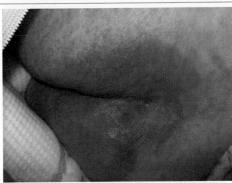

Stage 2: Partial-thickness skin loss with exposed dermis

Partial-thickness loss of skin with exposed dermis. The wound bed is viable, pink or red, moist, and may also present as an intact or ruptured serum-filled blister. Adipose (fat) and deeper tissues are not visible. Granulation tissue, slough, and eschar are not present. These injuries commonly result from adverse microclimate and shear in the skin over the pelvis and shear in the heel. This stage should not be used to describe moisture associated skin damage (MASD), including incontinence associated dermatitis (IAD), intertriginous dermatitis (ITD), medical adhesive related skin injury (MARSI), or traumatic wounds (skin tears, burns, abrasions).

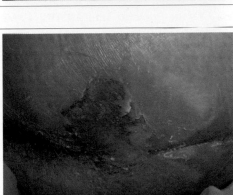

Stage 3: Full-thickness skin loss

Full-thickness loss of skin, in which adipose (fat) is visible in the ulcer and granulation tissue and epibole (rolled wound edges) are often present. Slough and/or eschar may be visible. The depth of tissue damage varies by anatomic location; areas of significant adiposity can develop deep wounds. Undermining and tunnelling may occur. Fascia, muscle, tendon, ligament, cartilage and/or bone are not exposed. If slough or eschar obscures the extent of tissue loss, this is an unstageable pressure injury.

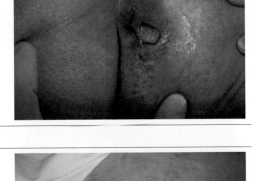

Stage 4: Full-thickness skin and tissue loss

Full-thickness skin and tissue loss with exposed or directly palpable fascia, muscle, tendon, ligament, cartilage, or bone in the ulcer. Slough and/or eschar may be visible. Epibole (rolled edges), undermining, and/or tunnelling often occur. Depth varies by anatomic location. If slough or eschar obscures the extent of tissue loss, this is an unstageable pressure injury.

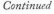

Continued

Table 20.2 STAGES OF PRESSURE INJURY—cont'd	
Definition	**Diagram**
Unstageable: Obscured full-thickness skin and tissue loss	
Full-thickness skin and tissue loss in which the extent of tissue damage within the ulcer cannot be confirmed because it is obscured by slough or eschar. If slough or eschar is removed, a stage-3 or stage-4 pressure injury will be revealed. Stable eschar (i.e., dry, adherent, intact, without erythema or fluctuance) on the heel or ischemic limb should not be softened or removed.	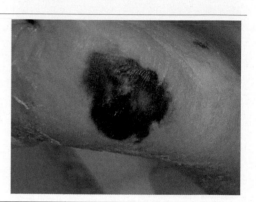
Deep Tissue Pressure Injury (DTPI): Persistent nonblanchable deep red, maroon, or purple discoloration	
Intact or nonintact skin with localized area of persistent nonblanchable deep red, maroon, or purple discoloration or epidermal separation revealing a dark wound bed or blood-filled blister. Pain and temperature change often precede skin color changes. Discoloration may appear different in darkly pigmented skin. This injury results from intense and/or prolonged pressure and shear forces at the bone-muscle interface. The wound may evolve rapidly to reveal the actual extent of tissue injury or may resolve without tissue loss. If necrotic tissue, subcutaneous tissue, granulation tissue, fascia, muscle, or other underlying structures are visible, this indicates a full-thickness pressure injury (unstageable, stage 3 or stage 4). Do not use DTPI to describe vascular, traumatic, neuropathic, or dermatologic conditions.	

From National Pressure Injury Advisory Panel (NPIAP): Updated staging system, 2016. Available at http://www.npuap.org/resources/educational-and-clinical-resources/pressure-injury-staging-illustrations. Used with permission of the National Pressure Injury Advisory Panel & date.

B. Dietary.
  1. Increased carbohydrates and protein.
  2. Increased vitamin C and zinc.

Nursing Interventions: Take Action

Goal: To prevent or relieve pressure, stimulate circulation.
A. Frequent change of position; turning frequency individualized based on risk factors, patient condition, and type of mattress; do not position directly on the trochanter.
B. Pressure-relieving mattress that provides for a continuous change in pressure across the mattress.
C. Memory foam mattresses or gel pads in chairs.
D. Avoid trauma to skin; use lift sheets and/or transfer devices.
E. Keep head of bed elevated less than 30 degrees when client is in bed.
F. Keep client's heels off the bed surface.

Goal: To keep skin clean and healthy and prevent the occurrence of a pressure injury.
A. Wash skin with mild soap and blot completely dry with a soft towel, especially after toileting.
B. Inspect skin frequently, especially over bony prominences and points of pressure.

C. Use moisturizer on dry skin.
D. Keep client well hydrated.
E. Use topical skin barrier creams, ointments, and pastes.
F. Avoid wrinkles in sheets or clothing that may serve as a source of irritation to the skin.

> **❗ NURSING PRIORITY** Avoid massage over bony prominences. When the side-lying position is used in bed, avoid positioning client directly on the trochanter; use the 30-degree lateral inclined position. Do not use donut-type devices. Maintain the head of the bed at or below 30 degrees or at the lowest degree of elevation. Teach able chair-bound persons to shift weight every 15 min.

Goal: To promote healing of pressure injury.
A. Specialized support surfaces such as mattresses and cushions.
B. Nutritional supplements. Ensure adequate fluid intake.
C. Wound care dressings.
D. Keep pressure injury area dry.
  1. Minimize skin exposure to moisture caused by incontinence, perspiration, or wound drainage.
  2. Use only underpads or briefs made of materials that absorb moisture and provide a quick-drying surface next to the skin.

3. Use skin barriers to decrease contamination and increase healing of a noninfected ulcer.
4. Observe the ulcer for signs of infection. Infected ulcers must be debrided for healing to occur.

SKIN INFECTIONS AND INFESTATIONS

Cellulitis

Cellulitis **is an inflammation of the subcutaneous tissues that often occurs after a break in the skin; it is most commonly caused by** *Staphylococcus aureus* **or** *Streptococcus.*

Assessment: Recognize Cues

A. Intense redness, edema with diffuse border, tenderness, localized warmth.
B. Chills, malaise, and fever.
C. Most common location is the lower legs.

Analyze Cues and Prioritize Hypotheses

The important problems include the potential for systemic infection.

Generate Solutions

Treatment
A. Medical.
  1. Moist heat, immobilization, elevation of affected extremity.
  2. Systemic antibiotic therapy.

Home Care

A. Teach the client and family the importance of good handwashing.
B. Encourage adherence to therapeutic regimen, especially taking the full course of antibiotics.

Viral infections

Viral infections **of the skin (similar to body infections) are difficult to treat.**

Assessment: Recognize Cues

A. Herpes simplex virus type 1 (HSV-1) (fever blister, cold sore).
  1. Painful local reaction consisting of vesicles with an erythematous base; most often appears around the mouth and/or nose.
  2. Contagious by direct contact; infection is lifelong and recurrent; there is no immunity.
  3. Chronic disorder that may be exacerbated by stress, trauma, menses, sunlight, fatigue, or systemic infection.
  4. Recurrent episodes are characterized by appearance of lesions in the same place.
  5. Not to be confused with HSV-2, which primarily occurs below the waist (genital herpes).
  6. It is possible for HSV-1 to cause genital lesions and for HSV-2 to cause oral lesions (see Chapter 18, Sexually Transmitted Infections).

B. Herpes zoster (shingles).
  1. Related to the chickenpox virus: varicella.
  2. Contagious to anyone who has not had chickenpox or who may be immunosuppressed.
  3. Linear patches of vesicles with an erythematous base are located along spinal and cranial nerve tracts, or dermatomes; zosteriform.
  4. Often unilateral and appears on the trunk; however, may also appear on the face.
  5. Pain, burning, and neuralgia occur at the site before outbreak of vesicles.
  6. Often precipitated by the same factors as herpes simplex infection; incidence increases with age.
  7. Postherpetic neuralgia is common in older adults.

Analyze Cues and Prioritize Hypotheses

The important problems include compromised tissue integrity, spread of infection to others, chronic nature of the herpes infections, and postherpetic neuralgia (herpes zoster).

Generate Solutions

Treatment
A. Usually symptomatic; application of soothing moist compresses.
B. Analgesics; gabapentin for postherpetic neuralgia; systemic corticosteroids may reduce symptoms.
C. Antiviral agents (see Appendix 20.2).
D. Herpes zoster vaccine (Shringrix) is recommended for adults over 50 years of age regardless of whether they report a prior episode of chickenpox or herpes zoster or received Zostavax (previous immunization that is no longer used).

Home Care

A. Alleviate pain by administering analgesics.
B. Antihistamines may be administered to control itching.
C. Usually, lesions heal without complications; herpes simplex usually heals without scarring, whereas herpes zoster may cause scarring.
D. If client is hospitalized, establish contact precautions for herpes zoster.

Neoplasms of the Integumentary System

Skin neoplasms **can be benign or malignant. Overexposure to sunlight is the major cause of skin cancer.**

Assessment: Recognize Cues

A. Risk factors/etiology.
  1. Overexposure to sunlight; indoor tanning.
  2. Fair skin type (blond or red hair and blue or green eyes).
  3. Exposure to chemicals.
  4. Family history of skin cancer.

B. Clinical manifestations.
1. Actinic keratosis.
   a. Most common of all premalignant conditions.
   b. Small macules or papules with dry, rough, adherent yellow or brown scales; irregular shape.
   c. Appears on face, neck, back of hand, and forearm.
   d. May slowly progress to squamous cell carcinoma.
2. Basal cell carcinoma.
   a. Most common type of skin malignancy.
   b. Appears as a small waxy nodule with a translucent pearly border.
   c. Appears more frequently on the face, usually between the hairline and upper lip.
   d. Rarely metastasizes.
3. Squamous cell carcinoma.
   a. Usually follows excessive sun exposure, irradiation, or trauma causing scarring.
   b. May metastasize.
   c. Appears as an opaque firm nodule (dome shaped) with an indistinct border, scaling, and ulceration.
   d. Increased risk in immunocompromised and those with kidney transplants.
4. Malignant melanoma (Fig. 20.1).
   a. Some genetic predisposition; also known to be related to UV exposure without protection or overexposure to artificial light (tanning beds).
   b. Highest mortality rate of any form of skin cancer.
   c. Common sites include legs, then back in women; and back, then chest in men.
   d. Characterized by a sudden or progressive change in size, symmetry, color, elevation, or shape of a mole.
   e. Often dark brown or black in color.
   f. Can metastasize to any organ, including brain and heart.

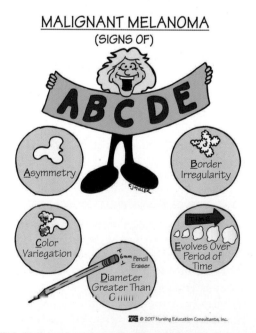

FIG. 20.1 Malignant melanoma. (From Zerwekh J, Garneau AJ, Miller CJ. Digital *Collection of the Memory Notebooks of Nursing*. 4th ed. Chandler, AZ: Nursing Education Consultants, Inc.; 2017.)

Analyze Cues and Prioritize Hypotheses

The important problems include compromised tissue integrity and the need for early recognition of whether the skin lesion is benign or malignant.

Generate Solutions

Treatment

A. Medical.
1. Radiation therapy.
2. Chemotherapy.
3. Biologic therapy.
B. Surgical.
1. Excisional surgery/skin grafts.
   a. All suspicious lesions should be biopsied.
   b. Mohs procedure: a specialized form of excision, used primarily to treat basal cell and squamous cell cancers; skin grafts may be required because of the extent of the excision.
2. Laser treatment.
3. Cryosurgery.

Nursing Interventions: Take Action

Goal: To help the client understand the disease process, importance of follow-up treatment, and measures to maintain health.

A. Teach the importance of avoiding unnecessary exposure to sunlight.
B. Apply protective sunscreen when outside.
C. Teach the warning signs of cancer.
D. Treat moles found in areas where there is friction or repeated irritation.

Goal: To support the client and promote psychological homeostasis.

A. Allow for verbalization of fear and anxiety.
B. Encourage verbalization relating to altered body image when large, wide, full-thickness excisions must be made to treat malignant melanoma.
C. Point out client's resources and support effective coping mechanisms.
D. Teach the importance of examining and checking moles and any new lesions.

Elective Cosmetic/Reconstruction Procedures

The purpose of cosmetic surgery is to improve self-image.

Assessment: Recognize Cues

A. Preoperative psychological assessment may be performed.
1. Assists in identifying unrealistic expectations.
B. Types of elective cosmetic surgery.
1. Chemical facelift or peel: superficial destruction of the upper layers of skin with a cauterant solution.
2. Tretinoin and alpha-hydroxy acids: topical application provides reversal of photodamaged skin and normal aging by influencing epithelial cell growth and differentiation.
3. Microdermabrasion: removal of epidermis to treat acne, scars, wrinkles, etc.

4. Botulinum toxin injection: neurotoxin that causes temporary interference with neuromuscular transmission, paralyzing the affected muscle.
5. Facelift (rhytidectomy): lifting and repositioning of facial and neck tissues.
6. Dermal fillers: injection of hyaluronic acid filler to smooth away wrinkles around mouth and nose.
7. Eyelid lift (blepharoplasty): removal of redundant (excess) eyelid tissue.
8. Liposuction: technique for removing subcutaneous fat from face and body.

Analyze Cues and Prioritize Hypotheses

The important problems are potential for infection and unrealistic expectations of the outcome.

Nursing Interventions: Take Action

Goal: To provide preoperative care.
A. Reinforce information from informed consent obtained by health care provider.
B. Instruct client to avoid taking vitamin E, aspirin, and other nonsteroidal anti-inflammatory agents at least 1 week before surgery to prevent bleeding.
C. Explain that wound healing and final results may not be complete until 1 year after procedure.

Goal: To provide postoperative care.
A. Administer analgesics for pain management.
B. Observe for bleeding.
C. Teach client about the signs and symptoms of infection.
D. Instruct client to avoid all tobacco products for several weeks after surgery because they constrict blood vessels and delay healing.
E. A reduction of melanin in the skin occurs as a result of the procedure; therefore, teach client who had a chemical peel to avoid the sun for 6 months to prevent hyperpigmentation.
F. Teach client who has had liposuction to wear spandex compression garments to reduce risk for bleeding and prevent fluid accumulation.

Burns

Burns are complex injuries involving loss of tissue integrity, which affects many body systems.
A. Types of burns.
1. Thermal injury: most common type of burn injury; results from flames, flash (explosion), scalding, or direct contact with hot object.
2. Electrical injury: intense heat is generated from electrical current and causes coagulation necrosis as current flows through the body.
3. Chemical injury: results from contact with a corrosive substance.
4. Smoke, inhalation injury, and noxious chemicals.
   a. Inhalation of smoke or superheated air causes swelling and/or occlusion of airway.
   b. Inhaled carbon monoxide combines with hemoglobin, thereby decreasing availability of oxygen to cells and resulting in hypoxia.

Assessment: Recognize Cues

A. Respiratory – determine circumstances surrounding injury: Did fire occur in an enclosed space? Is there risk for an inhalation injury?
1. Assess for burns on the face and in the mouth.
2. Examine mouth and sputum for black particles and the nasal septum for edema.
3. Assess for change in respiratory pattern indicating impending respiratory obstruction.
   a. Increased hoarseness.
   b. Drooling or difficulty swallowing.
   c. Audible wheezing, crackles, presence of stridor.
4. Assess for development of carbon monoxide poisoning.
   a. Mild: headache, decreased vision.
   b. Moderate: tinnitus, drowsiness, vertigo, altered mental state, decreased BP, skin has a "cherry red" color.
B. Evaluate cardiac output and peripheral circulation.
1. Hypovolemic shock may occur early.
2. Sludging (intravascular agglutination) may result from massive fluid shift.
3. Peripheral circulation may be impaired by circumferential burns or edema.
4. Assess these metrics: mean arterial pressure (MAP) greater than 65 mm Hg, systolic pressure above 90 mm Hg, and pulse less than 120 beats/min.
C. Determine hydration status.
1. Monitor for acute tubular necrosis.
2. Monitor urine output (should be at least 0.5-1 mL/kg/hr in older children and adults; 1-2 mL/kg/hr in children weighing less than 66 lb [30 kg]).
3. Fluid shift and edema formation occur within first 12 hrs after burn injury and can continue for 24 to 36 hrs.
4. Fluid mobilization and diuresis occur 48 to 72 hrs after burn injury when capillary integrity is restored.
D. Determine tetanus immunization status.

> **! NURSING PRIORITY** The client with a burn injury is often awake, mentally alert, and cooperative at first. The level of consciousness may change as respiratory status deteriorates or as the fluid shift occurs, precipitating hypovolemia.

E. Determine the severity of the burn injury (Box 20.2 and Fig. 20.2).
1. Extent of burn surface (burn surface area).
   a. Rule of nines: generally used for quick estimation in both adults and children.
   b. A more accurate determination uses charts that calculate the total body surface area burned and the depth of the burn based on client's age (e.g., Lund-Browder chart or Sage Burn Diagram).
2. Area of burn.
   a. Circumferential burns (burns surrounding an entire extremity) may cause severe reduction of circulation to an extremity as a result of edema formation and lack of elasticity of the eschar, leading to compartment syndrome.

Box 20.2 DEPTH OF BURNS

- *Superficial partial-thickness or first-degree burn*: Area is reddened and blanches with pressure; no edema is present; the area is generally painful to the touch.
- *Deep partial-thickness or second-degree burn*: Dermis and epidermis are affected; large, thick-walled blisters form; underlying skin is erythematous; these burns are painful.
- *Full-thickness or third- and fourth-degree burn*: All dermis skin layers are destroyed; subcutaneous tissue and muscle may be damaged; burn usually has a dry appearance, may be white or charred; will require skin grafting to cover the area; fourth degree involves underlying structures (fascia, tendons, and bones), which are severely damaged, usually blackened.

DEGREE OF BURN BY TISSUE LAYER

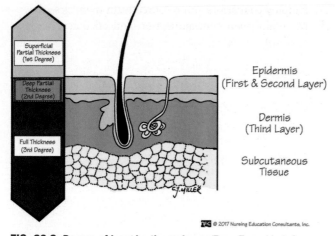

FIG. 20.2 Degree of burn by tissue layer. (From Zerwekh J, Garneau AJ, Miller CJ. *Digital Collection of the Memory Notebooks of Nursing.* 4th ed. Chandler, AZ: Nursing Education Consultants, Inc.; 2017.)

b. The location of the burn is related to the severity of the injury:
  (1) Face, neck, chest – respiratory obstruction.
  (2) Hands, feet, joints, eyes – difficulties with self-care.
  (3) Ears, nose, genital area – risk of infection.
3. Age.
  a. Infants have an immature immune system and poor body defense.
  b. Older adult clients heal more slowly and are more likely to have wound infection problems and pulmonary complications.
4. Presence of other health problems: diabetes and peripheral vascular disease delay wound healing.

Analyze Cues and Prioritize Hypotheses

The most important problems are alterations in fluid volume and nutrition, acute pain, risk of infection and contracture, change in body image, and coping with long-term rehabilitation.

Generate Solutions

Treatment

A. Respiratory status takes priority over treatment of the burn injury. Prophylactic intubation may be performed if inhalation injury is suspected.

B. If the burn area is small (less than approximately 10% of body surface area), apply cool compresses or immerse injured area in cool water to decrease heat; ice should not be directly applied to the burn area.

C. Administer tetanus immunization if more than 5 years since last injection.

D. Do not put any ointment or salve on the burn area.

E. If the cause of the burn is chemical, remove all clothing and brush all dry chemicals off the skin before thoroughly flushing the area with a large amounts of cool water.

F. Fluid resuscitation.
  1. Used for clients with burns on 15% to 20% or more of body surface area.
  2. Placement of large-bore intravenous catheters.
  3. Fluid replacement: calculation of fluid replacement begins from time of burn, not time of admission to the emergency department.
    a. One-half of first 24-hr fluid replacement amount is given during the first 8 hrs after burn injury.
    b. One-fourth of remaining amount is given during the second and third 8-hr periods.
    c. Urine output is the most sensitive indicator of fluid status; fluid replacement may be titrated to keep urine output adequate for client's age.

G. Maintain NPO (nothing by mouth) status; assess need for nasogastric tube.

H. Intravenous H_2 blockers and/or proton pump inhibitors started to prevent gastric (stress) ulcers.

I. Analgesics are given intravenously; do not give intramuscularly, subcutaneously, or orally, because they will not be absorbed effectively.

J. Methods of wound care (area is cleaned and debrided of necrotic burned tissue).
  1. Open method (exposure): burn is covered with a topical antibiotic cream and no dressing is applied.
  2. Closed method (dressing): fine mesh is used to cover the burned surface; may be impregnated with antibiotic ointment, or ointment may be applied before the dressing is placed.
  3. Escharotomy: procedure involves excision through the eschar to increase circulation to an extremity with circumferential burns.
  4. Enzymatic debriding agents: collagenase, fibrinolysin, and papain and urea may be used.
  5. Wound grafting: as eschar is debrided, and granulation tissue begins to form; grafts are used to protect the wound and promote healing.

K. Nutritional support.
  1. Diet should be high in calories and protein.
  2. In clients who have large burn surface areas, supplemental gastric tube feedings or hyperalimentation may be used.

Nursing Interventions: Take Action

Goal: To maintain patent airway and prevent hypoxia.

A. Anticipate respiratory difficulty if there are any indications of inhalation injury.

   1. Remain with client; assess respiratory status frequently.
   2. Provide supplemental oxygen.
   3. Be prepared to intubate client: airway edema can occur rapidly.
   4. Assess airway as fluid resuscitation begins; may precipitate more edema.

B. Assess for carbon monoxide poisoning.

C. Anticipate transfer to burn unit if burns cover more than 15% to 20% of body surface area, depending on depth of burn, age of client, and presence of other chronic illnesses.

Goal: To evaluate fluid status and determine circulatory status and adequacy of fluid replacement.

A. Obtain client's weight on admission.

B. Assess status and time frame of fluid resuscitation; *calculation of fluid replacement begins at time of burn injury, not on arrival at hospital.*

C. Evaluate kidney status and urine output; adequate output: adults 0.5 to 1 mL/kg/hr and children 1 to 2 mL/kg/hr.

Goal: To prevent or decrease infection.

A. Implement infection-control procedures to protect the client.

B. After eschar sloughs or is removed, assess wound for infection; infection is difficult to identify before the eschar sloughs.

Goal: To maintain nutrition and promote positive nitrogen balance for healing.

A. Work with dietitian to maintain nutritional intake.

B. Provide tube feedings as indicated.

C. Address total parenteral nutrition as indicated (see Appendix 14.5).

D. Monitor daily weight.

Goal: To prevent contractures and scarring.

A. Encourage client to attempt mobilization and ambulation as soon as possible.

B. Passive and active range of motion should be initiated from the beginning of burn therapy and continue throughout therapy.

C. Position client to prevent flexion contractures; position of comfort for the client may increase contracture formation.

D. Use splints and exercises to prevent flexion contractures.

E. Use pressure dressings and garments to contour the healing burn area and keep scars flat; prevent elevation and enlargement above the original burn injury area.

Goal: To promote acceptance and adaptation to alterations in body image.

A. Employ counselors and resource team members.

B. Maintain open communication and encourage expression of feelings.

C. Anticipate depression as a normal consequence of burn trauma; it should decrease as condition improves.

> **❗ NURSING PRIORITY** It is important to recognize that the client's anger is not a direct attack on the care provider; it is an expression of grief and sorrow.

Home Care

A. Physical therapy.

B. Continue high-calorie, high-protein diet.

C. Wound care management.

D. Avoid exposure of burn area to direct sunlight and irritating agents.

Appendix 20.1 SKIN DIAGNOSTIC STUDIES

Skin Testing

Purpose: to confirm sensitivity to a specific allergen by placing antigen on or directly below skin (intradermal) to check for presence of antibodies.

1. Three methods – allergen applied to arms or back and injected at a 15-degree angle.
   • Cutaneous scratch test (also known as a *tine* or *prick test*): allergen applied to a superficial scratch on skin.
   • Intradermal injection: small amount of the allergen is injected intradermally in rows; more accurate; high risk for severe allergic reaction; used only for those who do not react to cutaneous method.
   • Patch test: used to determine whether client is allergic to testing material (small amount applied on back) – client returns in 48 hrs for evaluation.
2. Interpreting results.
   • *Immediate* reaction: appears within minutes after the injection; marked by erythema and a wheal; denotes a positive reaction.
   • *Positive* reaction: indicates an antibody response to previous exposure; local wheal-and-flare response occurs.
   • *Negative* reaction: inconclusive; may indicate that antibodies have not formed yet or that antigen was deposited too deeply in skin (not an intradermal injection); may also indicate immunosuppression.
3. Complications: range from minor itching to anaphylaxis (see Chapter 6).

> **❗ NURSING PRIORITY** Never leave client alone during skin testing because of the risk of anaphylaxis. If a severe reaction occurs, plan to apply an anti-inflammatory topical cream to skin site (scratch test) or a tourniquet to the arm (intracutaneous test) and possible oral antihistamines and/or epinephrine injection.

Wood's Lamp (black light)

Purpose: examination of skin with long-wave ultraviolet light that causes specific substances or areas to fluoresce (e.g., *Pseudomonas* species, fungi, patches of vitiligo).

1. Test not painful.
2. Room is darkened.

Continued

❧ Practice & Next Generation NCLEX (NGN) Questions

Integumentary: Care of Adult Clients

1. An older adult client has an open wound over the coccyx that extends through the dermis and subcutaneous tissue, exposing the deep fascia. The wound edges are distinct, and the wound bed is a pink-red color. There is no bruising or sloughing. The nurse would correctly document this ulcer as what stage?
   1. Stage I.
   2. Stage II.
   3. Stage III.
   4. Stage IV.

2. Herpes zoster has been diagnosed in an older adult client. When planning nursing care for this client, what nursing action would be appropriate?
   1. Apply antifungal cream to the areas daily.
   2. Maintain client on contact precautions.
   3. Instruct on the need for sexual abstinence.
   4. Closely inspect the perineal area for lesions.

3. Which nursing interventions will the nurse take to reduce pressure points that may lead to pressure ulcers? **Select all that apply**.
   1. Position the client directly on the trochanter when side-lying.
   2. Avoid the use of donut-type devices.
   3. Massage bony prominences.
   4. Elevate the head of the bed no more than 30 degrees when possible.
   5. When the client is in side-lying position, use 30-degree lateral incline.
   6. Avoid uninterrupted sitting in any chair or wheelchair.

4. The nurse is teaching self-care to an older adult client. What would the nurse encourage the client to do for their dry, itchy skin?
   1. Apply a moisturizer on all dry areas daily.
   2. Shower twice a day with a mild soap.
   3. Use a pumice stone and exfoliating sponge on areas to remove dry scaly patches.
   4. Wear protective pads on areas that show the most dryness.

5. What is the **priority** assessment finding for a client who has sustained burns on the face and neck?
   1. Spreading, large, clear vesicles.
   2. Increased hoarseness.
   3. Difficulty with vision.
   4. Increased thirst.

6. A client has sustained a third-degree burn. What would the nurse expect to find during assessment of the burn?
   1. Area reddened, blanches with pressure, no edema.
   2. Blackened skin and underlying structures.
   3. Thick, clear blisters, underlying skin edematous and erythematous.
   4. Dry, white, and charred appearance; damage to subcutaneous tissues.

7. A client is prescribed bacitracin topical ointment for a skin lesion. The client **most likely** has what type of infection?
   1. Fungal infection.
   2. Viral infection.
   3. Parasitic infection.
   4. Bacterial infection.

8. When completing an assessment on a client with psoriasis, the nurse expects to find what type of skin appearance?
   1. Silvery scaling and plaques on the elbows with a red base when scraped.
   2. Inflammatory lesions or pustules, primarily on the face.
   3. Reddened lesions in the antecubital and popliteal space with pruritus.
   4. Pustule-like lesions with honey-colored crusts that are surrounded by erythema.

9. The nurse understands that melanomas tend to have the following characteristics. **Select all that apply**.
   1. Border irregularity.
   2. Diameter less than 6 mm.
   3. Asymmetric.
   4. Evolving or changing in some way.
   5. Differently colored areas.
   6. Clear or pearly translucent appearance.

10. Which assessment will require the most **immediate** action by the nurse for a client who had a rhytidectomy (i.e., facelift)?
    1. Identifies pain level at 3 on a 10-point scale.
    2. Heart rate 116 beats/min, BP 110/68 mm Hg, respirations 20 breaths/min.
    3. Scant amount of serosanguineous drainage on facial dressing.
    4. Skin around the left ear incision is pale and cool to palpation.

11. A client presents at the dermatology clinic.

| Health History | Nurses' Notes | Vital Signs | Laboratory Results |

1400: A 28-year-old female reports the sudden appearance of reddened areas with a silver-white scale on the elbows, which are somewhat painful and itchy. On exam, there are several large reddened and raised areas noted on both elbows that are covered with a silver plaque. Pinpoint bleeding is noted when the plaque is removed. Vitals signs are all within normal range. Client has never had a history of skin problems, is well nourished, and cooperative. Client relates that her mother has a long history of shingles.

For each client finding, use an X to specify whether the finding is consistent with the disease process of herpes zoster or psoriasis. Each finding may support more than one disease process.

CLIENT FINDING	HERPES ZOSTER	PSORIASIS
Raised red patches covered with silver scales		
Contagious		
Pruritis		
Small groups of vesicles on the skin		
Pinpoint bleeding		
Low-grade fever		
Pain in the area of the lesion		

12. An adult is admitted to the emergency department with burns.

| Health History | Nurses' Notes | Vital Signs | Laboratory Results |

2100: A 32-year-old client is admitted with burns to lower chest and arms from a flash of fire while lighting a fire in an outdoor firepit. Client is moaning with pain and reports pain at 9 on a scale of 10. Shirt appears adhered to the chest.

- Temperature: 99°F (37.2°C)
- BP: 102/68 mm Hg
- Heart rate: 120 beats/min and regular
- Respirations: 28 breaths/min
- SpO2: 95% on room air

Drag and drop the assessment findings from the choices below to fill in each blank in the following sentence.

The assessment findings that require **immediate** follow-up include _____, _____, _____, and _____.

ASSESSMENT FINDINGS

Moist blebs and blisters on lower chest and arms
Vital Signs: respirations 28, pulse 120 beats/min, BP 102/68 mm Hg
Clothing appears adhered to skin
Burn odor
Cherry-red appearance to skin
Pain of 9 on a scale of 10

Maternity Nursing Care

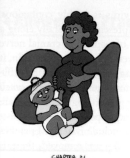

CHAPTER 21
MATERNITY/NEWBORN

ANTEPARTUM

Family Planning

Family planning *involves choosing when to have a family and includes contraception and methods to achieve pregnancy.*

Infertility

Infertility **is the inability to conceive a child after a year or more of regular unprotected intercourse or the inability to carry a pregnancy to live birth (recurrent spontaneous abortions).**

Assessment: Recognize Cues

A. Causes of infertility.
  1. Male.
    a. Coital difficulties, testicular abnormalities.
    b. Semen factors – low semen, autoantibodies.
    c. Structural abnormalities.
  2. Female.
    a. Hormonal dysfunction, structural abnormalities.
    b. Coital factors: use of lubricants should be avoided; douches negatively affect fertility.
    c. Chronic pelvic and vaginal infections.
    d. Isoimmunization to sperm: development of antibodies.

Analyze Cues and Prioritize Hypotheses

The most important problems are decreased self-esteem, feelings of hopelessness regarding inability to conceive, decreased ability to cope, and potential lack of understanding regarding conception and fertility.

Generate Solutions

Treatment
A. Surgery to correct structural defects.
B. Administration of fertility medications.
C. Therapeutic insemination.

Nursing Interventions: Take Action

Goal: To assist with the assessment and treatment of the couple's specific infertility problem.
Goal: To provide emotional support and encourage expression of feelings connected with infertility.
A. Promote expression of feelings related to sexuality, self-esteem, and body image.

B. Assess for common reactions of surprise, denial, anger, and guilt.
C. Promote a variety of coping strategies to help deal with the uncomfortable feelings.

Contraception

Contraception **is the voluntary prevention of pregnancy. Two important factors influence the selection of the type of contraceptive method: acceptability and effectiveness.**

TEST ALERT Determine the client's attitude toward and use of birth control methods and consider contraindications to chosen contraceptive method.

Assessment: Recognize Cues

A. Types of contraception.
  1. Temporary contraception: methods used to delay or avoid pregnancy.
  2. Permanent: voluntary sterilization.
B. Contraceptive methods (see Appendix 21.1).

Genetic Counseling

Genetic **(hereditary): describes any disorder or disease that is transmitted from generation to generation.**
Congenital: **describes any disorder present at birth or existing before birth that is caused by genetic or environmental factors or both.**

Assessment: Recognize Cues

A. Maternal and paternal factors.
  1. Increased age (35 years and older) and paternal (40-50 years of age).
  2. Presence of disease (e.g., diabetes mellitus, epilepsy).
  3. Reproductive history of spontaneous abortions, still-births, or birth defects in previous children.
B. Family history (e.g., hemophilia, spina bifida).
C. Ethnicity/racial background (e.g., sickle cell trait, Tay-Sachs disease).

Nursing Interventions: Take Action

Goal: To allow families to make informed decisions about reproduction.

A. Assist with detailed family history and pedigree chart.

B. Determine family's understanding of the information.

Goal: To provide information about available diagnostic tests and treatments.

A. Be precise and give detailed information.

B. Use familiar examples to illustrate probability of specific risks (e.g., flipping coins).

C. Emphasize the importance of the couple making an informed decision.

FETAL AND MATERNAL ASSESSMENT TESTING

Amniocentesis

An invasive procedure performed on the mother to obtain amniotic fluid.

A. An outpatient procedure performed at 14 to 16 weeks of pregnancy, although it may be performed later in the pregnancy for genetic testing if an ultrasound shows an anomaly.

B. Procedure: placenta is located by ultrasound examination; a needle is inserted through the abdomen (puncture site has been anesthetized); amniotic fluid is aspirated and sent to the laboratory for testing.

C. For Rh-negative women, $Rh_o(D)$ immune globulin (RhIG; also referred to as RhoGAM) is administered after the amniocentesis to prevent hemolysis of fetal blood cells.

! NURSING PRIORITY The fetal heart rate (FHR) is assessed before and after amniocentesis.

Ultrasonography

Ultrasonography is a noninvasive technique in which high-frequency pulse sound waves are transmitted by a transducer applied directly to the woman's abdomen or transvaginally.

A. Purpose.
1. Identifies placental location for amniocentesis or to determine placenta previa.
2. Determines gestational age; detects fetal anomalies and multifetal gestation.
3. Monitors fetal growth to assess for intrauterine growth restriction (IUGR).
4. Evaluates volume of amniotic fluid.

B. Procedure (abdominal).
1. Procedure may be done anytime during pregnancy.
2. Performed with a full bladder, except when ultrasonography is used to localize the placenta before amniocentesis.
3. Requires approximately 20 to 30 min to perform; client must lie flat on back, which may be uncomfortable.

C. Transvaginal is better tolerated because client is in lithotomy position and full bladder is not required.

Chorionic Villus Sampling

Chorionic villus sampling is a method of obtaining fetal tissue for genetic testing.

A. Purpose: to obtain fetal tissue to establish a genetic profile as a first trimester alternative to amniocentesis; use is declining with increased availability of noninvasive screening techniques.

B. Procedure.
1. An invasive procedure performed with ultrasound guidance between 10- and 13-weeks' gestation; technique may be transcervical or transabdominal.
2. Administer RhIG to Rh-negative mothers because of possibility of fetal-maternal hemorrhage.

Percutaneous Umbilical Blood Sampling

An invasive procedure, also called cordocentesis, percutaneous umbilical blood sampling (PUBS) is fetal blood sampling performed during the second and third trimesters.

A. Purpose: most widely used method for fetal blood sampling and transfusion.

B. Procedure.
1. Insertion of a needle directly into a fetal umbilical vessel under ultrasound guidance.
2. Continuous fetal heart rate (FHR) monitoring for up to 2 hrs after procedure to ensure that bleeding or hematoma formation did not occur.

Daily Fetal Movement Count

Performed by the mother to count daily fetal movements, also called "kick counts."

A. Purpose: to monitor the fetus when there may be complications affecting fetal oxygenation (e.g., preeclampsia, diabetes).

B. Procedure.
1. Count all fetal movements within a 12-hr period until a minimum of 10 movements are counted or count fetal activity two to three times daily (after meals and before bed) for 2 hrs until 10 movements are counted.
2. Less than 3 kicks in 30 minutes or less than 10 kicks in 3 hours requires further assessment and notification of the health care provider.

! NURSING PRIORITY Alcohol, depressant medications, and smoking temporarily reduce fetal movement, and obesity decreases the woman's ability to assess fetal movement. Fetal movement is not felt during fetal sleep cycle, and the movements *do not* decrease as the woman nears term.

Nonstress Test

This is a test to observe the response of the FHR to the stress of activity.

A. Procedure.

1. Requires approximately 20 min; client is placed in semi-Fowler position; external monitor is applied to document fetal activity; mother activates the "mark button" on the electronic fetal monitor when she feels fetal movement.
2. The client may be asked to drink juice or eat a light meal, because an increased blood glucose level may increase fetal activity.

B. Interpretation.
1. Reactive: shows two or more FHR accelerations of 15 beats/min or more lasting at least 15 sec for each acceleration within 20 min of beginning the test; indicates a healthy fetus; test may be rescheduled, as indicated by condition (15 x 15 criteria is for a fetus of at least 32 weeks' gestation).
2. Nonreactive: reactive criteria are not met. The accelerations are less than two in number, the accelerations are less than 15 beats/min, or there are no accelerations. If nonreactive, the test is extended another 20 min; if the tracing becomes reactive, the nonstress test (NST) is concluded. If still nonreactive after a second 20-min trial (total of 40 min), then additional testing, such as a biophysical profile, is considered. If gestation is near term, a contraction stress test (CST) may be done.

> **⚠ NURSING PRIORITY** Appearance of any decelerations of the FHR during an NST should be immediately evaluated by the health care provider.

C. Advantages of NST.
1. Simple; easy to perform; noninvasive.
2. Does not require hospitalization.
3. Has no contraindications.

Biophysical Profile

A *biophysical profile* is a noninvasive dynamic assessment of a fetus that is based on acute and chronic markers of fetal disease. It is an accurate indicator of impending fetal death.

A. First choice for follow-up fetal evaluation.
B. Assesses *five* fetal variables: fetal breathing movement, fetal body movement, muscle tone, amniotic fluid volume (AFV), and FHR; the first four are assessed by ultrasonography; the fifth is assessed by NST.
C. Each area has a possible score of 2, with a maximum score of 10. A score of 4 or less indicates need for immediate delivery.

Contraction Stress Test

The test is to observe the response of FHR to the stress of oxytocin-induced uterine contractions; means of evaluating respiratory function (oxygen and carbon dioxide exchange) of the placenta as an indicator of fetal health.

> **⚠ NURSING PRIORITY** Many facilities now use the breast self-stimulation CST, because endogenous oxytocin is produced in response to stimulation of the breasts or nipples.

A. Indications.
1. Preexisting maternal medical conditions: diabetes mellitus, heart disease, hypertension, sickle cell disease, hyperthyroidism, renal disease.
2. Postmaturity, IUGR, nonreactive NST results, preeclampsia.

B. Contraindications.
1. Third-trimester bleeding – placental previa.
2. Previous cesarean delivery with a classical incision.
3. Risk for preterm labor because of premature rupture of the membranes, incompetent cervical os, or multiple gestations.

C. Procedure: breast self-stimulation CST.
1. Semi-Fowler position, with fetal monitor in place.
2. Nipple stimulation begins with the woman massaging one nipple through her shirt or gown for 2 to 3 min, rest for 5 min; repeat until adequate contractions. Once contractions are adequate or if hyperstimulation occurs, nipple stimulation should stop.
3. Advantages: takes less time to perform, is less expensive, and causes less discomfort because no intravenous (IV) line is used.

D. Procedure: oxytocin challenge test.
1. Client must be nothing by mouth (NPO) status and be closely observed, either hospitalized or as an outpatient.
2. Place client in semi-Fowler position to avoid supine hypotension.
3. IV administration of oxytocin stimulates uterine contractions; uterine activity and FHR are recorded by means of external monitoring.
4. Hypoxia is reflected as late decelerations on monitor, which indicates a diminished fetal-placental reserve. Start oxygen with a mask and reposition.
5. IV oxytocin is delivered at a rate of 0.5 mU/min and *monitored by the registered nurse (RN)*.

E. Interpretation: oxytocin challenge test.
1. Negative (reassuring): shows no late decelerations after any contraction; implies that placental support is adequate.
2. Positive (nonreassuring; abnormal): shows late decelerations with 50% or more of contractions; may indicate the possibility of insufficient placental respiratory reserve.

> **⚠ NURSING PRIORITY** If the CST result is positive and there is no acceleration of FHR with fetal movement (nonreactive NST result), the positive CST result is an ominous sign, often indicating late fetal hypoxia. A negative CST result with a reactive NST result is desirable.

NORMAL PREGNANCY CYCLE: PHYSIOLOGIC CHANGES

Uterus

A. Increase in size caused by hypertrophy of the myometrial cells is a result of the stimulating influence of estrogen and the distention caused by the growing fetus.

B. Irregular, painless uterine contractions (Braxton Hicks) beginning after the fourth month; contraction and relaxation assist in accommodating the growing fetus.

C. Softening of the lower uterine segment (Hegar sign).

> **! NURSING PRIORITY** Multigravidas tend to report a greater incidence of Braxton Hicks contractions than primigravidas.

D. Cervical changes.
  1. Softening of the cervical tip caused by increased vascularity, hypertrophy, and hyperplasia of cervical glands (Goodell sign).
  2. Formation of the mucous plug to prevent bacterial contamination from the vagina.

Vagina

A. An increase in vaginal secretions.

B. A blue-purple hue of the vaginal walls is seen by the eighth week (Chadwick sign).

C. Vaginal secretions: acidic (pH is 3.5-6.0), thick, and white.

Breasts

A. Increase in breast size accompanied by feelings of fullness, tingling, and heaviness.

B. Superficial veins prominent; nipples erect; darkening and increase in diameter of the areolae.

Cardiovascular System

A. Blood volume increases progressively throughout pregnancy, peaking at approximately 40% to 50% greater than prepregnant levels.

B. Slight cardiac hypertrophy and systolic murmurs.

C. Increase in heart rate by 10 to 15 beats/min by the end of the first trimester.

D. Cardiac output increases 30% to 50%.

> **! NURSING PRIORITY** Blood pressure falls during the second trimester and rises slightly (no more than 15 mm in either systolic or diastolic) during the last trimester. It is important to have a baseline blood pressure measurement. Pulse rate increases by 10 to 15 beats/min. Respiratory rate remains unchanged or slightly increases.

E. Red blood cells (RBCs).
  1. The plasma volume increase is greater than the RBC increase, which leads to hemodilution, typically referred to as *physiologic anemia of pregnancy* (pseudoanemia).
  2. The hematocrit, the proportion of erythrocytes in whole blood, decreases by 4% to 7%.

F. White blood cells: 10,000 to 11,000/mm3 ($\times$ 109/L); may increase up to 30,000/mm3 (x 109/L) during labor and after delivery.

Respiratory System

A. Breathes deeper with no change in respiratory rate.

B. Oxygen consumption is increased by 20% to 40%.

C. Diaphragm is elevated; change from abdominal to thoracic breathing occurs around the 24th week.

D. Common complaints of nasal stuffiness and epistaxis caused by estrogen influence on nasal mucosa.

Urinary-Kidney System

A. Ureter and renal pelvis dilate (especially on the right side) as a result of the growing uterus.

B. Frequency of urination increases (first and last trimesters).

C. Decreased bladder tone (effect of progesterone); bladder capacity increases: 1300 to 1500 mL.

D. Ureter and renal pelvis dilation leads to urinary stasis and a potential stagnation of urine, which may result in an increased incidence of urinary tract infections (UTIs).

E. Frequent spilling of glucose in the urine (glycosuria), which leads to an increased incidence of urinary tract infections (UTIs).

Gastrointestinal System

A. Pregnancy gingivitis: gums redden, swell, and bleed easily.

B. Nausea and vomiting caused by elevated human chorionic gonadotropin (hCG) level during the first trimester; usually declines in second trimester.

C. Decreased tone and motility of smooth muscles; decreased emptying time of stomach; slowed peristalsis caused by increased progesterone level leads to complaints of bloating, heartburn (pyrosis), and constipation.

D. Pressure of expanding uterus leads to hemorrhoidal varicosities and contributes to continuing constipation.

E. Gallbladder: increased emptying time, slight hypercholesterolemia, and increased progesterone level may contribute to the development of gallstones during pregnancy.

Musculoskeletal System

A. Increase in the normal lumbosacral curve leads to backward tilt of the torso.

B. Center of gravity is changed, which often leads to leg and back strain and predisposes the client to falling.

C. Pelvis relaxes as a result of the hormone relaxin; leads to the characteristic "duck waddling" gait.

D. Abdominal wall stretches and loses tone.

Integumentary System

A. Increased skin pigmentation in various areas of the body.
  1. Facial: mask of pregnancy (chloasma).
  2. Abdomen: striae (red or purple stretch marks) and linea nigra (darkened vertical line from umbilicus to symphysis pubis).

B. Appearance of vascular spider nevi, especially on the neck, arms, and legs.

C. Acne may improve or worsen during pregnancy. Dermatitis and psoriasis usually improve during pregnancy.

Endocrine

A. Placenta.
1. Functions include transport of nutrients and removal of waste products from the fetus.
2. Produces hCG and human chorionic somatomammotropin (hCS), previously called human placental lactogen.
3. Produces estrogen and progesterone after 2 months of gestation.

B. Thyroid gland.
1. May increase in size and activity.
2. Increase in basal metabolic rate.
3. Parathyroid glands: increase in activity (especially in the last half of pregnancy) because of increased requirements for calcium and vitamin D.

C. Pituitary gland.
1. Enlargement greatest during the last month of gestation.
2. Prolactin levels start to rise in the 5th week; by 40 weeks, they have increased 10-fold.

> **! NURSING PRIORITY** Production of posterior pituitary hormones: oxytocin promotes uterine contractility and stimulation of milk let-down reflex, which are essential changes for postpartum lactation and uterine involution.

Metabolism

A. Weight gain: determined by prepregnancy weight-for-height, calculated using the body mass index (BMI); BMI of 18.5 to 24.9 is considered normal.
1. Normal weight gain: recommended 11.5 to 16 kg (~25-35 lb).
   a. Underweight: 12.5 to 18 kg (~27-39 lb).
   b. Overweight: 7 to 11 kg (~15-24 lb).
   c. Normal for multiple gestations: 17 to 25 kg (~37-55 lb).

> **! NURSING PRIORITY** The pattern of weight gain is important. Approximately 0.9 kg/week (~0.8 lb/week) for normal weight; 0.45 kg/week (~1.1 lb/week) for underweight; 0.3 kg/week (~0.6 lb/week) for overweight. Inadequate weight gain for a normal-weight woman would be less than 1 kg/month (~2.2 lb/month). Excessive weight gain is considered more than 3 kg/month (~6.6 lb/month) and should be evaluated, because this can indicate preeclampsia if it occurs after the 20th week of gestation.

2. Total weight gain is accounted for as follows:
   a. Fetus: 7 to 8.5 lb (3175-3856 g).
   b. Placenta and membranes: 2 to 2.5 lb (907-1134 g).
   c. Amniotic fluid: 2 lb (907 g).
   d. Uterus: 2 lb (907 g).
   e. Breasts: 1 to 4 lb (455-1814 g).
   f. Increased blood volume: 4 to 5 lb (1814-2268 g).
   g. Remaining 4 to 9 lb (1814-4082 g) is extravascular fluid and fat reserves.

B. Nutrient metabolism.
1. Increased intake of folic acid: 600 mcg daily (to prevent neural-tube defects).
2. Need for calcium is not increased over the dietary reference intakes (DRI) for nonpregnant women; however, many women do not consume the recommended amount.
3. Iron: approximately 30 mg daily.
4. Increased need for water (i.e., 3 L/day): normal is 2.3 L/day, so an increase of 700 mL/day is needed.

> **! NURSING PRIORITY** High levels of mercury can possibly harm the fetus' developing nervous system. Teach pregnant women to avoid fish high in mercury content and limit intake to no more than 12 oz in 2 meals/week. Avoid shark, swordfish, marlin, king mackerel, albacore or white tuna, and tilefish, because they have high levels of mercury (Fig. 21.1).

Prenatal Care

Assessment: Recognize Cues

A. Initial visit.
1. Complete history and physical examination.
2. Obstetric history.
   a. Past pregnancies (date, course of pregnancy, labor, and postpartum period; information about infant and neonatal course).
   b. Present pregnancy.

B. Schedule of return prenatal visits.
1. Frequency of return visits.
   a. Monthly for first 28 weeks.
   b. Every 2 weeks to the 36th week.
   c. After the 36th week, weekly until delivery.
   d. If a high-risk pregnancy, prenatal visits may be more often.
2. Subsequent assessment data follow-up.
   a. Vital signs.
   b. Urinalysis: check for protein and sugar.
   c. Monitor weight.
   d. Measure height of uterine fundus.
   e. Auscultation of FHR.

C. Definitions of common terms (Table 21.1).

D. Signs and symptoms of pregnancy (Table 21.2).

E. Summary of the antepartum period (Table 21.3).

Diagnostics

A. Pregnancy tests: all tests, including over-the-counter "home pregnancy" tests, are based on the presence of hCG as the biologic marker. A false-negative test result may be caused by testing too early. Whenever there is doubt about the results, further evaluation or retesting in a few days is appropriate.

B. Laboratory tests.
1. Urinalysis and/or urine culture.

ENVIRONMENTAL CONCERNS IN PREGNANCY

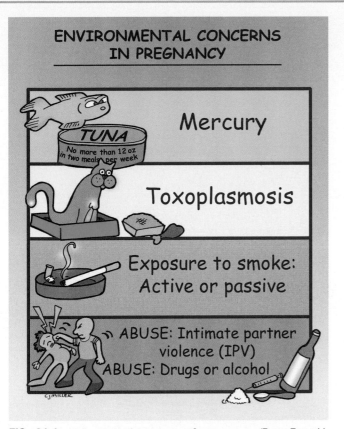

FIG. 21.1 Environmental concerns of pregnancy. (From Zerwekh J, Miller CJ. *Mosby's OB/PEDS & women's health memory notecards: visual, mnemonic, and memory aids for nurses.* St. Louis: Mosby; 2012.)

Table 21.1 DEFINITIONS OF COMMON TERMS

Common Term	Definition
Gravida	The number of pregnancies, regardless of the duration; includes the present pregnancy.
Para	The number of pregnancies in which the fetuses have reached 20 weeks' gestation when they are born.
Nulligravida	A woman who has never been pregnant.
Primigravida	Woman who is pregnant for the first time.
Multigravida	Woman who is pregnant for the second or subsequent time.
Nullipara (para 0)	Woman who has not completed a pregnancy with a fetus (or fetuses) who has reached 20 weeks' gestation.
Primipara (para I)	Woman who has completed one pregnancy with a fetus who has reached 20 weeks' gestation.
Multipara (para II, para III, para IV, etc.)	Woman who has completed two or more pregnancies to 20 or more weeks' gestation.
Parturient	A woman in labor.

[a]The terms *gravida* and *para* refer to the number of pregnancies, not the number of fetuses. The woman who delivers twins on her first pregnancy remains a para I, despite having two infants. She is also a para I if the fetus was stillborn or died soon after birth. The most common system used to describe reproductive status is the five-digit identification system characterized by the acronym GTPAL: G = total number of pregnancies, T = number of term infants (at least 37 weeks' gestation), P = number of preterm infants (before 37 weeks' gestation), A = number of spontaneous or therapeutic abortions, L = number of living children.

2. Complete blood count, electrolytes, blood urea nitrogen (BUN), creatinine.
3. Venereal Disease Research Laboratory (VDRL) test, rapid plasmin reagin (RPR) test, or fluorescent treponemal antibody-absorption (FTA-ABS) test: serologic screening for syphilis, human immunodeficiency virus (HIV) testing.
4. Rubella antibody titer.

> **! NURSING PRIORITY** It is important to understand the rubella titer and its significance to pregnancy. The rubella vaccination is not given during pregnancy, because it is a live virus and pregnancy should be prevented for at least 1 month after receiving the vaccination.

5. Blood type and Rh status.
   a. Administration of RhIG to prevent Rh sensitization in the pregnant woman.
      (1) RhIG is given at 28 weeks' gestation to an Rh-negative mother as a prophylactic measure.
      (2) A second dose of RhIG is given within the first 72 hrs after delivery to prevent the mother from producing antibodies to the fetal blood cells that may have entered her bloodstream during labor and delivery, if the infant is Rh positive.
      (3) A microdose of RhIG is administered after pregnancies that terminate before 13 weeks' gestation, after chorionic villus sampling, and after ectopic pregnancy.
6. Tuberculin skin testing; hepatitis B surface antigen (HBsAg); toxoplasmosis.
7. HIV antibody with client permission.
8. Maternal serum alpha-fetoprotein (MSAFP) at 15 to 20 weeks (ideally 16-18 weeks).
9. 1 hr glucose tolerance test, 3 hr glucose tolerance test (if indicated).
C. Pelvic examination.
   1. Pap smear of the cervix, gonorrhea and chlamydia testing, and vaginal/anal group B *Streptococcus* (GBS) culture.
   2. Pelvic measurements (pelvimetry).
D. Calculation of estimated date of birth (EDB).
   1. Nägele rule: count back 3 calendar months from the first day of the last menstrual period (LMP) and add 7 days.

Table 21.2   SIGNS AND SYMPTOMS OF PREGNANCY

Presumptive/Subjective	Probable/Objective	Positive/Diagnostic
1. Amenorrhea. 2. Nausea and vomiting. 3. Excessive fatigue. 4. Urinary frequency. 5. Breast changes: tenderness, fullness, increased pigmentation of areola, precolostrum discharge. 6. Quickening: active movements of the fetus felt by the mother.	1. Positive pregnancy test result (urine & serum). 2. Hegar sign: softening of lower uterine segment. 3. Chadwick sign: bluish discoloration of vagina. 4. Goodell sign: softening of cervical lip. 5. Ballottement: pushing on fetus (4th or 5th month) and feeling it rebound back. 6. Braxton Hicks contractions.	1. Fetal heart rate – 6th week; ultrasound 8th-17th week: Doppler ultrasound stethoscope 18th-19th week: fetal stethoscope. 2. Fetal movements felt by examiner. 3. Fetal sonography (5-6 weeks). 4. Fetal skeleton on x-ray film (not used often). 5. Fetal movements visible to examiner.

TEST ALERT   Be sure you are able to differentiate between presumptive, probable, and positive signs.

Table 21.3   SUMMARY OF NURSING MANAGEMENT DURING THE ANTEPARTUM PERIOD

Weeks' Gestation	Physical Signs and Symptoms	Characteristic Behaviors	Nursing Interventions
0-13	Amenorrhea Fatigue Nausea, vomiting Increased breast size and tenderness Urinary frequency Increased appetite	Ambivalence with mood swings. Anxiety related to confirmation of pregnancy. Telling selected close persons of pregnancy. *Couvade syndrome* refers to the presence of physical discomforts in the father during the pregnancy that mimic his partner's symptoms.	1. Obtain complete history, including gynecologic and obstetric histories. 2. Ascertain any maternal high-risk problems such as maternal age (greater than 35 years or less than 16 years), heart disease, diabetes, or potential neonatal high-risk problems such as history of congenital defects, premature births, etc. (See complete discussion in this chapter on high-risk problems.) 3. Identify maternal nutritional status by assessing height and weight and comparing with BMI chart. 4. Complete a diet history and instruction. Important to teach about necessary changes rather than all the concepts of good nutrition. 5. Food cravings are usually benign and may be indulged, providing a well-balanced diet is maintained. Pica is an abnormal eating pattern and requires treatment. 6. Encourage client to express feelings or ambivalence about pregnancy. 7. Anticipatory guidance and teaching (including family) related to OTC drugs, normal signs and symptoms of pregnancy, reportable signs of possible complications, and the normality of her mood swings.

14-26	Quickening
	 "Pregnant figure"
	 Increased energy
	 Feeling of well-being
	 Round ligament pain
		Wears maternity clothes.
		 Tells the world she's pregnant; begins to notice other pregnant women.
		 Interested in learning about birth and babies: reads books, seeks out and questions friends and family, attends classes.
		 Increased dependency as time goes on.
		 Promotes partner's involvement by allowing them to watch and feel fetal movement.
			1. Ongoing assessment of maternal and fetal status.
			 2. FHR; vital signs; fundal height.
			 3. Urine test for glucose (mild glycosuria is usually benign) and protein.
			 4. Finger stick for hemoglobin analysis (12-14 g/dL [120-140 g/L] normal).
			 5. Balanced diet.
			 6. Prevent or minimize activity intolerance and promote adequate rest by:
			    a. Encouraging 8 hrs of sleep each day, plus one nap.
			    b. Scheduling rest periods at place of employment.
			    c. Napping at home while other small children are sleeping.
			    d. Using left lateral position while resting or sleeping.
			 7. Promote adequate exercise (e.g., Kegels, pelvic rocking, modified sit-ups), sitting tailor-fashion (lotus position).
			 8. Anticipatory guidance/teaching (including family) related to libido changes, mood swings, increasing dependency, introversion, and reportable signs of possible complications.

Table 21.3   SUMMARY OF NURSING MANAGEMENT DURING THE ANTEPARTUM PERIOD—cont'd

Weeks' Gestation	Physical Signs and Symptoms	Characteristic Behaviors	Nursing Interventions
27-40	Dependent edema Pressure in lower abdomen Frequent urination Round ligament pain Backache Insomnia Clumsiness Fatigue Varicose veins	Introversion. Increased dependency (craves attention and tenderness). Altered responsiveness and spontaneity; abdominal bulk and fatigue; may decrease interest in genital sex. Intensifies study of labor and delivery. Increasingly feeling more vulnerable. Prepares nursery; buys baby things. Decides on feeding method for baby.	1. Ongoing continued physical assessment at more frequent intervals. 2. Reassure: provide emotional support related to attractiveness and self-worth. 3. Anticipatory guidance and teaching (including family) related to signs and symptoms of labor, environmental modification for coming infant, providing rest for mother, teaching associated with either breastfeeding or bottle-feeding, advising client concerning birthing and anesthesia options, and promoting the developing parent/child attachment (encourage family to verbalize mental picture of infant and concepts of selves as parents).

TEST ALERT Plan anticipatory guidance for developmental transitions. Pregnancy is considered a normal maturational crisis and developmental stage for the expectant couple.

BMI, body mass index; *FHR,* fetal heart rate, *OTC,* over the counter.

2. Examples.
   a. LMP, April 10: EDB, January 17.
   b. LMP, September 25: EDB, July 2.

Analyze Cues and Prioritize Hypotheses

The most important problems are the need for early prenatal care, preparation for parenthood, and monitoring for complications.

Nursing Interventions: Take Action

TEST ALERT Instruct client regarding antepartal care; modify approaches to care in accordance with client's developmental stage (adolescence).

Goal: To educate families regarding general health practices.
A. Hygiene: tub baths permitted but may be awkward during later weeks of gestation.
B. Clothing: loose, comfortable clothing with supportive brassiere; low-heeled shoes.
C. Breast and nipple care: client should avoid using excessive amounts of soap, ointment, alcohol-containing products, and tinctures, as this dries the nipple area and removes natural secretions; creams, lotions, and ointments are not needed on the nipple or areola and should be avoided.
D. Employment: no severe physical straining, heavy lifting, or prolonged periods of sitting or standing; wear support stockings. If sedentary job, client should get up and walk around several times a day.
E. Travel: client should avoid travel during the last month of pregnancy; when client is traveling by car or airplane, frequent walking and stretching are advised; seat belts (both lap and shoulder) should be used, with the lap belt positioned under the abdomen.
F. Rest and exercise: adequate amounts of exercise such as walking or swimming; client should stop exercising when she begins to feel tired; moderation is key.
G. Sexual activity: coital position may need to be altered to provide greater comfort; there is no contraindication to intercourse or any activity leading to orgasm, providing that membranes are intact, no vaginal bleeding exists, and there is no history of threatened abortion or premature labor.
H. Smoking: not advised; associated with infants who are small for gestational age.
I. Alcohol: no amount of alcohol use at any time during pregnancy is considered safe; fetal alcohol syndrome is a known risk.
J. Dental care: regular prophylactic care is encouraged; a soft-bristled toothbrush may be needed because of bleeding gums; x-ray examinations should be postponed, if possible.
K. Immunization: live, attenuated virus immunizations (e.g., measles-mumps-rubella [MMR] vaccine) are contraindicated during pregnancy; client is cautioned against getting pregnant for at least 28 days after receiving this type of immunization.
L. Medications: client advised to not take over-the-counter medications, especially during the first trimester because of possible teratogenic effects.
M. Advise against changing a cat litter box.

Goal: To promote relief of common discomforts through client education regarding self-care measures. (Table 21.4).

Goal: To promote adequate nutrition.
A. Obtain a complete diet history.

Table 21.4 SUMMARY OF COMMON DISCOMFORTS AND RELIEF MEASURES

Discomfort	Relief Measures
First Trimester	
Nausea and vomiting (morning sickness)	Frequent small meals; avoid empty and overloaded stomach; between meals eat crackers without fluid; take vitamin B6 and doxylamine.
Urinary frequency and urgency	Void frequently; decrease fluids before bedtime; avoid caffeinated or carbonated beverages; use perineal pads for leakage; perform Kegel exercises; report any pain or burning.
Breast tenderness	Wear a well-fitting supportive bra; alter sleep positions; avoid using soap on the nipple and areola area.
Increased vaginal discharge	Good hygiene; use perineal or panty liner pads; cotton underwear; no douching unless prescribed; report any pruritus, foul odor, or change in character or color.
Second and Third Trimesters	
Heartburn (pyrosis or acid indigestion)	Avoid fat and gas-producing foods; eat small, frequent meals; maintain good posture; sit upright.
Ankle edema	Need ample fluid intake; avoid prolonged sitting or standing; support stockings should be applied before rising; elevate feet while sitting.
Varicose veins	Avoid prolonged periods of standing; apply support hose before rising; elevate feet while sitting; do not cross legs at knees.
Hemorrhoids	Avoid constipation, do not strain; use ointments, bulk-producing laxatives, anesthetic suppositories as prescribed.
Constipation	Increase fluid intake (6-8 glasses/day); eat food and fruits high in fiber; exercise moderately; use stool softeners as prescribed.
Backache	Maintain correct posture; wear low-heeled shoes; perform pelvic tilt exercises.
Leg cramps	Stretch affected muscle and hold until it subsides; dorsiflex foot; supplement with calcium carbonate or lactate.
Faintness	Sit or lie down; avoid sudden changes in position; avoid prolonged standing.
Shortness of breath	Maintain correct posture; avoid overloading stomach; sleep with head elevated by several pillows.

TEST ALERT Instruct client on antepartum care.

1. Assess normal food intake.
2. Determine prepregnant nutritional status (existence of deficiency state; severity and time at gestation in which it occurs).
B. Dietary instructions and nutrient requirements (Fig. 21.2).
1. Increase calories for pregnancy (an additional 300 calories per day).
2. Increase calories for lactation (an additional 500 calories per day over prepregnant intake).
3. Increase protein (an additional 10g/day for pregnancy; an additional 5g/day for lactation); because the protein intake of many nonpregnant women is quite high, there may be little or no need to increase the protein intake during pregnancy.
4. Increase vitamins (generally, intake of all vitamins is increased, especially folic acid).
5. Increase amount of minerals (especially iron, calcium, and phosphorous).
6. Additional calories and protein may be recommended for the pregnant adolescent and multifetal pregnancies.

NURSING PRIORITY For a woman of normal prepregnancy weight with a singleton pregnancy, recommendations include 1800 kcal/day during the first trimester, 2200 kcal/day during the second trimester, and 2400 kcal/day during the third trimester.

Goal: To educate expectant family with regard to danger signs and symptoms requiring immediate attention (Box 21.1).
Goal: To provide education and preparation for childbirth.
A. Childbirth programs aim to dispel disinformation of pregnancy, labor, and delivery; promote a positive, healthy attitude; and teach students physical exercises and relaxation techniques.
B. Points about breathing recommendations during labor.
1. Slow-paced breathing or chest breathing is practiced for the first stage of labor.
2. Quick breathing is for the active and transitional phases of labor.
3. Panting or pursed-lip breathing is used to prevent pushing.

NUTRITION IN PREGNANCY

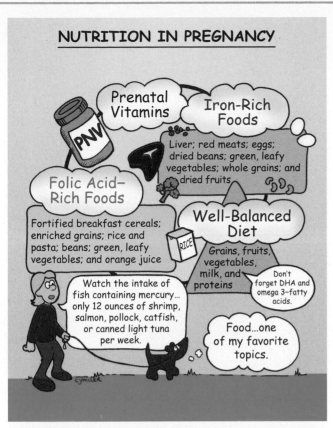

FIG. 21.2 Nutrition in pregnancy. (From Zerwekh J, Miller CJ. *Mosby's OB/PEDS & women's health memory notecards: visual, mnemonic, and memory aids for nurses.* St. Louis: Mosby; 2012.)

Box 21.1   DANGER SIGNS OF PREGNANCY

- Vaginal discharge of bloody or amniotic fluid
- Visual disturbances
- Swelling of face or fingers
- Fever and chills
- Severe continuous headache
- Pain in the abdomen
- Persistent vomiting
- Absence of fetal movement

🌳 FETAL DEVELOPMENT

Developmental Stages

A. Preembryonic stage: stage of the ovum.
   1. Conception to day 14.
   2. Fertilized ovum grows and differentiates; implants in the endometrial tissue.
   3. Formation of the three primary germ layers: endoderm, mesoderm, ectoderm.
B. Embryonic stage.
   1. Day 15 to end of eighth week.
   2. Period of organogenesis: differentiation of cells, organs, and organ systems.
   3. Highly vulnerable time; congenital anomalies are likely to occur during this period.

4. At the end of this period of development, embryo has features of the human body.
C. Fetal stage.
   1. Nine weeks to the time of birth.
   2. Characterized by growth and development of organs and organ systems.

Summary of Growth and Development

A. 4 weeks: heart begins beating.
B. 8 weeks: brain activity begins; fetus capable of some movement; 1 in (2.5 cm) long.
C. 16 weeks: fetus is 4.5 in (11.4 cm) long; sex clearly identifiable.
D. 20 weeks: hearing begins to develop; 6.7 in (17 cm) long.
E. 28 weeks: fetus can perceive light; senses are functional; sleep-wake periods; 10.6 in (27 cm) long; viable.
F. 30 to 40 weeks: increase in subcutaneous fat and weight.

> ❗ **NURSING PRIORITY** At week 36, there is sufficient surfactant production for the lungs, which are considered mature.

Multifetal Pregnancy

A. Incidence.
   1. 1%-1.5% of all natural conceptions result in twins.
   2. Twinning rates have stabilized in the United States; triplet and higher-order births have decreased as a result of advances in artificial reproductive techniques.
B. Dizygotic or fraternal twins.
   1. Fertilization of two separate ova.
   2. There are two placentas; however, they may be fused.
   3. Fraternal twins can be either the same sex or a different sex; fraternal twins may also have different gestational ages.
C. Monozygotic or identical twins.
   1. One ovum and one sperm; cells of the zygote separate and form two embryos.
   2. Same sex: resemble each other in appearance and structure.
   3. Usually one placenta, one chorion, and two amnions are present.

Placenta

A. Function.
   1. Transfer of oxygen, nutrients, and metabolites.
   2. Elimination of waste products from the fetus.
   3. Production of hormones: hCG, human placental lactogen, estrogen, and progesterone.
B. Development of the placenta.
   1. Fetal side is shiny and slightly grayish: *Schultze* (often called shiny Schultze).
   2. Maternal side is rough and beefy red: *Duncan* (often called dirty Duncan).
   3. Maternal and fetal bloodstreams are in close relationship to each other, but the circulations do not mix.

Fetal Circulation

A. Fetal lungs do not participate in respiratory gas exchange.

B. There are special fetal structures to bypass blood supply to the lungs.
1. Placenta.
2. One umbilical vein carries oxygenated blood from maternal circulation to fetus.
3. Two umbilical arteries carry unoxygenated (venous) blood from fetus to placenta.
4. Wharton jelly is a gelatinous substance that surrounds the three blood vessels, providing support.
5. Foramen ovale: an opening between the right atrium and the left atrium of the heart.
6. Ductus arteriosus: connects the pulmonary artery and the aorta.
7. Ductus venosus: connects the umbilical vein and the inferior vena cava.
C. At the time of birth, fetal circulation begins the transition to the adult pattern of circulation; a functional closure occurs within a few days; however, anatomic closure of the fetal vessels is not complete for several weeks or months.

> ⚠ **PEDIATRIC PRIORITY** A newborn heart murmur may not be significant because of incomplete closure of the ductus arteriosus.

COMPLICATIONS ASSOCIATED WITH PREGNANCY

> **TEST ALERT** Identify signs of potential prenatal complications.

📋 Abortion

Abortion **is termination of pregnancy before 20 weeks' gestation; abortions can be spontaneous (miscarriage) or induced (therapeutic or elective); approximately 75% to 80% of all spontaneous abortions occur during the second and third months of gestation.**

Assessment: Recognize Cues
A. Risk factors.
1. Maternal: chromosomal abnormalities, obesity, regular and heavy alcohol intake, and excessive caffeine intake.
2. Endocrine disturbance: poorly controlled diabetes, systemic lupus erythematosus, and thyroid disease.
3. Exposure to teratogens, environmental toxins, and increasing paternal age.
B. Clinical manifestations (types of spontaneous abortions).
1. Threatened abortion: slight bleeding, mild back and lower abdominal cramping, no cervical dilation, no passage of the products of conception.
2. Inevitable abortion: moderate amount of bleeding and mild to severe cramping; internal cervical os dilates, and membranes may rupture.
3. Incomplete abortion: only some of the products of conception are expelled.

4. Complete abortion: all the products of conception are expelled.
5. Missed abortion: fetus dies in utero, and the products of conception are retained from 4 to 8 weeks; symptoms of pregnancy subside; if fetus is retained past 6 weeks, complications of disseminated intravascular coagulation (DIC) may develop as a result of the release of thromboplastin from the fetal autolysis process.
6. Recurrent or habitual abortion: three or more successive, spontaneous abortions.

Analyze Cues and Prioritize Hypotheses
The most important problems are hemorrhage, acute pain, decreased self-esteem related to the inability to carry pregnancy to term, potential for infection, and grief or other emotional issues related to loss of pregnancy.

Generate Solutions
Treatment
Treatment varies according to type of abortion.
A. Threatened abortion: bed rest and acetaminophen-based analgesics.
B. Inevitable and incomplete abortion.
1. Fluid replacement: IV lines, type, and crossmatch for possible blood transfusion.
2. Medical management: administration of misoprostol.
3. Surgical management: dilation and curettage (D&C) or suction evacuation to remove products of conception.
4. Administration of RhIG if mother is Rh negative (given within 72 hrs).
C. Missed abortion.
1. Surgical management: suction evacuation or D&C will be performed, followed by oxytocin to prevent hemorrhage.
2. Medical management: induction of labor by IV oxytocin, prostaglandin.
D. Recurrent or habitual abortion: determination of cause, then specific therapy to correct.

Nursing Interventions: Take Action
Goal: To assess or control hemorrhage.
A. Monitoring of vital signs.
B. *Report any signs of increased bleeding to the RN.*
C. Assist in medical treatment: IV therapy, preparation for D&C.
Goal: To prevent complications.
A. Observe for shock, hypofibrinogenemia, and DIC.
B. Prevent isoimmunization by administration of RhIG.
C. Assess for infection and anemia.
Goal: To provide emotional support to the couple experiencing the loss of pregnancy.
A. Encourage verbalization of feelings.
B. Be available and actively listen.

📋 Ectopic Pregnancy

An *ectopic pregnancy* **is any pregnancy in which the gestational sac is implanted outside of the uterine cavity. Most**

(95%) ectopic pregnancies are tubal; they are more common on the right side.

Assessment: Recognize Cues

A. Risk factors: any condition that causes scarring or obstruction of the fallopian tubes (e.g., infections, surgery for prior tubal pregnancy, fertility restoration).
B. Clinical manifestations.
   1. If tube is unruptured, abdominal pain, delayed menses, and vaginal spotting.
   2. If a tube ruptures, sudden excruciating pain is felt in the lower abdomen, usually over the mass; referred shoulder pain is possible as the abdomen fills with blood; vaginal bleeding and shock may also occur.

Analyze Cues and Prioritize Hypotheses

The most important problems are hemorrhage, acute pain, grief resulting from loss of reproductive organ, and emotional issues related to loss of pregnancy.

Generate Solutions

Treatment
A. Surgical: laparoscopy, laparotomy, salpingectomy.
B. Medical: methotrexate used to dissolve residual tissue or as a one-time treatment for unruptured pregnancies.

Nursing Interventions: Take Action

Goal: To prevent and detect early complications.
A. Provision of nursing care for shock, as indicated.
B. Prepare for surgery (IV lines, oxygen, blood, etc.).
C. Administer RhIG if mother is Rh negative.
Goal: To provide emotional support (loss of pregnancy and reproductive organ).
A. Use a contraceptive method for 3 months to allow body to heal.

Cervical Insufficiency

Cervical insufficiency **is a defect related to trauma of the cervix or a congenitally short cervix, which leads to habitual abortion and premature labor.**

Assessment: Recognize Cues

A. Clinical manifestations.
   1. Cervical dilation or cervical effacement without painful uterine contractions.
   2. Membranes rupture, labor begins, and premature fetus is delivered.

Analyze Cues and Prioritize Hypotheses

The most important problems are potential loss of pregnancy and premature labor.

Generate Solutions

Treatment
A. Surgical.
   1. Reinforcement of the weakened cervix by a purse-string suture, which encircles the internal os.

2. McDonald cerclage: left in place until term, then removed around 37 weeks or left in place if a cesarean birth is anticipated.

Nursing Interventions: Take Action

Goal: To provide client education regarding presence of purse-string suture or cerclage.
A. Client should abstain from intercourse and douching and should reduce activity level for 2 weeks after surgery.
B. Physical activity and intercourse resumption is based on the status of the cervix and individualized for each woman.
C. During labor, the suture will be removed for a vaginal delivery, or it may be left in place for a cesarean delivery.

Hydatidiform Mole (molar pregnancy)

Gestational trophoblastic neoplasia **(GTN) is a spectrum of diseases resulting from abnormal fertilization (e.g., hydatidiform mole, placental site trophoblastic tumors, or gestational choriocarcinoma).**

Assessment: Recognize Cues

A. Clinical manifestations.
   1. Exaggerated symptoms of pregnancy: uterus large for week of pregnancy, excessive nausea and vomiting, early symptoms of preeclampsia.
   2. Discharge of brownish-red fluid (like prune juice) from vagina around 12 weeks; fluid may contain vesicles.
   3. Anemia and absence of FHR.
B. Diagnostics.
   1. Ultrasonography reveals a pattern of diffuse intra-uterine masses (snowstorm pattern).
   2. Elevated serum hCG level.
C. Complications – possible choriocarcinoma.

Analyze Cues and Prioritize Hypotheses

The most important problems are hemorrhage, acute pain, potential for taking chemotherapeutic medication, and grief or other emotional issues related to loss of pregnancy and fear of cancer.

Generate Solutions

Treatment
A. Surgical: D&C to empty uterus.
B. Medical: follow-up supervision for 1 year.
   1. Obtain β-hCG levels weekly, as rising titers of hCG indicate disease of choriocarcinoma, which is treated with methotrexate.
   2. Pregnancy should be avoided for at least 1 year during the follow-up assessment period.
   3. Oral contraceptive is preferred for birth control – no IUD.

Nursing Interventions: Take Action

Goal: To assess for complications associated with hemorrhage and the possibility of uterine rupture.

Goal: To provide emotional support and assist in selection of a contraceptive method.

📋 Hyperemesis Gravidarum

Hyperemesis gravidarum **is intractable vomiting during pregnancy that results in dehydration, electrolyte imbalance, nutritional deficiencies, and significant weight loss. It occurs in less than 0.3% to 3% of pregnancies. The cause is uncertain.**

Assessment: Recognize Cues

A. Clinical manifestations.
   1. Severe, persistent vomiting; dehydration, dry mucous membranes.
   2. Weight loss, decreased BP, increased pulse, poor skin turgor.

Analyze Cues and Prioritize Hypotheses

The most important problems are dehydration related to excessive vomiting as evidenced by fluid and electrolyte imbalance, inadequate weight gain related to nausea and persistent vomiting, and anxiety related to concern for fetal well-being.

Generate Solutions

Treatment

A. Medical: replacement of fluids and electrolytes, and vitamin B$_6$ (pyridoxine), along with doxylamine, dopamine antagonists, antihistamines, metoclopramide.
B. Dietary: client is NPO until vomiting stops; after condition improves, frequent small feedings of bland foods with limited fluids every 1 to 2 hrs; slowly progress as tolerated.
C. Most cases are managed at home, even if requiring IV or enteral therapy.

Nursing Interventions: Take Action

Goal: To assist with medical and dietary management.

A. Accurate recording of volume of vomitus.
B. Daily weight checks and maintenance of intake and output data.
C. Desired urine output is 1000 mL in 24 hrs; usually, administration of IV fluids at 3000 mL/hr in first 24 hrs after admission to correct hypovolemia.
D. Oral hygiene measures.
E. Provide a quiet, restful environment free of odors.

📋 Hypertensive Disorders

Hypertensive disorders **are common medical complications of pregnancy occurring in approximately 5% to 10% of pregnancies and the second leading cause of maternal and perinatal morbidity and mortality. Cause is multifactorial.**

Assessment: Recognize Cues

A. Risk factors.
   1. Diabetes mellitus, hypertension, renal disease, autoimmune diseases.
   2. History of preeclampsia, hydatidiform mole.
   3. Multifetal gestation, BMI greater than 30.
   4. Age (35 years or older).
   5. First pregnancy, family history of preeclampsia.
B. Clinical manifestations of preeclampsia (Table 21.5).

Table 21.5 CLINICAL MANIFESTATIONS OF PREECLAMPSIA AND ECLAMPSIA

Mild Preeclampsia	Preeclampsia with Severe Features	Eclampsia
Elevated BP: systolic increase to 140 mm Hg and diastolic increase of 90 mm Hg x 2 readings, 4-6 hrs apart, after 20 weeks gestation	Increased hypertension: systolic at 160 mm Hg; diastolic at 110 mm Hg or more on 2 separate occasions 4 hrs apart; pregnant woman is on bed rest	Convulsions appear suddenly and without warning. Increased hypertension and tonic contraction of all body muscles (arms flexed, hands clenched, legs inverted) precede the tonic-clonic convulsions. Hypotension follows. Disorientation, amnesia, and muscular twitching persist for a time.
Proteinuria: greater than 300 mg/24 hrs (1+ to 2+ proteinuria)	*Massive proteinuria is no longer used as a diagnostic criterion.* Elevated BUN, serum creatinine, uric acid levels, LDH, ALT, AST Oliguria: less than 500 mL/24 hrs Cerebral or visual disturbances Pulmonary edema Severe headache Vomiting Epigastric pain (caused by edema of liver capsule, usually indicative of impending seizure)	Coma (lasts from few minutes to several hours).

ALT, alanine aminotransferase; *AST*, aspartate aminotransferase; *BP*, blood pressure; *BUN*, blood urea nitrogen; *LDH*, lactate dehydrogenase.

HELLP SYNDROME

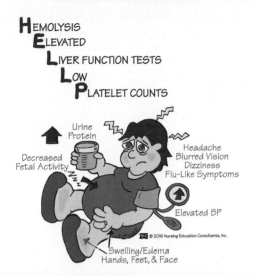

HEMOLYSIS
ELEVATED
LIVER FUNCTION TESTS
LOW **P**LATELET COUNTS

Urine Protein
Decreased Fetal Activity
Headache Blurred Vision Dizziness Flu-Like Symptoms
Elevated BP
Swelling/Edema Hands, Feet, & Face

© 2016 Nursing Education Consultants, Inc.

FIG. 21.3 HELLP (Hemolysis, Elevated Liver function tests, Low Platelet count). (From Zerwekh J, Garneau A, Miller CJ. *Digital collection of the memory notebooks of nursing.* 4th ed. Chandler, AZ: Nursing Education Consultants, Inc.; 2017.)

> **! NURSING PRIORITY** The hallmark symptoms of preeclampsia are hypertension and proteinuria.

C. Complications (severe preeclampsia): *maternal.*
   1. Retinal arteriolar spasm leads to scotoma (blind spots) and blurring.
   2. Cerebral edema and hemorrhages, with increased irritability (headache, hyperreflexia, positive ankle clonus, and seizures).
   3. **HELLP** (**H**emolysis, **E**levated **L**iver function tests, **L**ow **P**latelet count) syndrome (Fig. 21.3).
      a. Associated with severe preeclampsia and with hepatic dysfunction: epigastric pain, right upper quadrant pain.
D. Complications: *fetal.*
   1. Usually small for gestational age; born prematurely.
   2. Newborn may be born oversedated because of medications given to mother.

Analyze Cues and Prioritize Hypotheses

The most important problems are the need for health teaching in management of preeclampsia; potential for injury resulting from hypertension, central nervous system (CNS) irritability, vasospasm, and decreased renal perfusion; potential for fetal injury (placental abruption, preterm birth, intrauterine growth restriction), and disabled family coping.

Generate Solutions

Treatment
A. Medical.
   1. Preeclampsia: restricted activity with diversional activities and gentle exercise.
   2. Severe preeclampsia or HELLP syndrome: admitted to hospital, complete bed rest, antihypertensives

(hydralazine, labetalol, or nifedipine), anticonvulsants provide neuroprotection (magnesium sulfate); prepare for preterm delivery via cesarean delivery if HELLP syndrome begins.

> **! NURSING PRIORITY** Monitor for magnesium toxicity, characterized by loss of patellar reflexes, respiratory depression, oliguria, and decreased level of consciousness. When administering antihypertensives in preeclampsia associated with a contracted intravascular volume, give medications with caution and monitor client closely.

   3. Eclampsia: seizure precautions (padded bed rails, vital signs, oxygen, suction, positioning).
B. Dietary: high-protein diet, no added salt intake, and fluid intake of six to eight glasses of water per day.

Nursing Interventions: Take Action

Goal: To prevent worsening of preeclampsia.
A. Instruction for home care: encourage bed rest, provide dietary instruction, schedule regular prenatal checkups, teach symptoms of worsening of condition, provide meaningful activities to prevent boredom while on bed rest.
B. Tests to evaluate fetal status (e.g., fetal movement record, ultrasonography, NST, determination of estriol and creatinine levels).
C. Goals and nursing interventions for clients with severe preeclampsia and eclampsia are outlined in Box 21.2.

Cardiovascular Disease

Rheumatic heart disease (mitral valve problems) and *congenital heart defects* account for the greatest incidence of cardiac disease in pregnancy. Increasing numbers of heart transplant recipients are successfully completing pregnancies, with the recommendation that pregnancy be avoided for at least 1 year after the transplant.
A. Normal physiologic alterations of pregnancy that increase cardiovascular stress.
   1. Increase in oxygen requirements.
   2. Increase in cardiac output; peaks at 20 to 26 weeks' gestation.
   3. Weight gain.
   4. Hemodynamic changes during delivery.
B. As normal pregnancy advances, the cardiovascular system is unable to maintain adequate output to meet increasing demands.

Assessment: Recognize Cues

Clinical manifestations indicative of cardiac decompensation are those of impending heart failure (HF).
A. Frequent moist cough, progressive dyspnea with usual activities, orthopnea.
B. Progressive generalized edema.
C. Weak, irregular, and rapid pulse ($\geq$ 100 beats/min).
D. Rapid respirations ($\geq$ 25 breaths/min); crackles at base of lungs after two respirations and exhalations that do not clear after coughing.

Box 21.2 NURSING MANAGEMENT OF CLIENTS WITH GESTATIONAL HYPERTENSION AND PREECLAMPSIA

Goal: To recognize the early signs of gestational hypertension and increased BP.
1. Check BP and record Korotkoff phase IV (muffling of sound) and V (disappearance of sound) for diastolic reading. Take BP in left lateral recumbent position or seated. Allow 5 min of quiet rest before taking BP to encourage relaxation. Use proper size cuff; measure in right arm over brachial artery each time.

Goal: To recognize progression of gestational hypertension symptoms and minimize or control their sequelae.
1. Continue BP monitoring.
2. Regular diet with normal sodium intake.
3. Monitor for ominous signs of deteriorating condition: headache, visual disturbances, hyperreflexia, markedly decreased urine output, epigastric or right upper quadrant pain, dyspnea, vaginal bleeding (abruptio placentae), or any change in fetal activity.
4. Administer antihypertensives, as ordered; check maternal BP, pulse, and FHR.

Goal: To prevent or control seizures.
1. Administer IV magnesium sulfate. (Have calcium gluconate available as antidote for possible respiratory/neurologic depression.)
2. Have emergency equipment readily available (e.g., oxygen, suction, airway, sedatives).
3. Modify environment to ensure rest and quiet.
   a. Eliminate noise, bright lights, and other harsh stimuli.
   b. Minimize number of personnel giving care.
   c. Initiate painful and/or intrusive procedures after sedation.
   d. Promote comfort and total bed rest.
4. Monitor intake and output and edema for evidence of vasodilation and increased tissue perfusion.

Goal: To recognize alterations in fetal well-being and promote safe delivery of the infant.
1. Auscultate and record FHR pattern, noting presence of variability or accelerations, and report decelerations.
2. Instruct and support client during amniocentesis.
3. Collect specimen for estriol determination.
4. Assist with NST and/or oxytocin challenge test (contraction stress test).
5. Give instructions about induction of labor and electronic FHR monitoring.
6. Instruct client on the need for intravenous magnesium sulfate for 24 hrs after delivery to prevent seizures.

BP, blood pressure; *FHR,* fetal heart rate; *IV,* intravenous; *NST,* nonstress test; *OCT,* oxytocin challenge test.

E. Client reports palpitations (racing heart), feeling of smothering, and increasing fatigue and/or difficulty breathing with usual activities.
F. Cyanosis of lips and nailbeds.
G. Cardiac decompensation increases with length of gestation; *highest incidence* of HF is observed at 28 to 32 weeks' gestation.

Analyze Cues and Prioritize Hypotheses

The most important problems are decreased tissue perfusion related to hypotensive syndrome, reduced stamina related to cardiac condition, need for health teaching on cardiac condition and how pregnancy affects it, medication changes, requirements to alter self-care activities, reduced functional ability (bathing, dressing, toileting) related to fatigue or activity intolerance, and the need for bed rest and/or limited activity level.

Generate Solutions

Treatment
A. Management of the pregnant client.
   1. Balanced nutritional intake; iron and folic acid supplements.
   2. Limited physical activity; stop any activity that increases shortness of breath.
   3. Diuretics, digitalis, anticoagulants, antidysrhythmics, and prophylactic antibiotics (for clients with mitral valve disease from rheumatic fever) may be given.
   4. May be hospitalized at 28 to 32 weeks' gestation because of impending HF.
   5. If coagulation problems occur, heparin is usually used. because it does not cross the placenta.
B. Management of the client during labor and delivery.
   1. Supplemental oxygen.
   2. Epidural regional anesthesia is generally used for delivery.
C. Management of the client during the postpartum period: treated symptomatically according to status of cardiovascular system; the first 24 to 48 hrs postpartum is period of *highest risk* for HF in the mother.

Nursing Interventions: Take Action

Goal: To assist client to maintain homeostasis during pregnancy.
A. Provide information regarding nutritional needs (verbal and written).
B. Nursing assessment and client education regarding early symptoms of HF.
C. Frequent rest periods; activity may be severely restricted during the last trimester.

! NURSING PRIORITY One of the most effective means of decreasing the cardiac workload is to decrease activity; therefore, the pregnant client needs to avoid excessive fatigue to prevent or decrease cardiac decompensation.

Goal: To help client maintain homeostasis during labor and delivery.
A. Position client on side with head and shoulders elevated.
B. Observe for increasing dyspnea, cough, or adventitious breath sounds during labor.
C. Evaluate information from continuous fetal and maternal monitoring.
D. Encourage open glottis pushing during labor; prevent Valsalva maneuver.

E. Prepare for vaginal delivery.

F. Provide pain relief as indicated.

   1. Pain increases cardiac work.

   2. Evaluate effects of analgesia on fetus.

Goal: To maintain homeostasis in the postpartum period.

A. Assessment of cardiac adaptation to changes in hemodynamics.

   1. Increased blood flow resulting from decreased abdominal pressure may precipitate reflux bradycardia.

   2. Assess for chest pain and adequacy of cardiac output.

B. Maintain semi-Fowler position or side-lying position with the head elevated.

C. Gradual progression of activities (depending on cardiac status) as indicated by:

   1. Pulse rate.

   2. Respiratory status.

   3. Activity tolerance.

D. Progressive ambulation as soon as tolerated to prevent venous thrombosis.

E. Assist mother and family to prepare for discharge.

> ❗ **NURSING PRIORITY** Immediately after birth, the woman with cardiac dysfunction is at risk for heart failure, as blood volume increases significantly when extravascular fluid moves into the vascular compartment and creates a significant increase in the workload of the heart.

Diabetes

Diabetes mellitus **is a complex, multisystem disease characterized by the absence of, or a severe decrease in, the secretion or utilization of insulin.**

Assessment: Recognize Cues

A. Effects of pregnancy on diabetes.

   1. During the first trimester of pregnancy, there is an increase in the fetal need for glucose and amino acids; this lowers the maternal blood glucose level and decreases the maternal need for additional insulin.

   2. During the second and third trimesters, the need for insulin will increase as a result of insulin resistance from major hormone changes.

   3. Oral hypoglycemic agents are *not used* to control diabetes in the pregnant client who has **pregestational** diabetes.

   4. Metformin and glyburide are used with women who have gestational diabetes mellitus (GDM); however, insulin remains the preferred treatment.

B. Effects of diabetes on pregnancy.

   1. Increased tendency toward the development of metabolic acidosis caused by an increase in metabolic rate.

   2. Placental antagonist to insulin will decrease the effectiveness of insulin.

   3. Fetal antagonists to insulin decrease the utilization of glucose.

   4. Hormonal changes lead to decreased tolerance to glucose and increased insulin resistance (begins around 14-16 weeks).

C. Influence of pregnancy on diabetic control.

   1. Insulin requirements for pregestational diabetic mother.

      a. First trimester – insulin requirement decreased.

      b. Insulin resistance begins around weeks 14 to 16 gestation – insulin requirements increase to prevent hyperglycemia.

      c. Increase in insulin requirements continue during the second and third trimesters of pregnancy; may double or quadruple prepregnancy amounts.

      d. At week 36 gestation – insulin requirements plateau and often drop significantly on the day of birth.

      e. Breastfeeding mother maintains lower insulin requirements, as much as 25% less than those of prepregnancy.

   2. Insulin-dependent pregnant women are prone to hypoglycemia during the first trimester of pregnancy; may need to reduce insulin dosage.

   3. Tendency to intensify the existing complications of diabetes.

Analyze Cues and Prioritize Hypotheses

The most important problems are the need for health teaching on diabetic pregnancy, management, and potential effects on pregnant woman and fetus; insulin administration and its effects; potential for injury to fetus and mother related to improper insulin administration; episodes of hypoglycemia and hyperglycemia; possible cesarean or operative vaginal birth; and postpartum infection and other complications.

Generate Solutions

Treatment

A. Medication (insulin, oral hypoglycemics).

B. Diet – avoid simple carbohydrates, need a bedtime snack.

C. Exercise – preferably after meals when glucose level is higher.

Nursing Interventions: Take Action

Goal: To monitor fetal and maternal well-being during pregnancy, labor, and delivery.

1. Antepartum period for pregestational and GDM.

   a. For both pregestational and GDM mothers.

      (1) Home blood glucose monitoring.

      (2) Diet: well balanced, avoid refined sugar; no skipping meals or snacks.

      (3) Exercise as prescribed.

      (4) Labor induction at 38 to 40 weeks.

2. Intrapartum period.

   a. For pregestational diabetes, blood glucose levels are maintained with IV glucose and regular insulin.

   b. GDM mothers may need rapid-acting insulin IV; IV dextrose infusions are avoided.

   c. Fetal monitoring during labor.

3. Postpartum period.

   a. Insulin requirements for mother will be markedly decreased and fluctuate over next few weeks.

b. Pregestational diabetic mother must go through a period of diabetic reregulation.

c. GDM mothers' glucose returns to normal after delivery; however, some will continue to have impaired glucose metabolism and diabetes.

D. Presence of diabetes predisposes the mother to an increased incidence of:

1. Pregnancy-induced hypertension.
2. Hemorrhage.
3. Polyhydramnios (increase in volume of amniotic fluid).
4. Vaginal and urinary tract infections (UTIs).
5. Premature delivery.
6. Intrauterine death in third trimester.
7. Macrosomia (weight >4500 gm [9 lb 9 oz]).
8. Compromised newborn.
   a. Respiratory distress syndrome (RDS).
   b. Hypoglycemia.
   c. Extreme prematurity; intrauterine fetal demise.
   d. Congenital anomalies associated with pregestational diabetes.

Goal: To help the client with diabetes maintain homeostasis throughout pregnancy.

A. Prevent infection.

B. Frequent evaluation of glucose levels and monitoring of changes in insulin requirements.

C. Utilization of insulin rather than oral hypoglycemic agents for pregestational diabetic mother.

D. Maintain optimum level of weight gain; labor may be induced, or cesarean delivery may be required if complications are evident.

> **! NURSING PRIORITY** Advise client to stop exercising immediately if uterine contractions occur while exercising, drink two to three glasses of water, and lie down on her side for an hour. If contractions do not subside, have her contact her health care provider.

Goal: To help the client with diabetes maintain homeostasis throughout labor and delivery.

A. Fetal monitoring to identify early stages of fetal distress.

B. X-ray pelvimetry to identify cephalopelvic disproportion (CPD).

C. Increased incidence of dystocia because of large infants.

D. Frequent evaluation of serum glucose levels (every 2-3 hrs).

Goal: To help the client with diabetes return to homeostasis during the postpartum period.

A. Anticipate fluctuation in insulin requirements caused by:
1. Loss of fetal insulin.
2. Removal of placental influence on insulin.
3. Changes in metabolic activity.

B. Observe and monitor for rapid fluctuations in serum glucose levels.

C. Prevent postpartum infection.

INTRAPARTUM AND POSTPARTUM

Labor and Delivery

Intrapartal Factors

A. Common terms.
1. Bones of the fetal skull: one frontal, two parietal, two temporal, and one occipital.
2. Suture is the membranous tissue between the bones.
3. Anterior, large fontanel is diamond shaped; closes by 18 months.
4. Posterior, or small, fontanel closes at approximately 6 to 8 weeks after birth.
5. Fetal attitude: relationship of the various parts of the fetal body to one another in utero; characteristic uterine posture is one of moderate flexion of the head, extremities on the abdomen and chest.
6. Fetal lie: relationship of the fetal axis to the maternal axis – longitudinal or transverse.
7. Presentation and presenting parts: that part of the fetus that lies close to or has entered the true pelvis.
8. Cephalic: most common (97%).
9. Breech: buttocks or feet first.
10. Shoulder: most commonly seen with transverse lie.
11. Position: relationship of the landmark on the presenting part to a specific part of the maternal pelvis.
12. Station of the presenting part: the relationship between the presenting part and the maternal ischial spines (Fig. 21.4).

> **! NURSING PRIORITY** If presenting part is higher than the ischial spines (floating), a negative number is assigned, indicating the number of centimeters above 0 station. As labor progresses, the presenting part moves from the negative stations to the midpelvis at 0 station (engagement), then into the positive stations (sequence as follows: −5, −4, −3, −2, −1, 0, + 1, + 2, + 3, + 4, + 5).

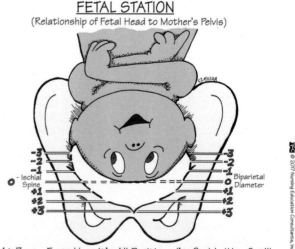

FETAL STATION
(Relationship of Fetal Head to Mother's Pelvis)

I'm At Zero... From Here It's All Positive... I'm On My Way Out!!!

FIG. 21.4 Stations of presenting part, or degree of descent. (From Zerwekh J, Garneau A, Miller CJ. *Digital collection of the memory notebooks of nursing.* 4th ed. Chandler, AZ: Nursing Education Consultants, Inc.; 2017.)

CLUE TO CONTRACTIONS

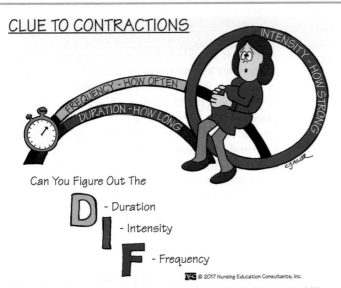

Can You Figure Out The

D - Duration
I - Intensity
F - Frequency

FIG. 21.5 Clue to contractions. (From Zerwekh J, Garneau A, Miller CJ. *Digital collection of the memory notebooks of nursing.* 4th ed. Chandler, AZ: Nursing Education Consultants, Inc.; 2017.)

Box 21.3 DIFFERENCE BETWEEN TRUE LABOR AND FALSE LABOR

True Labor
- Cervical dilation and effacement.
- Contractions occur at regular intervals and increase in duration and intensity; intensity usually increases with walking.
- Pain in the back that radiates around to the lower abdomen.
- Contractions continue despite comfort measures.

NURSING PRIORITY The two most important signs of *true labor* are cervical dilation and effacement (see Fig. 21.6).

False Labor
- Contractions are irregular or become regular temporarily.
- Contractions often stop with walking or position change.
- Pain felt in the back or abdomen above the umbilicus.
- Contractions often stopped through use of comfort measures.

B. The powers: involuntary, intermittent contractions of the uterine muscle (Fig. 21.5).
1. **Duration** of the contraction: the time between the first tightening sensation of the muscle and its subsequent complete relaxation.
2. **Frequency** of the contraction: time interval from the beginning of one contraction to the beginning of the next.
3. **Intensity** of the contraction: firmness of the uterine muscle during the contraction.
   a. Mild: slightly tense; easy to indent with fingertips (feels like touching finger to tip of nose).
   b. Moderate: firm fundus; difficult to indent with fingertips (feels like touching finger to chin).
   c. Strong: rigid, boardlike fundus; almost impossible to indent with fingertips (feels like touching finger to forehead).
4. **Resting tone:** relaxation of the uterine muscle between contractions.
5. Abdominal muscle and diaphragm contractions are the second power; during the second stage of labor, they push the fetus to the outside.

Assessment of the Labor Process
Maternal Assessment: Recognize Cues

A. Differentiate *true* labor from *false* labor (Box 21.3; Fig. 21.6).
B. Mechanism of labor: sequence of passive movements of the presenting part as it moves through the birth canal.
C. Engagement → descent → flexion → internal rotation → extension → external rotation *(restitution)* → expulsion.
D. Rupture of membranes.
1. If rupture occurs before onset of labor, it is called *premature rupture of the membranes*.
2. Delivery should occur within 24 hrs to decrease incidence of infection.

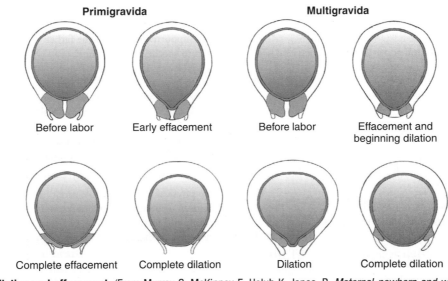

FIG. 21.6 Cervical dilation and effacement. (From Murray S, McKinney E, Holub K, Jones, R. *Maternal-newborn and women's health nursing.* 7th ed. Elsevier; 2019.)

A. Administer analgesic medication.
   1. Butorphanol tartrate or nalbuphine hydrochloride.
   2. Fentanyl: used with local anesthetic for induction of spinal block or epidural anesthesia.
   3. Sedatives (hydroxyzine and promethazine) are no longer used as adjuncts to analgesia to relieve tension and anxiety. The antiemetic metoclopramide potentiates analgesics and is a better choice.
B. Assist with regional or general anesthesia.
   1. Pudendal: administered late in second stage of labor.
      a. Perineal anesthesia of short duration (30 min).
      b. Indicated for client receiving an episiotomy or requiring forceps or a vacuum extractor during the birthing process.
   2. Epidural.
      a. Given in first and second stages of labor (no longer recommended that women reach a certain dilation or fetal station prior to receiving); intermittent or continuous administration; prehydrate with IV fluids.
      b. May cause maternal hypotension, labor dysfunction, and inability to push effectively.
   3. Spinal anesthesia (block).
      a. Used for delivery (vaginal or cesarean); not suitable for labor pain control.
      b. Postdural puncture headache (PDPH) can occur from leakage of cerebrospinal fluid (CSF) from site of puncture of the dura mater.
      c. Epidural blood patch: most rapid way to relieve a PDPH; inject 10 to 20 mL of client's blood into lumbar epidural space, creating a clot.

> **! NURSING PRIORITY** To reduce the risk for postpartum infection caused by the transmission of pathogens, it is recommended that masks be worn during the induction of intrathecal and epidural anesthesia/analgesia.

Fetal

Goal: To monitor fetal status and detect early complications (see Table 21.7).

Goal: To provide immediate care to the healthy newborn.

> **TEST ALERT** Assess newborn, provide care that meets the needs of the newborn, and contribute to newborn plan of care.

Table 21.7 SUMMARY OF FETAL HEART RATE: CHARACTERISTICS AND PATTERNS

Term	Definition	Therapeutic Interventions
Baseline rate: Approximate mean FHR rounded to increments of 5 beats/min during a 10-min segment, excluding periodic and episodic changes, periods of marked variability, and segments of baseline that differ by greater than 25 beats/min. During the 10-min time frame, the minimum baseline duration must be at least 2 min; otherwise, the baseline for that period is undetermined. Normal range at term is 110-160 beats/min.		
Variability: Irregular fluctuations in the baseline FHR of 2 cycles per minute or greater. It is considered reassuring to have variability.		

Baseline Changes

Term	Definition	Therapeutic Interventions
Tachycardia	Baseline rate >160 beats/min for 10 min or more *Pathophysiology:* Early fetal hypoxia Maternal fever Maternal hyperthyroidism Medications	1. Monitor maternal vital signs. 2. Change maternal position. 3. Continue to watch closely. 4. Administer oxygen and other provider orders.
Bradycardia	Baseline <110 beats/min lasting >10 min *Pathophysiology:* Viral infections Fetal structural defects Known to occur before fetal death	1. Inform neonatal personnel. 2. Change maternal position. 3. Administer oxygen to mother. 4. Prepare for immediate delivery.
Loss of variability	Smooth baseline as recorded by fetal monitor Can be: • Absent – amplitude range undetectable • Minimal – amplitude range detectable but ≤5 beats/min • Moderate – amplitude range 6-25 beats/min • Marked – amplitude range >25 beats/min *Pathophysiology:* Maternal medication Fetal acidosis and hypoxemia (especially if accompanied by late decelerations) Fetal neurologic immaturity	1. Note time and dose of medication on record. 2. See "late deceleration." 3. Change maternal position. 4. Temporary decrease in variability can occur when fetus is in a sleep state.

Table 21.7   SUMMARY OF FETAL HEART RATE: CHARACTERISTICS AND PATTERNS—cont'd

Term	Definition	Therapeutic Interventions
Periodic Changes		
Acceleration	Abrupt increase in FHR above the baseline rate of 15 beats/min or greater and lasting 15 sec or more *Pathophysiology:* Breech presentations; occur during fetal movement and are indications of fetal well-being	1. No specific intervention required.
Early deceleration	Visually apparent gradual decrease of the FHR with return to baseline associated with contractions Onset, maximal fall, and recovery coincide with onset, peak, and end of contraction, respectively *Pathophysiology:* Head compression	1. Distinguish from late deceleration. 2. Observe mother for progress in labor because these changes are usually indicative of cervical dilation of 4-6 cm or more. 3. Considered a reassuring pattern not associated with fetal hypoxemia, acidosis, or low Apgar.
Late deceleration	Visually apparent gradual decrease (onset to lowest point [nadir] ≥30 sec) of FHR below the baseline In general, the onset, nadir, and recovery of the deceleration occur after the onset, peak, and recovery of the contractions *Pathophysiology:* Uteroplacental insufficiency	1. Correct underlying cause – examples: 　• Supine hypotension – change maternal position. 　• Epidural or spinal anesthesia – elevate legs, increase hydration with IV fluids. 　• Uterine hyperactivity – reduce or discontinue dosage of oxytocin. 2. Considered a nonreassuring pattern. 3. Left lateral position during labor. 4. Administer oxygen to mother. 5. Be prepared for operative delivery if fetal condition warrants.
Variable deceleration	Visually apparent abrupt decrease (onset of nadir <30 sec) of the FHR below baseline Decrease is ≥15 secs and returns to baseline in <2 min *Pathophysiology:* Umbilical cord compression	1. Change maternal position (side to side, knee-chest). 2. Discontinue oxytocin if infusing. 3. Administer oxygen to mother; increase IV fluids. 4. Assist with birth if pattern not corrected.

> **⊞ NURSING PRIORITY** Reassuring FHR characterized by 110-160 beats/min with no periodic decelerations and moderate baseline variability; accelerations occur with fetal movement. Nonreassuring FHR is associated with fetal hypoxemia and includes increase or decrease in baseline rate, tachycardia (>160 beats/min), decrease in baseline variability, severe variable decelerations, late decelerations, absence of FHR variability, prolonged deceleration (>60-90 sec), or severe bradycardia (<70 beats/min).

FHR, fetal heart rate; *IV,* intravenous.

A. Airway: clear air passages to establish respirations.
B. Body temperature.
　1. For stable term newborn, place infant on mother's chest or abdomen for skin-to-skin contact. Dry infant with gentle rubbing, remove wet linens, and cover mother and infant with warm blanket. Apply cap to newborns' head to decrease heat loss by evaporation.
　2. For less than term or newborn requiring interventions, maintain warmth with a radiant heater during interventions and initial newborn assessment. Once stable, dry and wrap infant, place on mothers' chest for skin-to-skin contact, cover with warm blankets, and place cap on newborn's head.
C. Apgar scoring: immediate appraisal of newborn's condition taken at 1 min and again at 5 min. (Table 21.8).

> **TEST ALERT** Determine Apgar score of newborn.

D. Care of the umbilical cord: delayed cord clamping (cord clamped 1-5 min after birth or after pulsation ceases) is recommended standard of care. This allows transfusion of stem cells, RBCs, and whole blood from the placenta,

Assessment: Recognize Cues

A. Clinical manifestations.
 1. Contractions occurring in increasing frequency and intensity.
 2. Premature rupture of the membranes.
 3. Cervical dilation; cervical effacement.
 4. Cervical shortening in length.

Analyze Cues and Prioritize Hypotheses

The most important problems are the need for health teaching to recognize the symptoms of preterm labor, potential for maternal/fetal injury, anxiety about the potential birth of a premature neonate.

Generate Solutions

Treatment

A. Medications (see Appendix 21.2).
 1. Tocolytics: magnesium sulfate, beta-adrenergic agonist, prostaglandin synthetase inhibitors, and calcium channel blockers.
 2. Antenatal glucocorticoids: betamethasone or dexamethasone.

Nursing Interventions: Take Action

Goal: To assist in delivery if maternal complications are present.

A. Maternal complications: diabetes, pregnancy-induced hypertension, hemorrhage.
B. Prepare for delivery of premature infant: if indicated, administer betamethasone to minimize/prevent respiratory distress syndrome (RDS) in the newborn.

Goal: To provide emotional support.

A. Encourage expression of feelings related to anxiety and guilt.
B. Identify and support coping mechanisms for couple.

Goal: To minimize fetal complications.

A. Promote fetal oxygenation.
 1. Avoid supine position during labor: associated with risk of vena cava syndrome.
 2. Avoid maternal hyperventilation, which may decrease oxygen to fetus.

❗ NURSING PRIORITY Encourage left lateral Sims position, because it promotes placental perfusion.

📋 Dysfunctional Labor (dystocia)

Dysfunctional labor (dystocia) **is a long, difficult, or abnormal labor.**

Assessment: Recognize Cues

A. Dysfunctional labor.
 1. Hypotonic contractions: slow, infrequent, weak contractions occurring more than 3 min apart and lasting less than 40 sec.

 2. Hypertonic contractions: frequent, strong, painful contractions that are ineffective in causing cervical dilation or effacement.
B. Abnormal labor patterns.
 1. CPD: also called fetopelvic disproportion (FPD); related to excessive fetal size (4000 g or more).
 2. Abnormal fetal presentation: breech is most common.
 3. Multifetal pregnancy: higher risk than singleton births.
 4. Precipitous delivery: a very rapid, intense labor lasting less than 3 hrs from onset of contraction to time of birth.

Analyze Cues and Prioritize Hypotheses

The most important problems are potential maternal/fetal injury, anxiety related to loss of control, decreased ability to cope related to exhaustion secondary to a prolonged labor process, pain and discomfort, potential for impaired self-concept as parent related to separation from infant after emergency cesarean birth and/or emotional responses to a traumatic childbirth experience.

Generate Solutions

Treatment

A. Dysfunctional labor (dystocia) relating to CPD or malpresentation may be resolved by a cesarean delivery.
B. Prolonged labor or hypotonic uterine contractions are treated by IV administration of oxytocin.
C. Hypertonic uterine contractions are treated by sedation and rest.

Nursing Interventions: Take Action

Goal: To monitor level of fatigue and ability to cope with pain.

A. Provide basic comfort measures, back rubs, change of position, clean dry linen.
B. Provide emotional support to mother and significant other.
C. Give reassurance and stay with client continually.

Goal: To assist in the medical management of dysfunctional labor.

A. Explain procedures used to rule out cause of dystocia: sonogram, x-ray studies, etc.
B. Monitor oxytocin administration if indicated for hypotonic dysfunction or prolonged labor.
C. Prepare client for cesarean delivery (indicated in cases of CPD and/or malpresentation).
D. Administer broad-spectrum antibiotics to decrease incidence of infection.
E. Maintain hydration, monitor intake and output, and administer oxygen as needed.

Goal: To detect early complications associated with dysfunctional labor.

A. Monitor maternal vital signs.
B. Assess mother for signs of exhaustion, dehydration, increasing temperature, and acidosis.
C. Assess fetal heart tones frequently through fetal electronic monitoring.

Supine Hypotensive Syndrome

Supine hypotensive syndrome, or vena cava syndrome, occurs when the weight of the uterus causes partial occlusion of the vena cava, leading to decreased venous return to the heart.

Assessment: Recognize Cues

A. Shock-like symptoms seen when pregnant woman assumes a supine position.

B. Clients at greatest risk: gravidas with polyhydramnios or multifetal gestations, hypovolemia, dehydrated, and obese women.

Analyze Cues and Prioritize Hypotheses

The most important problem is the potential for maternal/fetal injury from a hypotensive episode and the need to change position (side-lying; left side preferable).

Nursing Interventions: Take Action

Goal: To decrease the duration of an episode of supine hypotensive syndrome.

A. Educate mother to turn to either right or left side with knees slightly flexed; preferred position because pressure is removed from vena cava.

B. Administer oxygen as necessary.

C. Assess FHR and *report any changes to the RN.*

Hemorrhage in the Pregnant Client

> **TEST ALERT** Recognize occurrence of a hemorrhage. It is important to plan nursing management for the pregnant client who has bleeding or hemorrhage (Table 21.9).

Types of Hemorrhage

A. *Placenta previa* is the abnormal implantation of placenta in the lower uterine segment near or over the internal cervical os.

B. *Abruptio placentae* is the premature separation of part or all of a normally implanted placenta, leading to hemorrhage.

C. A *ruptured uterus* is characterized by a tearing or splitting of the uterine wall during labor; it is usually a result of a thinned or weakened area that cannot withstand the strain and force of uterine contractions.

Analyze Cues and Prioritize Hypotheses

The most important problems are inadequate tissue perfusion related to excessive blood loss, dehydration, decreased placental perfusion related to hypovolemia and shunting of blood to central circulation, anxiety related to condition and pregnancy outcome, and grieving because of the actual or perceived threat to pregnancy.

Nursing Interventions: Take Action

Goal: To provide nursing management associated with hemorrhage (see Table 21.9).

Goal: To detect early complications.

Anaphylactoid Syndrome of Pregnancy (amniotic fluid embolism)

Anaphylactoid syndrome of pregnancy (amniotic fluid embolism) is rare and can occur during labor, birth, or within 30 min of delivery. It is a sudden respiratory and cardiovascular collapse, along with coagulopathy, as seen in anaphylaxis. The exact cause is unknown. It is diagnosed clinically. It is no longer thought to be an embolism or related to amniotic fluid. Neonatal prognosis is poor.

Assessment: Recognize Cues

A. Clinical manifestations.
   1. Sudden respiratory distress (dyspnea, cyanosis, pulmonary edema).
   2. Profound shock and vascular collapse.
   3. Bleeding from incisions, venipuncture sites, petechiae, ecchymosis.

Analyze Cues and Prioritize Hypotheses

The most important problems are hemorrhage, respiratory distress, potential coagulopathy, anxiety related to condition and pregnancy outcome, and grieving because of actual or perceived threat to pregnancy and fetus.

Generate Solutions

Treatment

A. Medical: management is similar to that for pulmonary embolism or respiratory distress.

Nursing Interventions: Take Action

Goal: To assist in emergency resuscitation.

Goal: To provide emotional support to father and significant others.

Abnormal Fetal Position

This is an *unfavorable fetal presentation* or position that may interfere with cervical dilation or fetal descent.

Assessment: Recognize Cues

A. Occiput: posterior position (most common).

B. Breech presentation.
   1. FHR is usually auscultated above the umbilicus.
   2. Passage of meconium is often seen.
   3. Increased danger of prolapsed umbilical cord, especially in incomplete breech presentation.

C. Transverse lie (shoulder presentation).

Analyze Cues and Prioritize Hypotheses

The most important problems are fetal distress and potential cesarean delivery.

Nursing Interventions: Take Action

Goal: To provide reassurance and explanations of procedures, as indicated.

A. Explanation of possible cesarean delivery.

Table 21.9 NURSING MANAGEMENT OF HEMORRHAGE IN THE PREGNANT CLIENT

Causes and Sources	Symptoms	Nursing Interventions
Antepartal Period		
Abortion Placenta previa Placental abruption (abruptio placentae)	Vaginal bleeding Intermittent uterine contractions Rupture of the membranes **Painless vaginal bleeding** Vaginal bleeding (dark red) Extreme tenderness in abdomen Rigid, boardlike abdomen **Increase in size of abdomen**	1. Obtain history of onset, duration, amount of bleeding, and associated symptoms. 2. Observe perineal pads for amount of bleeding (blood loss can be measured by weighing perineal pads, approximately 1 g = 1 mL of blood). 3. Monitor vital signs of mother and fetus (frequency is determined by severity of clinical symptoms).
	TEST ALERT Recognize the occurrence of hemorrhage and assess mother for complications.	
Intrapartal Period		
Placenta previa Placental abruption (abruptio placentae) Uterine atony in stage 3	Bright, painless vaginal bleeding Bright, red vaginal bleeding Ineffectual contractility	1. Start IV and provide volume replacement. 2. Request type and cross-match for blood. 3. Administer fluids and blood as prescribed. 4. Monitor intake and output. 5. Minimize chances for further bleeding. 6. *NO* vaginal or rectal examinations. 7. Bed rest in position of comfort. 8. Anticipate cesarean delivery.
Postpartum Period		
Uterine atony Retained placental fragments Lacerations of cervix or vagina	Boggy uterus Dark vaginal bleeding Presence of clots Firm uterus Bright red blood	1. Massage fundus of uterus. 2. Assess bladder status. 3. Anticipate administration of oxytocin for client with uterine atony. 4. Reduce anxiety. 5. Keep mother and family advised of treatment plan. 6. Record amount of bleeding in a specific amount of time. 7. Monitor vital signs: overt hypotension and shock will not be seen until the client has lost almost 30%-40% of her blood volume (1500-2000 mL); watch for tachycardia and orthostatic BP changes first.
	! NURSING PRIORITY Frequent, accurate assessment and documentation of blood loss are priorities in postpartum care.	

BP, blood pressure; *IV*, intravenous.

B. When fetus is in occiput-posterior position, encourage positioning of mother on the side or in a modified knee-chest position to decrease pressure on the sacral nerves.

C. Assess for complications related to prolonged labor and possible infection.

Multiple (multifetal) Pregnancy

The term *multifetal gestation* or pregnancy refers to more than one fetus in the uterus and can include twins (most common), triplets, and higher-order or number of fetuses (e.g., quadruplets [four], quintuplets [five], sextuplets [six], etc.).

Assessment: Recognize Cues

A. Clinical manifestations.
1. Increased experience of more physical discomfort: shortness of breath, dyspnea on exertion, backaches, and leg edema caused by excessive size of uterus.
2. Auscultation of two or more FHRs.
3. Measurement of fundal height exceeds gestational age.

Analyze Cues and Prioritize Hypotheses

The most important problems are preterm labor, potential for gestational diabetes, preeclampsia, postpartum hemorrhage, and premature newborn.

Generate Solutions

Treatment

A. Medical.
1. More frequent prenatal visits with frequent FHR monitoring.
2. Antiemetic for nausea and vomiting after the first trimester.
B. Dietary: increase of 1 serving from one of the following food groups: dairy, fruits, vegetables, grains.
C. Frequent ultrasound examinations, nonstress tests, and FHR monitoring.

Nursing Interventions: Take Action

Goal: To provide anticipatory guidance during the ante-partal period.
A. Nutrition: well-balanced diet with appropriate weight gain.
B. Management of discomforts of multifetal gestation.
C. Teach the signs of preterm labor.
Goal: To provide psychological support.
A. Provide assistance and advice regarding care of twins at home.
B. Because twins are apt to be small, anticipate nursing care for premature neonates.
C. *Assess for maternal complications (e.g., postpartum hemorrhage), and report to RN.*
D. Ensure correct identification: Baby A and Baby B.

Prolapsed Cord

A *prolapsed cord* occurs when the cord slips in front of the presenting part.

Assessment: Recognize Cues

A. Clinical manifestations.
1. Woman reports feeling cord after membranes rupture.
2. Visualization or palpation of the cord in the vagina.

Analyze Cues and Prioritize Hypotheses

The most important problems are fetal injury resulting from hypoxia from umbilical cord compression.

Generate Solutions

Treatment

A. Medical.
1. Administer oxygen to mother and *notify RN immediately.*
B. Surgical.
1. If dilation is incomplete, cesarean delivery is necessary.
2. Occasionally, if dilation is complete, vaginal delivery is possible.

Nursing Interventions: Take Action

Goal: To maintain fetal oxygenation and assist with immediate delivery.
A. Continuing assessment of FHR.

B. Insert a gloved finger into the vagina and lift the presenting part off the cord to relieve the pressure.
C. Place mother in side-lying position, knee-chest position, or in Trendelenburg position (head of bed or table is lowered).
D. Any prolapsed cord outside the vagina should be kept moistened with sterile towel soaked in warm saline solution.
E. Offer emotional support to the couple.

Severely Depressed Neonate

A neonate with hypoxia and significant acidosis is a severely depressed neonate (Apgar score is 0-3).

Assessment: Recognize Cues

A. Clinical manifestations.
1. Severe hypoxia and acidosis.
2. Pale, flaccid, apneic neonate.
3. Heart rate less than 100 beats/min.
4. Slightly reactive or unresponsive to stimulation.

Analyze Cues and Prioritize Hypotheses

The most important problems are neonatal hypoxia, the need for emergency resuscitative measures, and parental grieving in response to actual or perceived threat to neonate.

Nursing Interventions: Take Action

Goal: To identify appropriate treatment and initiate it quickly for the severely depressed neonate.
A. Assess for fetus at risk and be prepared for emergency measures at birth.
B. Initiate resuscitation procedures.

Intrauterine Fetal Death

Intrauterine fetal death is also called fetal demise.

Assessment: Recognize Cues

A. Absence of FHR and fetal movement.
B. Decreased maternal estriol level.
C. Diagnosis: ultrasound examination determines absence of FHR.
D. Monitor for complications: hypofibrinogenemia from fetal breakdown products.

Analyze Cues and Prioritize Hypotheses

The most important problems are death of the fetus, the potential for maternal hemorrhage, and parental grieving.

Nursing Interventions: Take Action

Goal: To support the couple through the grieving process.
A. Objectively listen; encourage expression of feelings; do not minimize the situation or event.
B. Anticipate the steps of the grieving process (denial, anger, bargaining, depression, and acceptance).
C. Provide an opportunity for the couple to spend time with the stillborn infant if they so desire.
D. Monitor for complications.

POSTPARTUM NURSING CARE

> **TEST ALERT** Collect postpartum data and monitor for complications. The puerperium or postpartum period spans the first 6 weeks after delivery. It is the period in which the body adjusts both physically and psychologically to the process of childbearing. Often referred to as the "fourth trimester."

Physiologic Changes

Assessment: Recognize Cues

A. Uterus.
  1. Uterine involution: process by which the uterus returns to its nonpregnant condition (Fig. 21.7).
  2. Immediately after delivery, top of fundus is 2 cm below (2 finger's width) the umbilicus.
  3. At 12 hrs after delivery, the fundus of the uterus is 1 cm above the umbilicus.
  4. Fundus recedes/descends into the pelvis approximately 1 to 2 cm per day.
  5. The uterus should not be palpable abdominally after 2 weeks.
  6. Afterpains: alternating contractions and relaxations of the uterine muscle.
    a. Occur primarily in multiparas.
    b. Usually subside within 3 to 7 days.
  7. Lochia.

> **! NURSING PRIORITY** Always chart the amount first, followed by the character (e.g., moderate amount of lochia rubra).

    a. Lochia rubra: bright red discharge; occurs the first 3 days.
    b. Lochia serosa: pinkish-brown, serosanguineous discharge; lasts approximately 4 to 10 days.
    c. Lochia alba: creamy or yellowish discharge; occurs after day 10 and may last 3 to 6 weeks.
    d. When lochia subsides, uterus is considered closed; postpartal infection is less likely.
B. Cervix.
  1. May be stretched and swollen.
  2. Small lacerations may be apparent.
  3. External os closes slowly; at the end of the first week after delivery, the opening is fingertip size.
C. Vagina.
  1. Does not return to its original prepregnant state.
  2. Labia majora and minora are flabbier.
D. Perineum.
  1. May be bruised and tender.
  2. Pelvic floor and ligaments are stretched.
  3. Muscle tone is restored by Kegel exercises.
E. Ovulation and menstruation.
  1. Nonlactating women.
    a. Menstruation resumes in 12 weeks.
    b. Ovulation: 7 to 9 weeks.
  2. Lactating women.
    a. The time that menses resumes varies.
    b. Mean time to resume ovulation is 6 months after delivery.

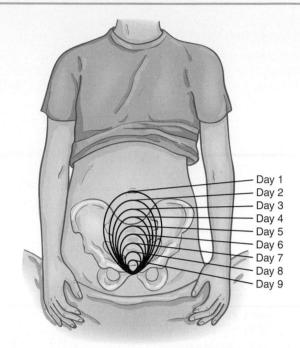

FIG. 21.7 Involution of uterus. (From Murray S, McKinney E, Holub K, Jones, R. *Maternal-newborn and women's health nursing.* 7th ed. Elsevier; 2019.)

F. Abdomen.
  1. Still pregnant appearance for the first days after delivery.
  2. Muscle tone can be restored within 6 weeks with exercise.
  3. Possible separation of the abdominal wall: diastasis recti.
G. Breasts.
  1. Anterior pituitary releases prolactin, which stimulates secretion of milk.
  2. Engorgement may occur approximately 3 to 5 days after delivery.
  3. Colostrum (thin, yellowish fluid) is released.
    a. Contains antibodies and is high in protein.
    b. Has a laxative effect on the newborn; promotes expulsion of bilirubin-laden meconium.
H. Gastrointestinal (GI) system.
  1. Immediately after delivery, hunger is common.
  2. GI tract is sluggish and hypoactive because of decreased muscle tone and peristalsis.
  3. Constipation may be a problem.
I. Urinary tract.
  1. Risk for UTI is increased if client was catheterized during labor and delivery.
  2. May have bruising and swelling caused by trauma around the urinary meatus.
  3. Increased bladder capacity, along with decreased sensitivity to pressure, leads to urinary retention.
  4. Assess for bladder distension, which displaces the uterus leading to a "boggy" uterus and increased bleeding.
  5. Urine will be mixed with lochia after birth, giving the appearance of hematuria.

6. Diuresis occurs during the first 2 to 3 days after delivery.

J. Integumentary system.
   1. Chloasma usually disappears in the postpartum period.
   2. Spider nevi generally regress, darker pigmentation of areolae, and linea nigra may persist. Dark red stretch-marks gradually fade.
   3. Fingernails return to normal.
   4. Profuse diaphoresis occurs at night for the first 2 to 3 days after birth.

K. Vital signs.
   1. Temperature may be slightly elevated (100.4 °F) (38°C) after a long labor; should return to normal within 24 hrs. *Report any elevated temperature to the RN.*
   2. BP may be slightly increased after delivery; however, it should remain stable.
   3. Pulse rate slows after delivery.

L. Blood values.
   1. Leukocytosis is present: white blood cell count of 30,000 mm3 (30 x 109/L) is common.
   2. Hemoglobin and hematocrit values and RBC count return to normal within 8 weeks.
   3. Rule of thumb: 4-point drop in hematocrit equals 1 pint of blood loss.
   4. Increased risk for development of thrombophlebitis and thromboembolism.

M. Weight loss.
   1. Initial 10 to 12 lb (4-5 kg) loss is from the weight of the infant, placenta, and amniotic fluid.
   2. Diuresis leads to an additional 5 lb (2 kg) weight loss.
   3. Six to 8 weeks after delivery: return to prepregnant weight if an average of 25 to 30 lb (11-13 kg) was gained.

Maternal Role Attainment

A. Phases.
   1. Dependent: taking-in phase.
      a. First 1 to 2 days after delivery.
      b. Characterized by passiveness and dependency.
      c. Mother is preoccupied with own needs: food, attention, and physical comforts and care.
      d. Talkative.
   2. Dependent-independent: taking-hold phase.
      a. Occurs approximately 2 to 3 days after delivery; characterized by increase in physical well-being.
      b. Emphasis on the present; woman takes hold of the task of mothering; requires reassurance.
      c. Very receptive to teaching.
   3. Interdependent: letting-go phase.
      a. Begins 10 days to several weeks after birth.
      b. Focus is on family unit moving forward: spouse, siblings.

B. Attachment behaviors.
   1. Exploration and identification pattern.
      a. Touch: begins by stroking the extremities and the outline of the head with the fingertips; gradually moves toward using the entire surface of the hand; touches and observes first at arm's length, then on lap, or slightly away from the body; finally enfolds infant close to body with both arms.
      b. Eye-to-eye contact: *en face position* (gazing into the eyes of the infant).
   2. Factors influencing maternal-infant attachment.
      a. Relationship with own parents.
      b. Previous experience with infants.
      c. Acceptance of pregnancy as a positive event.
      d. Amount of time of initial contact between mother and infant.
      e. Health and responsiveness of infant.
      f. Maternal age.

C. Postpartum blues.
   1. Transient period of depression (occurring during the puerperium).
   2. Complaints of anxiety; insomnia; tearfulness; a general let down, sad feeling.
   3. Cause is unknown.
   4. Mother needs support and reassurance that it is a transient and self-limiting experience.
   5. All severe depression and postpartum psychosis are hospitalized. Safety of both the mother and baby is a critically important priority if either of these conditions develops.

Analyze Cues and Prioritize Hypotheses

The most important issues are monitoring for postpartum complications (hemorrhage, bladder distention, infection, perineal lacerations) and teaching the mother about self-management (perineal care, breastfeeding) and infant care.

Postpartum Nursing Interventions: Take Action

> **TEST ALERT** Perform postpartum assessments and instruct client on postpartum care.

Goal: To initiate routine postpartum assessment (Fig. 21.8).

A. General observations of mood, activity level, and feelings of wellness; routine vital sign assessment.

B. Inspection of breasts: check for beginning engorgement and presence of cracks in nipples, any pain or tenderness, and progress of breastfeeding.

C. Check uterine fundus: determine height of fundus in relation to umbilicus; should feel firm and globular (Fig. 21.9).

D. Assess for bladder distention, especially during the first 24 to 48 hrs after delivery, and *report to RN if distended.*

E. Perineal area.
   1. Observe episiotomy or laceration site.
      a. Evaluate healing status of episiotomy or laceration.
      b. Apply anesthetic sprays or ointments to decrease pain.
   2. Determine whether hemorrhoids are present, and if so, provide relief measures.

POSTPARTUM ASSESSMENT

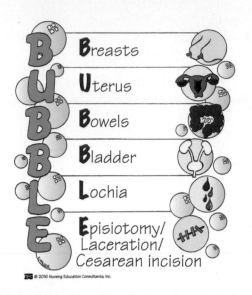

FIG. 21.8 Postpartum assessment. (From Zerwekh J, Garneau A, Miller CJ. *Digital collection of the memory notebooks of nursing.* 4th ed. Chandler, AZ: Nursing Education Consultants, Inc.; 2017.)

FUNDAL MASSAGE TECHNIQUE

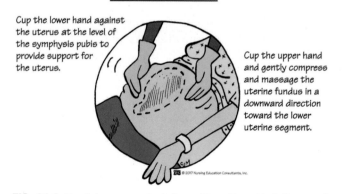

Cup the lower hand against the uterus at the level of the symphysis pubis to provide support for the uterus.

Cup the upper hand and gently compress and massage the uterine fundus in a downward direction toward the lower uterine segment.

FIG. 21.9 Fundal massage technique. (From Zerwekh J, Garneau A, Miller CJ. *Digital collection of the memory notebooks of nursing.* 4th ed. Chandler, AZ: Nursing Education Consultants, Inc.; 2017.)

F. Lochia: record color, odor, and amount of discharge. *Report any significant increase in amount or foul odor of lochia to the RN.*

G. Lower extremities: assess for venous thromboembolism; encourage ambulation as soon as possible to decrease venous stasis.

H. Abdomen and perineum.
1. Initiate strengthening exercises for both abdominal wall and perineum (e.g., buttock lifts and isometric Kegel exercises for strengthening pelvic floor).
2. Kegel exercises: practice trying to stop the passing of gas or pretending to stop the flow of urine midstream, which replicates the sensation of the pelvic muscles drawing upward and inward.

Goal: To provide comfort and relief of pain.

A. Episiotomy: ice packs for first 24 hrs; sitz baths.

B. Perineal care: use of "Peri bottles" to squirt warm water over perineum (front to back to prevent contamination); blot dry with toilet tissue.

C. Afterpains: use of analgesics (preferably 1 hr before feeding, especially for breastfeeding mothers).

D. Hemorrhoidal pain.
1. Sitz baths, anesthetic ointments, rectal suppositories, astringent wipes.
2. Encourage lying on side and avoidance of prolonged sitting.
3. Stool softeners or laxatives may be indicated; client usually has normal bowel movement by second or third day after delivery.

E. Breast engorgement (during lactation): well-fitting bra should be worn to provide support.

F. Lactation suppression: well-fitting bra or breast binder, ice packs to breasts; application of fresh cold cabbage leaves inside of bra.

Goal: To promote maternal-infant attachment and facilitate integration of the newborn into the family unit.

A. Use infant's name when talking about them.

B. Assist parents in problem solving and meeting their infant's needs. Explain ways to distinguish different types of cries – those related to hunger, illness, discomfort, etc.

C. Encourage parents to provide as much of the care to the infant as possible while still in the hospital.

D. Accept parents' emotions; encourage expression of feelings.

E. Help parents to understand sibling behavior and plan for the arrival of the new family member.

Goal: To establish successful infant feeding patterns.

A. Nonlactating mother.
1. Provide supportive bra.
2. Explain and demonstrate proper position for feeding.
3. Formulas: review formula recommended and how it is supplied.

B. Lactating mothers.
1. Teach mother to refrain from using soap to wash nipples or applying breast creams.
2. Application of expressed breast milk to nipples after each feeding has a bacteriostatic effect and may provide protection to damaged skin.
3. On first postpartum checkup, assess breasts for engorgement, nipple inversion, cracking, inflammation, or pain.
4. Explain process of lactation and refer mother to community resources such as a lactation consultant or La Leche League.

Goal: To prevent infection and detect potential complications.

Goal: To prepare and plan for discharge.

TEST ALERT Monitor client's ability to care for infant.

Box 21.5 BREASTFEEDING

Types of Feeding Positions
- Cradle position, side-lying, football or clutch position, and modified cradle position.

Teach mother to
- Bring infant to level of the breast: do not lean over.
- Turn infant completely on side with arms embracing the breast on either side.
- Bring infant in as close as possible with ears, shoulders, and hips in a straight line.
- Bring infant's lips to nipple; when infant opens mouth to its widest point, draw the infant the rest of the way on to the nipple for them to latch on (see Fig. 21.10).
- Break the suction by placing a clean finger in the side of the infant's mouth before removing the infant from the breast.
- Put infant to breast 8 to 12 times per day.
- Avoid the use of nipple shields or bottle nipples.
- Avoid use of pacifier until infant is well established on breastfeeding, usually approximately 4 to 6 weeks of age.

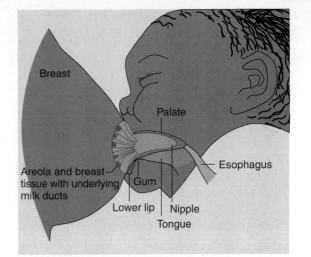

FIG. 21.10 Correct attachment (latch on) of infant at breast. (From Perry S, Hockenberry M, Lowdermilk D, et al. *Maternal child nursing care.* 5th ed. Elsevier/Mosby; 2014.)

Box 21.6 EVALUATING BREASTFEEDING

How do you know that an infant is getting enough breast milk?
- Hear infant swallow and make soft "ka" or "ah" sounds.
- Observe for smooth nutritive suckling – bursts of 15 to 20 sucks/swallows.
- Breast gets softer during the feeding.
- Infant is breastfeeding 8 to 12 times per day; more milk is produced with frequent breastfeeding.
- Infant has at least two to six wet diapers per day for first 2 days after birth; six to eight diapers per day by the 5th day.
- Infant has at least three bowel movements daily during the first month and often more.
- Infant is gaining weight and is satisfied after feedings.

A. Determine whether mother will need household help (especially important in birth of twins or after cesarean delivery).

B. *Assist the RN to explain and teach the following infant care skills.*
   1. Infant feeding (Box 21.5 and Fig. 21.10).
      a. Hold bottle so that air does not get into nipple.
      b. Method of making or preparing formula.
      c. How to break the infant's suction on the nipple.
      d. Positioning for burping and bubbling.
      e. Teach how to determine whether infant is getting enough milk (Box 21.6).
   2. Diapering.
      a. Frequent changing to prevent diaper rash.
      b. Protective ointment can be used to prevent irritation.
      c. Fold diaper below umbilical area.
   3. Bathing.
      a. Use of a neutral pH soap without preservatives.
      b. Daily bath is not necessary, no more than every other day.
      c. Non-alcohol-based lotions can be applied; best advice is to avoid use of powders.
   4. Umbilical cord.
      a. Wash with plain water and dry thoroughly.
      b. Stump usually falls off in 10 to 14 days.
   5. Nonnutritive sucking.
      a. Pacifiers may be used to meet infant's sucking need.
      b. There is evidence that pacifiers help prevent sudden infant death syndrome (SIDS).
      c. May be used up to age 4 years or when permanent teeth erupt.
   6. Sleeping.
      a. Place infant on back to sleep for the first year.
      b. Encourage mother to sleep while infant is sleeping to avoid sleep deprivation.
   7. Illness.
      a. Common behavior changes are vomiting, inconsolable crying, poor feeding, and fever.
      b. Explain how to take an infant's temperature.
   8. Taking the infant outside.
      a. Dress infant as you would dress yourself; do not overdress infant or "bundle up."
      b. Traveling: use a car seat.
   9. Explain importance of follow-up well-baby checkup visits with health care provider, usually scheduled within a week of discharge.

TEST ALERT Perform care for postpartum client and monitor for postpartum complications.

COMPLICATIONS ASSOCIATED WITH POSTPARTUM

📋 Hemorrhage

Postpartum hemorrhage is defined as the loss of 500 mL or more of blood after vaginal birth and 1000 mL or more after cesarean birth.

Assessment: Recognize Cues

A. Clinical manifestations (see Table 21.9).
1. Early postpartal hemorrhage: occurs within the first 24 hrs after delivery.
2. Late postpartal hemorrhage: occurs after the first 24 hrs but less than 6 weeks after birth.
3. Uterine fundus is difficult to locate or feels soft, "boggy", when located.
4. Bright red lochia, excessive clots expelled (with or without uterine massage).
5. Symptoms of shock: weak, rapid pulse; low BP; pallor; restlessness; etc.

Analyze Cues and Prioritize Hypotheses

The most important problems include a disrupted fluid balance related to bleeding, decreased tissue perfusion related to hypovolemia, and potential for infection related to blood loss and invasive procedures.

Generate Solutions

Treatment
A. Medical.
1. Uterine atony.
   a. Oxytocic medications.
   b. Bimanual compression of the uterus.

> ❗ **NURSING PRIORITY** The key to successful management of hemorrhage is prevention, which includes adequate nutrition, good prenatal care, early diagnosis and management of any complications as they arise, and avoidance of traumatic procedures.

B. Surgical.
1. Lacerations: suturing the bleeding edges.
2. Retained placenta: D&C to remove retained fragment(s).

Nursing Interventions: Take Action

Goal: To control and correct the cause of the hemorrhage.
A. Uterine atony.
1. Massage uterine fundus to stimulate contractions; make sure bladder is empty.
2. Administer oxytocic medications.
B. Lacerations.
1. Inspect perineal area.
2. Hematoma formation.
   a. *Any complaint of pain in the perineal area should prompt careful inspection and be reported to the RN.*
3. Do not administer rectal suppositories/enemas or perform rectal examinations.

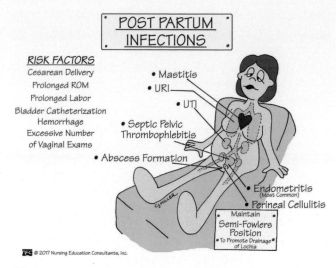

FIG. 21.11 Postpartum infections. (From Zerwekh J, Garneau A, Miller CJ. *Digital collection of the memory notebooks of nursing.* 4th ed. Chandler, AZ: Nursing Education Consultants, Inc.; 2017.)

> ❗ **NURSING PRIORITY** Careful observation of vaginal bleeding, by doing a pad count or weighing the perineal pads, is very important. Always check under client's buttocks, because blood may flow between buttocks onto linens under the client.

C. Retained placenta.
1. Inspect placenta at the time of delivery for intactness.
2. Never force the expulsion of the placenta.

📋 Postpartum Infection (puerperal infection)

Postpartum infection is any clinical infection of the genital canal that occurs within 28 days after miscarriage, abortion, or childbirth.

Assessment: Recognize Cues

A. Predisposing factors.
1. Antepartal infection.
2. Premature rupture of the membranes, prolonged labor.
3. Laceration.
4. Anemia; postpartum hemorrhage.
5. Poor aseptic technique.
B. Clinical manifestations (Fig. 21.11).
1. Temperature elevation 100.4°F (38°C), if taken at least four times daily on any 2 of the first 10 postpartum days, with the exception of the first 24 hrs after birth.
2. Symptoms vary depending on the system involved.
3. Area of involvement is characterized by five cardinal symptoms of inflammation (redness, pain, heat, edema, and loss of function).
4. Tachycardia, chills, and abdominal tenderness are common.
5. Headache, malaise, deep pelvic pain.
6. Profuse, foul-smelling lochia.
C. Area involved.

1. Uterus is most often affected: endometritis.
2. May have localized wound infection of the perineum, vulva, and vagina.
3. Local infection may extend via the lymphatics into the pelvic organs.
4. Urinary system: UTI.

Analyze Cues and Prioritize Hypotheses

The most important problems are delayed wound healing, acute pain, need for health teaching related to management of infection, transmission and prevention of infection, and fear of spreading infection to newborn.

Generate Solutions

Treatment

A. Medications: antibiotics, antipyretics.
B. Dietary.
   1. High-protein, high-calorie, high-vitamin diet.
   2. Encourage intake of 3000 to 4000 mL of fluid per day.

Nursing Interventions: Take Action

Goal: To prevent puerperal infection.

A. Maintain meticulous aseptic technique during labor and delivery.
B. Assess and treat antepartum infection and *report any significant elevation in temperature to the RN.*
C. Detect anemia: check hematocrit during prenatal visits. *Report any significant decrease in hematocrit to RN.*

Goal: To promote mother's resistance to infection.

> **! NURSING PRIORITY** The pathophysiology related to maintaining semi-Fowler position to localize infection is important to remember, not only for clients with obstetric complications, but also for others with contaminated drainage.

A. Administer antibiotic, antipyretic, and oxytocic medications.
B. Isolate client from other maternity clients.
C. Use semi-Fowler position to promote free drainage of lochia and prevent upward extension of infection into pelvis.

Mastitis

Mastitis is the invasion of the breast tissue by pathogenic organisms. It is usually unilateral and develops after the flow of milk is established.

Assessment: Recognize Cues

A. Predisposing factors.
   1. Fissured nipples.
   2. Inadequate breast emptying.
   3. Mastitis is most frequently caused by *Staphylococcus aureus*, which is transmitted from the nasopharynx of the nursing infant.
B. Clinical manifestations.
   1. Occurs most during the first 2 to 4 weeks postpartum.
   2. Chills, malaise, and body aches.

3. Red, swollen, painful breast(s); axillary adenopathy.
4. Fever of 103 °F (39.4°C) or 104°F (40°C).

Generate Solutions

Treatment

A. Medication.
   1. Antibiotics for 10 to 14 days.
   2. Antipyretics, analgesics.

Nursing Interventions: Take Action

Goal: To prevent the complication of mastitis.

A. Teach mother how to care for breasts and nipples.

> **! NURSING PRIORITY** Mother should continue to breastfeed on the affected side, because failure to do so increases the risk for abscess formation and relapse.

B. Explain the importance of wearing a bra that provides adequate support.

Goal: To promote comfort and maintain lactation.

A. Frequent breastfeeding, starting on the affected side.
B. Warm compresses to the breast before and during each feeding to thoroughly drain any blockages (a breast pump may be used as well).
C. Encourage good nutrition and adequate rest.
D. Warm showers; increased intake of fluids and vitamin C.
E. Administer antibiotics, as ordered.

Postpartum Mood Disorders

This is the predominant mental health disorder during the postpartum period and includes *postpartum blues (baby blues, most common), postpartum depression, and postpartum psychosis.*

Assessment: Recognize Cues

A. Postpartum blues ("baby blues").
   1. Normal functioning is not impaired.
   2. Mood swings, feelings of sadness and anxiety, crying, difficulty sleeping, and loss of appetite.
   3. Resolves within a few days.
   4. Treatment: none.
B. Postpartum depression.
   1. Similar to adult depression, except mother's ruminations of guilt and inadequacy feed worries of incompetence and inadequacy as a parent.
   2. Eventually cannot care for themselves or their newborn; often rejection of the infant occurs.
   3. Severe, labile mood swings.
   4. Intense fears, anger, anxiety, irritability, despondency.
   5. Obsessive thoughts about harming the infant.
   6. Treatment: antidepressant medication (selective serotonin reuptake inhibitors [SSRIs]).
C. Postpartum psychosis.
   1. Rare condition that has a rapid onset of bizarre behaviors.
   2. Associated with bipolar disorder.

3. Delusions, hallucinations, extreme deficits in judgment.
4. Suspiciousness, confusion, incoherence, irrational statements, obsessive concerns about infant.
5. Treatment: possible inpatient psychiatric care, antipsychotic and mood-stabilizing medications.

Analyze Cues and Prioritize Hypotheses

The most important problems are feeling sad, overwhelmed, mood changes, lack of sleep, and inability to cope with new parenthood.

Nursing Interventions: Take Action

Interventions are outlined in Chapter 7

> ❗ **NURSING PRIORITY** Mothers who have postpartum depression with psychotic symptoms may harm their infants, so early assessment and intervention are safety concerns.

Venous Thromboembolism (VTE)

VTE occurs in 1 in 1500 pregnancies, and the highest incidence is within the first 3 weeks after birth. The reason for the increased incidence is a change in blood coagulation during pregnancy and a decrease in partial thromboplastin time, along with engorgement of the veins of the lower extremities and pelvis, which leads to pooling of blood and venous stasis. Assessment and nursing interventions are discussed in Chapter 12.

Cystitis

Cystitis occurs as a result of trauma to the bladder mucosa, frequent pelvic examinations, and regional anesthesia. All three lead to distention and incomplete emptying of urine or introduction of pathogens into the urinary tract, predisposing the postpartum client to cystitis (see Chapter 19).

Parents' Reaction to Preterm Infant, Ill Newborn, or Infant With Congenital Anomaly

Assessment: Recognize Cues

A. Period of disorganization.
   1. Grief reaction characterized by guilt, anger, depression, and sorrow.
   2. Feelings of exhaustion, emptiness, and frequent crying.
B. Period of information seeking and resource utilization.
   1. Anxiety decreases; problem-solving begins.
   2. Begins to resolve the crisis.
   3. Often information seeking leads to further anger and sorrow, followed by a period of denial or disbelief.
C. Resolution of the crisis situation.
   1. Development of new coping strategies.
   2. Acceptance and coming to terms with the situation.

Nursing Interventions: Take Action

Goal: To provide emotional support to the parents.
A. Encourage verbalization of feelings and expression of grief.

B. Promote maternal-infant contact; point out normal characteristics.
C. Encourage parents to visit, touch, and care for their infant as much as possible.
D. Refer parents to social and community agencies.

HEALTHY NEWBORN

Biologic Adaptations in the Neonatal Period

Assessment: Recognize Cues

A. Respiratory system.
   1. Respirations are usually established within 1 min after birth, often within the first few seconds.
   2. Strong cry usually accompanies good respiratory effort.
   3. Newborn respiration should be quiet; no dyspnea or cyanosis.
   4. Cyanosis may be apparent in the hands and feet (acrocyanosis); circumoral cyanosis (around the mouth) may persist for an hour or two after birth but should subside.
   5. Average respiratory rate: 30 to 60 breaths/min.
   6. Respiratory movements: diaphragmatic and abdominal muscles are used; little thoracic movement.
   7. Neonate breathes through the nose (obligate nose-breather); consequently, nasal obstruction with mucus will lead to respiratory distress.
B. Circulatory system.
   1. Closure of the ductus arteriosus, the foramen ovale, and the ductus venosus.
   2. Circulatory changes are not always immediate and complete: usually complete in a few days; this period is often called *transitional circulation.*
   3. Pulse rate: 100 to 160 beats/min.
   4. Obtain baseline pulse oximetry before discharge.
   5. Normal BP at birth: systolic 60 to 80 mm Hg; diastolic 40 to 50 mm Hg.
C. Body temperature and heat production.
   1. Loss of body heat.
      a. Evaporation: heat loss as water evaporates from skin and from lungs; occurs when infant's body is wet with amniotic fluid at birth and during bath. Dry infant quickly.
      b. Convection: movement of body heat to cool air; infant loses heat to the cool air in the delivery room. Keep infant wrapped in blanket while in bassinette.
      c. Conduction: direct transfer of heat to a surface on which the infant is lying; infant loses heat to a cool sheet or blanket. Prewarm warmer and bassinette.
      d. Radiation: heat is lost from the infant's warm body as it travels through the air to cooler objects in the room; occurs when an unclothed infant is placed in an open crib or isolette. Avoid drafts.

> ❗ **NURSING PRIORITY** Excessive heat loss occurs from radiation and convection because of the newborn's larger surface area compared with body weight. It is important to remember that conduction loss occurs as a result of the marked difference between core body temperature and skin temperature.

2. Body temperature may drop to 94°F (34.4°C) or even as low as 92°F (33.3°C) after birth unless the infant is adequately protected.
3. Heat is generated immediately by *shivering*; infant shivering is characterized by increased muscular activity, restlessness, and crying.
4. Infant shivering activity is not as apparent as adult shivering activity.
5. Effect of chilling on the neonate.
   a. Increased heat production leads to increased oxygen consumption.
   b. When heat production is high, caloric need is high.
   c. Tendency to develop metabolic acidosis occurs.
   d. Production of surfactant is inhibited by cooling, and respiratory distress syndrome (RDS) may occur.
   e. Increased risk with smaller infants.

General Characteristics

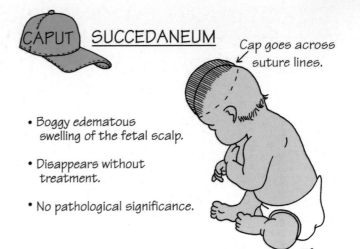

* Boggy edematous swelling of the fetal scalp.
* Disappears without treatment.
* No pathological significance.

© 2017 Nursing Education Consultants, Inc.

FIG. 21.12 Caput succedaneum. (From Zerwekh J, Garneau A, Miller CJ. *Digital collection of the memory notebooks of nursing.* 4th ed. Chandler, AZ: Nursing Education Consultants, Inc.; 2017.)

> **🔋 NURSING PRIORITY** Assess a newborn; monitor a newborn for complications.

A. Length.
   1. Average length of term neonate: 48 to 53 cm (19-21 in).
   2. To measure: infant is placed flat on the back on paper; a pencil is used to mark the locations of the infant's head and heels; after infant is removed from the paper, the distance between the two pencil marks is measured.
B. Weight.
   1. Average birth weight for a term neonate: 3400 g (7 lb 8 oz); average range is 2700 to 4000 g (6-9 lb).
   2. Low birth weight: 2500 g (5 lb 8 oz).
   3. Excessive weight: 4000 g (9 lb).
   4. Weight loss: between 5% and 10% of birth weight within the first few days of life; infant usually regains weight within 10 to 14 days.
C. Head.
   1. Molding.
      a. Head may appear elongated at birth; molding usually disappears within 24 to 48 hrs.
      b. Occurs as a result of abnormal fetal posture in utero and pressure during passage through the birth canal.
   2. Caput succedaneum (Fig. 21.12).
      a. Edema of the scalp caused by pressure occurring at the time of delivery.
      b. Disappears within 3 to 4 days.
      c. Edema goes across the cranial suture lines.
   3. Cephalhematoma.
      a. A collection of blood between the periosteum and the skull.
      b. Usually results from trauma during labor and delivery.
      c. Absorbed in a few weeks.

> **Box 21.7 FONTANELS**
>
> **Anterior**
> * Diamond shape approximately 3 x 2 cm.
> * Will increase as molding resolves.
> * Closes by 18 months of age.
>
> **Posterior**
> * Triangular shape approximately 1 x 2 cm.
> * Closes by 6 to 8 weeks; may be closed at birth.

   d. Does not cross cranial suture lines.
   4. Head measurement.
      a. Average head circumference of the term neonate: 34.2 cm; usual variation ranges from 33 to 35 cm (13-14 in).
      b. Head circumference is approximately 2 to 3 cm greater than the chest circumference; extremes in size may indicate microcephaly, hydrocephaly, or increased intracranial pressure.
   5. Fontanels (Box 21.7).
      a. Palpate for size and tension.
      b. Increase in tension may indicate tumor, hemorrhage, infection, or congenital anomaly.
      c. Decrease in tension (sunken fontanel) may indicate dehydration.
      d. Anterior fontanel closes by 18 months; posterior fontanel closes in 2 to 3 months.
D. Umbilical cord.
   1. Determine number of blood vessels; there should be two arteries and one vein surrounded by Wharton jelly.
   2. Cord atrophies and sloughs off in approximately 10 to 14 days.
   3. Should be no bleeding or oozing.

Table 21.10   MAJOR NEONATAL REFLEXES

Reflex	Disappears	How to Elicit	Response
Rooting	3-4 months; may persist during sleep until 7-8 months	Stroke cheek.	Head turns toward side that is touched.
Babinski	1 year	Lightly stroke lateral side of foot from heel to big toe across the ball of the foot.	Infant's toes fan, with dorsiflexion of great toe.
Sucking	10-12 months	Touch or stroke lips.	Infant sucks.
Moro (startle)	3-4 months	Make a loud noise or suddenly disturb infant's equilibrium.	Infant stiffens, briskly abducts, and extends arms with hands open and fingers extended to C shape. Infant's legs flex and abduct, and arms return to an embracing posture. Crying is usual.
Grasp palmar	3-4 months	Press a finger against infant's palm.	Infant's fingers momentarily close around object.
Asymmetric tonic neck (fencer's position)	3-4 months	Turn supine infant's head over the shoulder to one side.	Infant's arm and leg partially or completely extend on side to which head is turned; opposite arm and leg flex.

Behavioral Characteristics

A. Sleep and awake states.
  1. Newborn sleeps an average of 16 to 20 hrs a day during the first 2 weeks of life, with an average of 4 hrs at a time.
  2. May vary from a drowsy or semidozing state to an alert state to a crying state.
B. Infants vary a great deal in how they respond to stimuli.
  1. Infants move easily from one state of sleep to another state of consciousness.
  2. As the infant develops, they will reduce the total amount of sleeping time; wakeful periods will lengthen; sleeping will shift from daytime to nighttime.

Specific Body System Clinical Findings

A. Nervous system.
  1. Nervous system is relatively immature and characterized by the following:
    a. Poor nervous control; easily startled.
    b. Quivering chin.
    c. Tremors of the lower extremities of short duration.
  2. Reflex activity: the presence or absence of certain reflexes is indicative of ongoing normal development.
  3. Presence of positive Babinski sign.
    a. Normal finding until the age of 1 year.
    b. Dorsiflexion of big toe and fanning of the other toes.
  4. Neonatal reflexes (Table 21.10).

! NURSING PRIORITY Intactness of the neonate's nervous system is indicated by the state of alertness, resting posture, cry, and quality of muscle tone and motor activity.

B. Hematologic system.
  1. Anemia.
    a. Fetal hemoglobin has short life span; maternal/fetal iron stores sustain normal RBC production 4 to 5 months.
    b. *Physiologic anemia of the newborn* occurs as a result.
    c. Breastfed infants need iron supplements; formula should be iron fortified.
  2. Jaundice.
    a. *Physiologic jaundice*; increased incidence in breastfed infants; occurs on the second or third day of life as a result of an increase in the serum bilirubin level.
    b. *Pathologic jaundice* occurs within 24 hrs of birth (see hemolytic disease of the newborn).
    c. Treatment: phototherapy.
      (1) If bili lights are used, expose all areas to the light except for eyes and genitalia; cover infant's eyes with an opaque mask or eye patch and cover genitalia with a diaper or a disposable face mask (string bikini to expose more skin).

! NURSING PRIORITY If a face mask is used to cover genitalia, remove the metal nose strip to prevent burning the infant.

      (2) If a fiber-optic blanket is used, infant's eyes do not need to be covered; should have a covering pad between the infant's skin and the fiber-optic blanket; with this method, the infant may remain in the room with the mother or the fiber-optic blanket may be used at home.

(3) Monitor skin temperature: treatment may increase temperature.

(4) Reposition infant every 2 hrs to expose as much body surface as possible.

3. Transitory coagulation defects.
   a. Occur between the second and fifth postnatal days.
   b. Result from the lack of intestinal synthesis of vitamin K because of insufficient bacterial microbiota in the GI tract.
   c. Vitamin K (0.5-1.0 mg) is administered intramuscularly, usually at 1 hr of age, to prevent complications.

C. GI tract.
   1. Stomach produces hydrochloric acid immediately after birth.
   2. Stools.

> **! NURSING PRIORITY** Monitor passage of the first meconium stool.

   a. Meconium: sticky, black, odorless, sterile stool that is passed within the first 24 to 48 hrs after birth; if no stool is passed, further assessment is needed.
   b. Stools change according to type and number of feedings.
      (1) Transitional stools: occur during period between second and fourth day; consist of meconium and milk; greenish brown or greenish yellow; loose and often contain mucus.
      (2) Milk stools: usually occur by the fourth day; stools of formula-fed infant are drier, more formed, paler, and occur once or twice daily or one stool every 2 to 3 days.
      (3) Stools of breastfed infants are golden yellow, have a pasty consistency, and occur more frequently than stools of formula-fed infants, three to four stools in 24 hrs.

D. Genitourinary system.

> **! NURSING PRIORITY** Most newborns void within the first 24 to 48 hrs after birth. Weigh dry diaper before applying; then weigh wet diaper after infant voiding. Each gram of added weight equals 1 mL of urine.

   1. Approximately 30 to 60 mL is voided per day during the first 2 days of life; followed by 200 mL/day by the end of the first week.
   2. Frequency of voiding: average of two to six times per day, increasing up to 10 to 15 times per day.
   3. Female: labia majora are hypertrophied; small amount of bloody discharge from the vagina may be seen as a result of the presence of maternal hormones.
   4. Male: scrotum may be edematous; testes should have descended; assess the urethral opening.

E. Integumentary system.
   1. Vernix caseosa: a white cheesy-like material covers the skin at birth, particularly noted in the folds and creases.

2. Petechiae: pinpoint bluish discolorations primarily on the skin and face as a result of pressure from delivery; bruising of tissues may be seen.
3. Lanugo: downy, fine covering of hair that may be present on the shoulders, back, earlobes, and forehead; disappears during the first week.
4. Milia: sebaceous gland hyperplasia appears as pinpoint white bumps seen over the bridge of the nose and on the cheeks during the first 2 weeks of life.
5. Erythema toxicum: splotchy pink papular rash appearing anywhere on the body; disappears within the first few weeks of life; no treatment is necessary.
6. Mongolian spots: dark bluish pigmented areas commonly seen on the back or buttocks of infants of African American, Native American, and Mediterranean descent; usually disappear by school age.

F. Endocrine system.
   1. Because of the presence of maternal hormones in the bloodstream, neonate may have breast enlargement or vulvar enlargement.

G. Sensory system.
   1. Eyes appear large, and pupils appear small.
   2. All infants' eyes are blue, slate gray, or brown at birth; eyes become permanent color at approximately 6 to 12 months of age.
   3. Tears do not develop until 2 to 4 weeks of age.
   4. Eyes close in response to bright light; red reflex is present; pupils react to light.
   5. Sudden loud noises may elicit startle response.
   6. Usually able to locate the general direction of sounds.
   7. Hearing of all infants is screened before discharge from birthing facility.
   8. Differentiates between pleasant and unpleasant tastes.
   9. Searches for food when cheek is touched or begins sucking movement when lips are touched.

H. Musculoskeletal system.
   1. Assumes the position of comfort, which is usually the position assumed in utero.
   2. Normal palmar crease is present (simian crease is indicative of Down syndrome).
   3. Spine is straight and flat when in prone position.

Nursing Interventions: Take Action

> **TEST ALERT** Provide newborn care and reinforce parent education.

Goal: To establish and maintain a patent airway and promote oxygenation.

A. Position infant with head slightly lower than chest; may use postural drainage or side-lying position.
B. Suction nostrils and oropharynx with bulb syringe.
C. *Observe for periods of apnea lasting greater than 20 sec, cyanosis, and mucus collection, and report to RN.*

❗ NURSING PRIORITY During first 4 hrs after birth, the priority nursing goals are to maintain a clear airway, prevent heat loss, prevent hemorrhage and infection, and monitor transition. Bathing will be initiated when infant's temperature is stabilized; feeding may begin immediately if infant is interested.

Goal: To protect against heat loss.

A. Immediately after birth, wrap infant in warm blanket and dry off amniotic fluid.
B. Replace wet blanket with warm dry blanket.
C. Cover wet hair and head with a blanket or cap.
D. Immediately after birth, may provide for skin-to-skin contact with the mother; cover infant with warm blanket.
E. For initial physical assessment, place baby on a warm padded surface, preferably under a radiant heater.
F. Wrap infant securely in a warm blanket and give them to parents to cuddle and observe.
G. Avoid any unnecessary procedures until body temperature is stable.

Goal: To perform a newborn physical assessment and collect data on behavior.

A. Determine Apgar score at 1 min and again at 5 min (see Table 21.8 for Apgar scoring).

❗ NURSING PRIORITY Assess a newborn and determine Apgar scores.

1. The 1-min Apgar score is a rapid evaluation of the status of the neonate's intrauterine oxygenation.
2. The 5-min Apgar score is an evaluation of the neonate's response to cardiorespiratory adaptation after birth.

B. *Gestational age assessment within 2 hrs of birth completed by the RN.*
C. *Comprehensive physical assessment completed by the RN within 24 hrs of birth.*
D. Determine special needs and whether any significant risk factors are present.

Goal: To assess periods of reactivity.

A. First period of reactivity.
1. Lasts approximately 30 min.
2. Newborn is alert, awake, and usually hungry.

❗ NURSING PRIORITY Periods of reactivity are excellent opportunities for promoting attachment response.

B. Sleep phase.
1. First sleep usually occurs an average of 3 to 4 hrs after birth and may last from a few minutes to several hours.
2. Newborn is difficult to awaken during this phase.
C. Second period of reactivity.
1. Infant is alert and awake (good time to feed infant).
2. Lasts approximately 2 to 4 hrs.

❗ NURSING PRIORITY It is important to monitor the infant closely, because apnea, decreased heart rate, gagging, choking, and regurgitation may occur and require nursing intervention.

Goal: To protect against infection.

A. Follow guidelines for proper hand hygiene before handling infant.
B. Prevent ophthalmia neonatorum.
1. Administer prophylactic treatment to eyes soon after birth.
2. Place ophthalmic ointment or solution in the conjunctival sac.
C. Avoid exposure to people with possible upper respiratory tract, skin, or GI infections.

Goal: To prevent hemorrhagic disease.

A. Administer 0.5 to 1 mg of vitamin K intramuscularly into the upper third of the lateral aspect of the thigh.

Goal: To properly identify infant.

A. Secure identification bands to wrist or ankle of infant and wrist of mother in the delivery room. Father or support person may be banded.
B. Prints of infant's foot, palms, or fingers may be obtained according to hospital policy; mother's palm prints or fingerprints may also be obtained.
C. Advise parents not to release the infant to anyone who does not have proper unit identification.

❗ NURSING PRIORITY Always check the infant's identification band with the mother's identification band every time the infant and mother have been separated; monitor area for anyone who does not have security clearance to be in the newborn area; security of the newborn is a priority! Electronic tags may be placed on the infant that ring when the infant is carried out of the newborn area. Teach family to carefully monitor identification badges of individuals/nursing staff who come in contact with their newborn, especially if they are wanting to remove the infant. Remind them not to give the infant to anyone without proper identification.

Goal: To promote parental attachment to infant immediately after birth.

A. Place skin to skin after delivery and cover both mother and newborn with warm blanket. Or, wrap infant snugly in warm blanket and encourage parents to hold infant. Do not allow chilling to occur.
B. Encourage touching and holding during periods of reactivity.

Goal: To initiate feeding and evaluate parents' ability to feed infant and provide nutrition.

A. Encourage breastfeeding, if desired, immediately after delivery or in recovery area; breast milk is bacteriologically safe.
B. First formula feeding or test feeding: Feed newborn slowly with head slightly elevated. Burp the newborn after feeding 30 to 45 mL.
C. Considerations in infant feeding.
1. An infant should always be placed on the right side after feeding to avoid aspiration and prevent regurgitation and distention.
2. Infant will require more frequent feedings initially; will generally establish a routine of feeding every 3 to 4 hrs.
   a. Breastfed infants feed 8 to 12 times per 24 hrs (every 2-3 hrs).

b. Formula-fed infants feed six to eight times per 24 hrs.

Goal: To provide daily general care.

A. Care of the umbilical cord stump.
  1. Hospital protocol directs routine cord care; initial cleaning with sterile water; subsequent cleaning with plain water is recommended.
  2. Clean the umbilical cord stump several times a day with plain water, especially after infant voids.
  3. To encourage drying of the cord, expose umbilical area to air frequently and position diaper below umbilicus.
  4. Observe for bleeding, oozing, or foul odor. Average cord separation time is 10 to 14 days.

B. Circumcision care.
  1. Keep area clean; change diaper frequently.
  2. Observe for bleeding: check site hourly for 12 hrs postprocedure.
  3. A small sterile petrolatum gauze dressing may be applied to the area during the first 2 to 3 days (if Gomco or Mogen clamp are used for procedure).
  4. If a PlastiBell was used, keep area clean; application of petrolatum jelly is not necessary; plastic ring will dislodge when area has healed (5-7 days).

> **! NURSING PRIORITY** Teach the parents that a whitish-yellow exudate around the glans is granulation tissue and is normal and not indicative of infection. It may be observed for 2 to 3 days and should not be removed.

C. Neonate's bath.
  1. Bath is delayed until vital signs and temperature stabilize.
  2. Warm water is used for the first 4 days; do not immerse infant in water until umbilical cord stump has been released.
  3. When bathing neonate, apply principles of clean-to-dirty areas; wash areas in the following order: eyes, face, ears, head, body, genitals, buttocks.
  4. Head is an area of significant heat loss; keep it covered.

D. Determine weight loss over first 24 hrs after birth – monitor wet diapers.

E. Assess stools.
  1. Meconium stools.
  2. Transitional stools.

Goal: To detect complications and provide early treatment.

A. If infant is discharged before 24 hrs, explain to parents the importance of returning to health care provider for newborn checkup and screening tests. A newborn screen for phenylketonuria (PKU) should be done after the first 24 hrs for a formula-fed infant; if mother is breastfeeding, the newborn screen should be done when infant is 1 week old. National newborn screening requires PKU and thyroid screens. Many states require additional newborn screens.

B. Administration of first hepatitis B vaccine before discharge.

1. Encourage follow-up visits for second and third doses of hepatitis B vaccine and other immunizations.
2. Infants are tested at 9 months for HBsAg and anti-HBsAg.

> **! NURSING PRIORITY** Explain to parents the importance of returning for a well-baby check when the infant is 2 to 4 weeks old.

Goal: To promote infant feeding.

A. Breastfeeding.
  1. First feeding should occur immediately or within a few hours after birth.
  2. Assess the mother's knowledge of breastfeeding during the first feeding and provide teaching.
  3. Initially, frequent feedings are important to establish milk production, often every 1.5 to 2 hrs.
  4. Encourage mother not to offer the infant a bottle until lactation is well established, generally after approximately 4 weeks.
  5. Engorgement and nipple soreness are the most common problems the mother experiences.

B. Bottle-feeding.
  1. It is not necessary to sterilize the water used to reconstitute infant's formula.
  2. The infant should be placed in a semiupright position for feeding.
  3. Never prop the bottle; always hold the infant.
  4. Mother should not coax infant to finish all of the bottle every time; any unused formula should be discarded.
  5. Do not warm bottles or any food for infants in the microwave, because formula or food gets excessively hot, and the temperature is not uniform.

> **! NURSING PRIORITY** Proportions of formula must not be altered. Teach mother not to dilute or expand the amount of formula and not to concentrate it to provide more calories.

Disorders Acquired During and After Birth

See Table 21.11.

HIGH-RISK NEWBORN

Gestational Age Variation

Assessment: Recognize Cues

A. Gestational age assessment (Table 21.12).
B. Clinical estimation of gestational age assessed using visual Ballard scale (see Fig. 21.13).
C. Respiratory parameters.
  1. Observe respiratory rate, rhythm, and depth.
    a. Initially, rate increases without a change in rhythm.
    b. Flaring of nares and expiratory grunting are early signs of respiratory distress.
  2. Increase in apical pulse rate.
  3. Subcostal and xiphoid retractions progress to intercostal, substernal, and clavicular retractions.

Table 21.11 DISORDERS ACQUIRED DURING AND AFTER BIRTH

	Trauma	Peripheral Nerve Injuries	Neonatal Sepsis
Data collection	Soft tissue injury Caput succedaneum	Temporary paralysis of the facial nerve is the most common.	Apathy, lethargy, low-grade temperature
	Cephalhematoma	Affected side of the face is smooth.	Poor feeding, abdominal distention, diarrhea
	Injury to bone: fractured clavicle is the most common; often occurs with a large-sized infant	Eye may stay open. Mouth droops at the corner. Forehead cannot be wrinkled. Possible difficulty sucking.	Cyanosis, irregular respirations, apnea Hyperbilirubinemia
		Brachial palsy: A partial or complete paralysis of the nerve fibers of the brachial plexus.	Infant often described as "not acting right."
		Cannot elevate or abduct the arm.	CBC, chest x-ray film, and viral studies TORCH syndrome blood screening
		Abnormal arm position or diminished arm movements.	
Nursing interventions	*Fractured clavicle* 1. Place affected arm against chest wall with hand lying across chest. 2. Position is held by a Fig. 8 stockinette around the arm and chest. 3. Pick infant up carefully; shoulder should not be pressed toward middle of body. 4. Affected side should not be placed in gown or undershirt.	*Facial nerve palsy* 1. Apply eye patch; may use artificial tears to prevent corneal irritation. 2. Provide support during feeding; infant may not latch on to nipple well. *Brachial nerve palsy* 1. Keep arm abducted and externally rotated with elbow flexed. 2. Arm is raised to shoulder height, and elbow is flexed 90 degrees.	1. Prenatal prevention, maternal screening for STDs, and assessment of rubella titers 2. Maintenance of sterile technique 3. Prophylactic antibiotic treatment 4. Possible cesarean delivery for mother with genital herpes

CBC, complete blood count; *STDs*, sexually transmitted diseases; *TORCH*, toxoplasmosis, other (congenital syphilis and viruses) rubella, cytomegalovirus, and herpes virus.

4. Color.
   a. Progresses from pink to circumoral pallor to circumoral cyanosis to generalized cyanosis.
   b. Increased intensity of acrocyanosis.
5. Progressive respiratory distress.
   a. Respiratory rate increases to 80 to 120 breaths/min; accessory muscles of respiration are used; nasal flaring.
   b. Abdominal seesaw breathing patterns; central cyanosis.
   c. Distinguish between apneic episodes (15 sec or longer) and periodic breathing (cessation of breathing for 5-10 sec, followed by 10-15 sec of compensatory rapid respirations).
6. Progressing anoxia leading to cardiac decompensation and failure.
7. Increased muscle flaccidity: froglike position.
D. Nutrition.
   1. Assess readiness and ability to feed: swallowing, gag reflexes.

2. Screen for hypoglycemia.
3. Observe for congenital dysfunction and anomalies related to tracheoesophageal fistula (TEF), anal atresia, and metabolic disorders.
4. Check amount and frequency of elimination.
5. Assess for vomiting or regurgitation; a preterm infant's stomach capacity is small, and overfeeding can occur.
6. Check mucous membranes, urine output, and skin turgor to identify fluid and electrolyte imbalances.
   a. Skin turgor over abdomen and inner thighs.
   b. Sunken fontanel.
   c. Urinary output of less than 30 mL/day.
E. Temperature regulation.
   1. Monitor infant's temperature: frequently done with a skin probe for continuous monitoring of temperature in infants at high risk for complications.
   2. Check coolness or warmth of body and extremities.
   3. Detect early signs of cold stress.
      a. Increased physical activity and crying.

Table 21.12 GESTATIONAL AGE ASSESSMENT: RECOGNIZE CUES

By Weight	By Age
Large for gestational age (LGA): Greater than the 90th percentile for estimated weeks of gestation; weight of 4000 g or more at birth.	Postterm or postmature: Born after completion of 42 weeks' gestation.
Appropriate for gestational age (AGA): Weight between 10th and 90th percentile for infant's age.	
Small for gestational age (SGA) or small for date (SFD): Weight less than the 10th percentile for estimated weeks of gestation.	Full term: Born between the beginning of week 38 and the end of week 42 of gestation.
Low birth weight (LBW): Weight less than 2500 g (5.5 lb), regardless of gestational age.	
Very low birth weight (VLBW): Weight of 1500 g (3.3 lb) or less at birth.	Late preterm: Born between 34 and 36 weeks' gestation.
Extremely low birth weight (ELBW): Weight less than 1000 g (2.2 lb).	
Intrauterine growth restriction (IUGR): Growth of fetus does not meet expected norms.	Preterm or premature: Born before completion of 37 weeks' gestation, regardless of birth weight.

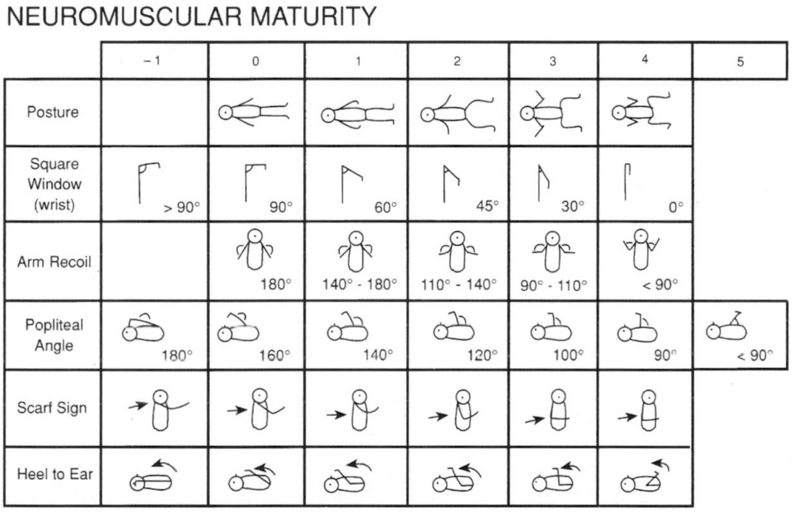

NEUROMUSCULAR MATURITY

PHYSICAL MATURITY

MATURITY RATING

score	weeks
-10	20
-5	22
0	24
5	26
10	28
15	30
20	32
25	34
30	36
35	38
40	40
45	42
50	44

FIG. 21.13 Estimation of gestational age. (From Lowdermilk D, Perry S. *Maternity and women's health care.* 11th ed. Mosby; 2016.)

b. Increased respiratory rate.

c. Increased acrocyanosis or generalized cyanosis along with mottling of the skin (cutis marmorata).

d. Male with descended testes: presence of cremasteric reflex (testes are pulled back up into the inguinal canal on exposure to cold).

4. Monitor infant's temperature.

a. Axillary temperature: 36.5°C to 37.2°C (average: 37°C or 97.7°F).

b. Place a temperature skin probe on infant while they are in the radiant warmer or isolette.

> ⓘ **NURSING PRIORITY** Maintain desired temperature of newborn by using external devices.

Analyze Cues and Prioritize Hypotheses

The most important problems are respiratory effort, temperature regulation, initiation of first feeding, and passage of first meconium stool.

Nursing Interventions: Take Action

Goal: To maintain respiratory functioning.

A. Provide gentle physical stimulation to remind infant to breathe.

1. Gently rub the infant's back.

2. Lightly tap the infant's feet.

> ⓘ **NURSING PRIORITY** Physically stimulate a newborn to breathe; administer oxygen; monitor newborn's gas exchange by obtaining arterial blood gas values, pulse oximetry readings, etc.

B. Ensure patency of respiratory tract.

1. Maintain open airway by means of nasal, oral, or pharyngeal suctioning.

2. Position to promote oxygenation.

a. Elevate head 10 degrees with neck slightly extended by placement of a small folded towel under the shoulders.

b. Flex and abduct infant's arms and place at sides.

c. Avoid diapers or adhere them loosely.

d. Turn side to side every 1 to 2 hrs.

> ⓘ **NURSING PRIORITY** Do not place newborn in prone position.

C. Assist infant's respiratory efforts.

1. Monitor oxygen pressure.

a. Anywhere from 21% to 100% oxygen is administered.

b. Avoid high concentrations of oxygen for prolonged periods; may lead to complication of bronchopulmonary dysplasia.

2. Continuous positive airway pressure (CPAP) counteracts the tendency of the alveoli to collapse by providing continuous distending airway pressure.

a. CPAP is administered either by endotracheal tube or nasal prongs.

b. Cluster activities to prevent prolong stimulation that increases oxygen needs.

Goal: To provide adequate nutrition.

A. Detect hypoglycemia and treat immediately: administer 5% dextrose in water intravenously if infant is unable to tolerate oral feeding.

B. Oral feeding: initial feeding.

1. Use sterile water: 1 to 2 mL for a small infant.

2. Use preemie nipple to conserve infant's energy.

3. Because of small size of infant's stomach, feedings are small in amount and increased in frequency.

C. Orogastric tube feedings.

1. Usually administered by continuous flow of formula with an infusion pump (kangaroo pump) when the infant is:

a. Having severe respiratory distress.

b. Too immature and weak to suck.

c. Tired and fatigues easily when a preemie nipple is used.

2. Placement and insertion of orogastric feeding tube.

a. Position infant on the back or toward the right side with the head and chest slightly elevated.

b. Measure correct length of insertion by marking on the catheter the distance from the tip of the nose to the ear lobe to the tip of the sternum.

c. Lubricate tube with sterile water and slowly insert catheter into mouth and down the esophagus into the stomach.

d. Test for placement of the tube by aspirating stomach contents or injecting 0.5 to 1.0 mL of air for the premature infant (up to 5 mL for larger infants) and auscultating the abdomen for the sound.

e. Before infusing a feeding by gravity into the stomach, check for residual; this is done by aspirating and measuring amount left in stomach from previous feeding; feeding is usually held if residual is greater than 50% of feeding.

f. If feeding is not continuous, remove tubing by pinching or clamping it and withdrawing it rapidly.

g. Burp infant after feeding by turning head or positioning them on the right side.

h. Check to see whether mother wants to pump her breast to provide the milk supply to the infant for gavage.

Goal: To maintain warmth and temperature control (see maintaining temperature of healthy newborn).

A. Oxygen and air should be warmed and humidified.

B. Maintain abdominal skin temperature at 36.1°C to 36.7°C (97°F to 98°F); axillary temperature 36.5°C to 37.2°C (97.7°F to 99.0°F).

C. Monitor infant's temperature continuously; make sure that temperature probe is set on control panel, probe is on infant's abdomen, and all safety precautions are maintained.

D. Prevent rapid warming or cooling, because this may cause apnea and acidosis; warming process is increased gradually over a period of 2 to 4 hrs.

E. Infant may need extra clothing or to be wrapped in an extra blanket for additional warmth.

Respiratory Distress

Neonates can experience respiratory distress from a variety of factors. *Respiratory distress syndrome* (RDS) occurs as a result of a deficiency of surfactant, which lines the alveoli; alveoli collapse at the end of each expiration, retaining little or no residual air, leading to generalized atelectasis. *Meconium aspiration syndrome* occurs when the fetus passes meconium in utero and the meconium enters the fetal lungs and plugs small air passages, which leads to inflammation and areas of atelectasis, causing obstruction in the small airway passages and, frequently, a secondary infection.

Assessment: Recognize Cues

A. Usually appears within 6 hrs after birth.
B. Tachypnea: more than 60 breaths/min.
C. Apneic spells (in excess of 15 sec).
D. Abnormal breath sounds: rales and rhonchi.
E. Chest retraction.
F. Flaring of the nares.
G. Expiratory grunting.

NURSING PRIORITY Grunting is an ominous sign and indicates impending need for respiratory assistance; most often, mucus needs to be cleared from airway.

H. Complications.
1. Hypoxia and respiratory acidosis caused by alveolar hypoventilation.
2. Retinopathy of prematurity caused by high levels of oxygen.
3. Bronchopulmonary dysplasia: chronic stiff, noncompliant lungs.

Analyze Cues and Prioritize Hypotheses

The most important problems are hypoxia, acid-base imbalance, and reducing long-term effects of retinopathy, prematurity, and bronchopulmonary dysplasia.

Generate Solutions

Treatment
A. RDS.
1. CPAP is the primary treatment.
2. Administration of surfactant through the airway into the infant's lungs.
B. Meconium aspiration.
1. Administration of oxygen with humidification.
2. Postural drainage and percussion.
3. Antibiotic therapy and correction of acid-base imbalance.

Nursing Interventions: Take Action

Goal: To promote oxygenation and respiratory functioning.

A. Administer antenatal steroids to mothers between 24 and 34 weeks if preterm birth is threatened and administer surfactant to neonate after delivery to stimulate surfactant production.
B. Refer to nursing intervention for the high-risk newborn.

Cleft Lip and Cleft Palate

Cleft lip is a fissure of the upper lip to the side of the midline, which may vary from a slight notch to a complete separation extending into the nostril; may be unilateral or bilateral. *Cleft palate* is a fissure or a split in the roof of the mouth (palate).

Assessment: Recognize Cues

A. Visible at birth as an incompletely formed lip.
B. Opening in roof of mouth; may be isolated or associated with a cleft lip.
C. Sucking difficulties; breathing problems.
D. Later problems include increased incidence of upper respiratory tract infection and otitis media.
E. Later problems are related to speech and hearing difficulties and self-esteem issues.

Analyze Cues and Prioritize Hypotheses

The most important problems are feeding difficulties and visible defect.

Generate Solutions

Treatment
A. Surgical.
1. Closure of lip defect is usually done between 2 and 3 months after birth.
2. Surgery may be done in stages; closure of palate defect typically performed between 6 to 12 months of age.
B. Long-term care management.
1. Extensive orthodontics to correct problems of malpositioned teeth and maxillary arches.
2. Speech therapy.
3. Hearing problems related to chronic, recurrent otitis media; varying degrees of hearing loss may occur.

Nursing Interventions: Take Action

Goal: To provide preoperative care.
A. Maintain nutrition.
1. Use modified nipple to increase infant's ability to obtain milk without sucking and allow feeder to provide assistance (e.g., Haberman feeder).
2. Feed slowly.
3. Burp frequently (after every 15-30 mL).
4. Feed with infant's head in an upright position.
B. Prepare parents for newborn's surgery.
1. Address psychosocial needs of the parents.
2. Encourage parents to position infant flat on back in upright position or on side to accustom infant to the postoperative positioning.
3. Encourage parents to feed infant with the same method that will be used after surgery.

Goal: To provide postoperative care.
A. Prevent trauma to suture line.
   1. Position infant on back or side and elevate head (infant seat).
   2. Restrain arms with soft elbow restraints, although benefit is questionable.
   3. Cleanse lip suture line gently after each feeding; use cotton-tipped applicator with prescribed solution and roll along the suture line; may apply antibiotic ointment.
   4. Prevent any crust or scab formation on lip and suture line.
B. Maintain a patent airway and facilitate breathing.
   1. Assess for respiratory distress.
   2. Observe for swelling of the nose, tongue, or lips.
C. Provide adequate nutrition.
   1. Feed in an upright, sitting position using a modified nipple.
   2. Avoid use of any objects in the mouth (e.g., straws, suction catheters, tongue depressors, pacifiers, spoons, or certain toys).
D. Provide discharge teaching to parents.
   1. Encourage parents to cuddle and play with infant to decrease crying and prevent trauma to suture line.
   2. Teach feeding, cleansing, and restraining procedures.

Esophageal Atresia and Tracheoesophageal Fistula

Esophageal atresia (EA) and *tracheoesophageal fistula* (TEF) are rare malformations that represent a failure of the esophagus to develop as a continuous passage and a failure of the trachea and esophagus to separate into distinct structures.

Assessment: Recognize Cues

A. Characterized by the classic *three Cs: choking, coughing,* and *cyanosis*.
B. Excessive frothy saliva and constant drooling.
C. Aspiration is a complication, especially during feeding.

Analyze Cues and Prioritize Hypotheses

The most important problems are hypoxia and feeding difficulties.

Generate Solutions

Treatment
A. Surgical correction (for EA with TEF).
   1. Thoracotomy.
   2. Surgical repair is done in stages.

Nursing Interventions: Take Action

> ⚠️ **NURSING PRIORITY** When there is any suspicion of possible esophageal problems, infant should receive nothing by mouth (NPO status) until further evaluation can be done.

Goal: To provide preoperative care.

A. Maintain patent airway.

1. Supine position with head elevated on an inclined plane of at least 30 degrees.
2. Suction nasopharynx.
3. Observe for symptoms of respiratory distress.
4. Maintain NPO status.
B. Prepare parents for infant's surgery.

Goal: To provide postoperative care.
A. Maintain respirations and prevent respiratory complications.
   1. Administer oxygen.
   2. Oral suction of secretions and position for optimum ventilation.
   3. Maintain care of chest tubes.
   4. Administer antibiotics.
   5. Place in warm, high-humidity isolette.
   6. Maintain nasogastric suctioning.
B. Provide adequate nutrition.
   1. Gastrostomy feedings may be started on the second or third postoperative day.
   2. Oral feedings are frequently delayed after surgery or until the esophageal anastomosis is healed.
   3. Meet oral sucking needs by offering infant a pacifier.

Imperforate Anus

Imperforate anus is a type of anorectal malformation caused by abnormal development.

Assessment: Recognize Cues

A. No anal opening.
B. Absence of meconium or meconium in urine.
C. Gradual increase in abdominal distention.

Analyze Cues and Prioritize Hypotheses

The most important problem is inability to eliminate or pass first meconium stool.

Generate Solutions

Treatment
A. Surgery.
   1. Anoplasty: reconstruction of the anus.
   2. Abdominal-perineal pull-through with colostomy.
   3. Colostomy (often done initially until full repair is done at 1-2 months of age for more complicated types).

Nursing Interventions: Take Action

Goal: To identify anal malformation.
A. Detect increasing abdominal distention.
B. Inspect anal area for opening.

> ⚠️ **NURSING PRIORITY** Record the first passage of meconium stool. If infant does not pass stool within 24 hrs after birth, further assessment is required.

Goal: To provide postoperative care.
A. Prevent infection by maintaining good perineal care and keeping operative site clean and dry, especially after passage of stool and urine.

B. Instruct parents in care of colostomy (e.g., frequent dressing changes, meticulous skin care, placement of collection device, avoidance of tight diapers and clothes around stoma).

C. Anal dilations may be necessary; observe stooling patterns.

Neural Tube Defects

A *neural tube defect* (spina bifida) results in midline defects and closure of the spinal cord (may be noncystic or cystic); most common site is lumbosacral area.

Assessment: Recognize Cues

A. Types.
1. Spina bifida occulta.
   a. Bone of spine does not cover the spinal cord.
   b. Infant may have no apparent clinical manifestations.
2. Spina bifida cystica.
   a. Meningocele: a saclike cyst of meninges filled with spinal fluid that protrudes through a defect in the bony part of the spine.
   b. Myelomeningocele: a saclike cyst containing meninges, spinal fluid, and a portion of the spinal cord with its nerves that protrudes through a defect in the vertebral column; other defect most frequently associated with this is hydrocephalus.

Analyze Cues and Prioritize Hypotheses

The most important problems are prevention of spinal-sac drying and the need for proper positioning.

Generate Solutions

Treatment

A. Surgical: closure of defect within 24 to 48 hrs to decrease risk of infection, relieve pressure, repair sac, and possibly insert a shunt; closure at 12 to 18 hrs if sac is leaking.

B. Prophylactic: a decrease in the incidence of neural tube defects is associated with an increase in folic acid intake during pregnancy.

Nursing Interventions: Take Action

> ❗ **NURSING PRIORITY** Correct positioning of the infant is critical in preventing damage to the sac and providing nursing care after surgery.

Goal: To provide preoperative care.

A. Prevent and protect sac from drying, rupturing, and infection.
1. Position infant prone on abdomen.
2. Avoid touching sac.
3. Provide meticulous skin care after voiding and bowel movements.
4. Often, sterile, normal saline soaks on a nonadherent dressing may be used to prevent drying.

B. Detect early development of hydrocephalus.
1. Measure head and check circumference frequently.
2. Check fontanels for bulging and separation of suture line.

C. Monitor elimination function.
1. Note whether urine is dripping or is retained.
2. Indwelling catheter may be inserted, or intermittent catheterization may be used at regular intervals to ensure regular bladder emptying.
3. Assess for bowel function: glycerin suppository may be ordered to stimulate meconium passage.

Goal: To provide postoperative care.

A. Prevent trauma and infection at the surgical site.
1. Place infant in same position (prone on abdomen) as before surgery.
2. Continue to provide scrupulous skin care as described under preoperative goal.
3. Maintain good perineal care, as there is frequent continuous urinary drainage.

B. Assess neurologic status frequently for indications of increasing intracranial pressure, development of hydrocephalus, or early signs of infection and *report any signs immediately to the RN.*
1. Continue to measure head circumference daily.
2. Perform frequent neurologic checks.

C. Provide parents with education in regard to positioning, feeding, skin care, elimination procedures, and range-of-motion exercises.
1. Encourage and facilitate parental bonding.
2. Refer to community and social agencies for financial and social support.
3. Encourage long-range planning and support of parents for long-term rehabilitation of infant.

Necrotizing Enterocolitis

The condition is an acute inflammatory disease of the bowel; increased incidence in preterm infants; cause is unknown. It is characterized by ischemic necrosis of the GI tract, which leads to perforation.

Assessment: Recognize Cues

A. Problems occur within 4 to 10 days of initiating feeding but may be evident as early as 4 hrs of age and, in preterm infants, may be delayed for up to 30 days; it usually occurs in the first 10 days of life in full-term infants.

B. Abdominal distention and rigidity may be seen.

C. Bowel sounds may be absent.

D. Bile-stained emesis and blood-streaked diarrhea or guaiac-positive stool.

Analyze Cues and Prioritize Hypotheses

The most important problems are infection, possible ileus, and potential for abdominal perforation.

Generate Solutions

Treatment

A. Medical.
1. All enteric feedings are discontinued.
2. Nasogastric suctioning is initiated.
3. IV therapy and total parenteral nutrition.

B. Medications: antibiotics.

B. Minimize trauma to heel site by performing heel stick correctly (Fig. 21.14).
   1. Warm heel for 5 to 10 min before sticking.
   2. Cleanse site with alcohol and dry before sticking.
   3. The lateral heel is the site of choice.

Drug-Exposed Infants (neonatal abstinence syndrome)

Infants born to mothers dependent on opioids exhibit neonatal abstinence syndrome. Many of the mothers often use several drugs, such as tranquilizers, nicotine, sedatives, narcotics, amphetamines, phencyclidine (PCP), marijuana, and other psychotropic agents.

Assessment: Recognize Cues

A. Clinical manifestations.
   1. Signs of withdrawal within 12 to 24 hrs after birth, depending on the substance and pattern of mother's use; symptoms more pronounced at 48 to 72 hrs and may last from 6 days to 8 weeks.
   2. If mother is on methadone, withdrawal occurs from 1 to 2 days to 2 to 3 weeks after birth.
   3. Increased muscle tone, increased respiratory rate, disturbed sleep, fever, excessive sucking; loose, watery stools, generalized perspiring (unusual in newborns).
   4. Projectile vomiting, mottling, crying, nasal stuffiness, hyperactive Moro reflex, tremors.

Analyze Cues and Prioritize Hypotheses

The most important problems are the neonate's withdrawal symptoms and possible long-term effects (e.g., fetal alcohol syndrome).

Generate Solutions

Treatment

A. Appropriate withdrawal medications and support based on the particular drug.

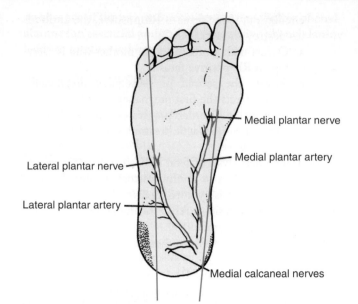

FIG. 21.14 Heel-Stick Sites. Use shaded areas on infant's foot for obtaining capillary blood. (From Lowdermilk D, Perry S. *Maternity and women's health care*. 12th ed. Mosby; 2020.)

Nursing Interventions: Take Action

Goal: To reduce external stimuli to avoid triggering hyperactivity and irritability.

A. Dim lights and decrease noise.
B. Swaddle infant; rocking and holding the infant tightly limits his or her ability to self-stimulate.
C. Provide adequate nutrition and hydration.
D. Monitor frequently with various scoring tools to evaluate level and severity of withdrawal.

Appendix 21.1 CONTRACEPTIVE METHODS

METHODS/DESCRIPTION	NURSING IMPLICATIONS/CLIENT TEACHING

Natural Family Planning Methods

Calendar (rhythm) or Standard Days Method (SDM)

1. Calendar (rhythm) method: calculate the days of fertility; considered to be days 10-17 of a 28-day menstrual cycle.
2. CycleBeads: red beads mark first day of menstrual cycle; white beads are fertile days; brown beads are when ovulation is unlikely.
3. Basal body temperature (BBT) method: a slight decrease (0.5 degree) at ovulation, then an increase of approximately 0.2-0.5 degree in temperature after ovulation occurs; fertile period is day the temperature drops through 3 consecutive days of temperature elevation; need a special BBT thermometer.
4. Cervical mucus method: before ovulation, mucus becomes clear and stringy; nonfertile period occurs when mucus becomes thick, cloudy, and sticky or when no mucus is apparent.
5. Symptothermal method: combines two methods, usually cervical mucus and BBT.
6. Home Predictor Test Kits: urine test is used to determine ovulation; test monitors and identifies a luteinizing hormone (LH) surge in a color change.

Intrauterine Device (IUD)

Hormonal intrauterine system IUD; Copper T 380 A IUD

1. Discuss the technique and the experience of IUD insertion and removal.
2. Emphasize the need for yearly Pap smears.
3. Encourage client to check IUD string, especially after each period.
4. Make sure the woman understands which type of IUD she has and when to return to have it checked or replaced. Copper IUD is approved for 10 years. The hormonal intrauterine system IUD is effective for up to 5 years, and uterine cramping and bleeding are diminished compared with the copper IUD.
5. Review common side effects and serious complications. Report any of the symptoms (PAINS) shown in Fig. 21.15.

Hormonal Methods

Combined oral contraceptive: the "pill" is a combination of estrogen and progestin

Progestin only: norethindrone; medroxyprogesterone

Transdermal contraceptive patch: applied once a week; has both hormones

Vaginal contraceptive ring: a ring inserted into the vagina for 3 weeks; removed for 1 week, then new ring inserted

1. Instruct as to correct use of medication, the need for follow-up in 3 months, and importance of taking the pill at same time each day; effectiveness is close to 100% when used correctly.
2. If using a 28-day cycle product (21 active pills and 7 inactive pills) (except Natazia), provide the following instructions regarding missed doses.
   - If *one or more pills* are missed in the *first* week, take one pill as soon as possible and then continue with the pack. Use an additional form of contraception for 7 days.
   - If *one or two pills* are missed during the *second* or *third week*, take one pill as soon as possible and then continue with the active pills in the pack – but skip the inactive pills and go straight to a new pack once all the active pills have been taken.
   - If *three or more pills* are missed during the *second* or *third week*, follow the same instructions given for missing one or two pills, but use an additional form of contraception for 7 days.[a]
3. Review common side effects and serious complications. Report any of the symptoms (**ACHES**) shown in Fig. 21.16.
4. Progestin-only pill causes more menstrual irregularity (breakthrough bleeding, variation in blood flow, etc.).

Injectable/Implantable Progestins

Injectable (Depot medroxyprogesterone acetate: IM or subQ)

1. Started during the first 5 days of menstrual cycle and requires injections only four times per year (every 11-13 weeks).

> ⚠ **NURSING PRIORITY** *Do not massage* the site after the injection because it may speed up absorption and decrease duration of effectiveness; effectiveness rate is comparable with that of oral contraceptives.

Continued

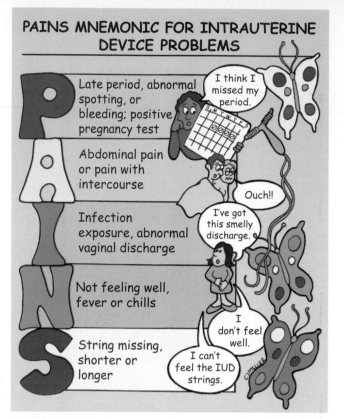

FIG. 21.15 PAINS mnemonic for intrauterine device. (From Zerwekh J, Miller CJ. *Mosby's OB/PEDS & women's health memory notecards: visual, mnemonic, and memory aids for nurses.* St. Louis: Mosby; 2012.)

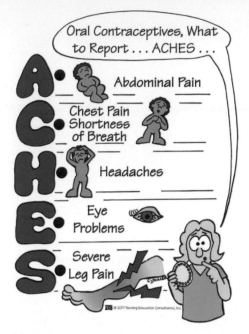

FIG. 21.16 ACHES mnemonic for oral contraceptive complications. (From Zerwekh J, Garneau A, Miller CJ. *Digital collection of the memory notebooks of nursing.* 4th ed. Chandler, AZ: Nursing Education Consultants, Inc.; 2017.)

METHODS/DESCRIPTION	NURSING IMPLICATIONS/CLIENT TEACHING
	2. Disadvantages include weight gain, prolonged amenorrhea, and breakthrough uterine bleeding.
	3. Because of loss of bone mineral density, women should be advised to ensure adequate calcium intake and exercise regularly.
Implantable: single rod implant	1. Requires a small incision in the inner aspect of the nondominant upper arm with a local anesthetic; provides up to 3 years of contraception.
	2. The most common side effect is irregular menstrual bleeding.

Barrier Methods

Diaphragm: a dome-shaped rubber device that fits over the cervix Cervical caps: a rubber or latex- silicone cap that fits snuggly over the cervix	1. Should be refitted after every pregnancy or when there is a weight gain or loss of 10-20 lb (4.54-9.09 kg) or a 20% weight fluctuation; replaced every 2 years.
	2. Instruct client to use spermicidal jelly or cream around diaphragm rim and in the dome.
	3. Instruct client to inspect diaphragm before use for any holes or punctures and leave diaphragm in place 6-8 hrs after intercourse.
	4. Explain the proper method for cleansing (use mild soap only), storing (dry thoroughly and dust with cornstarch, not baby powder), and checking for defects or holes in the diaphragm.
	5. Allow for sufficient practice of insertion/removal techniques and use with a spermicide, such as nonoxynol-9 (N-9).
	6. Risk of toxic shock syndrome with both devices if left in place longer than 8 hrs.

Appendix 21.1 CONTRACEPTIVE METHODS—cont'd

METHODS/DESCRIPTION	NURSING IMPLICATIONS/CLIENT TEACHING
Condoms are thin sheaths of rubber that fit over an erect penis Female condom: disposable	1. Advise client to apply condom to erect penis by rolling the sheath along the entire shaft and leaving enough slack at the end of the penis to receive the semen. 2. Explain importance of holding the condom in place while withdrawing the penis to prevent emptying of sperm into the vagina. 3. Condom should be applied before any penetration, because the preejaculatory seminal fluid may contain sperm. 4. Ask client about allergy to latex. **! NURSING PRIORITY** Use of nonoxynol-9 with diaphragms or condoms is not a recommended method for preventing STDs or HIV.

Unreliable Practices

Withdrawal (coitus interruptus): withdrawal of penis before ejaculation	1. Requires absolute cooperation and control of partner. 2. Good choice for couples who do not have any other contraceptive methods available.
Douching: the act of washing the semen out of the vagina	1. Douching may actually move the sperm upward in the vagina. 2. Encourage use of a more reliable contraceptive practice.

Emergency Contraception

Plan B: One-step dose of high-dose progestin *Other options:* High-dose oral estrogen Insertion of copper IUD	1. Available without a prescription; prescription required if under age 18. 2. Should be taken within 72 hrs of unprotected intercourse; may be effective up to 5 days after intercourse. 3. Plan B will not terminate an existing pregnancy or harm a fetus; hence, it does not cause abortion because it acts prior to fertilization and implantation. 4. To prevent nausea with high-dose estrogen, take an over-the-counter antiemetic 1 hr before each dose. 5. IUD must be inserted within 5 days of unprotected intercourse.

Permanent Sterilization

Tubal ligation (minilaparotomy)	1. Discuss the permanence of the sterilization procedure – informed consent required for all procedures. 2. Explain that the woman may experience sensation of tugging but not pain during procedure, which is carried out via local anesthetic.
Essure system (transcervical sterilization)	1. Insertion of an occlusive agent (small metallic implants) into the uterine tubes, which stimulate scar tissue formation that occludes the tubes. 2. Procedure does not provide immediate contraception – need to use another form of contraception until tubal blockage is proven, which may take up to 3 months. 3. Instruct client to report any unusual vaginal bleeding, spotting, purulent drainage, persistent abdominal pain, fever, or chills to health care provider.
Vasectomy: surgical ligation and resection bilaterally of the vas deferens	1. Discuss the permanence of vasectomy (informed consent required); even if the vas deferens is reconnected, fertility varies between 5% and 60%. 2. Activity level should be moderate for 2 days; skin sutures are usually removed within a week. 3. Encourage use of a scrotal support and application of ice for scrotal pain or swelling. 4. Follow-up visit for sperm sample is usually done in 4-6 weeks. 5. Advise client to use another form of birth control until it is verified that two ejaculate sperm counts contain no sperm.

[a]Burchum JR, Rosenthal LD. *Lehne's pharmacology for nursing care.* 9th ed. St. Louis: Elsevier/Saunders; 2016:766.
BBT, basal body temperature; *HIV,* human immunodeficiency virus; *IM,* intramuscularly; *IUD,* intrauterine device; *STD,* sexually transmitted diseases; *subQ,* subcutaneously.

Appendix 21.2   MEDICATIONS

MEDICATIONS	SIDE EFFECTS	NURSING IMPLICATIONS
Anticonvulsants		

▲Magnesium Sulfate: IV; given via an IV pump, piggybacked to primary infusion. A bolus dose (4-6 g over 15-20 min) is routinely given, followed by a maintenance infusion (1-4 g/hr).	*Maternal:* Sweating, flushing, muscle weakness, depressed or absent reflexes, oliguria, respiratory paralysis
	Fetal: Crosses placenta; lethargy, hypotonia, weakness
	Contraindications: Maternal – impaired renal function
		1. Criteria for continuing administration:
		  a. Respirations: greater than 12 breaths/min.
		  b. Presence of patellar knee-jerk movement.
		  c. Urinary output: greater than 30 mL/hr.
		2. Check BP frequently for symptoms of hypotension.
		3. Antidote for magnesium sulfate is *calcium gluconate;* should be available at bedside in case of respiratory paralysis.
		4. Monitor FHR and serum magnesium levels.
		5. Administration of magnesium sulfate is continued at least 24 hrs after delivery to reduce risk for seizure activity.
		6. *Never* abbreviate magnesium sulfate in the medical record as MgSO4.
		7. *Uses:* Prevention or control of eclampsia and as a tocolytic.

Oxytocic Medications and Prostaglandins to Cause Uterine Contractions
Oxytocic Medications: Stimulate contraction of uterine muscle fibers; have a mild antidiuretic effect; stimulate postpartum milk flow but do not affect amount.

MEDICATIONS	SIDE EFFECTS	NURSING IMPLICATIONS

▲Oxytocin: IM, IV, intranasal
Ergonovine: PO, IM, IV
Methylergonovine: PO, IM, IV
	Maternal: Tetanic uterine contractions, hypertension, tachycardia
	Fetal: Hypoxia, irregularity and decrease in FHR, possible hyperbilirubinemia
	Contraindications:
	Severe preeclampsia or eclampsia
	Predisposition to uterine rupture or CPD
	Preterm infant or presence of fetal distress
		1. Apply fetal monitor: assess FHR pattern throughout oxytocin administration.
		2. Assess maternal vital signs before increasing oxytocin infusion rate.
		3. Discontinue IV oxytocin, turn on primary IV solution, and *notify the RN if any of the following occur:*
		  a. Nonreassuring FHR pattern; absent variability; abnormal baseline rate.
		  b. Sustained uterine contractions lasting more than 90 sec.
		  c. Insufficient relaxation of the uterus between contractions.
		  d. Contractions occurring more often than every 2 min.
		  e. Repeated late decelerations or prolonged decelerations.
		4. Oxytocin is the only oxytocic used to induce labor; others (ergonovine and methylergonovine) are used after delivery to control bleeding.
		5. *Uses:* Uterine dystocia; induction of labor, control of hemorrhage, and uterine atony: uterine involution.

Prostaglandin F2α: IM	Contraindications: Asthma	1. Used to contract the uterus in situations of postpartum hemorrhage.

Tocolytic Agents to Suppress Labor
Tocolytic Agents: Relax myometrial cells of the uterus leading to inhibition of labor. Also result in bronchial dilation and cardiac output.

MEDICATIONS	SIDE EFFECTS	NURSING IMPLICATIONS
Beta-Adrenergic Agonists (betamimetics) Terbutaline	*Rarely used and are being replaced by safer medications because of adverse reactions related to stimulation of beta-receptors.* *Maternal:* Tachycardia (very little effect on BP), nervousness and tremors, headache, and possible pulmonary edema *Fetal:* Tachycardia, hypoglycemia	If used: 1. Assess maternal (especially pulse) and fetal vital signs frequently; fetal monitoring is necessary; notify health care provider if maternal pulse is greater than 120 beats/min or FHR is greater than *180 beats/min.* 2. Strict I&O, daily weight. 3. Encourage lateral position (Sims) to decrease hypotension and increase placental perfusion. 4. IV: Use a pump for continuous infusion; infusion is continued for 12 hrs after labor has stopped. 5. *Use:* Premature labor.
Calcium Channel Blockers Nifedipine: PO	*Maternal:* Facial flushing, mild hypotension, reflex tachycardia, headache, nausea *Fetal:* Rare problems	1. No reported fetal side effects. 2. Not commonly used as a tocolytic agent. 3. Monitor blood pressure for hypotension. 4. Do not use sublingual route.

Appendix 21.2 MEDICATIONS—cont'd

MEDICATIONS	SIDE EFFECTS	NURSING IMPLICATIONS
Prostaglandin synthesis inhibitors Indomethacin: PO or rectally	*Maternal:* Nausea, vomiting, dyspepsia *Fetal:* Oligohydramnios, premature closure of the ductus arteriosus in utero syndrome, respiratory distress syndrome	1. Used when other methods fail and gestational age is less than 30 weeks. 2. Administer for 48-72 hrs or less, as may close the fetal patent ductus. 3. Administer with food or use rectal route to decrease gastrointestinal distress.
Magnesium sulfate	*Maternal:* Promotes relaxation of smooth muscles *Fetal:* Nonreactive NST, decreased breathing, reduced FHR variability	1. *Most commonly used tocolytic agent* because maternal and fetal/neonatal adverse reactions are less common than with the other tocolytic agents, especially the beta-adrenergic agonist (terbutaline). 2. Monitor serum magnesium levels. 3. Have antidote of calcium gluconate available.

Rho(D) Immune Globulin (RhIG; also referred to as RhoGAM): Prevents Rho(D) sensitization in nonsensitized individuals (Fig. 21.17).

Rh-negative mothers after pregnancy or accidental transfusion; "tricks" the body into thinking it has already made antibodies.

RhIG: IM	*Maternal:* Pain and soreness at injection site *Contraindications:* sensitized Rh-negative woman	1. Is administered twice, at 28 weeks injection site gestation and within 72 hrs of delivery, or after an abortion, miscarriage, or transfusion to Rh-negative women. 2. Do not administer this to the infant. 3. *Uses:* prevention of hemolytic disease of the newborn. 4. *Contraindications:* sensitized Rh-negative woman.

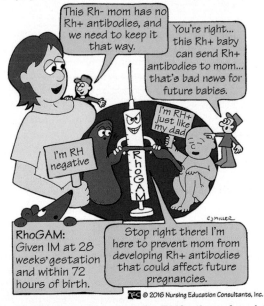

FIG. 21.17 Rho(D) immune globulin (RhIG; also referred to as RhoGAM). (From Zerwekh J. *Mosby's pharmacology notecards: visual, mnemonic, and memory aids for nurses.* 5th ed. St. Louis: Elsevier/Mosby; 2019.)

▲High-alert medications.
BP, blood pressure; *CPD,* cephalopelvic disproportion; *FHR,* fetal heart rate; *NST,* nonstress test; *I&O,* intake and output; *IM,* intramuscularly; *IV,* intravenously; *NSAIDs,* nonsteroidal antiinflammatory drugs; *PO,* by mouth (orally); *subQ,* subcutaneously.

Practice & Next Generation NCLEX (NGN) Questions

Maternity Nursing Care

More questions on **evolve**

1. When reinforcing the teaching of clients in a prenatal clinic, the nurse includes all of the following areas. What is the **most** important area of discussion for clients in their first trimester?
   1. Diet to promote fetal development and maternal well-being.
   2. Postpartum care with emphasis on hygiene and breast care.
   3. Anticipation and points on how to deal with sibling rivalry.
   4. Signs of beginning labor and instructions to come to the hospital as soon as the membranes rupture.

2. The nurse is checking a postpartum client the day after her delivery and notes the lochia has a foul smell. What is the **best** nursing intervention?
   1. Report the foul-smelling lochia to the RN or health care provider.
   2. Do nothing; this is normal during the first few days after delivery.
   3. Begin vaginal irrigations to decrease the odor and increase client comfort.
   4. Stop the use of perineal pads for the next few days.

3. While assessing a prenatal client, the nurse would be alert to symptoms of preeclampsia, which include:
   1. Oliguria, hypotension.
   2. Hypertension, tachycardia.
   3. Edema, tachycardia.
   4. Hypertension, proteinuria.

4. What signs would a nurse observe in a newborn with respiratory distress?
   1. Flaring of the nares, grunting, and intercostal retractions.
   2. Lusty crying, heaving chest wall, and flailing arms.
   3. Respiratory rate of 50 breaths/min, pulse rate of 166 beats/min, and sneezing.
   4. Uncontrolled crying, acrocyanosis, and respiratory rate of 60 breaths/min.

5. To meet the goal of promoting infant feeding in a breastfed baby, what would the nurse reinforce in the teaching plan for the mother? **Select all that apply.**
   1. Feed the baby on a 3- to 4-hr schedule.
   2. Alternate breastfeeding and formula for each feeding.
   3. Stop breastfeeding if her nipples get sore.
   4. Make sure there are 8 to 12 breastfeedings every 24 hrs.
   5. Drink lots of fluids and get adequate rest.
   6. Offer a pacifier between feedings to meet sucking needs.

6. The nurse is observing a new mother use formula to bottle feed her infant. To decrease the amount of regurgitation and vomiting after feedings, the nurse reinforces which of the following with the parent?
   1. Place the newborn on the back with the head turned to the left.
   2. Offer the infant the pacifier after each feeding.
   3. Burp the infant every few minutes of feeding.
   4. Limit the infant to only 10 min at one feeding.

7. A client is having an early postpartum hemorrhage with an estimate of 600 mL of blood loss. What would be the **most** important nursing intervention?
   1. Give a stat dose of oxytocin as ordered.
   2. Place a stat call to the primary health care provider.
   3. Evaluate vital signs and watch for hypovolemic shock.
   4. Palpate the uterus and massage it if it is boggy.

8. A woman (gravida 4, para 3) delivered a 10-lb 9-oz (4790 g) infant after 24 hrs of labor. During the immediate postpartum period, what complication would this client be at an increased risk of developing?
   1. Urinary retention
   2. Puerperal infection
   3. Thrombophlebitis
   4. Postpartum hemorrhage

9. Which of these birth defects require the newborn to be placed in the prone position?
   1. Cleft palate
   2. Imperforate anus
   3. Meningocele
   4. Tracheoesophageal fistula

10. A newborn weighing 4 lb 6 oz (1985 gm) is born at 31 weeks of gestation. During an assessment 12 hrs after birth, the nurse notices hyperactivity, a persistent shrill cry, frequent yawning and sneezing, and jitteriness. In analyzing the symptoms, the nurse would be most concerned regarding the development of what condition?
    1. Sepsis
    2. Hydrocephalus
    3. Drug dependence
    4. Hypoglycemia

11. The nurse is caring for a 28-year-old new client who presents to the clinic for her first prenatal visit after a positive home pregnancy test. The nurse reviews the client's nurses' notes.

| Health History | Nurses' Notes | Provider Orders | Laboratory Results |

1000: Client presents to clinic for confirmation of pregnancy after a missed menstrual period and a positive home pregnancy test. Client reports nausea with vomiting for several days, breast tenderness, and frequent urination. Urine sample provided, and clinic HCG test is positive. Client awaits confirmation of pregnancy by ultrasound.

- Temperature: 98.8°F (37.1°C)
- BP: 120/70 mm Hg
- Heart rate: 80 beats/min and regular
- Respirations: 20 breaths/min
- SpO2: 98% on room air

1100: Ultrasound and health care provider provide confirmation of an 8-week gestation pregnancy. Routine prenatal lab work ordered. Client verbalizes excitement with pregnancy and reports this is her first pregnancy.

The client inquires what changes to expect in the first trimester of pregnancy. Which of the following are common experiences in the first trimester of pregnancy? **Select four clinical findings.**

1. Linea nigra
2. Heartburn
3. Fetal movement
4. Evening nausea
5. Adjustment to the reality of pregnancy
6. Constipation
7. Leg cramps
8. Backache

---

12. A term newborn born 1 hr ago is undergoing a physical and gestational age assessment by the admitting nurse. The LPN/LVN is preparing to assist with this care.

| Health History | Nurses' Notes | Vital Signs | Laboratory Results |

0907: Delivery of viable female term newborn, spontaneous cry at delivery, delayed cord clamping initiated, and newborn placed skin to skin with mother.

0915: Modified newborn assessment and vital signs completed while skin to skin. Pediatric health care provider updated on birth.

0930: Newborn remains skin to skin, color pink centrally acrocyanosis present in extremities; no respiratory distress noted. Vital signs completed.

0945: Newborn remains skin to skin, color pink centrally acrocyanosis present in extremities; no respiratory distress noted. Vital signs completed. Breastfeeding assistance provided with successful newborn latch accomplished.

1000: Newborn to infant radiant warmer at the bedside to complete full physical, gestational age assessment and administer prophylactic medications.

Complete the following sentence. Drag and drop the words from the options below to fill in each blank.

During the physical assessment, the nurse identifies _____, _____, and _____ as normal newborn findings at 1 hr of age.

ASSESSMENT FINDINGS

Nasal flaring
Molding
Jaundice
Acrocyanosis
Moro reflex

13. The nurse is assisting to care for a term newborn client who was delivered 8 hrs ago and is planning to administer the first newborn bath. The nurse plans to involve the parents in this first bath to help them learn newborn care.

When providing a newborn bath, which actions should the nurse take? **Select all that apply**.
1. Clean newborn from cleanest to soiled areas.
2. Wash the vulva from back to front.
3. Dry after washing each area.
4. Use clean corners of the washcloth for each eye.
5. Test the temperature of bath water with the wrist before bathing.
6. Only expose the area being washed to keep the baby warm.
7. Bathe the newborn around the same time each day.
8. Complete shampooing the hair first so the hair can dry while body is washed.

⚡Answers to Practice & Next Generation NCLEX (NGN) Questions

1. 1
Client Needs: Health Promotion and Maintenance
Clinical Judgment/Cognitive Skill: Prioritize Hypotheses
Item Type: Multiple Choice
Rationale & Test Taking Strategy: Note the **key** word, "most." This is a priority test item asking about what is most important to discuss with the client during the first trimester. Ideally, counseling about nutrition begins at the first prenatal visit, starting with the assessment of dietary intake. Labor and postpartum needs are appropriate teaching for the third trimester, along with preparing younger children about the arrival of the newborn.

2. 1
Client Needs: Health Promotion and Maintenance
Clinical Judgment/Cognitive Skill: Take Action
Item Type: Multiple choice
Rationale & Test Taking Strategy: Note the key word, "most." This test item focuses on a priority nursing intervention for a client who has a foul-smelling lochia. Lochia that has a foul odor may indicate the presence of an infection and *should be reported to the registered nurse or the health care provider*. The health care provider will probably start antibiotics. Vaginal irrigations would not be indicated. The client would need to continue to use perineal pads, as an internal tampon would not be indicated.

3. 4
Client Needs: Health Promotion and Maintenance
Clinical Judgment/Cognitive Skill: Recognize Cues
Item Type: Multiple Choice
Rationale & Test Taking Strategy: Recall the two cardinal signs and symptoms of preeclampsia. Proteinuria and increased blood pressure are the classic indications of the development of early problems with preeclampsia. The other symptoms (oliguria, hypotension, tachycardia, edema) are not indicators of preeclampsia.

4. 1
Client Needs: Health Promotion and Maintenance
Clinical Judgment/Cognitive Skill: Recognize Cues
Item Type: Multiple Choice
Rationale & Test Taking Strategy: Review each option and remember the normal vital signs for the newborn, especially respiratory rate. These three factors—grunting, flaring nares, intercostal and sternal retractions—are classic symptoms of respiratory distress in infants. A lusty cry, heaving chest wall, flailing arms, respiratory rate of 30 to 60 breaths/min, pulse rate of 110 to 160 beats/min, sneezing, crying, and acrocyanosis are normal findings in the newborn.

5. 4, 5
Client Needs: Physiological Integrity/Basic Care and Comfort
Clinical Judgment/Cognitive Skill: Generate Solutions
Item Type: Select All That Apply
Rationale & Test Taking Strategy: Review each of the options and determine if they are appropriate for a mother who is breastfeeding. The mother should feed the infant 8 to 12 times each day until the infant is satisfied. Typically, this is breastfeeding every 1.5 to 3 hours. Adequate rest and good fluid intake help to promote milk production. This is most important during the early days after birth. Feeding only breast milk frequently stimulates milk production. Nipple soreness is one of the most common problems and teaching the mother proper positioning will greatly reduce nipple soreness. Offering a pacifier is not recommended for the breastfeeding mother.

6. 3
Client Needs: Physiological Integrity/Basic Care and Comfort
Clinical Judgment/Cognitive Skill: Take Action
Item Type: Multiple Choice
Rationale & Test Taking Strategy: Think about why a newborn regurgitates and/or vomits after a formula feeding. Because of the immaturity of the gastrointestinal system in the neonate, regurgitation and vomiting are common events. To decrease the incidence of regurgitation and vomiting, instruct the parents to avoid overfeeding the infant, burp the infant every few minutes during the feeding, and position the infant with their head slightly elevated after feeding. Pacifiers are discouraged during the first month so that feeding routines (both bottle- and breastfed infants) are established.

7. 4
Client Needs: Physiological Integrity/Physiological Adaptation
Clinical Judgment/Cognitive Skill: Take Action
Item Type: Multiple Choice
Rationale & Test Taking Strategy: Note the **key** word, "most." This is a priority test item concerned about the most important nursing intervention for a client experiencing postpartum hemorrhage. Although all of these are appropriate interventions, the nurse needs to determine if a boggy uterus is causing the bleeding. Early postpartum hemorrhage is often the result of uterine atony. The initial management and treatment of uterine atony is fundal massage.

8. 4
Client Needs: Physiological Integrity/Physiological Adaptation
Clinical Judgment/Cognitive Skill: Analyze Cues
Item Type: Multiple Choice
Rationale & Test Taking Strategy: The question is asking about the mother's increased risk for developing a complication. Hemorrhage is always a consideration with a large baby and numerous past pregnancies because the uterine wall muscles may contract poorly. Urinary retention may occur in any client during the immediate postpartum period. Thrombophlebitis and puerperal infection may develop several days after delivery but not in the immediate postpartum period.

9. 3
Client Needs: Physiological Integrity/Basic Care and Comfort
Clinical Judgment/Cognitive Skill: Prioritize Hypotheses
Item Type: Multiple Choice
Rationale & Test Taking Strategy: Remember that prone position places the infant on the abdomen. Recall which of these conditions would require this type of positioning. Meningocele is a form of spina bifida cystica where a saclike cyst protrudes through a defect in the spine. The infant is placed prone to prevent cyst rupture. A child with cleft palate should be placed supine with the head elevated. The child with imperforate anus should be placed in a side-lying position. The infant with tracheoesophageal fistula should be placed supine with the head elevated to 30 degrees to prevent aspiration and maintain a patent airway.

10. 3
Client Needs: Health Promotion and Maintenance
Clinical Judgment/Cognitive Skill: Analyze Cues
Item Type: Multiple Choice

Rationale & Test Taking Strategy: Think about the newborn's symptoms—are they normal or do they indicate some complication? These classic symptoms of drug dependency usually appear within the first 24 hours after birth. Sepsis is indicated by increased temperature, tachypnea, and tachycardia. Hydrocephalus is characterized by an increase in frontal-occipital circumference and a changing level of consciousness (signs of intracranial pressure). Signs of hypoglycemia include hypothermia, muscle twitching, diaphoresis, and respiratory distress.

11. 1, 2, 5, 6
Client Needs: Health Promotion and Maintenance
Clinical Judgment/Cognitive Skill: Recognize Cues
Item Type: Extended Multiple Response: Select N
Rationale & Test Taking Strategy: The question asks you to select four common findings that occur during the first trimester. Common changes in the first trimester of pregnancy include linea nigra, which is a deepening pigmentation on the abdomen due to hormone changes, frequently referred to as the "line of pregnancy." Heartburn may occur in the first trimester and can be attributed to decreased gastric motility due to elevated hormone levels. Constipation can also occur secondary to a decrease in gastric motility. A psychological adjustment to pregnancy may include feelings of ambivalence. This often resolves in the second trimester when the pregnancy becomes more visually apparent with increased uterine size. Evening nausea is not as common as morning sickness (nausea and vomiting) in the first trimester. Fetal movement felt by the client does not typically occur until the second trimester. Leg cramps and backache are more common in the second and third trimesters.

12. A term newborn born 1 hour ago is undergoing a physical and gestational-age assessment by the admitting nurse. The licensed practical nurse/licensed vocational nurse is preparing to assist with this care.

Health History	Nurses' Notes	Vital Signs	Laboratory Results

0907: Delivery of viable female term newborn, spontaneous cry at delivery, delayed cord clamping initiated, and newborn placed skin to skin with mother.

0915: Modified newborn assessment and vital signs completed while skin to skin. Pediatric health care provider updated on birth.

0930: Newborn remains skin to skin, color pink, centrally acrocyanosis present in extremities; no respiratory distress noted. Vital signs completed.

0945: Newborn remains skin to skin, color pink, centrally acrocyanosis present in extremities; no respiratory distress noted. Vital signs completed. Breastfeeding assistance provided with successful newborn latch accomplished.

1000: Newborn to infant radiant warmer at the bedside to complete full physical, gestational age assessment and administer prophylactic medications.

Complete the following sentence. Drag and drop the words from the options below to fill in each blank.

During the physical assessment, the nurse identifies *molding*, *acrocyanosis*, and *Moro reflex* as normal newborn findings at 1 hour of age.

Client Needs: Health Promotion and Maintenance
Clinical Judgment/Cognitive Skill: Analyze Cues
Item Type: Drag-and-Drop Cloze
Rationale & Test Taking Strategy: At 1 hour of age, molding is common to observe, as the fetal head has conformed to fit the size and shape of the maternal birth canal. Molding recedes rapidly in the hours following vaginal delivery. Acrocyanosis is another common finding in the newborn. This is due to circulation priorities being central and the extremities taking longer to become pink. The Moro "startle" reflex is elicited when the newborn reacts to a noise or sudden movement. It is a protective reflex where the infant suddenly draws up the legs and extends the arms. Nasal flaring is often accompanied by rapid breathing and can signal respiratory distress. Further assessment is required. Jaundice that is apparent within the first 24 hours following delivery can be related to an ABO-Rh incompatibility and should be documented and reported to the pediatric health care provider.

13. **1, 3, 4**
Client Needs: Physiological Integrity/Basic Care and Comfort
Clinical Judgment/Cognitive Skill: Take Action
Item Type: Extended Multiple Response: Select All That Apply
Rationale & Test Taking Strategy: The principles of care that should be emphasized when providing a newborn bath include cleaning the newborn from cleanest to soiled areas, using separate clean areas of a washcloth to cleanse the eyes, ears, and nose. After each area is cleansed, it should be dried and only the area being washed should be exposed. This will help keep the newborn from losing heat and lowering the body temperature during the sponge bath. When providing care to the newborn genitals, the vulva should be washed from front to back to prevent possible transfer of rectal content. Shampooing the hair should be done last as newborns lose heat quickly with a wet head. The wet hair should be dried with a washcloth and a clean hat can also be applied. Before bathing, the temperature of the bath should be confirmed with a thermometer and the water should be between 37.2° and 38°C (99° and 100.4°F). The newborn does not need a daily bath; two to three times a week is sufficient.

CHAPTER TWENTY-TWO

Pediatric Nursing Care

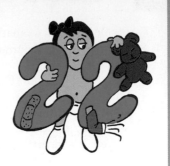

EYE

Visual Impairment in Children

Assessment: Recognize Cues

A. Refractory problems: same as those of an adult (see Appendix 8.1).

B. Amblyopia: reduced visual acuity in one eye; preventable if primary problem is corrected before 6 years of age.

C. Strabismus (misalignment of eyes) may result if amblyopia is not corrected.

D. Retinopathy of prematurity: originally known as *retrolental fibroplasia*; results in vasoconstriction of retina vessels, causing retinal damage.

Analyze Cues and Prioritize Hypotheses

The most important problems are safety (poor vision) and growth and development deficits (poor school performance due to inability to see).

Nursing Intervention: Take Action

A. Promote discovery of the problem as early as possible.
1. Identify children at increased risk because of history (prematurity).
2. Assess children for behaviors that indicate poor vision.
3. Encourage screening for visual acuity (schools, clinics).

B. Educate parents regarding importance of therapy and continued medical follow-up.

Conjunctivitis

Conjunctivitis **is an inflammation of the conjunctiva.**

Assessment: Recognize Cues

A. Exposure to bacterial or viral infections, allergens, or chemical irritants.

B. Redness, edema, tearing, and mucopurulent drainage.

Analyze Cues and Prioritize Hypotheses

The most important problems are infection and transmission to others.

Generate Solutions

Treatment

A. Antibiotic eyedrops for infections: instill after the eye has been cleaned.

B. Antihistamines and corticosteroids for allergic conjunctivitis.

C. Warm, moist compresses are used to remove crust and exudates.

Nursing Intervention: Take Action

Goal: To prevent the transmission of organisms to the uninfected eye and to others.

A. Always clean eye from inner canthus downward and outward to prevent contamination of the other lacrimal duct. Do not contaminate other eye.

B. Highly contagious; spreads easily from one eye to other.

C. Encourage good handwashing and instruct not to share washclothes with others.

EAR

Otitis Media

Otitis media **is an infection of the middle ear caused by a viral or bacterial agent. Infants and young children are predisposed to the development of acute otitis media because of the physiologic characteristics of the ear—the eustachian tube is shorter, wider, and straighter in children than in adults.**

Assessment: Recognize Cues

A. Acute otitis media (AOM).
1. May be purulent (pus filled) or suppurative (capable of producing pus).
2. Symptoms vary with the severity of the infection.

B. Repeated or persistent acute infections may lead to perforation of the tympanic membrane or more severe complications such as mastoiditis.

C. Chronic otitis media with effusion (OME): a collection of fluid in the middle ear without infection or acute symptoms that results from a blocked eustachian tube; may persist for weeks to months; most common cause of conductive hearing loss.

D. Risk factors.
1. Age: increased incidence from 6 months to 20 months; decreases with age.
2. Upper respiratory tract infection.
3. Allergies, asthma.
4. Exposure to tobacco smoke.
5. Out-of-home day care and exposure to siblings or parents with chronic otitis media.
6. Feeding bottle to infant/toddler in the supine position.

589

7. Pacifier use past 6 months of age.
8. Not receiving immunization with pneumococcal conjugate vaccine (PCV).
E. Clinical manifestations (Fig. 22.1).
 1. Otalgia (pain from pressure in the middle ear).
  a. Infants are irritable; may pull at their ears or cry; sucking exacerbates pain.
  b. Young children verbally complain of severe ear pain.
 2. Fever as high as 104°F (40°C) is not uncommon with AOM.
 3. Otoscopic examination.
  a. AOM—tympanic membrane is immobile, bright red, and bulging, with purulent effusion and no light reflex.
  b. OME—tympanic membrane is immobile, dull gray, and may have fluid behind it.
 4. Postauricular and cervical lymph node enlargement.
 5. If tympanic membrane ruptures, purulent drainage or blood may be present in the outer ear; pain will decrease temporarily (AOM and OME).
 6. Conductive hearing loss may occur with recurrent rupture.
 7. Speech and language development may be delayed.

Analyze Cues and Prioritize Hypotheses

The most important problems are acute pain from the infection and permanent hearing loss due to scarring of the tympanic membrane rupture.

Generate Solutions

Treatment
A. Medications.
 1. Antibiotics, analgesics, antipyretics.

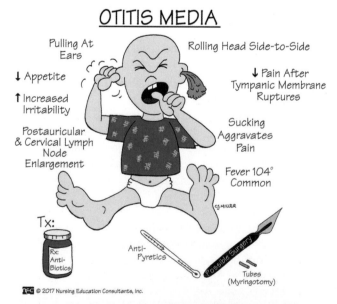

FIG. 22.1 Otitis Media. (From Zerwekh, J., Garneau, A., & Miller, C. J. [2017]. *Digital collection of the memory notebooks of nursing* [4th ed.]. Nursing Education Consultants.)

 2. Eardrops (antibiotic and steroid combination) (see Fig. 8.3 in Chapter 8).
 3. Decongestants and antihistamines.
 4. Corticosteroids for eustachian tube edema as needed.
 5. OME does not require antibiotic therapy.
B. Surgical—myringotomy: drainage of the middle ear with insertion of tubes or grommets (or tympanostomy myringotomy) to relieve pressure and promote healing; used for recurrent cases that do not respond to medication; tubes are also known as pressure-equalizing tubes (PE tubes or myringotomy tubes).

> **⚠ NURSING PRIORITY** Teach the parents to administer the full course of the antibiotic.

Nursing Intervention: Take Action

Goal: To enable parents of clients to describe problem, handle medication schedule, and cope with home care.
A. Recurrent infections cause an increased risk for permanent hearing loss or mastoiditis with potential intracranial spread of infection.
B. Antibiotics should be continued until all prescribed medication is taken, even after all symptoms are relieved.
C. Administer acetaminophen or ibuprofen for pain and fever. There should be relief of symptoms within 24 to 72 hours; if not, the health care provider should be contacted.
D. Pain-relieving ear drops (antipyrine, benzocaine, and glycerin) should be used only when there is no tympanostomy tube or rupture of the tympanic membrane.

> **⚠ NURSING PRIORITY** Aspirin should not be used for fever or pain in children 18 years of age or younger.

E. Control allergies and upper respiratory congestion, including decreased exposure to those with respiratory infections.
F. The child should be discouraged from forcefully blowing the nose or holding the nose closed when sneezing.
G. Decrease risk for recurrence by preventing fluids from pooling around eustachian tube.
 1. Hold or elevate infant's head while feeding.
 2. Do not prop bottle or allow infant to fall asleep with a bottle.
 3. Encourage intake of water before sleeping.
Goal: Care for child after placement of tympanostomy tubes (myringotomy tubes or grommets).
A. Do not allow any water to get into the child's ears; use of earplugs is currently controversial following tympanoplasty.
B. Assure parents that if the ear grommet or tube falls out, it is not a significant problem and to notify the health care provider.

🌳 External Otitis

External otitis **is an inflammation or infection of the skin of the auricle of the ear and/or the ear canal.**

Assessment: Recognize Cues

A. Risk factors/etiology.
1. Swimming, especially when the water is contaminated or contains chemicals.
2. Trauma to the ear, such as piercing.
B. Clinical manifestations.
1. Ear pain, fever; disturbances of hearing.
2. Drainage from the ear: blood-tinged or white to green-colored fluid.

Analyze Cues and Prioritize Hypotheses

The most important problem is acute pain from the infection.

Generate Solutions

Treatment

A. Antibiotics (typically given as an eardrop; oral preparations for severe cases).

Nursing Intervention: Take Action

Goal: To prevent and reduce risk factors.
A. Encourage an eardrop drying agent (isopropyl alcohol and glycerin) after swimming, showering, or bathing to dry external ear canal and/or use of earplugs when child goes swimming.
B. Use earplugs if swimming or performing any activities that may precipitate water getting into the ears.
C. Do not use a cotton-tipped applicator to remove water from the ears.

IMMUNE

🍦 Pediatric Acquired Immunodeficiency Syndrome

The majority of children with AIDS were infected in the perinatal period. Cases related to blood transfusions are relatively rare.

> ❗ **NURSING PRIORITY** HIV-positive mothers should not breastfeed their infants.

Assessment: Recognize Cues

A. Risk factors.
1. Sexual activity and IV drug use are the major causes of HIV infection in adolescents.
2. Infants born to mothers who are HIV positive account for the majority of children with HIV infection; antiretroviral therapy during pregnancy reduces risk for transmission to fetus.
3. Children rarely have Kaposi sarcoma.
4. *Pneumocystis jiroveci* pneumonia (PJP; or *Pneumocystis* pneumonia [PCP]) is the most common opportunistic infection.
B. Clinical manifestations.
1. Infants affected during the prenatal period have rapid disease progression.
2. HIV-positive infants usually have symptoms by 18 to 24 months of age.

3. Infants diagnosed within the first year of life have a poor prognosis, as do those who develop PJP and progressive encephalopathy.
4. Symptoms include lymphadenopathy, hepatosplenomegaly, oral candidiasis, chronic diarrhea, failure to thrive, developmental delay, and parotitis.
5. Severe symptoms in adolescents include AIDS-defining illnesses such as PJP, wasting syndrome, HIV encephalopathy, *Candida* esophagitis, and cryptosporidiosis.
6. Immune categories are based on CD4+ T-cell counts; these are age adjusted.
C. Diagnostics:
1. Enzyme-linked immunoassay (ELISA), also known as enzyme immunoassay (EIA), and Western blot (WB) for children 18 months or older.
2. Newborn: polymerase chain reaction (PCR); p24 antigen detection; majority of infants who are HIV positive can be identified by 3 months of age.
3. Maternal antibodies to HIV may persist for up to 18 months, then the infant may seroconvert to a negative status.
4. Positive results on two separate occasions and from separate blood specimens for p24 antigen detection, PCR, and virus culture are required to confirm diagnosis of HIV infection.

Analyze Cues and Prioritize Hypotheses

The most important problems are potential for infection, inadequate gas exchange and nutrition, pain, diarrhea, and reduced tissue integrity.

Treatment

Treatment for children is essentially the same as that for an adult.

Nursing Interventions Specific to Children: Take Action

Goal: To maintain homeostasis.
A. Infants and children should receive the standard immunizations against childhood diseases. Measles–mumps–rubella (MMR) and varicella (chickenpox) vaccines may be given if the child is not severely immunocompromised or HIV positive.
B. Pneumococcal and influenza vaccines are recommended.
C. Nutritional support; high-calorie, high-protein diet.
D. Antifungal medications to prevent fungal infections.
E. Educate adolescents regarding safe sex.

🔆 Home Care

A. Teach parent(s) how to care for the child.
1. How to administer medications and importance of administering medications as scheduled.
2. Symptoms of complications: PJP, *Candida*, failure to thrive.
3. Teach parents standard precautions, including proper handling of diapers and avoidance of contact with blood and body fluids.

4. Prevent biting behaviors in young children.
5. Help parents deal with child's pain—multiple procedures, infections (abscessed tooth, otitis media).
   a. Aggressive management of pain with nonsteroidal antiinflammatory drugs (NSAIDs), opioids, muscle relaxants.
   b. Ongoing assessment of pain in nonverbal children—irritability, lack of interaction, lack of play.
B. Teach parents how to prevent transmission of disease.
C. Course of disease in infants and children is unpredictable.
D. Work with school personnel to maintain privacy/confidentiality.
E. Promote normal growth and development.

PSYCHOSOCIAL

Child Abuse

Assessment: Recognize Cues

A. Child neglect: the failure to provide a child with the basic necessities; this may be classified as physical or emotional neglect.
   1. Failure to thrive: Infant or child is below the normal ranges on the growth chart.
   2. Infant or child does not appear to be physically cared for. Inappropriate diapering, diaper rash, or a strong urine smell to the body may be seen in infants who have been neglected.
   3. Evidence of malnutrition.
   4. Lack of adequate supervision; child is allowed to engage in dangerous play activities and sustains frequent injuries.
   5. Language development may be delayed.
   6. Withdrawal; inappropriate fearfulness.
   7. Parents may be apathetic and unresponsive to the child's needs. The nurse is most often able to observe the parent–child interaction in school situations, in a doctor's office, or in the emergency department (ED).
B. Physical child abuse.
   1. Symptoms.
      a. Bruises and welts from being beaten with a belt, strap, stick, or coat hanger or from being slapped repeatedly in the face.
      b. Rope burns from being tied up or beaten with a rope.
      c. Human bite marks.
      d. Burns.
         (1) Burns on the buttocks from being immersed in hot water.
         (2) Pattern of burns: round, small burns from cigarettes; patterns that suggest an object was used.
         (3) Burns are frequently on the buttocks, in the genital area, or on the soles of the feet.
      e. Evidence of various fractures in different stages of healing.
      f. Internal injuries from being hit repeatedly in the abdomen.
      g. Head injuries: skull, facial fractures.

2. Behavior symptoms.
   a. Withdrawal from physical contact with adults.
   b. Inappropriate response to pain or injury; failure to cry or seek comfort from parents.
   c. Infant may stiffen when held; child may stiffen when approached by adult or parent.
   d. Little eye contact with adults.
   e. Child may try to protect abusing parent for fear of punishment if abuse is discovered.
3. Parents or caretakers.
   a. Conflicting stories regarding accident or injury.
   b. Explanation of accident is inconsistent with injuries sustained (fractured skull and broken leg from "falling out of bed").
   c. Initial complaint is not associated with child's injury (child is brought to the ED with complaints of the "flu" and there is evidence of a skull fracture).
   d. Exaggerated concern or lack of concern related to level of child's injury.
   e. Refusal to allow further tests or additional medical care.
   f. Lack of nurturing response to injured or ill child; no cuddling, touching, or comforting child in distress.
   g. Repeated visits to various medical emergency facilities.
   h. Unrealistic expectations of the child; lack of understanding about stages of growth and development (e.g., severely spanking or beating a 1-year-old for lack of response to toilet training).

Analyze Cues and Prioritize Hypotheses

The most important problems are trauma and injury to the child, neglect or emotional abuse, and family dysfunction.

Nursing Interventions: Take Action

Goal: To establish a safe environment.
A. It is important for the nurse to be knowledgeable of the legal responsibilities in regard to state practice acts and child abuse laws (Box 22.1).
B. All 50 states have a designated agency that is available on a 24-hour basis for reporting child abuse.
C. All states have mechanisms for removing the child from the immediate abusive environment.
Goal: To educate the parents and help them identify assistance for long-term supportive care.
A. Educate parents in regard to normal growth and development of children, the role of discipline, and the necessity for having realistic expectations.
B. Become familiar with available community resources such as crisis centers, crisis hotlines, parent effectiveness training groups, Parents Anonymous groups, etc.

Incest

Assessment: Recognize Cues

A. Victim is usually female; the perpetrator of abuse is primarily male, usually between age 30 and 50, and often the victim's father or other member of the immediate family.

Box 22.1   DOCUMENTATION FOR SUSPECTED CHILD ABUSE

Procedure

1. Obtain the client's or parent's permission before photographing the victim.
2. Do not make assumptions about the identity of the perpetrator.
3. Chart the exact words used by the client/child to describe the abuser.
4. Record information very objectively; do not record your feelings, assumptions, or opinions of the incident or how it occurred.

History

1. Specify the time, date, and location as described by the client.
2. Report the sequence of events before the abuse/attack.
3. Identify and explain the period of time between the abuse/attack and initiation of medical attention.
4. List other people/children in the immediate vicinity of the abuse/attack.
5. Include quotations from the client.
6. Use objective, specific documentation when recording observations of the client and the person who brought the client to the ED.
7. Observe and record the interaction of the child and the parents.
8. Do conduct the interview in private.

Physical Examination

1. Be very specific in describing the location, size, and shape of bruises and lacerations. If possible, photograph the client to demonstrate the extent of the injuries.
2. If possible, describe the location and extent of injuries on an anatomic diagram.
3. Identify the presence of other injuries.
4. Describe the victim's reaction to pain, level of pain, and location of pain.

B. Incest is a symptom of severe dysfunction in an individual and within the family.
C. Perpetrators of sexual exploitation.
 1. Emotionally dependent men.
 2. Feelings of inferiority and low self-esteem.
 3. Perpetrators frequently seduce their victims by being endearing and "good" to the child.
 4. Often, these men are pillars of the community and are involved in many youth activities.
 5. Frequently, the mother is unaware of the problem. If she suspects it, she may feel guilty for having such ideas.
D. Sexually exploited child.
 1. Child may fear retaliation if anyone finds out; she may fear that she will not be believed if she tells anyone.
 2. Child may feel guilty for participating in the sexual activity and afraid of disruption of the family if it is revealed.
 3. Violence rarely accompanies incest relationship.
 4. The child may be emotionally and physically dependent on the abusing parent.

Analyze Cues and Prioritize Hypotheses

The most important problems are emotional trauma and injury to the exploited individual and family dysfunction.

Nursing Interventions: Take Action

Goal: To educate children that their bodies belong to themselves and are private.

A. Instruct children to report any type of touching, fondling, or caressing that makes them feel uncomfortable.
B. Provide educational material to help parents talk about sexual assault and inappropriate fondling with their children.

Goal: To support the parents and the child and to help them identify assistance for long-term supportive care.

A. Provide support and the opportunity for the child and family members to discuss their feelings.
B. Assist the family to identify community resources; strongly encourage involvement in family counseling.

Sex Trafficking

Assessment: Recognize Cues

A. Victim is younger than 18 years of age and engaged in sexual activity in which there is an exchange for something of value.
B. Risk factors placing children at higher risk for sex trafficking abuse.
 1. Unstable living situation.
 2. History of experiencing either sexual or domestic violence or both.
 3. Runaway.
 4. Involved in the juvenile justice or child welfare system.
 5. Undocumented immigrant.
 6. Family in poverty or economic need.
 7. Caregiver or family member with substance abuse addiction.
 8. Child is addicted to drugs or alcohol.
 9. Members of the LGBTQ+ (lesbian, gay, bisexual, transgender, queer/questioning) community.
C. Perpetrators of sex trafficking.
 1. No evidence supporting a specific race, nationality, gender, or sexual orientation.
 2. Perpetrators are sometimes strangers and others are peers, friends, or family members.
D. Sex-trafficked child.
 1. Children who are being sex trafficked may show some of the following signs.
  a. Absent from school; failing grades.
  b. New onset substance abuse.
  c. Change in dress; change in friends.
  d. Age-inappropriate romantic partner.
  e. Repeat runaway.
  f. Inability to speak for self.
  g. Evidence of being controlled.
  h. Wears inappropriate clothing for weather.

Analyze Cues and Prioritize Hypotheses

The most important problems are emotional trauma and injury to the exploited individual and potential missing person from family unit.

Nursing Interventions: Take Action

Goal: To keep the child safe.

A. Know and follow your state's mandatory reporting requirements.

B. Never confront a suspected trafficker as it places your client and yourself in danger.

Goal: To screen for sex trafficking.

A. Record activities the client reported they were required to perform.

B. Use client quotes as much as possible. When paraphrasing or summarizing, use care and accuracy.

Intellectual Developmental Disorder

A child who has an *intellectual disability* has deficits in three areas: intellectual functioning, social functioning, and practical aspects of daily living. This was previously called *mental retardation*.

Assessment: Recognize Cues

A. Causes.
   1. Down syndrome, fragile X syndrome, phenylketonuria, rubella.
   2. Kernicterus (elevated bilirubin level), anoxia, fetal alcohol syndrome.
   3. Lead poisoning, meningitis, encephalitis.
   4. Neoplasms; Tay-Sachs disease.
B. Additional characteristics.
   1. Irritability, temper tantrums, stereotyped movements.
   2. Multiple neurologic abnormalities: dysfunction in vision or hearing or seizure activity.

Analyze Cues and Prioritize Hypotheses

The most important problems are intellectual disability, disturbances in social functioning, and possible neurologic abnormalities.

Nursing Interventions: Take Action

Goal: To promote optimum development within a family and community setting.

A. Promote feelings of self-esteem, worth, and security.

B. Educate the parents about developmental stages and tasks; deal with child's developmental, *not* chronologic, age.

Goal: To promote independence by setting realistic goals.

A. Teach basic skills in simple terms, with steps outlined.

B. Use behavior modification as a method for behavior control.

C. Use the principles of *repetition*, *reinforcement*, and *routine* when providing information for understanding and learning.

Down Syndrome

Down syndrome **is a common chromosomal abnormality characterized by an extra chromosome 21 (trisomy 21); incidence increases with maternal age.**

Assessment: Recognize Cues

A. Physical characteristics criteria.
   1. Head: small in size; face has flat profile, sparse hair.
   2. Eyes: inner epicanthal folds; short and sparse eyelashes.
   3. Nose: small and depressed nasal bridge (saddle nose).
   4. Ears: small and sometimes low-set.
   5. Mouth: protruding tongue; high arched palate.
   6. Neck: short and broad.
   7. Abdomen: protruding; umbilical hernia.
   8. Genitalia: small penis, cryptorchidism.
   9. Hands: short, stubby fingers; simian crease (transverse palmar crease).
   10. Muscles: hypotonic.
B. Mental characteristics.
   1. Cognitive impairment.
   2. Developmental delay.

Analyze Cues and Prioritize Hypotheses

The most important problems are potential intellectual disability, developmental delay, potential disturbance in social functioning, and physical abnormalities.

Nursing Interventions: Take Action

Goal: To promote optimal development

A. Involve child and parents in early stimulation program.

B. Promote self-care skills.

C. Help parents identify realistic goals for child.

D. Encourage parents to enroll child in special day care programs and education classes.

E. Emphasize to parents that their child has the same needs of play, discipline, and social interaction as all children.

Goal: To encourage early identification of Down syndrome.

A. It is common for pregnant women at risk (older than 35 years, family history of Down syndrome, or previous birth of a child with Down syndrome) to have an amniocentesis before the 16th week to rule out Down syndrome.

Home Care

A. Prevent respiratory tract infections by teaching parents about postural drainage and percussion.

B. Encourage use of cool-mist vaporizer.

C. Stress importance of changing infant's position frequently; swaddle infant to prevent heat loss.

D. Explain to parents about feeding difficulties and the need for direct supervision; encourage small, frequent feedings; feed solid food by pushing food back inside of mouth; provide foods that will form bulk to prevent constipation.

E. Discuss alternative options to home care with parents.

F. Individuals with Down syndrome develop a clinical syndrome of dementia that has almost identical clinical and neuropathologic characteristics of Alzheimer disease as described in individuals without Down syndrome.
   1. The main difference is the age of onset of Alzheimer disease in individuals with Down syndrome.
   2. These clients present with clinical symptoms in their late 40s or early 50s.

Attention-Deficit/Hyperactivity Disorder

Attention-deficit/hyperactivity disorder (ADHD) **is a developmental disorder characterized by inappropriate inattention and impulsivity, which usually appears between 3 and 7 years of age. Names previously used include** *hyperkinetic syndrome,* *minimal brain damage,* **and** *minimal brain dysfunction.*

Assessment: Recognize Cues

A. Diagnostic criteria.
1. Inattention.
   a. Fails to finish things they start.
   b. Often does not seem to listen when spoken to.
   c. Is easily distracted.
   d. Has difficulty concentrating.
   e. Has difficulty sticking to play activity.
2. Impulsivity.
   a. Often acts before thinking.
   b. Shifts excessively from one activity to another.
   c. Has difficulty organizing work.
   d. Needs frequent supervision.
   e. Frequently calls out in class.
   f. Has difficulty waiting for their turn in games or group activities.
3. Hyperactivity.
   a. Runs about or climbs on things.
   b. Has difficulty sitting still; fidgets.
   c. Has difficulty staying seated.
   d. Moves about excessively during sleep.
   e. Is always "on the go."
4. Onset before 7 years of age.
5. Duration of at least 6 months.

Analyze Cues and Prioritize Hypotheses

The most important problems are inappropriate attention, impulsivity, and hyperactivity that can interfere with school and social activities.

Nursing Interventions: Take Action

Goal: To keep child from harming self or others.
A. Assist child to recognize when feeling angry.
B. Help child accept feelings of anger.
C. Teach child appropriate expression of angry feelings.
D. Redirect violent behavior with physical outlets for child's anxiety (e.g., use of punching bag, jogging).
E. Confront child; withdraw attention when interactions with others are manipulative or exploitative.
F. Use time-out, isolation room, and restraints only when other interventions are unsuccessful.
Note: The nurse should review and be aware of the agency's policies related to the use of chemical and physical restraints.
Goal: To encourage age-appropriate, socially acceptable coping skills.
A. If child is hyperactive, make environment safe for continuous large muscle movement.
B. Provide large motor skill activities for child to participate in.
C. Provide frequent, nutritious snacks for child to "eat on the run."

Goal: To decrease anxiety and increase self-esteem.
A. Encourage child to seek out staff to discuss true feelings.
B. Offer support during times of increased anxiety; ensure physical and psychological safety.
Goal: To administer prescribed medication.
A. Methylphenidate hydrochloride or dextroamphetamine sulfate may be used; not recommended for children younger than 6 years of age.
B. Prolonged administration may produce a temporary suppression of normal weight gain.
Administer in morning (to prevent insomnia) and 30 to 45 minutes before meals.

Autism Spectrum Disorders (Autism)

Infantile *autism* **is characterized by a lack of responsiveness to other people, a lack of involvement with others, a lack of verbal communication, a preoccupation with inanimate objects, and ritualistic behavior.**

Assessment: Recognize Cues

A. Diagnostic criteria.
1. Onset before 3 years of age.
2. Impairment in social interactions—lack of responsiveness and involvement with others; difficulty maintaining eye contact.
3. Impairment in communication and imaginative activity.
   a. Gross deficits in language development: speech is characterized by echolalia, parrot speech (i.e., automatic repetition of words).
   b. Pronominal reversal (tendency to use *you* for *I*).
   c. Lack of spontaneous make-believe play.
4. Markedly restricted, stereotypical patterns of behavior, interest, and activities.
   a. Rigid adherence to routines and rituals.
   b. Repetitive motor mannerisms—hand flapping, clapping, rocking, or rhythmic body movements.
5. *Absence* of delusions, hallucinations, and associative looseness, which are characteristics of childhood schizophrenia.

Analyze Cues and Prioritize Hypotheses

The most important problems are difficulty with social communication (absent or delayed speech), interaction, and behavior.

Nursing Interventions: Take Action

Goal: To increase social awareness.
A. Encourage a significant one-to-one relationship with an adult.
B. Promote and engage in peer interaction.
C. Develop play and self-care skills.
D. Do not force interactions. Begin with positive reinforcement for eye contact. Gradually introduce touch, smiling, and hugging.
Goal: To teach verbal (oral) communication.
A. Respond to verbalization by telling the child what you do not understand.

B. Respond to nonverbal cues with verbal (oral) interpretation.

C. Observe and record context in which lack of clarity of spoken word occurred.

D. Use *en face* approach (face-to-face, eye-to-eye) to convey correct nonverbal expressions by example.

Goal: To decrease unacceptable behavior.

A. Encourage child to recognize and respond to own physiologic needs and urges.

B. Encourage verbalization of body needs but do not make an issue of it.

C. Offer fluids and encourage exercise to prevent constipation.

D. Offer the bathroom at appropriate intervals throughout the day.

E. Prevent the child from hurting self or others by setting firm limits and recognizing feelings of anger, fear, and frustration.

♣ Separation Anxiety Disorder

When a child demonstrates persistent and excessive anxiety on separation from parent or familiar surroundings, it is called *separation anxiety disorder*.

Assessment: Recognize Cues

A. Diagnostic criteria.
1. Excessive distress when separated from home or parents.
2. Unrealistic worry about harm occurring.
3. Refusal to sleep unless near parent.
4. Refusal to attend school or other activities without parent.
5. Physical symptoms as a response to anxiety (e.g., upset stomach, vomiting, headache, etc.).

B. Additional characteristics.
1. Depressed mood.
2. Excessive conformity; often demonstrates need for constant attention; may be demanding.
3. Usual age of onset any time between preschool years and 11 or 12 years.

Analyze Cues and Prioritize Hypotheses

The most important problem is excessive anxiety when separated from parent or familiar surroundings.

Nursing Interventions: Take Action

Goal: To reduce the level of anxiety in anxiety-provoking situations.

A. Identify factors that produce anxiety.

B. Turn on nightlights to allay night fears.

C. Offer calm reassurance.

Goal: To differentiate between normal separation anxiety, which is seen in early childhood, and excessive anxiety, which is seen in separation anxiety disorder.

♣ Specific Disorders with Physical Symptoms

Assessment: Recognize Cues

A. Dysfluency (stuttering).
1. Frequent repetitions or prolongations of sounds, syllables, or words.

2. Unusual hesitations and pauses that disrupt the flow of speech.
3. Speech may be rapid or slow.
4. Stuttering is often absent during singing or talking to inanimate objects.

B. Enuresis (bed-wetting).
1. Repeated involuntary voiding during the day or night.
2. The involuntary voiding occurs after the age at which it is expected and is not due to any physical disorder.

C. Encopresis (fecal incontinence).
1. Repeated voluntary or involuntary passage of feces of normal consistency in inappropriate places.
2. Smearing feces, which should be differentiated from the smearing that takes place involuntarily and in the younger child (1 or 2 years of age).

Analyze Cues and Prioritize Hypotheses

The most important problems are associated with physical symptoms, such as stuttering, bed-wetting, and fecal incontinence.

Nursing Interventions: Take Action

Goal: To assess and medically evaluate for any physiologic cause related to stuttering, enuresis, or encopresis.

Goal: To promote a positive self-concept by helping the child overcome feelings of shame and guilt associated with the disorder.

Goal: To identify various approaches to controlling enuresis.

A. Administer imipramine.

B. Restrict fluids before going to bed.

C. Encourage behavioral intervention therapies (a buzzer that wakes child when starting to urinate; bladder training programs).

Goal: To identify various approaches to controlling fecal incontinence.

A. If child is retaining feces, initiate a bowel-cleaning regimen.

B. If child has loose stools, a daily bulk laxative is needed.

C. If soiling is deliberate, help child express feelings through other means.

D. Educate child about bodily signals (rectal pressure).

E. Teach child to sit on toilet for 10 to 15 minutes after eating to establish regular elimination pattern.

> **TEST ALERT** Initiate a toileting schedule.

♣ Specific Developmental Disorders

Assessment: Recognize Cues

A. Developmental reading disorder.
1. Impairment in the development of reading skills.
2. Often referred to as *dyslexia*.
3. Slow reading speed and reduced comprehension.

B. Developmental arithmetic disorder: impairment in the development of arithmetic skills.

C. Developmental language disorder.
1. Three major types.

a. Failure to acquire any language.

b. Acquired language disability.

c. Delayed language acquisition.

2. Often the result of trauma or a neurologic disorder.

Analyze Cues and Prioritize Hypotheses

The most important problems relate to developmental disorders and are associated with the skills of reading, writing, and arithmetic.

Nursing Interventions: Take Action

Goal: To identify specific developmental disorders in relationship to chronologic age in preschool testing.

Goal: To refer child to appropriate developmental program in school.

INTEGUMENTARY

🍦 Acne Vulgaris

Acne is an inflammatory disorder of the sebaceous glands and their hair follicles.

Assessment: Recognize Cues

A. Risk factors/etiology.

1. More common in teenagers; may persist into adulthood.

2. Under hormonal influence during puberty; affected by presence of androgen, which stimulates the sebaceous glands to secrete sebum.

B. Clinical manifestations.

1. Inflammatory papules or pustules; noninflammatory lesions such as open comedones (blackheads) and closed comedones (whiteheads).

2. Cysts: deep nodules that may produce scarring.

3. Most common on the face, neck, and upper back.

Analyze Cues and Prioritize Hypotheses

The most important problems are body image disturbance due to the appearance of the skin lesions and monitoring for infection.

Generate Solutions

Treatment

A. Medical: topical or systemic therapy.

1. Antibacterial and peeling agents: benzoyl peroxide and glycolic acid.

2. Long-term oral antibiotic therapy.

3. Combination therapy (both oral and topical is common).

4. Isotretinoin—derivative of vitamin A, may cause serious side effects; may be teratogenic; contraindicated during pregnancy. Client will require two forms of birth control during course of therapy and monitoring (e.g., liver, triglycerides, symptoms of depression).

🕯️Home Care

A. Instruct client to cleanse face twice daily but to avoid overcleansing.

B. May use a polyester sponge pad to cleanse because it provides mechanical removal of the epidermal layer.

C. Instruct client to keep hands away from face and to avoid any friction or trauma to the area; avoid propping hands against face, rubbing face, etc. Make sure client recognizes that picking and squeezing lesions will worsen condition.

D. Emphasize the importance of a nutritious diet; encourage adequate food intake and use of vitamin A.

E. Avoid the use of cosmetics, shaving creams, and lotions because they may exacerbate acne; if cosmetics are to be used, water-based makeup is preferable.

F. Instruct the client to administer medication appropriately: topical application; avoid sunlight while using medications, etc.

🍦 Atopic Dermatitis

Atopic dermatitis (also called *eczema*) is a superficial, chronic inflammatory disorder associated with allergy, with a hereditary tendency. The condition commonly occurs during infancy, usually between 2 and 6 months of age, and often persists into adulthood.

Assessment: Recognize Cues

A. Symptoms are similar with both adults and children: reddened lesions occur on the cheeks, arms, and legs in infants and children and in the antecubital and popliteal space in adults; lesions may have oozing vesicles.

B. Intense itching (worse at night).

C. As the child gets older, the lesions tend to be dry with a thickening of the skin (lichenification).

D. Infants with eczema are more likely to have allergies as children and adults and are at increased risk for developing asthma.

Analyze Cues and Prioritize Hypotheses

The most important problems are intense itching and potential for infection.

Generate Solutions

Treatment

A. Milk, eggs, wheat, and peanuts are the most commonly suspected causes in children; food allergies are not associated with adult atopic dermatitis.

B. Pruritus is treated with oral antihistamines, topical steroids, and topical immunomodulators.

C. Systemic steroids are prescribed if condition is severe.

D. Antibiotics may be needed if secondary infection occurs.

🕯️Home Care

A. Teach parents about dietary restrictions; provide them with written guidelines.

B. Keep fingernails and toenails cut short.

C. Feed the child when well rested and not itching.

D. Assist parents to identify foods that contain eggs, milk, and other "hidden" allergenic foods.

E. Avoid overheating; decrease likelihood of perspiration (no nylon clothing).

F. Child should avoid contact with persons who have the chickenpox virus or herpes simplex.

G. Monitor client receiving immunizations with live vaccines because of the possibility of severe reactions.

H. Child should wear nonirritating clothing; wool and abrasive fabrics should be avoided.

I. Tepid bath with mild soap or an emulsifying oil followed immediately by application of an emollient; cool compresses decrease itching.

J. Teach adults to avoid things that cause a flare-up of the condition and to treat symptoms with topical medication when they occur.

> ❗ **NURSING PRIORITY** Apply emollients (medications) to treat dry skin immediately after bathing while skin is slightly moist.

Contact Dermatitis

Contact dermatitis is an inflammatory skin reaction that results because the skin has come in contact with a specific irritant or allergen. Diaper dermatitis occurs after prolonged contact with urine, feces, ointments, soaps, or friction. Allergic contact dermatitis is usually a symptom of delayed hypersensitivity.

Assessment: Recognize Cues

A. Risk factors/etiology.
   1. Poison ivy, poison sumac, and poison oak; fabrics such as wool, polyester.
   2. Cosmetics; household products such as detergents, soap, hair dye.
   3. Industrial substances: paints, dyes, insecticides, rubber compounds, etc.
   4. Prolonged contact with diaper wetness, fecal enzymes, increased skin pH due to urine, friction/irritation.

B. Clinical manifestations.
   1. Pruritus; hive-like red papules, vesicles, and plaques (more chronic).
   2. Sharply circumscribed areas (with occasional vesicle formation) that crust and ooze.
   3. Often pruritic.

C. Diagnostics.
   1. Skin testing to determine allergen.

Analyze Cues and Prioritize Hypotheses

The most important problems are itching, discomfort, and potential for infection.

Generate Solutions
Treatment

A. Medical.
   1. Eliminate allergen.
   2. Topical steroids; oral steroids for severe cases.
   3. Antihistamines, antipruritic agents, and antifungals (diaper dermatitis).
   4. Skin lubrication.

Home Care

A. Teach importance of washing exposed skin with cool water and soap as soon as possible after exposure (within 15 minutes is best).

B. Provide cool, tepid bath; trim fingernails; and use measures to control itching.

C. Teach about fallacy of blister fluid spreading the disease.

D. Change diaper frequently, keep skin dry, and use protective ointment (zinc oxide or petrolatum).

> ❗ **PEDIATRIC PRIORITY** Talc powders may keep skin dry, but they are harmful if breathed. Plain cornstarch is safer to use.

Impetigo

Impetigo is a bacterial skin infection caused by invasion of the epidermis by pathogenic Staphylococcus aureus and/ or group A beta-hemolytic streptococci and occurring most often in children age 2 to 5 years.

Assessment: Recognize Cues

A. Pustule-like lesions with moist honey-colored crusts surrounded by redness.

B. Pruritus; spreads to surrounding areas.

C. May appear anywhere on the body but most commonly on the face, especially around the mouth.

Analyze Cues and Prioritize Hypotheses

The most important problems are contagiousness of the lesion and discomfort.

Generate Solutions
Treatment

A. Medical.
   1. Local: topical treatment.
      a. Warm soaks with water or aluminum acetate solution. Gently wash two to three times a day to remove crusts.
      b. Use topical mupirocin antibiotic cream if only a couple of lesions are found.
   2. Systemic antibiotic therapy is the treatment of choice with extensive lesions.

Home Care

A. Teach the client and family the importance of good handwashing and assure them that lesions heal without scarring.

B. Encourage adherence to therapeutic regimen, especially taking the full course of antibiotics.

C. Untreated impetigo may result in systemic infection and glomerulonephritis.

D. Empirically treat the nares of *Staphylococcus* carriers with mupirocin to prevent spread/reinfection.

Fungal (Dermatophyte) Infections

The nails, skin, and hair can become infected with fungi because there is a large number of fungi present in the environment.

Assessment: Recognize Cues

A. Types.
   1. Tinea corporis (ringworm): causes a ring-shaped lesion on the skin; temporary hair loss may occur if scalp is affected; seen when there is close physical contact (i.e., wrestlers).

2. Tinea capitis: scaly patches on scalp; areas of alopecia; pruritus; most common fungal infection in pediatrics.
3. Tinea cruris (jock itch): small, red, scaly patches in the groin area.
4. Tinea pedis (athlete's foot): scaling, maceration, erythema, blistering, and pruritus; usually found between the toes; may be painful.
5. Tinea unguium (onychomycosis): thickened, crumbling nails (usually toes) with yellowish discoloration.
6. Candidiasis: caused by *Candida albicans*, known as moniliasis or thrush and often called a yeast infection; may affect oral mucosa, vulvovaginal, and rectal areas; causes white plaques in mouth; diffuse red rash with pinpoint satellite lesions on skin.

Analyze Cues and Prioritize Hypotheses

The most important problems are transmission of fungal infection, itching, and discomfort.

Generate Solutions

Treatment
A. Topical antifungal cream (see Appendix 13.2).
B. Oral antifungal medication.
C. Systemic therapy: griseofulvin; used primarily for extensive cases.

Home Care

A. To prevent athlete's foot, client should be instructed to keep feet as dry as possible and wear socks made of absorbent cotton.
   1. Talcum powder or antifungal powder may be used; tolnaftate may be applied twice daily.
   2. Encourage aeration of shoes to allow them to completely dry out.
B. Client should maintain hygienic measures to prevent the spread of fungal diseases, specifically ringworm of the scalp.
   1. Family members should avoid using the same comb or hairbrush.
   2. Scarves and hats should be washed thoroughly.
   3. Examine family and household pets frequently for symptoms of the disease.

Parasite Infestations

Parasites **are organisms that live off other organisms, or hosts, to survive and obtain their food from or at the expense of the host. Some parasite infections/infestations are easy to treat and others are not.**

Assessment: Recognize Cues

A. Pediculosis.
   1. Types.
      a. *Pediculus humanus capitis:* head lice.
      b. *Pediculus humanus corporis:* body lice.
      c. *Phthirus pubis:* pubic lice or crabs.
   2. Clinical manifestations.
      a. Intense pruritus, which may lead to secondary excoriation and infection.
      b. Lesions vary by species: head lice (red, noninflammatory papules), body lice (urticarial papule), and pubic lice (gray-blue lesions).
      c. Eggs (nits) of both head and body lice are often attached to the hair shafts.
      d. Pubic lice are often spread by sexual contact.
B. Scabies: an infestation of the skin by *Sarcoptes scabiei* mites.
   1. Intense itching, especially at night.
   2. Burrows are seen, especially between fingers, on the surfaces of wrists, and in axillary folds.
   3. Redness, swelling, and vesicular formation may be noted.
C. Bedbugs: an infestation caused by the *Cimex lectularius*.
   1. Does not live on the human body but survives by feeding on human blood.
   2. Bites resemble a mosquito or flea bite, wheal surrounded by a flare, and cause intense itching.
   3. Often grouped in threes appearing on uncovered parts of the body.

Analyze Cues and Prioritize Hypotheses

The most important problems are transmission of the parasite infection, itching, and discomfort.

Generate Solutions

Treatment
A. Pediculosis.
   1. Permethrin 1% liquid: effective against nits and lice with just one application; shampoo hair first, leave Nix on hair for 10 minutes, rinse off; may repeat in 7 days.
   2. Pyrethrin compounds for pubic and head lice.
B. Scabies.
   1. Permethrin 5% cream; cream is applied to the skin from head to soles of feet and left on for 8 to 14 hours, then washed off, with a repeat application in 7 days.
C. Bedbugs.
   1. Treatment of the bite area is with topical or systemic antihistamines, depending on the extent of the bites.
   2. Bedding should be inspected for infestation of the bugs (about the same size, shape, and color of an apple seed).
   3. Eradication is by washing clothing and linens in hot water and drying on the hot setting.
   4. Bedding and furniture that cannot be washed must be treated by a pest control professional or disposed of.

Home Care

A. All family members and close contacts need to be treated for parasitic disorders; lice can survive up to 48 hours; nits can hatch in 7 to 10 days when shed in the environment.
B. Bedding and clothing that may have lice or nits should be washed or dry cleaned; furniture and rugs should be vacuumed or treated.
C. Nonwashable items should be sealed in a plastic bag for 14 days if unable to dry clean or vacuum.

D. Nurses should wear gloves when examining scalp to prevent spread to others.

E. When shampooing hair, use a fine-tooth comb or tweezers to remove remaining nits.

🎈 Burns

See Chapter 20; pediatric implications are noted with a balloon.

ENDOCRINE

🎈 Congenital Hypothyroidism

Congenital hypothyroidism (formerly known as cretinism) is a deficiency of thyroid hormones present at birth. Symptoms depend on the number of thyroid hormones present at birth.

Assessment: Recognize Cues

A. Condition is not generally evident in the newborn because of thyroid hormones received through the maternal circulation; symptoms usually appear after 6 weeks.

B. Early clinical manifestations.
1. Lethargy; thick, dry, mottled skin.
2. Bradycardia, hypothermia, hypotension, hypotonia, hyporeflexia.
3. Poor feeding.
4. Hypotonic abdominal musculature.
   a. Constipation.
   b. Protruding abdomen (umbilical hernia).

C. Diagnostics.
1. Filter-paper blood-spot thyroxine (T_4) test; if result is low, then a TSH test is done.
2. Mandatory test in all states; should be done within 24 to 48 hours after birth and repeated at 2 weeks of age.

Analyze Cues and Prioritize Hypotheses

The most important problems are early recognition of hormone deficiency and replacement of the hormone to prevent intellectual disability.

Generate Solutions

Treatment

Medical management includes replacement of thyroid hormones. (If replacement is accomplished shortly after birth, it is possible that the child will have normal physical growth and intellectual development.)

Nursing Interventions: Take Action

Goal: To identify neonates experiencing congenital hypothyroidism.

Goal: To assist parents to understand the implications of the disease and requirements for continued health maintenance.

A. Child will require lifelong medication.

B. Continue medical care to evaluate changes in thyroid replacement as the child grows.

🎈 Diabetes Mellitus

See Chapter 9; pediatric implications are noted with a balloon.

HEMATOLOGY

🎈 Sickle Cell Anemia

Sickle cell anemia is an inherited autosomal recessive disorder characterized by the sickling effect of the erythrocytes.

A. Basic defect of the erythrocyte is in the globulin portion of the hemoglobin.

B. Sickling is not apparent until around 6 months of age; the increased levels of fetal hemoglobin up to that age prevent serious sickling problems.

C. Predominantly a problem of children and adolescents. A child may be asymptomatic between crises. The problems from childhood may cause long-term complications as they become adults.

D. Pathologic changes of sickle cell (elongated, crescent-shaped red blood cells [RBCs]) disease result from:
1. Increased blood viscosity.
2. Increased RBC destruction.
3. Increased viscosity of the blood and sickling eventually precipitates ischemia and tissue necrosis caused by capillary stasis and thrombosis.
4. Cycle of occlusion, ischemia, and infarction to vascular organs, especially the spleen, liver, and kidneys.

E. Conditions precipitating sickling effect triggered by low oxygen tension in the blood.
1. Dehydration, acidosis, hypoxia.
2. Viral or bacterial infection (most common).
3. High altitude; extremes in environmental and body temperatures.
4. Emotional or physical stress or surgery.
5. Nicotine use.

F. Pathologic effects of sickle cell disease on pregnancy.
1. Mother.
   a. Increased anemia problems.
   b. Increase in thromboembolic problems.
   c. Increased risk for preeclampsia.
2. Infant.
   a. Small for gestational age (SGA).
   b. Spontaneous abortion.
   c. Fetal distress caused by hypoxia.

G. Multiple body systems are involved.

> **⧗ NURSING PRIORITY** Because pregnant women with sickle cell anemia are not iron deficient, they should avoid taking iron supplements, even those found in prenatal vitamins.

Assessment: Recognize Cues

A. Risk factors/etiology.
1. Autosomal recessive disorder (see Chapter 26).
   a. Normal hemoglobin (HgbA) is replaced by abnormal sickle hemoglobin (HgbS).
   b. Presence of HgbS in 35 to 45% of hemoglobin indicates sickle cell trait.
2. May occur in persons of African American, Mediterranean, Caribbean, Arabian, East Indian, and Hispanic descent.

B. Clinical manifestations: primarily the result of obstruction caused by sickled RBCs and by increased RBC destruction.

SICKLE CELL ANEMIA CRISIS
(Inherited Red Blood Cell Disorder)

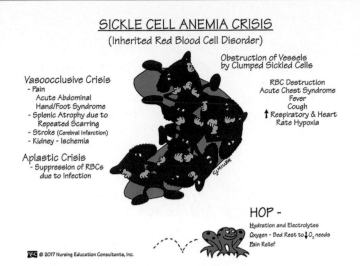

Vasoocclusive Crisis
- Pain
  Acute Abdominal
  Hand/Foot Syndrome
- Splenic Atrophy due to
  Repeated Scarring
- Stroke (Cerebral Infarction)
- Kidney - Ischemia

Aplastic Crisis
- Suppression of RBCs
  due to Infection

Obstruction of Vessels
by Clumped Sickled Cells

RBC Destruction
Acute Chest Syndrome
Fever
Cough
↑ Respiratory & Heart
Rate Hypoxia

HOP -
Hydration and Electrolytes
Oxygen - Bed Rest to ↓ O₂ needs
Pain Relief

© 2017 Nursing Education Consultants, Inc.

FIG. 22.2 Sickle Cell Anemia Crisis. (From Zerwekh, J., Garneau, A., & Miller, C. J. [2017]. *Digital collection of the memory notebooks of nursing* [4th ed.]. Nursing Education Consultants.)

1. Splenomegaly: caused by congestion and engorgement with sickled cells; decreases immune response.
2. Liver failure, hepatomegaly, and necrosis from severe impairment of hepatic blood flow.
3. Jaundice, pale mucous membranes, fatigue, fever, and intense pain.
4. Kidney damage caused by the congestion of glomerular capillaries and tubular arterioles.
5. Skeletal changes caused by hyperplasia and congestion of bone marrow.

C. Crisis: often precipitated by an infection or dehydration; can occur spontaneously (Fig. 22.2).
   1. Vaso-occlusive crisis: blood flow is impaired by sickled cells, causing ischemia and pain.
      a. Extremities: occlusions in the small distal vessels of the hands and the feet, characterized by pain, swelling, and decreased function (hand–foot syndrome).
      b. Abdomen: severe abdominal pain.
      c. Pulmonary: symptoms of pneumonia.
      d. Renal: hematuria.
      e. Central nervous system: visual problems.
   2. Sequestration crisis: pooling of the blood in the liver and spleen, with decreased blood volume.

> **TEST ALERT** Recognize occurrence of a hemorrhage; plan and implement nursing care to prevent complications; notify health care provider regarding signs of potential complications.

D. Diagnostics: early diagnosis, before 2 months of age, helps minimize complications.
   1. Hemoglobin electrophoresis indicates the presence and percentage of HgbS.
   2. Sickle turbidity tests (SICKLEDEX) used for screening.

Analyze Cues and Prioritize Hypotheses

The most important problems are pain, joint destruction, potential for infection, multiple organ dysfunction syndrome, and death.

Generate Solutions

Treatment

A. Prevention of the sickling problem.
   1. Adequate hydration.
   2. Prevent infections, especially respiratory tract infections; pneumococcal and influenza vaccines are recommended.
   3. Clients generally do not require iron because of increased resorption.
   4. Daily folic acid supplement.
   5. Hydroxyurea to increase the production of HgbF, thereby reducing hemolysis and the number of sickled cells.
   6. Oxygen: assists in preventing a crisis in clients with respiratory problems, but it does not reverse a sickling crisis or reduce pain; client should avoid high altitudes.
B. Treatment of crisis.
   1. Bed rest, deep vein thrombosis prophylaxis (using anticoagulants), hydration, antibiotics.
   2. Analgesics for pain; supplemental oxygen as needed.
   3. Blood transfusions and/or exchange transfusions (see Appendix 16.3).
C. Surgery: splenectomy for severe splenic sequestration.

Complications

A. With repeated sickling episodes, organs that have high need for oxygen are most affected.
B. Infection, especially pneumonia.

Nursing Interventions: Take Action

Goal: To prevent sickle cell disease.
A. Participate in community screening programs and education for high-risk population.
B. Refer persons who are carriers (autosomal recessive trait) for genetic counseling.

Goal: To prevent sickling crisis.
A. Maintain adequate hydration; intravenous (IV) fluids may be necessary.
B. Promote respiratory health and tissue oxygenation; avoiding crowds, inhaling irritants, and routine exercise.
C. Prevent infection; promote thorough hand hygiene.
D. Hydroxyurea: reduces sickling episodes; a long-term complication is leukemia.

Goal: To control pain.
A. Assessment of involved area (severity scale 1–10, location, quality).
B. Appropriate analgesics: meperidine is not recommended; morphine, hydromorphone, fentanyl, or methadone may be used; patient-controlled analgesia (PCA) devices are frequently used to control pain.
C. NSAIDs and antiseizure medications may also be used for pain control.
D. Allow client to assume a position of comfort.
   1. Passive range of motion may be beneficial.
   2. No active or passive range of motion if client is actively bleeding into joints.
E. Maintain rest if movement exacerbates pain.

TEST ALERT Determine effectiveness of pain control. Care of the child with sickle cell disease frequently centers around this (see Chapter 3).

Goal: To maintain adequate hydration and oxygenation.

A. Evaluate adequacy of hydration; assess skin turgor; monitor urine output, thirst mechanism.

B. Low urine specific gravity may not be indicative of fluid balance if there is renal involvement; monitor blood urea nitrogen (BUN), creatinine, and urine specific gravity.

C. Monitor IV fluid administration; normal saline often given first in crises.

D. Maintain accurate intake and output records; assess daily weight, signs of fluid overload with replacement.

E. Evaluate electrolyte balance; monitor laboratory values, replace deficiencies.

F. Administer oxygen as indicated; monitor arterial blood gases (ABGs) and/or O_2 saturation.

G. Provide good pulmonary hygiene.

H. Assess for metabolic acidosis.

TEST ALERT Monitor hydration status; evaluate client's response to parenteral administration of fluids.

Goal: To identify complication of affected organs—systematic evaluation of client to identify problems discussed in section on clinical manifestations.

Home Care

A. Increase fluids with physical activity and/or if living in excessively hot or cold climates.

B. Seek early intervention for symptoms of infection, especially respiratory tract infection; report temperature elevations, coughing, or pain.

C. Encourage normal growth and developmental activities as tolerated by the child.

D. Client with sickle cell disease should avoid situations that may precipitate hypoxia.
   1. Traveling to high-altitude areas.
   2. Flying in an unpressurized aircraft.
   3. Participating in overly strenuous exercise.

E. Inform family that child should wear medic-alert bracelet.

TEST ALERT Compare physical development of client with normal development. Chronically ill children are frequently slower in growth and development; care is provided for the developmental level, not the chronologic age.

Hemophilia

Hemophilia is a genetic disorder caused by a defect in the clotting mechanism. Classically, there are two types, distinguishable only by laboratory tests. Clinically, the two types are the same, but both may occur in varying degrees of severity. The disease is most often recognized during the toddler stage (Fig. 22.3).

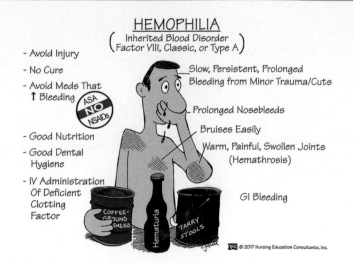

FIG. 22.3 Hemophilia. (From Zerwekh, J., Garneau, A., & Miller, C. J. [2017]. *Digital collection of the memory notebooks of nursing* [4th ed.]. Nursing Education Consultants.)

A. Hemophilia A: factor VIII deficiency (classic hemophilia).

B. Hemophilia B: factor IX deficiency (Christmas disease).

Assessment: Recognize Cues

A. Risk factors/etiology: both types of hemophilia are sex-linked recessive disorders.
   1. Family history of hemophilia.
   2. Primarily affects males; females are carriers.

B. Clinical manifestations.
   1. Persistent or prolonged bleeding that occurs from minor trauma/insults.
   2. Hemarthrosis: bleeding into joint cavities.
   3. Spontaneous hematuria.
   4. Hematoma.
   5. Intracranial hemorrhage may be fatal.
   6. Petechiae are uncommon because platelet count is normal.

C. Diagnostics.
   1. History of bleeding episodes.
   2. Family inheritance pattern.
   3. Identification of deficient factor (factor assay).
   4. Partial thromboplastin time (PTT), bleeding time.

Analyze Cues and Prioritize Hypotheses

The most important problems are prolonged bleeding due to missing clotting factor, hemarthrosis, potential intracranial hemorrhage, anemia due to bleeding into gastrointestinal (GI) tract, and paralysis due to hematomas in the spinal cord.

Generate Solutions

Treatment

A. Intravenous administration of the specific coagulation factor the client is lacking. Monitor the client for signs and symptoms of possible mild or severe (anaphylactic) allergic reaction.

B. Desmopressin (DDAVP): synthetic vasopressin used to treat mild cases; given IV or intranasally.

C. Aminocaproic acid and tranexamic acid—antifibrinolytic agents used to prevent recurrent bleeds rather than treat acute, ongoing bleeds.

D. Treatment may be carried out at home.

Nursing Interventions: Take Action

Goal: To prevent spontaneous bleeding episodes (see Box 16.1).

A. Decrease risk for injury.
   1. Make environment as safe as possible without hampering motor development.
   2. Instruct client to avoid contact sports but encourage noncontact sports (e.g., swimming).
   3. Regular exercise and physical therapy to promote muscle strength around joints and decrease bleeding episodes.
B. Preventive dental care and prevent oral infections.
C. Maintain normal weight; increased weight causes increased strain on the joints.
D. Avoid any aspirin compounds or NSAIDs.
E. Administer clotting factors before, during, and after invasive medical procedures.
F. Child with a bleeding disorder should wear medic-alert bracelet.

Goal: To recognize and treat bleeding episodes.

A. Apply pressure to the area.
B. Immobilize and elevate the joints involved.
C. Do not perform passive range of motion on affected joints.
D. Apply cold pack to promote vasoconstriction.
E. Observe for signs of internal bleeding: tarry stools, slurred speech, headache.
F. Administer clotting factors in a timely manner.

Goal: To prepare client and family to administer clotting factors intravenously at home.

A. Correct technique for venipuncture.
B. Indications for use.
C. Encourage child to learn self-administration, generally around age 9 to 12 years.

Goal: To prevent permanent joint degeneration.

A. Elevate joint and immobilize during acute bleeding episode.
B. Encourage active range of motion so child will limit movement based on pain tolerance.
C. Physical therapy after the acute phase, no weight bearing until swelling has resolved.
D. Maintain pain relief during physical therapy.

> ! **NURSING PRIORITY** Apply RICE to the affected joints: rest, ice, compression, elevation.

Home Care

A. Have client and family demonstrate ability to perform IV initiation and administration.
B. Have client and family discuss situations that call for use of IV infusion of deficient factor: endoscopy, dental work, etc.

C. Discuss with family the importance of routine prophylactic dental checkups.
D. Encourage venting of feelings regarding diagnosis of the disease.
E. Encourage counseling for parents regarding concern and guilt over hereditary disorder.

> **TEST ALERT** Modify approaches in care based on child's development; determine family's understanding of the causes and/or consequences of the client's illness and ability to provide care; assist family in crisis.

🎈 Iron Deficiency Anemia, Leukemia

See Chapter 16; pediatric implications are noted with a balloon.

RESPIRATORY

🎈 Croup Syndromes

The term *croup* describes a group of conditions characterized by edema and inflammation of the upper respiratory tract.

Assessment: Recognize Cues

A. Acute epiglottitis: a severe bacterial infection of the epiglottis characterized by rapid inflammation and edema of the area; generally occurs in children age 2 to 5 years; may rapidly cause airway obstruction.
   1. Cause: most commonly *Haemophilus influenzae*.
   2. Clinical manifestations: hypoxia.
      a. Rapid, abrupt onset.
      b. Sore throat, difficulty swallowing.
      c. Inflamed epiglottis.
      d. Symptoms of increasing respiratory tract obstruction.
         (1) Characteristic position: sitting with the neck hyperextended (sniffing position) and mouth open (tripod position), drooling.
         (2) Inspiratory stridor (crowing).
         (3) Suprasternal and substernal retractions.
         (4) Increased restlessness and apprehension.
      e. High fever (greater than 102°F).

> ! **NURSING PRIORITY** The absence of spontaneous cough and the presence of drooling and agitation are cardinal signs distinctive of epiglottitis. Do not put tongue blade or culture swab into the mouth or throat; can cause airway obstruction.

   3. Treatment.
      a. Endotracheal intubation for obstruction (see Appendix 17.5).
      b. Humidified oxygen, IV fluids.
      c. Antibiotics: IV and then by mouth (PO).
B. Acute laryngotracheobronchitis (croup): inflammation of the larynx and trachea, most often in children under 5 years of age.
   1. Cause: viral agents (influenza and parainfluenza viruses, respiratory syncytial virus).

Table 22.1 SYMPTOMS OF RESPIRATORY DISTRESS AND HYPOXIA IN PEDIATRICS

Early Symptoms	Late Symptoms
Restlessness	Cyanosis (peripheral or central)
Flaring nares (infants)	
Substernal, suprasternal, supraclavicular, and intercostal retractions	Mottling, pallor, and cyanosis
	Sudden increase or sudden decrease in agitation
Stridor—expiratory and inspiratory	Inaudible breath sounds
	Altered level of consciousness
Increased agitation	Inability to cry or to speak
Disorientation	

2. Slow onset, frequently preceded by upper respiratory tract infection.
3. Respiratory distress (see Table 22.1).
    a. Inspiratory stridor when disturbed, progressing to continuous stridor.
    b. Flaring of nares, use of accessory muscles of respiration.
    c. "Seal bark" cough is classic sign.
4. Low-grade fever (usually less than 102°F [38.8°C]).
5. Signs of impending obstruction.
    a. Retractions (intercostals, suprasternal, and substernal) at rest.
    b. Increased anxiety and restlessness.
    c. Tachypnea (rate may be greater than 60 breaths/min).
    d. Pallor and diaphoresis.
    e. Nasal flaring.

TEST ALERT Intervene when vital signs are abnormal; position client to prevent complications; interpret client data that need to be reported immediately.

6. Treatment.
    a. Maintain patent airway.
    b. Bronchodilators, racemic epinephrine (for moderate to severe croup) by inhalation.
    c. Cool-mist humidification.
    d. No sedatives.
    e. Heliox (mixture of oxygen and helium) for moderate to severe croup.
    f. Corticosteroids, administered intravenously, intramuscularly, or orally.
C. Acute spasmodic laryngitis: mildest form of croup; generally occurs in children 1 to 3 years old.
    1. Cause: viral with an allergy component.
    2. Clinical manifestations.
        a. Characterized by paroxysmal attacks.
        b. Characteristically occurs suddenly at night.
        c. Mild respiratory distress (see Table 22.1).
        d. No fever.
        e. After the attack, the child appears well.
    3. Treatment:
        a. Child is generally cared for at home.

b. Usually self-limiting.
c. Cool mist or humidity may decrease spasm.

Analyze Cues and Prioritize Hypotheses
The most important problems are hypoxemia, tachypnea, and inadequate oral fluid intake.

Nursing Interventions: Take Action
Goal: To maintain patent airway in hospitalized child.
A. Tracheotomy set or endotracheal intubation equipment readily available.

! NURSING PRIORITY For a child with suspected epiglottitis, do not examine the throat with a tongue depressor or take a throat culture; have child seen by primary care provider immediately. Resuscitation equipment and suction should be readily available.

B. Suction endotracheal tube or tracheotomy only as necessary.
C. Position for comfort; do not force child to lie down.
D. If child is intubated, do not leave unattended.
E. If obstruction is impending, maintain ventilation with a bag-valve-mask resuscitator until child can be intubated.
F. If transport is required, allow the child to sit upright in parent's lap, if possible.
Goal: To evaluate and maintain adequate ventilation.
A. Assess for increasing hypoxia.
B. Provide humidified O$_2$; closely evaluate because cyanosis is a late sign of hypoxia.
C. Conserve energy; prevent crying.
D. Monitor pulse oximetry for adequate oxygenation.
Goal: To maintain hydration and nutrition.
A. Administer IV fluids.
B. Do not give oral fluids until danger of aspiration is past.

TEST ALERT Identify client potential for aspiration. In children with severe respiratory distress (rate greater than 60), do not give anything by mouth because of increased risk for aspiration.

C. Give IV fluids during acute episodes.
D. Provide high-calorie liquids when danger of aspiration is over.
E. Suction nares of infant before feeding.
F. Assess for adequate hydration.

Home Care

A. Teach parents to recognize symptoms of increasing respiratory problems and when to notify health care provider.
B. Cool mist may assist to decrease edema and/or spasms of airway.
C. Maintain adequate fluid intake.
D. Immunization with *H. influenza* type B vaccine.

Bronchiolitis (Respiratory Syncytial Virus)
Bronchiolitis is an inflammation of the bronchioles; alveoli are usually normal.

A. Respiratory syncytial virus (RSV) infection is most common in winter and spring (November to March); peaks in children 2 to 12 months old, rare after 2 years.

B. RSV is transmitted by direct contact with respiratory secretions.

C. RSV is considered the single most important respiratory pathogen of infancy and early childhood.

Assessment: Recognize Cues

A. Cause: usually begins after an upper respiratory tract infection; incubation period of 2 to 8 days.

B. Reinfection is common; severity tends to decrease with age and repeated infections.

C. Clinical manifestations.
1. Initial.
   a. Rhinorrhea and low-grade fever commonly occur first.
   b. Coughing, wheezing.
2. Acute phase.
   a. Lethargic.
   b. Tachypnea, air hunger, retractions.
   c. Increased wheezing and coughing.
   d. Periods of apnea; poor air exchange.

D. Diagnostics: nasal secretions for RSV antigens.

Analyze Cues and Prioritize Hypotheses

The most important problems are hypoxemia, tachypnea, and inadequate oral fluid intake.

Generate Solutions

Treatment

A. Rest, fluids, and high-humidity environment.

B. Oxygen via heated, high-flow nasal cannula (HHFNC), which adds extra humidity; can add positive pressure.

C. Prevention—medication: palivizumab (once every 30 days for high-risk children).

D. Treatment—medication: ribavirin (high cost, potentially toxic to caregivers, controversial).

Nursing Interventions: Take Action

Goal: To promote effective breathing patterns.

A. Frequent assessment for development of hypoxia; close monitoring of O$_2$ saturation (oximetry) levels.

B. Increase in respiratory rate and audible crackles in the lungs are indications of cardiac failure and should be reported immediately.

C. Maintain airway via position and removal of secretions.

D. Maintain adequate hydration to facilitate removal of respiratory secretions.

E. Conserve energy; avoid unnecessary procedures but encourage parents to console and cuddle infant.

Goal: To prevent transmission of organisms.

A. If hospitalized, the child should be placed in a private room or a room with another RSV child, with contact precautions in place (see Appendix 9.3).

B. Decrease number of health care personnel in client's room.

C. Nurses assigned to care for these children should not be assigned the care of other children who are at high risk for respiratory tract infections.

D. Prophylaxis medication with palivizumab for high-risk infants.

Home Care

A. Decreased energy level; will tire easily.

B. Small, frequent feedings.

C. Teach parents how to assess for respiratory difficulty.

D. Teach parents care implications if child is receiving prophylactic medications (see Appendix 17.2).

Tonsillitis

Tonsillitis **is an inflammation and infection of the palatine tonsils.**

Assessment: Recognize Cues

A. Risk factors/etiology.
1. More common in children.
2. Increased severity in adults.

B. Clinical manifestations.
1. Edematous, enlarged tonsils; exudate on tonsils.
2. Difficulty swallowing and breathing.
3. Frequently precipitates otitis media or difficulty hearing.
4. Mouth breathing, persistent cough, fever.

C. Diagnostics: throat culture for group A beta-hemolytic streptococci.

Analyze Cues and Prioritize Hypotheses

The most important problems are hemorrhage, potential airway obstruction, and inadequate nutrition and oral fluid intake.

Generate Solutions

Treatment

A. Antibiotic for identified organism.

B. Surgery: tonsillectomy for severe repeated episodes of tonsillitis once acute infectious episode is resolved.

Nursing Interventions: Take Action

Goal: To promote comfort and healing in home environment (Fig. 22.4).

A. Nonirritating soft or liquid diet.

B. Cool-mist vaporizer to maintain moisture in mucous membranes.

C. Throat lozenges, warm gargles to soothe the throat.

D. Antibiotics: important to give child all of the medication prescribed to prevent reoccurrence.

E. Analgesics, antipyretic (acetaminophen).

Goal: To provide preoperative nursing measures if surgery is indicated (see Chapter 3).

Goal: To maintain patent airway and evaluate for bleeding after tonsillectomy.

A. No fluids until child is fully awake; then cool, clear liquids initially. Avoid brown- or red-colored fluids and milk products.

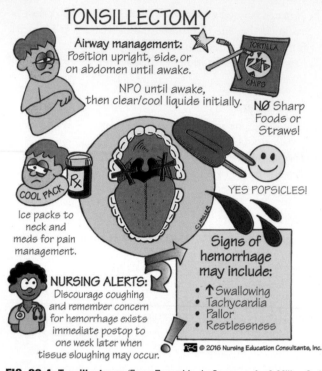

FIG. 22.4 Tonsillectomy. (From Zerwekh, J., Garneau, A., & Miller, C. J. [2017]. *Digital collection of the memory notebooks of nursing* [4th ed.]. Nursing Education Consultants.)

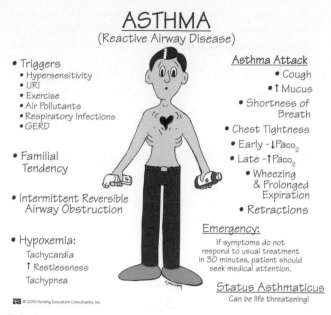

FIG. 22.5 Asthma. (From Zerwekh, J., Garneau, A., & Miller, C. J. [2017]. *Digital collection of the memory notebooks of nursing* [4th ed.]. Nursing Education Consultants.)

B. Position child on side or abdomen to facilitate drainage until fully awake; when awake and alert, child may assume position of comfort but needs to remain in bed for the day.

C. Evaluate for frequent or continuous swallowing or clearing of throat caused by bleeding; check throat with flashlight for bleeding.

D. Have nasopharyngeal suction equipment available.

E. Monitor for tachycardia, pallor, and increasing restlessness.

F. Apply ice collar to decrease edema.

G. Give oral acetaminophen (with codeine or hydrocodone, if needed) for pain; aspirin is contraindicated.

H. Discourage coughing.

I. Do not use straws for drinks.

> **⚠ NURSING PRIORITY** Before the child is fully awake, position on side or abdomen to prevent aspiration from bloody drainage or vomitus. Always consider the client who has had a tonsillectomy to be nauseated as a result of swallowing blood.

Home Care

A. Child will have sore throat for several days; discourage coughing and excessive activity.

B. Symptoms of bleeding are especially significant on the fifth to tenth postoperative days, when tissue sloughing may occur as a result of healing and/or infection.

C. Maintain adequate hydration; encourage intake of soft foods and nonirritating fluids.

D. A gray membrane on the sides of the throat is normal and should disappear in 1 to 2 weeks.

Asthma

Asthma **is an intermittent, reversible obstructive airway problem. It is characterized by exacerbations and remissions. Between attacks the client is generally asymptomatic. It is a common disorder of childhood but may also cause problems throughout adult life (Fig. 22.5).**

A. A chronic inflammatory process producing bronchial wall edema and inflammation, increased mucus secretion, and smooth muscle contraction.

B. Intermittent narrowing of the airway is caused by:
  1. Constriction of the smooth muscles of the bronchi and the bronchioles (bronchospasm).
  2. Excessive mucus production.
  3. Mucosal edema of the respiratory tract.

C. Constriction of the smooth muscle causes significant increase in airway resistance, thereby trapping air in the lungs.

D. Emotional factors are known to play an important role in precipitating childhood asthma attacks.

E. Exercise-induced asthma: initially after exercise there is an improvement in the respiratory status, followed by a significant decline; occurs in the majority of clients; may be worse in cold, dry air and better in warm, moist air.

Assessment: Recognize Cues

A. Risk factors/etiology.
  1. Hypersensitivity (allergens) and airway inflammation.
  2. Exercise.
  3. Air pollutants and occupational factors.
  4. Pediatric implications.

a. *Reactive airway disease* is the term used to describe asthma in children.

b. General onset before age 3 years.

c. Children are more likely to have airway obstruction.

B. Diagnostics (see Appendix 17.1).

1. Pulmonary function studies/tests (PFTs).

2. History of hypersensitivity reactions (history of eczema in children).

3. Increased serum eosinophil count.

C. Clinical manifestations: *early-phase reactions* occur immediately and last about an hour; *late-phase reactions* do not begin until 4 to 8 hours after exposure and may last for hours or as long as 2 days; attacks may begin gradually or abruptly.

1. Episodic wheezing, chest tightness, shortness of breath, persistent cough.

2. Use of accessory muscles in breathing; orthopnea.

3. Symptoms of hypoxia; cyanosis occurs late.

4. Increased anxiety, restlessness, diaphoresis.

5. Difficulty speaking; thick tenacious sputum.

PEDIATRIC PRIORITY Children who are sweating profusely and refuse to lie down are more ill than children who lie quietly. Parents should seek immediate medical attention if a child does not respond to early treatment of an asthma attack.

D. Complications: status asthmaticus is severe asthma unresponsive to initial or conventional treatment.

Analyze Cues and Prioritize Hypotheses

The most important problems are airway obstruction, bronchial hyperresponsiveness, and recurring symptoms.

Generate Solutions

Treatment

A. Medications (see Appendix 17.2).

1. Beta$_2$-adrenergic agonists (short-acting and long-acting) administered by nebulizer or metered-dose inhaler.

2. Antibiotics, if infection is present.

3. Bronchodilators, expectorants.

4. Inhaled steroids and antiinflammatory drugs to prevent and/or decrease edema.

5. Supplemental O$_2$ to maintain Sao$_2$ at 90%.

B. Status asthmaticus.

1. Oxygen, IV fluids for hydration.

2. May require intubation and mechanical ventilation (Appendix 17.8).

3. IV bronchodilators and steroids.

C. Medications to avoid for the client with asthma.

1. Beta-adrenergic blockers cause bronchoconstriction.

2. Cough suppressants, antihistamines.

NURSING PRIORITY Using a spacer device allows more medication to reach its site of action in the lungs with less deposited in the mouth and throat.

Nursing Interventions: Take Action

See Nursing Interventions for hypoxia.

Goal: To relieve asthma attacks.

A. Position for comfort: usually high-Fowler position or tripod position.

B. Close monitoring of response to O$_2$ therapy: Sao$_2$ levels and changes in respiratory status.

C. Assess response to bronchodilators and aerosol therapy.

D. Carefully monitor ability to take PO fluids; risk for aspiration is increased.

E. Observe for sudden increase or decrease in restlessness; either may indicate an abrupt decrease in oxygenation.

F. Assess for side effects of medications, such as tremors and tachycardia.

NURSING PRIORITY Determine changes in a client's respiratory status: the inability to hear wheezing breath sounds in the client with asthma in acute respiratory distress may be an indication of impending respiratory obstruction.

Home Care

A. Assess emotional factors precipitating asthma attacks.

B. Educate client and family regarding identifying and avoiding allergens.

C. Implement therapeutic measures before attack becomes severe.

D. Explain purposes of prescribed medications and how to use them correctly (see Appendix 17.2).

E. Administer bronchodilators before performing postural drainage.

F. Use bronchodilators and warm up before exercise to prevent exercise-induced asthma.

G. Encourage participation in "quiet" activities according to developmental level.

Cystic Fibrosis

Cystic fibrosis **is a chromosomal abnormality characterized by a generalized dysfunction of the exocrine glands. The disease primarily affects the lungs, pancreas, and sweat glands.**

A. The factor responsible for the multiple clinical manifestations of the disease process is the mechanical obstruction caused by thick mucus secretions.

B. Effects of disease process.

1. Pulmonary system: bronchial and bronchiolar obstruction by thick mucus, causing atelectasis and reduced area for gas exchange; the thick mucus provides an excellent medium for bacterial growth and secondary respiratory tract infections.

2. Pancreas: decreased absorption of nutrients caused by the obstruction of pancreatic ducts and lack of adequate enzymes for digestion.

3. Sweat glands: excretion of excess amounts of sodium and chloride.

Assessment: Recognize Cues

A. Risk factors/etiology.

1. Inherited as an autosomal recessive trait.
2. Most common in Caucasians.
B. Clinical manifestations.
   1. Wide variation in severity and extent of manifestations, as well as period of onset.
   2. GI tract.
      a. May present with meconium ileus in the newborn.
      b. Increased bulk in feces from undigested foods.
      c. Increased fat in stools (steatorrhea); foul smelling.
      d. Decreased absorption of nutrients: weight loss or failure to thrive.
      e. Increased appetite caused by decreased absorption of nutrients.
      f. Abdominal distention.
      g. Rectal prolapse related to the large bulky stools and loss of supportive tissue around rectum.
      h. Vitamin A, D, E, and K deficiency.
   3. Genital tract.
      a. In females the increased viscosity of cervical mucus may lead to decreased fertility due to blockage of sperm.
      b. Males are generally sterile because of absence or obstruction of the vas deferens.
   4. Respiratory tract.
      a. Evidence of respiratory tract involvement generally occurs in early childhood.
      b. Increasing dyspnea, tachypnea.
      c. Paroxysmal, chronic productive cough.
      d. Pulmonary inflammation: chronic bronchiolitis and bronchitis.
      e. Symptoms of chronic hypoxia: clubbing, barrel chest.
      f. Mucus provides excellent medium for bacteria growth and chronic infections.
   5. Excessive salt on the skin: "salty taste when kissed."
C. Diagnostics (see Appendix 17.1).
   1. Sweat chloride test: normal chloride concentration range is less than 40 mEq/L (mmol/L), with a mean of 18 mEq/L (mmol/L); chloride concentration 40 to 60 mEq/L (mmol/L) is suggestive of a diagnosis of cystic fibrosis.
   2. Pancreatic enzymes: decrease or absence of trypsin and chymotrypsin.
   3. Fat absorption in intestines is impaired.
D. Complications.
   1. Frequent pulmonary infections; pneumothorax.
   2. Diabetes secondary to destruction of pancreatic tissue.
   3. Cor pulmonale and respiratory failure are late complications.
   4. Gastroesophageal reflux disease (GERD).

Analyze Cues and Prioritize Hypotheses

The most important problems are abnormal mucus secretion and obstruction in the bronchi, small intestine, pancreatic and bile ducts.

Generate Solutions

Treatment

Child is usually cared for at home unless complications are present.

A. Diet: balanced, high-calorie, high-protein, fats as tolerated, increased salt intake.
B. Fat-soluble vitamins A, D, E, and K in water-soluble forms.
C. Pancreatic enzyme replacement with meals (see Appendix 15.2).
D. Antibiotics are given prophylactically and when there is evidence of infection; tobramycin.
E. Pulmonary therapy.
   1. Physical therapy: postural drainage, breathing exercises.
   2. Aerosol therapy and chest physiotherapy (CPT).
   3. Percussion and vibration.
   4. Expectorants (see Appendix 17.2).

Nursing Interventions: Take Action

Goal: To promote optimum home care for child (see Chapter 2 for care of chronically ill child).
A. Identify community resources for family.
B. Assist family to identify problems and solutions congruent with their lifestyle.
C. Encourage verbalization regarding effect of child's problem on the family and the family's ability to cope with the child at home.

> **TEST ALERT** Determine family needs, evaluate family's emotional response and adaptation; evaluate family resources and ability to comply with therapy.

D. When appropriate, teach child about disease and treatment and encourage active participation in planning of care.
E. Assist parents to identify activities to promote normal growth and development.

Goal: To maintain nutrition.
A. Minimum restriction of fats; need to increase intake of pancreatic enzyme with increased fat intake.
B. Pancreatic enzymes with meals and snacks.
C. Vitamins A, D, E, and K in water-soluble form.
D. Good oral hygiene after postural drainage.
E. Postural drainage 1 to 2 hours before meals or 3 hours after meals.

Goal: To prevent or minimize pulmonary complications.
A. Assist child to mobilize secretions.
   1. CPT: postural drainage, breathing exercises, nebulization treatments.
   2. Encourage active exercises appropriate to child's capacity and developmental level.
B. Prevent respiratory tract infections.
C. Prevent pneumothorax: no power lifting, intensive isometric exercises, scuba diving.

Pneumonia and Tuberculosis

See Chapter 17; pediatric implications are noted with a balloon.

CARDIAC

Rheumatic Fever and Heart Disease

Rheumatic fever is an inflammatory disease that is usually self-limiting. *Rheumatic heart disease* is the term used to

describe the cardiac value damage that occurs as a complication from rheumatic fever.

A. Usually preceded by a group A beta-hemolytic streptococcal (GABHS) infection.

> **! NURSING PRIORITY** Prevention and adequate treatment of streptococcal (GABHS) infections prevent the development of rheumatic heart disease.

B. Inflammatory hemorrhagic lesions called *Aschoff bodies* form, causing swelling, fragmentation, and alterations of connective tissue in the heart, joints, skin, and the central nervous system.

C. Myocardial involvement is characterized by the development of valvulitis, pericarditis, and myocarditis.
1. Valvulitis produces scarring of the cardiac valves.
2. Rheumatic carditis is the only symptom that produces permanent damage; most often involves damage to the endocardium and primarily to the mitral valve.
3. Rheumatic fever usually occurs during childhood, but manifestations of cardiac damage may not be evident for years.

Assessment: Recognize Cues

A. Risk factors/etiology: previous infection by GABHS.
B. Clinical manifestations: symptoms vary; no specific symptom or laboratory test is diagnostic of rheumatic fever. Criteria for the diagnosis require a combination of symptoms to be present.
1. Carditis.
   a. Tachycardia out of proportion to fever.
   b. Long, high-pitched apical systolic murmur beginning with S_1 and continuing throughout cycle.
   c. Pericarditis, pericardial friction rub, and complaints of chest pain.
2. Migratory polyarthritis.
3. Chorea—of gradual onset; a sudden aimless, irregular movement of the extremities, involuntary facial grimacing, speech disturbance, weakness.
4. Erythema marginatum—nonpruritic macule found on trunk and proximal portion of extremities.
5. Subcutaneous nodules over bony prominences.
6. History of a recent streptococcal infection.

Analyze Cues and Prioritize Hypotheses

The most important problems include an abnormal immune response to a group A *streptococci* infection, heart valve damage, inflammation of connective tissues (i.e., joints, skin, brain, and heart).

Generate Solutions

Treatment

A. Adequate antibiotic treatment of initial streptococcal infection.
B. Rest and decreased activity until tachycardia subsides.
C. Salicylates to reduce fever and discomfort and control the inflammatory process, especially in the joints.

D. Prophylactic treatment: client is susceptible to reoccurrence of rheumatic fever.
1. Begin after immediate therapy is complete.
2. Monthly administration of penicillin over extended period, depending on extent of cardiac involvement.
3. Additional prophylactic antibiotics are given when invasive procedures are necessary (genitourinary procedures, dental work, etc.).

Complications

A. Severe valvular damage precipitates the development of heart failure (HF) and may require open heart surgery for replacement of diseased valve.
B. HF.

Nursing Interventions: Take Action

Child is generally cared for in the home environment.
Goal: To assist parents and family to provide home environment conducive to healing and recovery.

A. Decrease activity if pulse rate is increased or if child is febrile.
B. Friends may visit for short periods; child is not contagious.
C. Maintain adequate nutrition.
1. May be anorexic during the febrile phase.
2. Provide soft or liquid foods as tolerated.
3. Assist child with feeding if choreiform movements are severe.
4. Maintain adequate hydration.
D. Salicylates to control inflammatory process and as analgesics for arthralgia.
E. Reassure child that chorea and joint involvement are only temporary and there will be no residual damage.
F. Teach signs of HF and when to seek medical attention.
Goal: To help parents understand need for long-term prophylactic antibiotic therapy.

A. Importance of preventing recurring infections.
B. Include child in planning, especially when numerous injections are involved.
C. Importance of prophylactic therapy before invasive procedures.
D. Continued medical follow-up for the development of valvular problems as child grows.
E. Follow-up required with females; cardiac problems may not be manifested until woman is pregnant.

🌳 Kawasaki Disease

Kawasaki disease **(mucocutaneous lymph node syndrome) is an acute systemic vasculitis of unknown cause that is self-limiting but can lead to a complication of coronary artery aneurysm in early childhood (6 months to 5 years of age) (Fig. 22.6).**

Assessment: Recognize Cues

A. Clinical manifestations.
1. High fever unresponsive to antipyretics and antibiotics.
2. Conjunctiva of eye.

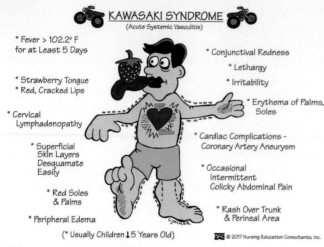

FIG. 22.6 Kawasaki Syndrome. (From Zerwekh, J., Garneau, A., & Miller, C. J. [2017]. *Digital collection of the memory notebooks of nursing* [4th ed.]. Nursing Education Consultants.)

3. Inflammation of pharynx.
4. Red cracked lips, "strawberry tongue"—sloughing of outer coating of tongue, leaving large papillae exposed.
5. Rash; cervical lymphadenopathy.
6. Erythema of palms and soles; edema of hands and feet.
7. Myocarditis, tachycardia, gallop rhythm.

B. Diagnostics.
  1. Anemia; leukocytosis (shift to the left).
  2. Elevated sedimentation rate, CRP.
  3. Echocardiogram to monitor cardiac function.

C. Complications.
  1. Coronary artery aneurysm.
  2. Myocardial infarction.

Analyze Cues and Prioritize Hypotheses

The most important problems are high fever and potential coronary aneurysm and/or myocardial infarction.

Generate Solutions

Treatment

A. High-dose IV immunoglobulin G (IVIG) for 7 to 10 days.
B. Salicylate therapy initially at higher dosages followed by low-dose therapy.
C. Anticoagulant therapy for heart enlargement or with coronary aneurysms.

Nursing Interventions: Take Action

Goal: To ensure early diagnosis and treatment.
Goal: To prevent cardiovascular complications.
Goal: To provide discharge teaching regarding medications, potential complication of myocardial infarction and signs of cardiac ischemia, delay of MMR and varicella vaccine for 11 months after IVIG administration.

🌳 Congenital Heart Disease

Congenital heart defects are malformations of the heart, which are not a problem for the fetus because of the fetal-maternal circulation that compensates for all fetal oxygen

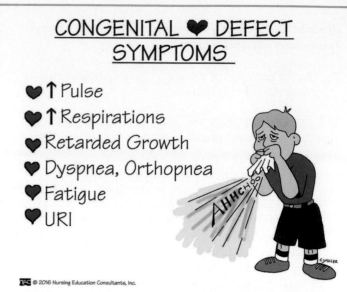

FIG. 22.7 Congenital Heart Defect Symptoms. (From Zerwekh, J., Garneau, A. J., & Miller, C. J. [2017]. *Digital collection of the memory notebooks of nursing* [4th ed.]. Nursing Education Consultants.)

needs. **However, at birth when the infant's circulatory system takes over, then symptoms occur.** *Selected cardiac heart defects are described below.*

Assessment: Recognize Cues

A. Clinical manifestations depend on the severity of the defect and the adequacy of pulmonary blood flow.
B. Normal pressure in the right side of the heart is significantly lower than pressure in the left side; there is an increased blood flow from an area of high pressure to an area of low pressure.
  1. When there is an opening between the right and left sides of the heart, oxygenated blood will shunt from the left side of the heart to the right side (right-to-left shunt).
  2. When the pressures on the right side of the heart exceed the pressure on the left side of the heart, unoxygenated blood from the right side will flow into the left side, and unoxygenated blood will flow into the systemic circulation (left-to-right shunt).
C. Physical consequences of congenital heart defects (Fig. 22.7).
  1. Delayed physical development.
    a. Failure to gain weight, caused by anorexia and/or inability to maintain adequate caloric intake to meet increased metabolic demands.
    b. Tachycardia and tachypnea precipitate increase in caloric requirements.
  2. Excessive fatigue, especially during feedings.
  3. Frequent upper respiratory tract infections.
  4. Dyspnea, tachycardia, tachypnea.
  5. Hypercyanotic spells (called "blue" spells or "tet" spells): infant suddenly becomes acutely cyanotic and hyperpneic; occur most often in children 2 months to 1 year of age.
D. Diagnostics—cardiac catheterization, echocardiography, magnetic resonance imaging (MRI).

❗ **NURSING PRIORITY** Infants and children less than 2 years with congenital heart disease should receive a monthly RSV prophylaxis during RSV season.

Defects with Increased Pulmonary Artery Blood Flow

Increased blood volume on the right side of the heart increases the flow of blood through the pulmonary artery. This may decrease the systemic blood flow.

A. Atrial septal defect (ASD): opening in the septum between the atrium; blood shunts from left to right; often caused by failure of foramen ovale to close.

B. Ventricular septal defect (VSD): opening in the septum between the ventricles; blood shunts from left side to right side, allowing oxygenated blood to mix with unoxygenated blood.

C. Patent ductus arteriosus (PDA): failure of the fetal ductus arteriosus to close after birth; blood is shunted from the left side to the right side; may be treated with indomethacin (prostaglandin inhibitor) or ibuprofen, NSAIDs that change the oxygen concentration of the tissue and enhance tissue changes that close the defect.

D. Clinical manifestations.
  1. May be asymptomatic.
  2. Signs of HF are common.
  3. Characteristic "machinery-type" murmurs.

Obstructive Defects with Decreased Pulmonary Artery Blood Flow

Problems occur when the normal blood flow through the heart meets an obstruction. The pressure in the ventricle and in the artery before the obstruction is increased; pressure beyond the obstruction is decreased.

A. Coarctation of the aorta (narrowing of the aortic arch); specific symptoms depend on the location of the coarctation in relation to arteries coming off the aortic arch.
  1. Clinical manifestations.
    a. Marked differences in blood pressure in the upper and lower extremities; area proximal to the defect (upper extremities) has high pressure and a bounding pulse.
      (1) Epistaxis.
      (2) Headaches.
      (3) Bounding radial and temporal pulses.
      (4) Dizziness and fainting.
    b. Area distal to defect has decreased blood pressure and weaker pulse.
      (1) Lower extremities are cooler; mottling is present.
      (2) Weak peripheral and femoral pulses.
    c. May develop HF, especially in infants.
  2. Increased risk for hypertension, ruptured aorta, aortic aneurysm, and stroke.

Defects with Decreased Pulmonary Blood Flow

An anatomic defect is present between the right and left sides of the heart (ASD or VSD). There is increased pulmonary artery resistance to blood flow, therefore pressure increases in the right side of the heart. As the resistance in the pulmonary circulation increases, pressure in the right ventricle increases. This pressure increases until it is greater than pressure on the left side of the heart and unoxygenated (unsaturated) blood moves into the left side of the heart (right-to-left shunt).

A. Tetralogy of Fallot: consists of four defects—VSD, pulmonic stenosis, overriding aorta, and right-ventricular hypertrophy.
  1. Clinical manifestations depend on the size of the VSD and the pressures in the heart.
    a. May be acutely cyanotic at birth or may have minimal cyanosis due to patent ductus arteriosus.
    b. Child may have mild cyanosis that progresses.
    c. Infant may experience acute episodes of hypoxia (blue spells, tet spells); may occur during agitation or crying.
    d. Posturing or squatting in the older child.
    e. HF does not usually develop because overload of right ventricle flows into the aorta and the left ventricle; therefore, pulmonary congestion does not occur. HR may occur postoperatively.
  2. At risk for emboli, seizures, changes in level of consciousness, or sudden death from anoxia.

Mixed Defects

Mixed defects are present when the survival of the infant depends on the mixing of oxygenated and unoxygenated blood for survival. Pulmonary congestion occurs as a result of the increased flow of blood into pulmonary vasculature.

A. Transposition of great vessels: the pulmonary artery receives blood from the left ventricle, and the aorta receives blood from the right ventricle. A communicated defect—ASD, VSD, or patent ductus arteriosus—must be present to provide for mixing of oxygenated and unoxygenated blood.
  1. Clinical manifestations depend on size of associated defects and mixing of blood.
    a. Newborns with minimal communication defects are cyanotic at birth.
    b. Symptoms of HF.
    c. Cardiomegaly develops shortly after birth.
  2. Prostaglandins may be given to maintain patency of ductus arteriosus to promote mixing of blood.

Analyze Cues and Prioritize Hypotheses

The most important problems are potential HF and hypoxemia that may occur both prior and after surgical repair.

Nursing Interventions: Take Action

Goal: To evaluate infant's response to cardiac defect.

A. Evaluate infant's Apgar scores at birth.
B. Evaluate adequacy of weight gain in first few months.
C. Assess feeding problems.
  1. Poor sucking reflex.
  2. Poor coordination of sucking, swallowing, and breathing.
  3. Fatigues easily during feeding.

D. Frequency of upper respiratory tract infections.

E. Determine whether cyanosis occurs at rest or is precipitated by activity.

F. Presence and quality of pulses in extremities.

G. Bacterial endocarditis is a primary concern before and after correction of a congenital defect; all fevers should be reported.

Goal: To promote oxygenation.

A. Effectively cope with hypercyanotic spells (blue spells, tet spells).

1. Occurs suddenly, often when the infant is agitated.

2. Hold the infant upright in a knee-chest position; this reduces the venous return and increases systemic vascular resistance, which increases pressure on the right side of the heart and diverts more blood flow through the pulmonary artery.

3. Administer 100% O_2 via face mask until respirations are improved.

4. Maintain good hydration and carefully monitor hemoglobin levels.

5. Older child may assume squatting position to increase peripheral resistance and decrease right-to-left shunting.

B. Supplemental oxygen, good pulmonary hygiene, and chest physiotherapy to maintain oxygen saturation levels.

C. Prevent overexertion, decrease excessive crying, and promote rest to conserve energy and caloric expenditure.

D. Maintain hydration for pulmonary hygiene and to prevent embolic problems and stroke.

E. Infants may require gavage feeding if respiratory distress limits oral feeding.

Goal: To assist parents in adjusting to diagnosis.

A. Allow family to grieve over loss of perfect infant.

B. Evaluate parents' level of understanding of the child's problem.

C. Foster early parent–infant attachment; encourage touching, holding, feeding, and general physical contact.

D. Help the family develop a relationship that fosters optimum growth and development of all family members. (See Chapter 2 for psychosocial aspects of caring for chronically ill children.)

E. Discharge teaching subjects should include medication administration (digoxin), activity level, diet, wound care, prophylaxis for infective endocarditis, follow-up appointments, and instructions on when to contact health care provider.

> **TEST ALERT** Provide emotional support to family; assist family members in managing care of a child with a chronic illness.

Goal: To detect, prevent, and treat HF.

Goal: To provide appropriate nursing interventions for the client undergoing open heart surgery for repair of a defect.

GASTROINTESTINAL

🍀 Appendicitis

Appendicitis is the inflammation and obstruction of the appendix, leading to bacterial infection. If appendicitis is not treated, the appendix can become gangrenous and

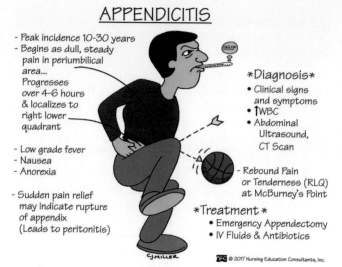

FIG. 22.8 Appendicitis. (From Zerwekh, J., Garneau, A., & Miller, C. J. [2017]. *Digital collection of the memory notebooks of nursing* [4th ed.]. Nursing Education Consultants.)

burst, causing peritonitis and septicemia, which could progress to death. It is the most common cause of acute abdominal pain.

Assessment: Recognize Cues

A. Risk factors/etiology.

1. Age: peak at 10 to 12 years of age; uncommon in children younger than 2 years.

2. Diet: risk associated with a diet low in fiber and high in refined sugars and carbohydrates.

3. Obstruction to opening of appendix: hardened fecal matter, foreign bodies, or microorganisms.

B. Clinical manifestations (Fig. 22.8).

1. Abdominal cramping and pain, beginning near the navel and then migrating toward McBurney's point (right lower quadrant); pain worsens with time.

2. Rovsing sign: pain in right lower quadrant when palpating or percussing other quadrants.

3. Anorexia, nausea, vomiting, diarrhea.

4. Low-grade fever.

5. Side-lying position with knees flexed.

6. Client complains of pain when asked to cough; asking client to cough is a better assessment method than palpating for rebound tenderness.

7. Sudden, temporary relief from pain may indicate rupture of appendix.

C. Diagnostics—no specific diagnostic tool; diagnosis made from compilation of findings.

1. Clinical manifestations.

2. Urinalysis to rule out urinary tract infection (UTI).

3. Abdominal ultrasonography and computed tomography (CT) to differentiate from other abdominal problems.

4. CBC with differential reveals elevated white blood cell (WBC) count.

5. Pregnancy test for adolescent females to rule out ectopic pregnancy.

D. Complications: rupture and peritonitis.

Analyze Cues and Prioritize Hypotheses

The most important problems are acute abdominal pain and the potential for peritonitis due to rupture of the appendix.

Generate Solutions

Treatment

A. Presurgery: NPO, fluid resuscitation, prophylactic antibiotic therapy; after diagnosis of appendicitis has been established, pain management with analgesics.
B. Open appendectomy or laparoscopic appendectomy.
C. Abdominal laparotomy and peritoneal lavage if appendix has ruptured.

Nursing Interventions: Take Action

Goal: To assess clinical manifestations and to prepare for surgery.
A. Careful nursing assessment for clinical manifestations.
B. Maintain NPO status until otherwise indicated.
C. Maintain bed rest in position of comfort.

TEST ALERT Determine need for administration of pain medications. Do not give opioids for pain control before a diagnosis of appendicitis is confirmed because this could mask symptoms.

D. Do not apply heat to the abdomen; cold applications may provide some relief or comfort.
E. Do not administer enemas or laxatives.
F. Avoid unnecessary palpation of abdomen.

! PEDIATRIC NURSING PRIORITY Because children associate the stethoscope with listening, use the bell piece for initial palpation of the abdomen for tenderness. Children tolerate this type of pressure rather than palpation and probing with the fingers. Follow this initial approach, with manual palpation while carefully watching child's face for signs of discomfort.

TEST ALERT Determine whether client is prepared for surgery or procedures. Appendicitis is a common problem; know how to care for client during diagnostic phase.

Goal: To maintain homeostasis and healing after appendectomy (see Chapter 3).
Goal: To prevent abdominal distention and to assess bowel function after abdominal laparotomy.
A. Maintain NPO status; then begin clear liquid diet, progressing to soft diet as tolerated.
B. Gastric decompression by nasogastric (NG) tube; maintain patency and suction.
C. Monitor abdomen for distention and increased pain.
D. Assess peristaltic activity.
E. Evaluate and record character of bowel movements.
Goal: To decrease infection and promote healing after abdominal laparotomy.
A. Place client in semi-Fowler position to localize and prevent spread of infection and reduce abdominal tension.
B. Antibiotics are usually administered via IV infusion; monitor response to antibiotics and status of IV infusion site.

C. Monitor vital signs frequently (every 2–4 hours) and evaluate for escalation of infectious process.
D. Provide appropriate wound care; evaluate drainage from abdominal Penrose drains and incisional area.
Goal: To maintain adequate hydration and nutrition and to promote comfort after abdominal laparotomy.
A. Maintain adequate hydration via IV infusion.
B. Evaluate tolerance of oral liquids when NG tube is removed.
C. Begin oral administration of clear liquids when peristalsis returns.
D. Progress diet as tolerated.
E. Administer analgesics as indicated.

TEST ALERT Identify infection; peritonitis is common after surgery for a ruptured appendix.

Hypertrophic Pyloric Stenosis

Hypertrophic pyloric stenosis (HPS) is the obstruction of the pyloric sphincter by hypertrophy and hyperplasia of the circular muscle of the pylorus. Symptoms usually present in the first few weeks of life.

Assessment: Recognize Cues

A. Risk factors/etiology.
   1. Occurs most often in firstborn, full-term male infants (infantile hypertrophic pyloric stenosis).
   2. Seen more frequently in Caucasian infants.
B. Clinical manifestations.
   1. Onset of vomiting may be gradual; usually occurs at 3 weeks or as late as 5 months; is progressive and may be projectile.
   2. Emesis is not bile stained but may be curdled or bloody.
   3. Vomiting occurs shortly after feeding.
   4. Infant is hungry and irritable; wants to eat after vomiting.
   5. Infant does not appear to be in pain or acute distress.
   6. Weight loss occurs, if untreated.
   7. Stools decrease in number and in size.
   8. Dehydration occurs as condition progresses; hypochloremia and hypokalemia occur as vomiting continues.
   9. Upper abdomen is distended and an "olive-shaped" mass may be palpated in the right epigastric area.
C. Diagnostics—ultrasound of abdomen, upper GI radiography.

Analyze Cues and Prioritize Hypotheses

The most important problems are dehydration, metabolic alkalosis, electrolyte imbalance, and failure to thrive.

Generate Solutions

Treatment

A. Surgical release of the pyloric muscle (pyloromyotomy).

Nursing Interventions: Take Action

Goal: To maintain hydration and gastric decompression; to initiate appropriate preoperative nursing activities (see Appendix 14.4).

A. Maintain nasogastric decompression if NG tube is in place and record type and amount of drainage.
B. Assess hydration status and electrolyte balance, especially serum calcium, sodium, and potassium levels.
C. NPO status with continuous IV infusion (most often saline solutions) may be required.
D. Accurate intake and output records: complete description of all vomitus and stools.
E. Monitor vital signs and check for signs of peritonitis.
F. Preoperative teaching for parents.

Goal: To maintain adequate hydration and promote healing after pyloromyotomy.

A. Postoperative vomiting in the first 24 to 48 hours is not uncommon; maintain IV fluids until infant tolerates adequate oral intake.
B. Continue to monitor infant in the same manner as in the preoperative period.
C. Feedings are initiated early; bottle-fed infant may begin with clear liquids containing glucose and electrolytes, small amounts offered frequently.
D. Breast-fed infants: mother can express breast milk and offer small amounts in a bottle or initially limit nursing time.

Goal: To help parents provide appropriate home care after pyloromyotomy.

A. No residual problems are anticipated after surgery.
B. Instruct parents regarding care of the incisional area.

🎈 Hirschsprung's Disease

Hirschsprung's disease (congenital aganglionic megacolon) is characterized by a congenital absence of ganglionic cells that innervate a segment of the colon wall.

A. Clinical symptoms vary depending on the age when symptoms are recognized, the length of the affected bowel, and presence of inflammation.
B. Most common site is the rectosigmoid colon; colon proximal to the area dilates (i.e., megacolon).

Assessment: Recognize Cues

A. Risk factors/etiology: congenital anomaly.
B. Clinical manifestations.
1. May be acute and life threatening or may be a chronic presentation.
2. Internal sphincter loses ability to relax for defecation.
3. Newborn.
   a. Failure to pass meconium within 48 hours after birth.
   b. Vomiting; abdominal distention.
   c. Reluctance to take fluids.
4. Older infant and child.
   a. Chronic constipation, impactions.
   b. Passage of ribbon-like, foul-smelling stools and diarrhea.
   c. Failure to thrive.
   d. Lack of appetite.
C. Diagnostics—rectal biopsy to confirm.

Analyze Cues and Prioritize Hypotheses

The most important problems are distended abdomen, feeding intolerance, delay in passage of meconium, and possible intestinal obstruction.

Generate Solutions

Treatment

A. Surgical correction usually involves resection of aganglionic bowel with creation of a temporary colostomy to relieve the obstruction.
B. The final repair closes the colostomy, and the bowel is reanastomosed.

Nursing Interventions: Take Action

Goal: To promote normal attachment and prepare infant and parents for surgery.

A. Allow parents to vent feelings regarding congenital defect of infant.
B. Foster infant–parent attachment.
C. General preoperative preparation of the infant; neonate does not require any bowel preparation.
D. Careful explanation of colostomy to parents.

Goal: See Nursing Interventions for client who has undergone abdominal surgery in the Intestinal Obstruction section of this chapter.

Goal: To help parents understand and provide appropriate home care for their infant/child after colostomy (see Appendix 14.8).

A. Colostomy is most often temporary.
B. Parents should be actively involved in colostomy care before discharge.

🎈 Hepatitis, Intussusception, Celiac Disease

See Chapter 20; pediatric implications are noted with a balloon.

NEUROLOGY

🎈 Hydrocephalus

Hydrocephalus is a condition caused by an imbalance in the production and absorption of cerebrospinal fluid (CSF) in the ventricles of the brain.

Classification: Primary

A. Noncommunicating (obstructive): circulation of CSF is blocked within the ventricular system of the brain.
B. Communicating: CSF flows freely within the ventricular system but is not adequately absorbed by arachnoid villi.

Classification: Secondary

A. Congenital.
B. Acquired—possibly from trauma, infection, or tumor.

Assessment: Recognize Cues

A. Risk factors/etiology.
1. Neonate: usually the result of a congenital malformation.
2. Older child, adult.

a. Space-occupying lesion.
b. Preexisting developmental defects.

B. Clinical manifestations: infant.
1. Head enlargement: increasing circumference in excess of normal 2 cm per month for first 3 months.
2. Separation of cranial suture lines.
3. Fontanel becomes tense and bulging.
4. Dilated scalp veins.
5. Frontal enlargement, bulging "sunset eyes."
6. Symptoms of increasing intracranial pressure (ICP).

C. Clinical manifestations: older child, adult.
1. Symptoms of increasing ICP.
2. Specific manifestations related to site of the lesion.

D. Diagnostics
1. Increasing head circumference is diagnostic in infants.

Analyze Cues and Prioritize Hypotheses

The most important problems are head enlargement and symptoms of increasing ICP.

Generate Solutions

Treatment

A. Noncommunicating and communicating: ventriculoperitoneal shunt; CSF is shunted into the peritoneum.
B. Obstructive: removal of the obstruction (cyst, hematoma, tumor).

Nursing Interventions: Take Action

Goal: To monitor for the development of increasing ICP.

A. Daily measurement of the frontal–occipital circumference of the head in infants.
B. Assess for symptoms of increasing ICP (see Box 22.2; Table 22.1).
C. Infant is often difficult to feed; administer small feedings at frequent intervals because vomiting may be a problem.

Goal: To maintain patency of the shunt and monitor ICP after shunt procedure.

A. Position flat turned to unoperated side to prevent pressure on shunt valve.
B. Position is not a problem with children who are having a shunt revision; they have not had an increase in ventricular pressure.
C. Monitor for increasing ICP and compare with previous data.
D. Monitor for infection, especially meningitis or encephalitis.

Home Care

A. Teach parents symptoms of increasing ICP and shunt infection.
B. Have parents participate in care of the shunt before client's discharge.
C. Encourage parents and family to express feelings regarding client's condition.
D. Refer client to appropriate community agencies.

Reye Syndrome

Reye syndrome **is a rare acute illness occurring after a viral illness (frequently after aspirin has been consumed) and results in fatty infiltration of the liver and subsequent liver degeneration and increased ICP.**

A. Damaged liver cells no longer adequately convert ammonia to urea for excretion from the body.
B. Circulating ammonia crosses the blood-brain barrier to produce acute neurologic effects.

Assessment: Recognize Cues

A. Risk factors/etiology.
1. Most often preceded by an acute viral infection.
2. Primarily affects children from the age of 6 months to adolescence.
3. Frequently, the affected child has received salicylate (aspirin) for control of fever during the preceding viral infection.
4. With warning labels now on aspirin, problem has significantly decreased.

B. Clinical manifestations.
1. Stage 1.
a. Initial symptom may be severe persistent vomiting.
b. Lethargy; listlessness.
2. Stage 2.
a. Irritability; disorientation.
b. Progresses to state of increased ICP with deepening coma and abnormal posturing.

C. Diagnostics.
1. Definitive diagnosis is a liver biopsy.
2. Prolonged prothrombin time.
3. Elevated blood ammonia levels.
4. Elevated serum aspartate aminotransferase (AST) and alanine aminotransferase (ALT) levels.

Analyze Cues and Prioritize Hypotheses

The most important problems are an impaired level of consciousness, electrolyte imbalance, and hepatic dysfunction.

Generate Solutions

Treatment

A. Primarily supportive, based on stage of disease; mechanical ventilation, fluid, and electrolyte balance.
B. Measures to decrease ICP.
C. Early intervention critical to successful treatment.

Nursing Interventions: Take Action

Goal: To monitor progress of disease state and maintain homeostasis.

A. IV fluids, frequent monitoring of intake and output to adjust fluid volume.
B. Monitor serum electrolytes and liver function studies.
C. Maintain respiratory status; prevent hypoxia.
D. Assess for problems of impaired coagulation.
E. Decrease stress, anxiety: child may not remember events before the critical phase.

2. Frequently difficult to diagnose in early months; condition may not be evident until child attempts to sit alone or walk (up to 2 years old).
3. Gait laboratory analysis: evaluates walking ability.

Analyze Cues and Prioritize Hypotheses

The most important problems are motor abnormalities, alteration in muscle tone, abnormal posture, seizures, cognitive deficits that include issues with communication and behavior.

Generate Solutions

Treatment
A. Maintain and promote mobility with orthotic/assistive devices and physical therapy.
B. Skeletal muscle relaxants.
C. Anticonvulsants, as indicated.

Nursing Interventions: Take Action

Child is frequently cared for at home and on an outpatient basis unless complications occur.
Goal: To assist child to become as independent and self-sufficient as possible.
A. Physical and occupational therapy designed to assist child to gain maximum function.
B. Assist child to progress according to developmental level and functional abilities; encourage crawling, sitting, and balancing appropriate to developmental level.
C. Assist child to carry out activities of daily living (ADLs) as age and capacities permit.
D. Speech therapy, as indicated.
E. Encourage play appropriate for age.
F. Encourage appropriate educational activities.
G. Bowel and bladder training may be difficult because of poor control.
Goal: To maintain physiologic homeostasis.
A. Maintain adequate nutrition.
   1. May experience difficulty eating because of spasticity; may drool excessively; use of manual jaw control when feeding.
   2. Encourage independence in eating and use of self-help devices.
   3. Provide a balanced diet with increased caloric intake to meet extra energy demands.
B. Maintain safety precautions to prevent injury.
C. Increased susceptibility to infections, especially respiratory tract infections because of poor control of intercostal muscles and diaphragm.
D. Increased incidence of dental problems; schedule frequent dental checkups.
Goal: To promote a positive self-image in the child and provide support to the family.
A. Use positive reinforcement frequently.
B. Assist parents to set realistic goals.
C. Encourage recreation and educational activities, especially those involving other children with CP.
D. Encourage child to express feelings regarding the disorder.

E. Do not "talk down" to child; communicate at appropriate developmental level.
F. Assist parents in problem solving in home environment.
G. Identify available community resources.
H. Utilize principles in caring for chronically ill pediatric client (see Chapter 2).

Seizure Disorder, Head Injury, Spinal Cord Injury

See Chapter 16; *pediatric implications are noted with a balloon.*

MUSCULOSKELETAL

Developmental Dysplasia of the Hip

Developmental dysplasia of the hip (DDH) **is the correct terminology for a variety of disorders related to abnormal development of the hip. The older term,** *congenital hip dysplasia,* **has been replaced by DDH, which includes various hip problems, such as a shallow acetabulum, subluxation, or dislocation.**

Assessment: Recognize Cues

A. Risk factors/etiology.
   1. Frequently associated with other congenital deformities.
   2. Prenatal factors.
      a. Maternal hormone secretion.
      b. Intrauterine posture, especially frank breech position.
      c. Genetic—higher incidence in siblings of affected children.
B. Clinical manifestations (newborn).
   1. Ortolani sign: infant supine, knees flexed, hips fully abducted; a click is heard or felt as the hip is reduced by abduction.

> **! NURSING PRIORITY** The Ortolani and Barlow tests should only be performed by experienced nurses trained in these tests.

   2. Asymmetric gluteal and thigh folds.
   3. Shortening of the leg on the affected side; one knee is lower than the other (Galeazzi sign).
   4. Positive Barlow maneuver—adducting the infant's hips while applying light pressure on the knee posteriorly. If the hip is at risk for dislocation or unstable, the test is considered positive.
C. Diagnostics (see Appendix 17.1).

Analyze Cues and Prioritize Hypotheses

The most important problems are hip instability and potential for hip deformity if treatment is not initiated early.

Generate Solutions

Treatment
A. Treatment is initiated as soon as condition is identified.
B. For the newborn, the dislocated hip is securely held in a full abduction position. This keeps the femur in the acetabulum and stabilizes the area.
   1. Abduction devices.

a. Pavlik harness: a fabric strap harness that is secured around the infant's shoulders and chest and is connected to straps around the lower legs. The harness acts as a brace to maintain the legs in a flexed, abducted position at the hip. The harness may be removed for bathing but should be worn 23 hours a day until the hip is stable.

b. Hip spica cast: most often used when adduction contracture is present. After the removal of the cast, a protective abduction brace is fitted.

2. Closed reduction: performed in older children, 6 to 24 months old.

3. Open reduction: performed if hip is not reducible with traction or closed reduction.

C. Successful reduction becomes increasingly difficult after the age of 4 years.

Nursing Interventions: Take Action

Goal: To identify hip dysplasia in the newborn before discharge.

Goal: To assist parents to understand mechanism to maintain reduction.

A. Pavlik harness.
1. Teach parents proper application of harness.
2. Undershirts should be worn beneath the brace.
3. Check skin under brace for irritation or pressure areas at least two or three times a day.
4. No oils or lotions should be applied to skin that will be under the brace.
5. Reposition the child frequently and lightly massage skin under straps to improve circulation at least once a day.
6. Always place the diaper under the straps.

> ⚠ **NURSING PRIORITY** Because of rapid growth of infants, straps should be checked and adjusted every 1 to 2 weeks to prevent vascular or nerve injury.

B. Spica cast.
1. Teach parents cast care if hip spica cast is applied (e.g., keep cast dry, do not insert foreign objects into the cast).
2. Assess for and reduce skin irritation by maintaining cleanliness of the cast and the child.
3. Elevate the child's head during feedings to prevent choking.
4. If the child is being breast-fed, elevating the child on pillows and using the "football" hold is recommended.

Goal: To facilitate developmental progress.

A. Provide stimuli and activity appropriate for developmental level.

B. Encourage parents to hold and cuddle child.

C. Maintain normal home routine.

🎈 Congenital Clubfoot (Talipes Equinovarus)

Congenital clubfoot (talipes equinovarus) **is a deformity of the ankle and foot in which adduction, plantar flexion, and inversion of the foot occur in varying degrees of severity. The unilateral form occurs more commonly than the bilateral form.** *Talipes equinovarus (TEV)* **involves bone deformity. Metatarsus adductus (***metatarsus varus***), which is often confused with congenital clubfoot, occurs as a result of abnormal intrauterine positioning and involves medial adduction of the toes and forefoot and inversion (kidney-shaped foot); ankle range of motion (ROM) is normal.**

Assessment: Recognize Cues

A. Risk factors/etiology (inconclusive).
1. Familial tendency.
2. Arrested fetal development of the skeletal and soft tissue of the foot.
3. Intrauterine positioning/compression.

B. Clinical manifestations.
1. Condition is apparent at birth.
2. In true clubfoot, there is severe limitation of ROM.

C. Diagnostics—clinical manifestations.

Analyze Cues and Prioritize Hypotheses

The most important problems are potential for bone deformity if treatment is not initiated early.

Generate Solutions

Treatment

Treatment begins immediately and most often requires three stages for correction.

A. Correction of deformity: casts are applied in series for gradual stretching and straightening; massage accompanied by special bandaging may also be used.

B. Surgical intervention followed by casting.

C. After cast(s) removal, varus prevention brace to maintain correction.

D. Maintenance of correction: orthopedic shoes.

E. Follow-up observations.

Nursing Interventions: Take Action

Goal: To assist parents to understand mechanism of treatment to achieve correction.

A. Appropriate care of cast or brace at home.

B. Follow-up care and importance of frequent cast changes.

Goal: To facilitate developmental progress and adapt nurturing activities to meet infant's and parents' needs (same as for developmental dysplasia of the hip).

🎈 Scoliosis

Scoliosis **is a lateral curvature of the spine. If it is allowed to progress without treatment, it will severely affect the shape of the thoracic cavity and impair ventilation.**

A. Idiopathic (predominant type) occurs primarily in adolescent girls.

B. Most noticeable at beginning of growth spurt, around 10 years of age.

Assessment: Recognize Cues

A. Clinical manifestations.
1. Uneven hips and shoulders.
2. Visible curvature of the spinal column; head and hips are not in alignment.

Assessment: Recognize Cues

A. Risk factors/etiology.
   1. Familial history of the disease (X-linked recessive disorders).
   2. Onset generally occurs between the ages of 3 and 5 years.
B. Clinical manifestations.
   1. Bilateral symmetric muscle wasting.
   2. Ataxic or waddling gait with frequent falls and lordosis.
   3. Progressive weakening of muscles around the trunk.
   4. Difficulty rising from the floor and climbing stairs.
   5. Toe-walking children older than 3 years.
   6. Ambulation is frequently impossible by 12 years of age.
   7. Difficulty raising arms over head.
C. Diagnostics (see Appendix 17.1).
   1. Serum muscle enzymes (especially creatine kinase, aldolase).
   2. Electromyogram (EMG) testing.
   3. Genetic testing for Duchene.
D. Complications
   1. Contractures; disuse atrophy.
   2. Infections; obesity.
   3. Respiratory and cardiopulmonary problems.

Analyze Cues and Prioritize Hypotheses

The most important problems are muscle weakness, gait disturbances, mild to moderate mental impairment, and the potential for pulmonary infections and obesity.

Generate Solutions

Treatment
A. No definitive therapy is available to stop the progressive wasting of MD.

Nursing Interventions: Take Action

Child is frequently cared for at home and hospitalized only when complications occur.
Goal: To preserve mobility and independence in ADLs through physical therapy and orthopedic appliances.
A. Prevent injuries and deformities; regular physical therapy to stretch and strengthen muscles and prevent contractures.
B. Avoid prolonged bed rest that may lead to further muscle wasting.
C. Assist family to identify resources, adapt physiologic barriers within the home, and promote child's mobility and independence in ADLs.
D. Teach family to monitor for respiratory problems and to identify methods of preventing respiratory tract infection.
E. Breathing exercises and incentive spirometry.
F. Provide psychosocial support for client and caregivers.
G. Counseling to assist family and child with chronic illness and child's eventual death.

Fractures

See Chapter 17; pediatric implications are noted with a balloon.

REPRODUCTIVE

Undescended Testes (Cryptorchidism)

Cryptorchidism is a condition of failure of one or both testes to descend into the scrotal sac.

Assessment: Recognize Cues

A. Clinical manifestations.
   1. Inability to palpate the testes in the scrotal sac.
   2. Testicle may be absent or small or may be located in the abdomen.
   3. Cremasteric reflex is normal retraction of the testes when stimulated by stroking the thigh on affected side downward; may present a problem in attempting to determine whether there is an undescended testicle or if a testicle is retractable.

Analyze Cues and Prioritize Hypotheses

The most important problem is the potential for sterility and testicular cancer if the condition is not treated early.

Generate Solutions

Treatment
A. Medical: condition may be observed for 1 year; most cases descend spontaneously; if undescended after 1 year, surgery may be required.
B. Surgical: testis is brought into the scrotal sac and secured (orchiopexy).
   1. Usually done between the ages of 6 and 24 months; fewer complications are encountered if repair is done before 6 years of age.
   2. Individuals with a history of cryptorchidism are at increased risk for fertility problems and development of testicular cancer in adulthood, especially if the testes have not descended by age 6.

Nursing Interventions: Take Action

Home Care

A. Long-term follow-up regarding fertility.
B. Prevent infection by careful cleansing after defecation and urination because of the close proximity of the scrotum.
C. Teach parents to show the child how to do testicular self-examinations when he is old enough.

Testicular Tumors (Cancer)

Tumors of the testicles are often malignant and tend to metastasize quickly.

Assessment: Recognize Cues

A. Risk factors/etiology.

1. Most common cancer in males age 15 to 35 years.
2. More common in clients who have had cryptorchidism and frequent reproductive organ infections.
3. For clients 40 to 60 years of age, determine, if possible, whether mother was given diethylstilbestrol (DES) during pregnancy. There is a significant increase in the risk for testicular cancer among these clients.

B. Clinical manifestations.
1. A painless lump (typically pea sized) is palpated in the scrotum.
2. Most men experience "heaviness" in the scrotum.
3. Significant enlargement of or shrinking of one testicle.

C. Diagnostics.
1. Levels of alpha-fetoprotein (AFP) and human chorionic gonadotropin (hCG) are increased.
2. CT and MRI to identify metastases.
3. Ultrasound.
4. Biopsy is not recommended because of the risk for spreading cancer locally.

Analyze Cues and Prioritize Hypotheses

The most important problems are sterility following surgery and the potential for metastasis.

Generate Solutions

Treatment

A. Medical.
1. Postoperative irradiation to the lymphatic drainage pathways.
2. Multiple chemotherapy medications.
3. Sperm banking prior to surgery to preserve and store semen.

B. Surgical.
1. Orchiectomy (removal of the testicle) is performed as soon as possible to remove the tumor and make a definite diagnosis.
2. If there is lymph node involvement, a retroperitoneal lymph node dissection is performed.

Nursing Interventions: Take Action

Goal: To detect any abnormality of the testes through client self-examination (Box 22.3).

> **TEST ALERT** Participate in health promotion programs. Teach men how to perform self-examinations.

A. Teach clients, especially those between the ages 15 and 35 years, to self-examine monthly while showering or bathing to detect any abnormality of the testes.
B. Emphasize importance of follow-up for clients with a history of undescended testes or a previous testicular tumor.

Testicular Torsion

Testicular torsion involves a twisting of the spermatic cord that supplies blood to the testes and epididymis.

Box 22.3   TESTICULAR SELF-EXAMINATION

- Examine the testicles at same time every month to help you remember to do it.
- Visually inspect scrotum in front of a mirror, observing for swelling.
- Perform the examination after a warm bath or shower because this is when the testes are lower in the scrotal sac.
- Examine each testicle individually by placing index and middle fingers of both hands under one testicle at a time with thumbs on top of testicle. Roll the testicle between the thumbs and fingers. This should *not* cause pain. The tissue should feel smooth.
- Locate the epididymis, which is a tubular sac behind the testicle. This sac should not be confused with a lump.
- Also assess for any "heaviness" or dull ache in the groin or abdomen or significant increase or decrease in size of either testicle.
- If there is any lump or irregularity on either testicle, report it to the health care provider as soon as possible.

Assessment: Recognize Cues

A. Risk factors/etiology.
1. Occurs in men under age 25; peak incidence 14 years of age.
B. Clinical manifestations.
1. Scrotal pain, tenderness, swelling, redness; nausea, vomiting.
2. Absent cremasteric reflex.

Analyze Cues and Prioritize Hypotheses

The most important problems are pain and the potential for sterility if the condition is not treated early.

Generate Solutions

Treatment

A. Surgical.
1. Emergency surgery to preserve testicle.

Nursing Interventions: Take Action

A. Provide preoperative and postoperative care if indicated (see Chapter 3).

Sexually Transmitted Infections

See Chapter 18; pediatric implications are noted with a balloon.

URINARY-RENAL

Hypospadias and Epispadias

Hypospadias is a common congenital anomaly of a urethral opening located behind the glans penis or along the penile shaft. *Epispadias* is a rare problem of a urethral opening located on the dorsal or upper side of the penis.

Assessment: Recognize Cues

A. Clinical manifestations.
1. Visualization of defect.

2. Circulatory overload (pulmonary edema) and congestive heart failure.
3. Hypertensive episodes.
4. In children, hypertensive encephalopathy, acute renal failure, or cardiac failure may occur.

Analyze Cues and Prioritize Hypotheses

The most important problems are hypertension, edema, oliguria, and possible HF.

Generate Solutions

Treatment
A. Medical.
   1. Diuretics for severe edema and fluid overload.
   2. Antihypertensives.
   3. Antibiotics if the streptococcal infection is still present.
   4. Plasmapheresis for filtering out immune complexes (antigens and antibodies).
B. Dietary.
   1. Decrease sodium intake.
   2. Protein restriction if client is azotemic; however, the anorexia that a child experiences frequently limits sufficient protein intake.
   3. Foods containing large amounts of potassium are often restricted during the oliguric phase.
C. Children with normal blood pressure, adequate urine output, and mild symptoms are cared for at home.
D. Fluid restriction may be implemented if urinary output is decreased.

Nursing Interventions: Take Action

Goal: To protect client's kidneys by preventing secondary infections.
A. Antibiotic therapy if cultures are positive.
B. Encourage rest until signs of glomerular inflammation (proteinuria, hematuria) and hypertension subside.
C. Avoid medications that are nephrotoxic, especially aminoglycosides.
Goal: To maintain fluid balance.
A. Monitor intake and output; maintain diet and fluid restrictions.
B. Monitor renal function: check proteinuria, specific gravity, and color of urine; weigh client daily; if client has hypertension, check blood pressure every 2 to 4 hours.
C. Monitor serum potassium levels.
D. Frequently, the first sign of improvement is an increase in the urine output, which may progress to profuse diuresis.
Goal: To prevent complications and promote comfort.
A. Encourage verbalization of fears.
B. Decrease anxiety by explaining treatments and reassuring client and family that the majority of clients recover fully.
C. Most children recover spontaneously, and recurrences are uncommon.

Home Care

A. Teach parents or client symptoms to be reported to health care provider: fatigue, nausea, vomiting, decrease in urinary output, and symptoms of infection.
B. Explain the need for rest, good nutrition, and avoidance of people with respiratory tract infections.
C. Teach measures to prevent UTIs.
D. Instruct client in regard to diet, fluid needs, and medication therapy.
E. Teach client to perform dipstick urine test to monitor for protein.

Wilms Tumor (Nephroblastoma)

Nephroblastoma (Wilms tumor) is one of the most common intraabdominal tumors of childhood and is associated with congenital anomalies, especially those of the genitourinary tract. The treatment and survival rate are based on the stage of the tumor at the time it is diagnosed. Five stages are used to maximize the effectiveness of treatment protocols.

Assessment: Recognize Cues

A. Risk factors/etiology.
   1. Family history of cancer.
   2. Associated with genitourinary anomalies.
   3. Majority of children (80%) diagnosed are younger than 5 years; peak incidence at 3 years.
B. Clinical manifestations.
   1. Swelling or mass within the abdomen: firm, confined to one side of the abdomen, causing vague or no pain.
   2. Abdominal pain as tumor enlarges.
   3. Hematuria, pallor, anorexia, weight loss, and malaise occur as condition progresses.
   4. Hypertension (63%).
C. Diagnostics—CT, MRI, abdominal x-ray.

Analyze Cues and Prioritize Hypotheses

The most important problems are abdominal pain, hypertension, weight loss, and potential for metastasis of the tumor cells if the abdomen is palpated.

Generate Solutions

Treatment
The survival rate greatly depends on the stage of the tumor at the time of diagnosis. If the tumor is diagnosed and treated in the early stages, there is a high survival rate.
A. Surgery.
   1. Surgery is frequently scheduled within 24 to 48 hours after the diagnosis.
   2. Nephrectomy: kidney is removed, but the adrenal gland may be spared, depending on the invasiveness of the tumor.
   3. If both kidneys are involved, the less affected kidney is retained and the more involved one is removed. Bilateral nephrectomy is a last resort.
D. Medical.

1. Preoperative and postoperative radiation therapy for large tumors.
2. Postoperative chemotherapy.

Nursing Interventions: Take Action

Goal: To provide safe preoperative care.

> **⛔ NURSING PRIORITY** Post a sign above the bed that reads "Do Not Palpate Abdomen."

A. Handle child carefully to prevent trauma to the tumor site.
B. Prepare child and family for the surgery, including anticipation of a large incision and dressing. Intensive care unit care immediately after surgery.
C. Assess vital signs, especially blood pressure, for indications of hypertension. If adrenal gland is removed, blood pressure may be labile.

Goal:. To assess kidney function and to prevent infection.
A. Usual postoperative care for abdominal surgery.
B. Monitor for GI complications.
C. Provide good pulmonary hygiene because child is at increased risk for pulmonary infections postoperatively.

D. Vincristine is frequently used in chemotherapy; observe the child closely for the development of paralytic ileus. Another choice is actinomycin D, while doxorubicin and cyclophosphamide may be used in advanced-stage disease.
E. Child is at risk for intestinal obstruction from the vincristine-induced adynamic ileus, edema caused by radiation, or postsurgical adhesions.

Home Care

A. Teach parents management of the effects of chemotherapy.
B. Child has only one kidney; teach parents how to protect renal function.
   1. Signs and symptoms of UTI and ways to prevent the occurrence.
   2. Advise all health care providers of compromised renal function.
   3. Prompt treatment of other infections.
   4. Encourage noncontact sports when older.

⚡ Practice & Next Generation NCLEX (NGN) Questions

Pediatric Nursing Care

1. A client in sickle cell crisis is admitted to the ED. What are the **priorities** of care in order of importance?
   1. Nutrition, hydration, electrolyte balance
   2. Hydration, pain management, electrolyte balance
   3. Hydration, oxygenation, pain management
   4. Hydration, oxygenation, electrolyte balance

2. What assessment finding would indicate a positive response in the adolescent who is being treated for an acute asthmatic problem?
   1. Respiratory rate of 18 breaths per minute
   2. Pulse oximetry of 90%
   3. Pulse rate of 110 beats per minute
   4. Nonproductive cough

3. Which laboratory test would the nurse identify as indicative of improvement in a child with rheumatic heart disease?
   1. Positive C-reactive protein
   2. Hemoglobin, 14.0 g/100 mL (140 g/L) blood
   3. White blood cell count, 11,000/mm³ (11×10^9/L)
   4. Decreasing erythrocyte sedimentation rate

4. The nurse is caring for a 9-year-old who is being prepared for surgery for appendicitis. What is the preoperative preparation?
   1. Ambulate to decrease problems with distention.
   2. Administer morphine for pain.
   3. Allow position of comfort; maintain NPO.
   4. Put a warm pad on abdomen; offer clear liquids.

5. The nurse is assigned a school-age child. The child was in a diving accident and has tetraplegia (quadriplegia). What would the nurse expect to find when assessing the child?
   1. One side of the child's body is paralyzed.
   2. The child is paralyzed with no sensation from the waist down.
   3. The child experiences no sensation to pain below the waist.
   4. There is minimal voluntary muscle response from the child's arms down.

6. A child comes to the outpatient clinic and is diagnosed with impetigo on the left arm. What information would the nurse give to the parent of this child?
   1. Apply antibiotic ointment to the crusted lesions.
   2. Wash the lesions with soap and water and then apply a steroid ointment.
   3. Soak the scabs off the lesions and apply an antibiotic ointment.
   4. Wash the lesions with hydrogen peroxide and apply an antifungal cream.

7. A teacher notifies the school nurse that many of the students in the third-grade class have been scratching their heads and reporting intense itching of the scalp. The nurse notices tiny white material at the base of a student's hair shaft. What condition is **most** likely occurring?
   1. Tinea capitis
   2. Pediculosis capitis
   3. Dandruff
   4. Scabies

8. A parent and an 8-month-old child come into the clinic for a well-child checkup. The parent tells the nurse the child has been crying more than usual. What information obtained during the nursing assessment would cause the nurse the **most** concern?
   1. Crying when sucking on the bottle
   2. Crying when placed in crib at night
   3. On-and-off crying throughout the day
   4. Crying when left at the child care center

9. The nurse is caring for an infant with a tentative diagnosis of hypertrophic pyloric stenosis. The nurse would anticipate what test would be done to confirm this diagnosis?
   1. Barium enema
   2. Colonoscopy with biopsy
   3. Hemodilution with increased sodium and potassium
   4. Ultrasound of abdomen

10. The nurse is caring for a child who is currently experiencing a generalized seizure. Which nursing intervention takes **highest priority** when caring for this child?
    1. Protect the child from injury.
    2. Use a padded tongue blade to protect the airway.
    3. Assess for patent airway.
    4. Allow seizure activity to end without interference.

11. The nurse reviews the ED admission documentation.

    Highlight the assessment findings that require immediate follow-up by the nurse.

Health History	Nurses' Notes	Provider Orders	Laboratory Results

    0600: A 12-year-old client presents to the ED with a fever that has persisted for several days, along with dizziness and severe pain. The child has a history of sickle cell disease. The child states that the pain is a 9 on a scale of 10. The child states their abdomen hurts as well as the legs and feet. The feet are swollen bilaterally.

    - Temperature: 101.7°F (38.7°C)
    - BP: 111/55 mm Hg
    - Heart rate: 125 bpm and regular
    - Respirations: 32 breaths/min
    - SpO2: 97% on room air
    - Capillary refill: 3 seconds
    - Extremity pulses: + 3

12. The nurse is assigned to a newly admitted 19-month-old toddler. The nurse is reviewing the toddler's assessment data to prepare the plan of care.

Health History	Nurses' Notes	Provider Orders	Laboratory Results

1900: The toddler was admitted to the acute care unit from the ED for lethargy, abdominal pain, diarrhea, and irritability. The toddler has had decreased oral intake, one episode of vomiting about 4 hours ago, small amounts of "jelly"-like diarrhea, and has not had a wet diaper in 14 hours. The mother states that the pain seems to come and go. The toddler has an unremarkable past medical history.

Assessment findings:

- Lung sounds clear bilaterally
- Diffuse abdominal tenderness upon palpation with small palpable mass
- Abdomen distended
- Capillary refill delayed
- Client appears lethargic and in pain, difficult to console
- Bilious vomit noted in emesis basin
- Pallor noted

1930

- Temperature: 99.3°F (37.4°C)
- BP: 96/48 mm Hg
- Heart rate: 124 bpm
- Respirations: 28 breaths/minute
- SpO2: 98% on room air
- FLACC Pain Scale Score: 6

Complete the diagram by dragging from the choices below to specify what condition the client is most likely experiencing, two actions the nurse should take to address that condition, and two parameters the nurse should monitor to assess the client's progress.

Actions to Take		Parameters to Monitor
Actions to Take	Condition Most Likely Experiencing	Parameters to Monitor

ACTIONS TO TAKE	POTENTIAL CONDITIONS	PARAMETERS TO MONITOR
Prepare toddler for ultrasound	Intussusception	Sepsis
Do not palpate the abdomen	Hirschsprung' disease	Oxygen saturation
Start prescribed IV fluids	Wilms tumor	Pain level
Start BRAT diet	Fluid overload	Vital signs
Administer oxygen at 4 L/minute via nasal cannula		PO intake

⚡Answers to Practice & Next Generation NCLEX (NGN) Questions

1. 3
Client Needs: Physiological Integrity/Physiological Adaptation
Clinical Judgment/Cognitive Skill: Prioritize Hypotheses
Item Type: Multiple Choice
Rationale & Test Taking Strategy: Note the **key** word, "priorities." Remember all of the entries for each option must be correct for it to be a correct answer and the need to be in order of priority or importance. The priorities for care of a client in sickle cell crisis are focused on providing fluid (hydration), oxygen, and pain control during the crisis to reduce sickling and prevent complications. Electrolyte management is not a priority nor is nutrition.

2. 1
Client Needs: Physiological Integrity/Physiological Adaptation
Clinical Judgment/Cognitive Skill: Evaluate Outcomes
Item Type: Multiple Choice
Rationale & Test Taking Strategy: Review each option and consider if it is normal or abnormal. The respiratory rate is within normal limits—16 to 20 breaths/min for the adolescent. The increased pulse rate and the low oximetry levels correlate with respiratory difficulty and are not indicative of an improvement in the client. Secretions should mobilize as the client improves.

3. 4
Client Needs: Physiological Integrity/Reduction of Risk Potential
Clinical Judgment/Cognitive Skill: Evaluate Outcomes
Item Type: Multiple Choice
Rationale & Test Taking Strategy: An immune response causes an inflammatory condition in the body, which can result in heart valve damage. What tests monitor the inflammatory response? A decrease in the ESR indicates that the inflammatory process is resolving. The C-reactive protein also measures levels of inflammation, but it is not recorded as positive or negative; it is recorded as a level (less than 0.3 mg is normal; 1 mg to 10 mg is indicative of an inflammatory response). The white blood cell count is elevated when there is an inflammatory or infectious problem. The hemoglobin is within normal limits and is not affected by rheumatic heart disease.

4. 3
Client Needs: Physiological Integrity/Physiological Adaptation
Clinical Judgment/Cognitive Skill: Generate Solutions
Item Type: Multiple Choice
Rationale & Test Taking Strategy: Before an appendectomy, the child is usually maintained in a position of comfort and kept NPO;

no heat is applied to the abdomen. Opioid analgesics are used sparingly. It is important to be able to identify changes in the character of the client's pain.

5. 4
Client Needs: Physiological Integrity/Physiological Adaptation
Clinical Judgment/Cognitive Skill: Analyze Cues
Item Type: Multiple Choice
Rationale & Test Taking Strategy: It may be helpful to break the word *tetraplegia* down to its components. *Tetra* means "four" and so does *quadri*. The term *tetraplegia* (formerly called quadriplegia) refers to an injury involving the cervical vertebrae and involves all four extremities. The severity of the damage depends on the cervical vertebrae affected and determines what responses or movement the client will eventually be able to achieve. The degree of impairment in the arms following cervical injury depends on the level of injury. The lower the level, the more function is retained in the arms. It is important to understand that with complete cord involvement there is a total loss of sensory and motor function below the level of injury. With incomplete cord involvement there is a mixed loss of voluntary motor activity and sensation that leaves some tracts intact. The degree of sensory and motor loss depends on the level of injury and reflects specific damaged nerve tracts. Paralysis and loss of sensation on one side of the body is referred to as hemiplegia.

6. 3
Client Needs: Physiological Integrity/Physiological Adaptation
Clinical Judgment/Cognitive Skill: Take Action
Item Type: Multiple Choice
Rationale & Test Taking Strategy: Think about what you know regarding impetigo. Teaching should include the use of warm saline or aluminum acetate soaks followed by soap-and-water removal of crusts and application of a suitable antibiotic ointment, such as mupirocin (Bactroban). Hydrogen peroxide has little ability to reduce bacteria in wounds and can inflame healthy skin cells that surround a lesion, increasing the amount of time the wounds take to heal. Impetigo is caused by group A beta-hemolytic *Streptococci* or *Staphylococcus* species, which are bacterial and would not be treated by an antifungal cream or a steroid ointment. If lesions are on the face, a systemic antibiotic may also be given.

7. 2
Client Needs: Physiological Integrity/Physiological Adaptation
Clinical Judgment/Cognitive Skill: Prioritize Hypotheses
Item Type: Multiple Choice
Rationale & Test Taking Strategy: Consider the symptoms of each of the four conditions listed. Pediculosis capitis (head lice) is characterized by tiny white nits (eggs) that attach to the base of the hair shaft and are highly contagious, which is what the students have. Tinea capitis is characterized by a red, scaly rash with central clearing in the well-defined margins. Dandruff is often mistaken for head lice, but dandruff can be easily removed from the hair shaft. Nits adhere to the hair shaft and are not easy to remove. Scabies form burrows under the skin and cause intense nighttime itching.

8. 1
Client Needs: Physiological Integrity/Physiological Adaptation
Clinical Judgment/Cognitive Skill: Prioritize Hypotheses
Item Type: Multiple Choice

Rationale & Test Taking Strategy: Note the **key** word, "most." This is a priority question asking about what assessment finding is of most concern. Pain during feeding may indicate increased inner ear pain during sucking. With effusion in the middle ear space, negative pressure draws mucus into the middle ear in response to a child crying or sucking on a nipple, resulting in increased pressure and pain. Crying when placed in a crib and on and off during the day is normal in childhood development. Separation anxiety is a common problem.

9. 4
Client Needs: Physiological Integrity/Physiological Adaptation
Clinical Judgment/Cognitive Skill: Analyze Cues
Item Type: Multiple Choice
Rationale & Test Taking Strategy: Think about what signs and symptoms an infant with HPS may have (i.e., forceful, projectile vomiting). An ultrasound is a noninvasive test that can diagnose HPS. If ultrasonography does not demonstrate a hypertrophied pylorus, upper gastrointestinal radiography would be done to rule out other causes of vomiting. Hemoconcentration (not hemodilution) is frequently present because of the dehydration status of the infant. With HPS there is a severe narrowing of the pyloric canal between the stomach and the duodenum. Colonoscopy is not indicated. A barium enema detects abnormalities in the large intestine (colon, rectum, and anus).

10. 1
Client Needs: Physiological Integrity/Physiological Adaptation
Clinical Judgment/Cognitive Skill: Prioritize Hypotheses
Item Type: Multiple Choice
Rationale & Test Taking Strategy: Note the **key** words, "highest priority." This is a priority question asking what intervention would be done during a generalized seizure. The nurse should protect the child from injury by preventing the child from hitting the side rails or falling. A padded tongue blade should never be used because it can cause damage to the mouth and airway. The airway cannot be effectively assessed during the seizure. Allowing the seizure activity to end without interference may cause the child injury. The nurse should position the child on the side to prevent aspiration and place the child on the ground if the client is likely to fall and sustain injury.

11. The nurse reviews the emergency department (ED) admission documentation.

Highlight the assessment findings that require immediate follow-up by the nurse.

Health History	Nurses' Notes	Provider Orders	Laboratory Results

0600: A 12-year-old client presents to the ED with a fever that has persisted for several days, along with dizziness and severe pain. The child has a history of sickle cell disease. The child states that the pain is a 9 on a scale of 10. The child states the abdomen hurts as well as the legs and feet. The feet are swollen bilaterally

- Temperature: 101.7°F (38.7°C)
- BP: 111/55 mmHg
- Heart rate: 125 bpm and regular
- Respirations: 32 breaths/min
- SpO2: 97% on room air
- Capillary refill: 3 seconds
- Extremity pulses: +3

Client Needs: Physiological Integrity/Physiological Adaptation
Clinical Judgment/Cognitive Skill: Recognize Cues
Item Type: Highlight in Table
Rationale & Test Taking Strategy: Sickle cell crisis or vaso-occlusive crisis often presents with a low-grade fever, tachycardia, tachypnea, and pain. Treatment should be based both on support and symptoms. Analgesics should be provided for pain and fever. Children with severe pain may require narcotics, such as morphine. Analgesics and fluids, for dehydration, will help improve the child's vital signs and symptoms.

12. The nurse is assigned to a newly admitted 19-month-old male toddler. The nurse is reviewing the toddler's assessment data to prepare the plan of care.

Health History	Nurses' Notes	Provider Orders	Laboratory Results

1900: The toddler was admitted to the acute care unit from the emergency department for lethargy, abdominal pain, diarrhea, and irritability. The toddler has had decreased oral intake, one episode of vomiting about 4 hours ago, and small amounts of "jelly"-like diarrhea and has not had a wet diaper in 14 hours. The mother states that the pain seems to come and go. The toddler has an unremarkable past medical history.

Assessment findings:

Lung sounds clear bilaterally
Diffuse abdominal tenderness upon palpation with small palpable mass
Abdomen distended
Capillary refill delayed
Client appears lethargic and in pain, difficult to console
Bilious vomit noted in emesis basin
Pallor noted

1930

- Temperature: 99.3°F (37.4°C)
- BP: 96/48 mmHg
- Heart rate: 124 bpm
- Respirations: 28 breaths/minute
- SpO2: 98% on room air
- FLACC Pain Scale Score: 6

Complete the diagram by dragging from the choices below to specify what condition the client is most likely experiencing, two actions the nurse should take to address that condition, and two parameters the nurse should monitor to assess the client's progress.

Action to Take		Parameter to Monitor
Prepare toddler for ultrasound		Sepsis

Action to Take	Condition	Parameter to Monitor
Start prescribed IV fluids	**Most Likely Experiencing** Intussusception	Vital signs

ACTIONS TO TAKE	POTENTIAL CONDITIONS	PARAMETERS TO MONITOR
Prepare toddler for ultrasound.	Intussusception	Sepsis
Do not palpate the abdomen.	Hirschsprung's disease	Oxygen saturation
Start prescribed IV fluids.	Wilms tumor	Pain level
Start BRAT diet.	Fluid overload	Vital signs
Administer oxygen at 4L/minute via nasal cannula.		PO intake

Client Needs: Physiological Integrity/Physiological Adaptation
Clinical Judgment/Cognitive Skill: Recognize Cues, Analyze Cues, Take Action
Item Type: Bow-tie
Rationale & Test Taking Strategy: Children with intussusception typically present with vomiting, mucus ("currant jelly") stools or diarrhea, lethargy, and decreased oral intake. A small palpable mass may be felt. Bowel edema and loss of blood supply to the intestines can lead to necrosis and later possible sepsis. Dehydration is commonly seen with intussusception and should be treated with IV hydration while maintaining NPO (nothing by mouth) status. Intussusception is an emergent situation due to the possibility of bowel necrosis. It is diagnosed with an ultrasound and an ultrasound-guided hydrostatic reduction or air enema is the first-line treatment. If surgery is needed, then a bowel resection will be performed. Sepsis is high possibility with bowel necrosis and should be monitored for closely. FLACC is a behavioral pain assessment scale used for nonverbal or preverbal clients (age 2 months and on) who are unable to self-report their level of pain. Pain is assessed through observation of five categories—face, legs, activity, cry, and consolability—and scored as a 0, 1, or 2. A zero is relaxed and comfortable; 1 to 3 mild discomfort, 4 to 6 moderate pain, and 7 to 10 severe discomfort, pain, or both.

Normal Laboratory Data

Test	Normal Adult Values
Blood Serum Values	
Activated partial thromboplastin time (aPTT)	30–45 sec
Alanine aminotransferase (ALT)	10–40 units/L (0.17–0.68 µkat/L)
Albumin	3.4–5.0 g/dL (35–50 g/L)
Alkaline phosphatase	30–120 units/L (0.5–2.0 µkat/L)
Ammonia	15–45 mcg N/dL (11–32 µmol N/L)
Amylase	30–122 U/L [method dependent] (0.51–2.07 µkat/L)
Aspartate aminotransferase (AST)	10–30 units/L (0.17–0.51 ukat/L)
Bleeding time	Ivy method: 2–7 minutes
Blood urea nitrogen (BUN)	10–20 mg/dL (3.57–7.14 mmol/L)
Calcium (ionized) serum	4.5–5.5 mg/dL (1.13–1.38 mmol/L)
Calcium, total serum	8.6–10.2 mg/dL (2.15–2.55 mmol/L)
Carbon dioxide (venous CO_2)	20–30 mEq/L (20–30 mmol/L)
Chloride (serum)	95–105 mEq/L (95–105 mmol/L)
Cholesterol	<200 mg/dL
High-density lipoprotein (HDL), low-density lipoprotein (LDL), triglycerides (*see Vascular chapter*)	
Complete white blood cell (WBC) count	4.0–11 10³/mcL (× 10⁹/L)
Differential WBC count	Expressed as a percentage of total WBCs
Segmented neutrophils	50–70%
Band neutrophils	0–8%
Eosinophils	0–4%
Basophils	0–2%
Monocytes	4–8%
Lymphocytes	20–40%
C-reactive protein (highly sensitive-hs-CRP)	Less than 1.0 mg/dL (<9.52 nmol/L)
Creatinine (serum)	Men: 0.6–1.2 mg/dL (53–106 umol/L) Women: 0.5–1.1 mg/dL (445-97 umol/L)
Creatinine kinase (CK)	20–200 U/L (20–200 U/L)
D-Dimer	<250 ng/mL (<250 mcg/L)
Erythrocyte sedimentation rate (ESR)	<30 mm/hr (some gender variation)
Fibrin split-products (FSP)	Less than 10 mcg/mL (<10 mg/L)

Test	Normal Adult Values
Fibrinogen	Quantitative: 200–400 mg/dL (2–4 g/L)
Glucose (baseline fasting)	70–99 mg/dL (3.9–5.5 mmol/L)
Glucose 2-hour postprandial	Less than 140 mg/dL (7.77 mmol/L)
Glycosylated hemoglobin assay (A1c)	4–6%
Hematocrit	Men: 39–50% (0.39–0.54) Women: 35–47% (0.35–0.47)
Hemoglobin	Men: 14–18 g/dL (140–180 g/L) Women: 12–16 g/dL (120–160 g/L)
International normalized ratio (INR)	2–3 prophylaxis for deep venous thrombosis 2.5–3.5 prosthetic cardiac valves
Iron-binding capacity	250–425 mcg/dL (44.8–76.1 µmol/L)
Iron, total serum	50–175 mcg/dL (9.0–31.3 µmol/L)
Lactic acid dehydrogenase (LDH)	140–280 units/L (0.83–2.5 ukat/L)
Magnesium (serum)	1.5–2.5 mEq/L (0.75–1.25 mmol/L)
Partial thromboplastin time (PTT)	60–70 sec
Phosphorus serum	2.8–4.5 mg/dL (0.9–1.45 mmol/L)
Platelets	150–400 × 10³ units/L (150–350 × 10⁹/L)
Potassium (plasma)	3.5–5.0 mEq/L (3.5–5.0 mmol/L)
Prostate-specific antigen	Less than 4 ng/mL (4 ug/L)
Prothrombin time	11–16 sec
Red blood cell (RBC) count	Men: 4.3–5.7 × 10⁶/mcL (4.3–5.7 × 10¹²/L) Women: 3.8–5.1 × 10⁶/mcL (3.8–5.1 × 10¹²/L)
Serum osmolarity	275–295 mOsm/kg (275–295 mmol/kg)
Sodium (serum or plasma)	135–145 mEq/L (135–145 mmol/L)
T4 (thyroxine), total	4.6–11.0 mcg/dL (59–142 nmo/L)
T4 (thyroxine), free	0.8–2.7 ng/dL (10–35 pmol/L)
T3 uptake	24–34% (0.24–0.34)
T3 (triiodothyronine), total	Age 20–50: 70–204 ng/dL (1.08–3.14 nmol/L) Age >50: 40–181 ng/dL (0.62–2.79 nmol/L)
Thyroid-stimulating hormone (TSH)	0.4–4.2 µU/mL (0.4–4.2 mU/L)
Uric acid (serum)	Men: 4.0–8.5 mg/dL (240–505.62 µmol/L) Women: 2.7–7.3 mg/dL (160.61–434.24 µmol/L)

Test	Normal Adult Values
Bilirubin	
Direct bilirubin	0.1–0.3 mg/dL (1.7–5.1 µmol/L)
Indirect bilirubin	0.1–1.0 mg/dL (1.7–17.10 µmol/L)
Total bilirubin	0.2–1.2 mg/dL (3–21 µmol/L)
Cerebral Spinal Fluid (CSF) Analysis	
Albumin	56–76%
Blood	Negative
Color	Clear and colorless
Glucose	40–70 mg/dL (2.2–3.9 mmol/L)
Pressure	Less than 20 cm H_2O
Protein	15–45 mg/dL (0.15–0.45 g/L) (higher in older adults and children) (up to 0.7 g/L in older adults and children)
WBCs	Adults: 5000–10,000 mm^3 (5–10 cells × 10^9 /L)
Normal Arterial Blood Gas Values	
Acidity index (pH)	7.35–7.45
Bicarbonate (HCO_3^-)	22–26 mEq/L (mmol/L)
Partial pressure of dissolved carbon dioxide ($Paco_2$)	35–45 mm Hg
Partial pressure of dissolved oxygen (Pao_2)	80–100 mm Hg
Percentage of hemoglobin saturated with oxygen (O_2 saturation)	95% or above

Test	Normal Adult Values
Urine Values	
Creatinine clearance (24-hour urine collection)	59–137 mL/min (59–137 mL/s/m^2)
Microscopic urinalysis	Negative
Bacteria	None present
Casts	Negative
Crystals	Less than 2
RBCs	0–4 per low-power field
WBCs	
Specific gravity	Adult: 1.005–1.030; Older adult: values decrease
Ketones	24-hr specimen—20–50 mg/dL
Uric acid (urine)	250–750 mg/24 hr (1.48–4.43 mmol/day)
Urinalysis	0.2–1.9 mg/dL (2.0–19.0 mcg/24 hr)
Microalbumin	Negative
Bilirubin	Clear, golden yellow
Color	Negative
Glucose	70-99 mg/dL (3.9–5.5 mmol/L)
Urine electrolytes (24-hour urine collection)	40–250 mEq/24 hr (mmol/day) (varies with dietary intake)
Sodium	100–250 mg/day (2.5–6.3 mmol/day)
Calcium	
Urine osmolarity	300–1300 mOsm/kg H_2O (mmol/kg H_2O) (random sample)

Anticoagulants

These drugs (e.g., warfarin) prolong coagulation by inactivating clotting factors (heparin) and decreasing the synthesis of clotting factors.

GENERAL NURSING IMPLICATIONS

• Increased risk for bleeding when used concurrently with other drugs, herbal remedies, or foods affecting coagulation.
• Maintain bleeding precautions.
• Review laboratory results—complete blood count (CBC) with attention to hemoglobin and hematocrit (H & H) and platelets.

• A second health care provider should always check order, calculation of dosage, and/or infusion pump settings when medications are being administered intravenously.
• Do not automatically discontinue according to "automatic stop" policies (procedures, surgery) without verifying the order; reevaluate all clients whose anticoagulants are being held for procedures; and assess the need to reorder the anticoagulant therapy.
• Client should wear a medical alert bracelet.

> ■ **NURSING PRIORITY** Clarify all anticoagulant dosing for clients. Caution to be taken with reading labels for heparin concentrations, especially for intravenous bolus doses.

▲Heparin: IV, SQ May not be given PO Short-term anticoagulation	Visible or occult blood in emesis, urine, stool, or sputum Bleeding from trauma site, surgical site, or intracranially Heparin-induced thrombocytopenia: associated with increase in thrombosis	1. Check the activated partial thromboplastin time (APTT) for normal levels versus therapeutic levels. 2. Protamine sulfate is the antidote. 3. Intravenous administration should occur via infusion pump to ensure accurate dosage. 4. Will not dissolve established clots. 5. Evaluate client for decreased platelet count. 6. Effective immediately after administration; anticoagulation effect has short half-life. 7. Before starting infusion and with each change of the container or rate of infusion, have second practitioner check drug, dosage, route, and rate. 8. Do not store in same area as insulin; both are given by units.

Low-Molecular-Weight Heparin (LMWH)

Enoxaparin: SQ Dalteparin: SQ Tinzaparin: SQ	Similar to those with heparin	1. **Use:** prophylaxis for thromboembolic problems in high-risk clients (immobility, hip, or knee replacement). 2. Dosage is not interchangeable with heparin. 3. Leave the air lock in the prefilled syringe to prevent leakage. 4. Should be injected into the "love handles" of the abdomen.

▲Warfarin sodium: PO
Long-term
  anticoagulation
	Bleeding ranging from bruising to major hemorrhage	1. Check the prothrombin time (PT) and international normalized ratio (INR) to evaluate level of anticoagulation; INR greater than 3 may indicate adverse drug reaction.
		2. Vitamin K is the antidote.
		3. Client teaching:
		  a. Bleeding precautions.
		  b. Advise all health care providers of medication.
		  c. Not recommended if client is pregnant or lactating.
		  d. Maintain routine checks on coagulation studies.
		  e. Client must not stop taking medication unless told to do so by health care provider.
		4. Check drug literature when administering with other medications; drug interactions are common.
		5. Oral contraceptives may decrease effectiveness.
		6. Half-life is 3–5 days; discontinue 3 days before an invasive procedure

Direct Thrombin Inhibitors

Argatroban: IV Dabigatran: PO	Bleeding, dizziness, shortness of breath, fever, urticaria, dyspepsia	1. Due to potential breakdown and loss of potency from moisture, should not be stored in pillboxes or organizers. 2. Does not require INR/PT monitoring. 3. Idarucizumab is an antidote to reverse bleeding caused by dabigatran. 4. Do not double up on doses at the same time if a dose is missed.

Factor Xa Inhibitors

Apixaban: PO Rivaroxaban: PO	Has same potential for bleeding, as with warfarin Does not have the dietary and drug interactions that warfarin has	1. Inform health care provider if client is having surgery or dental surgery. 2. Does not require INR/PT monitoring. 3. Andexanet Alfa is an antidote to reverse bleeding for apixaban or rivaroxaban.

TEST ALERT Questions about anticoagulant medications are consistently found on the examination. Antiplatelet Medications: Inhibit platelet aggregation and prolong bleeding time. Used to prevent and treat thromboembolism events such as stroke, MI, and peripheral artery disease.

References and Resources

Commission on Graduates of Foreign Nursing Schools (CGFNS). https://www.cgfns.org

Cooper, K., & Gosnell, K. (2023). *Foundations and adult health nursing* (9 ed.). Elsevier.

Halter, M. J. (2022). *Varcarolis' foundations of psychiatric mental health nursing* (9th ed.). Elsevier.

Harding, M., Kwong, J., Hagler, D., & Reinisch, C. (2023). *Lewis's medical-surgical nursing: Assessment and management of clinical problems* (12th ed.). Mosby.

Ignatavicius, D. D., Workman, M. L., Rebar, C., & Heimgartner, N. M. (2021). *Medical-surgical nursing: Patient-centered collaborative care* (10th ed.). Elsevier.

The Joint Commission, One Renaissance Blvd. Oakbrook Terrace, IL 60181.

Leifer, G. (2019). *Introduction to maternity and pediatric nursing* (8th ed.). Elsevier.

Lilley, L. L., Collins, S. R., & Snyder, J. S. (2023). *Pharmacology and the nursing process* (10th ed.). Elsevier.

National Council of State Boards of Nursing. (2019a, Fall). Approved NGN item types. *Next Generation NCLEX News.* https://www.ncsbn.org/NGN_Fall19_ENG_final.pdf

National Council of State Boards of Nursing. (2019b, Winter). Clinical judgment measurement model. *Next Generation NCLEX News.* https://www.ncsbn.org/NGN_Winter19.pdf

National Council of State Boards of Nursing. (2019c, Spring). Clinical judgment measurement model and task model. *Next Generation NCLEX News.* https://www.ncsbn.org/NGN_Spring19_Eng_04_Final.pdf

National Council of State Boards of Nursing. (2020a, Fall). Licensed practical/vocational nurses. *Next Generation NCLEX News.* https://www.ncsbn.org/public-files/NGN_Fall20_Eng_03_FINAL.pdf

National Council of State Boards of Nursing. (2020b, Spring). The NGN case study. *Next Generation NCLEX News.* https://www.ncsbn.org/NGN_Spring20_Eng_02.pdf.

National Council of State Boards of Nursing. (2021a). *2022 NCLEX information flyer.* https://www.ncsbn.org/public-files/2022_NCLEX_factsheet_English.pdf

National Council of State Boards of Nursing. (2021b, Fall). Next Generation NCLEX: Comparison between case studies and stand-alone items. *Next Generation NCLEX News.* https://www.ncsbn.org/public-files/NGN_Fall21_English_Final.pdf

National Council of State Boards of Nursing. (2021c, Spring). Next Generation NCLEX: Stand-alone items. *Next Generation NCLEX News.* https://www.ncsbn.org/NGN_Spring21_Eng.pdf

National Council of State Boards of Nursing. (2022a). *2021 LPN/VN practice analysis: Linking the NCLEX-PN examination to practice* (Vol. 82). https://www.ncsbn.org/public-files/21_NCLEX_PN_PA.pdf

National Council of State Boards of Nursing. (2022b, Summer). Overview of the 2021 PN Practice Analysis. *Next Generation NCLEX News.* https://www.ncsbn.org/public-files/NGN_Summer22_ENG_FINAL.pdf

National Council of State Boards of Nursing. (2023a). *2023 NCLEX-PN test plan.* https://www.ncsbn.org/public-files/2023_PN_Test%20Plan_FINAL.pdf

National Council of State Boards of Nursing. (2023b). *Frequently asked questions about NCLEX.* https://www.ncsbn.org/nclex-faqs.htm

National Council of State Boards of Nursing. (2023c). *NCLEX Examination Candidate Bulletin.* https://www.ncsbn.org/public-files/2022_NCLEX_Candidate_Bulletin_English.pdf *Note: this changes yearly and may be updated throughout the year; navigate to* https://www.ncsbn.org/exams/before-the-exam/candidate-bulletin-information.page

National Council of State Boards of Nursing. (2023d). *Next Generation NCLEX project.* https://www.ncsbn.org/next-generation-nclex.htm

National Council of State Boards of Nursing. (2023e). *NGN FAQs for candidates.* https://www.ncsbn.org/11436.htm

National Council of State Boards of Nursing. (2023f). *NGN FAQs for educators.* https://www.ncsbn.org/11447.htm

Nielsen, A., Gonzalez, L., Jessee, M., Monagle, J., Dickison, P., & Lasater, K. (2022). Current practices for teaching clinical judgment. *Nurse Educator, 48*(1), 7–12. https://doi.org/10.1097/NNE.0000000000001268.

Pagana, K. D., & Pagana, T. J. (2022). *Mosby's manual of diagnostic and laboratory tests* (7th ed.). Elsevier.

Potter, P. A., Perry, A. G., Stockert, P. A., Hall, A. M., & Ostendorf, W. R. (2023). *Fundamentals of nursing* (11th ed.). Mosby.

Steele, D. (2023). *Keltner's psychiatric nursing* (9th ed.). Elsevier.

Stromberg, H. (2023). *Medical-surgical nursing: Concepts and practice* (5th ed.). Elsevier.

Williams, P. (2022). *Fundamental concepts and skills for nursing* (6th ed.). Elsevier.

Willihnganz, M. J., Gurevitz, S. L., & Clayton, B. D. (2022). *Basic pharmacology for nurses* (19th ed.). Elsevier.

Zerwekh, J., & Garneau, A. (2023). *Nursing today: Transitions and trends* (11th ed.). Elsevier.

Index

Note: Page numbers followed by "*f*" indicate figures; "*t*", tables; "*b*", boxes.